全国高等中医药院校中药学类专业双语规划教材

Bilingual Planned Textbooks for Chinese Materia Medica Majors in TCM Colleges and Universities

系统中药学

Systematic Chinese Materia Medica

（供中药学类、中医学、药学类及相关专业用）

(For Chinese Materia Medica, Traditional Chinese Medicine, Pharmacy and Other Related Majors)

U0265118

主 编　彭　成

副主编　邱智东　余林中　彭代银　裴　瑾

编　者（以姓氏笔画为序）

王寒冰（成都中医药大学）　　　孟　江（广东药科大学）

叶　冰（云南中医药大学）　　　赵云生（河北中医学院）

史亚军（陕西中医药大学）　　　贾艾玲（长春中医药大学）

代　敏（成都医学院）　　　　　黄林芳（中国医学科学院

　　　　　　　　　　　　　　　　　　　药用植物研究所）

刘俊珊（南方医科大学）

李芸霞（成都中医药大学）　　　彭　成（成都中医药大学）

吴红梅（贵州中医药大学）　　　彭代银（安徽中医药大学）

邱智东（长春中医药大学）　　　谢晓芳（成都中医药大学）

余林中（南方医科大学）　　　　蔡　玥（安徽中医药大学）

邹　亮（成都大学）　　　　　　裴　瑾（成都中医药大学）

邵　晶（甘肃中医药大学）　　　薛淑娟（河南中医药大学）

学术秘书（兼）　谢晓芳（成都中医药大学）

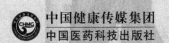

中国健康传媒集团
中国医药科技出版社

内 容 提 要

本书是"全国高等中医药院校中药学类专业双语教材"之一，根据双语教材的编写要求，并遵照教材编写大纲和课程特点编写而成，内容上涵盖总论和各论两部分。总论重点介绍系统中药学和系统中药学关键要素的科学内涵、认知过程和现代研究；各论选择临床常用中药，从品种、品质、制药、性能、功效和应用六方面进行阐释。本书是全新学科教材，具有系统性、科学性、创新性、实用性、前瞻性等突出特点，英文翻译但求准确、恰当。

本书供普通高等中医药院校中药学类、中医学、药学类及相关专业使用。

图书在版编目（CIP）数据

系统中药学：汉、英 / 彭成主编 . —北京：中国医药科技出版社，2021.12

全国高等中医药院校中药学类专业双语规划教材

ISBN 978-7-5214-2713-4

Ⅰ . ①系… Ⅱ . ①彭… Ⅲ . ①中药学 – 双语教学 – 中医学院 – 教材 – 汉、英 Ⅳ . ① R28

中国版本图书馆 CIP 数据核字（2021）第 202019 号

美术编辑 陈君杞

版式设计 辰轩文化

出版　**中国健康传媒集团** | 中国医药科技出版社

地址　北京市海淀区文慧园北路甲 22 号

邮编　100082

电话　发行：010-62227427　邮购：010-62236938

网址　www.cmstp.com

规格　889 × 1194 mm ¹/₁₆

印张　28¹/₂

字数　835 千字

版次　2021 年 12 月第 1 版

印次　2021 年 12 月第 2 次印刷

印刷　三河市万龙印装有限公司

经销　全国各地新华书店

书号　ISBN 978-7-5214-2713-4

定价　88.00 元

获取新书信息、投稿、为图书纠错，请扫码联系我们。

近些年随着世界范围的中医药热潮的涌动，来中国学习中医药学的留学生逐年增多，走出国门的中医药学人才也在增加。为了适应中医药国际交流与合作的需要，加快中医药国际化进程，提高来中国留学生和国际班学生的教学质量，满足双语教学的需要和中医药对外交流需求，培养优秀的国际化中医药人才，进一步推动中医药国际化进程，根据教育部、国家中医药管理局、国家药品监督管理局等部门的有关精神，在本套教材建设指导委员会主任委员成都中医药大学彭成教授等专家的指导和顶层设计下，中国医药科技出版社组织全国 50 余所高等中医药院校及附属医疗机构约 420 名专家、教师精心编撰了全国高等中医药院校中药学类专业双语规划教材，该套教材即将付梓出版。

本套教材共计 23 门，主要供全国高等中医药院校中药学类专业教学使用。本套教材定位清晰、特色鲜明，主要体现在以下方面。

一、立足双语教学实际，培养复合应用型人才

本套教材以高校双语教学课程建设要求为依据，以满足国内医药院校开展留学生教学和双语教学的需求为目标，突出中医药文化特色鲜明、中医药专业术语规范的特点，注重培养中医药技能、反映中医药传承和现代研究成果，旨在优化教育质量，培养优秀的国际化中医药人才，推进中医药对外交流。

本套教材建设围绕目前中医药院校本科教育教学改革方向对教材体系进行科学规划、合理设计，坚持以培养创新型和复合型人才为宗旨，以社会需求为导向，以培养适应中药开发、利用、管理、服务等各个领域需求的高素质应用型人才为目标的教材建设思路与原则。

二、遵循教材编写规律，整体优化，紧跟学科发展步伐

本套教材的编写遵循"三基、五性、三特定"的教材编写规律；以"必需、够用"为度；坚持与时俱进，注意吸收新技术和新方法，适当拓展知识面，为学生后续发展奠定必要的基础。实验教材密切结合主干教材内容，体现理实一体，注重培养学生实践技能训练的同时，按照教育部相关精神，增加设计性实验部分，以现实问题作为驱动力来培养学生自主获取和应用新知识的能力，从而培养学生独立思考能力、实验设计能力、实践操作能力和可持续发展能力，满足培养应用型和复合型人才的要求。强调全套教材内容的整体优化，并注重不同教材内容的联系与衔接，避免遗漏和不必要的交叉重复。

三、对接职业资格考试，"教考""理实"密切融合

本套教材的内容和结构设计紧密对接国家执业中药师职业资格考试大纲要求，实现教学与考试、理论与实践的密切融合，并且在教材编写过程中，吸收具有丰富实践经验的企业人员参与教材的编写，确保教材的内容密切结合应用，更加体现高等教育的实践性和开放性，为学生参加考试和实践工作打下坚实基础。

四、创新教材呈现形式，书网融合，使教与学更便捷更轻松

全套教材为书网融合教材，即纸质教材与数字教材、配套教学资源、题库系统、数字化教学服务有机融合。通过"一书一码"的强关联，为读者提供全免费增值服务。按教材封底的提示激活教材后，读者可通过 PC、手机阅读电子教材和配套课程资源（PPT、微课、视频等），并可在线进行同步练习，实时收到答案反馈和解析。同时，读者也可以直接扫描书中二维码，阅读与教材内容关联的课程资源，从而丰富学习体验，使学习更便捷。教师可通过 PC 在线创建课程，与学生互动，开展在线课程内容定制、布置和批改作业、在线组织考试、讨论与答疑等教学活动，学生通过 PC、手机均可实现在线作业、在线考试，提升学习效率，使教与学更轻松。此外，平台尚有数据分析、教学诊断等功能，可为教学研究与管理提供技术和数据支撑。需要特殊说明的是，有些专业基础课程，例如《药理学》等9种教材，起源于西方医学，因篇幅所限，在本次双语教材建设中纸质教材以英语为主，仅将专业词汇对照了中文翻译，同时在中国医药科技出版社数字平台"医药大学堂"上配套了中文电子教材供学生学习参考。

编写出版本套高质量教材，得到了全国知名专家的精心指导和各有关院校领导与编者的大力支持，在此一并表示衷心感谢。希望广大师生在教学中积极使用本套教材和提出宝贵意见，以便修订完善，共同打造精品教材，为促进我国高等中医药院校中药学类专业教育教学改革和人才培养做出积极贡献。

全国高等中医药院校中药学类专业双语规划教材
建设指导委员会

在中华民族浩瀚的历史长河中，中医药护佑着中华儿女，虽然经历无数灾难瘟疫，中华儿女依然屹立，繁荣兴旺，生生不息。无数中医药前辈如神农、华佗、张仲景、李时珍等中医药大家，发现大自然赋予人类的宝藏——中药，中药在世世代代中华儿女抗击疾病的过程中，展现出了神奇的功效：清热解毒，祛风除湿，扶正祛邪，延年益寿……对急、慢性病的治疗效果绝佳。但是中药功效是如何产生的，中药、方剂和中成药中含有什么样的物质，需要用什么样的方法才能更为直观地揭示其发挥作用的物质基础和作用原理等，中外科学家、医药学家和各国人民都翘首期盼能解开中药瑰宝的奥秘。

一味中药是一个系统吗？一个方剂是否是由多个子系统构成的复杂系统？复杂系统科学能否用于研究中药和方剂？系统中药学团队将复杂系统科学引入中药学，在凌一揆教授提出的"大中药"理论基础之上，提出中药是中药生态环境系统和人体复杂系统相互作用的复杂系统，并提出六要素系统是影响中药复杂系统的关键因素，反映中药和中药方剂产生作用的奇妙机制，从而形成"系统中药学"。

系统中药学是世代中药人智慧的结晶，是对凌一揆教授"大中药"思想的传承和创新。在"大中药"思想指导下，创办了中药学本科专业，中药人才辈出，系列中药学教材先后出版。这为系统中药学的发展奠定了坚实的基础。

系统中药学的诞生是对所有对中药学发展做出卓越贡献的前辈科学家的致敬。为了更好地传承和创新"大中药"思想，持续发展先辈科学家的成果，深度揭示中药的作用机理以及相关影响因素，彭成教授于 2000 年以来，在国家 973 计划、国家自然科学基金重点项目等国家级项目的支持下带领其研究团队，以附子作为研究对象，传承"大中药"思想，并充分结合现代"系统科学"的理论和方法，针对中药品种的多样性、化学成分的复杂性、药效作用的多向性、临床应用的广泛性，研究附子不同来源，不同炮制品种，不同制备工艺，不同化学层次的空间特征、生态特征、数量特征、化学特征和生物学特征，试图阐明附子空间、时间、剂量与效应之间的动态变化过程，揭示中药附子的物质基础、生物效应和应用规律，在此基础上，形成了系统中药学的三个子系统，提炼并形成了系统中药学的核心"品、质、制、性、效、用"及"多维评价"方法。自此，系统中药学的理论技术体系和实践方法日渐成熟。

2019 年，彭成教授组织全国 14 所高校的中医学和中药学专家组成编委会，成功编著了全国中医药行业高等教育"十三五"创新教材《系统中药学》。为了让中外科学家和医学家深刻理解中药产生效果的机制，并在药物的研发和创新中更大地发挥中药的价值，激发世界医药界的学术争鸣、国际间深入的学术探讨和合作，让中医药 5000 年的发展成果贡献于世界人民的健康保健事业，更加广泛、畅通地为世界医药事业的发展，为人民的健康福祉做贡献，在已出版的《系统中药学》创新教材基础上，经进一步修订、翻译，编写成本教材（双语教材）。

本教材分总论和各论两部分。总论重点介绍系统中药学和系统中药学关键要素的科学内涵、认知过程和现代研究。各论按中药功效分类，对临床常用中药的基本特点、品种品质、制药、性能功效、应用进行阐释。教材编写，力求做到六方面　①系统性：根据系统中药学学科知识技术体系，总论按照概述、中药的品种、中药的品质、中药的制药、中药的药性、中药的功效、中药的应用七个方面布局；各论按照药物的基本概述、品种品质、制药、性能功效、应用展开，全面系统阐释系统中药学知识技术体系。②科学性：深入研究和厘清中药理论、技术、方法，充分体现特色，写作中表述力求客观、公正、平和，避免引起歧义和争议。同时，本教材中凡涉及基原、质量标准限定、性能、功效和主治，均以《中华人民共和国药典》2020年版为准。③创新性：教材不仅构建了系统中药学的知识技术体系，而且将中药系统研究的最新成果写进教材，体现知识更新和进步。④实用性：针对目前教材存在知识点多、小、乱和前后重复的现状，写作上力求紧密结合"学科前沿、实际应用、执业需求"，达到"教师好教、学生好学、用者好用"的目的。⑤前瞻性：本教材不仅与时俱进，体现学科发展的新知识、新技术、新成果，而且为学科的交叉融合奠定了基础，体现前瞻性。⑥翻译的准确性：本教材具有较强的专业性，在英文翻译中针对古籍书名、中药名称、方剂名称的翻译，及中医药专业术语的翻译力求符合国际标准，并附有附录，以方便读者查询。在翻译中强调本土化，主要以《中医基本名词术语中英对照国际标准》（李振吉，2008）和《中华人民共和国药典》英文版等为参考，并编写五个附录便于读者查找。古文的翻译力求"信达雅"。

本教材由成都中医药大学牵头，联合长春中医药大学、安徽中医药大学、南方医科大学、陕西中医药大学、云南中医药大学、广东药科大学、中国医学科学院药用植物研究所、河南中医药大学、贵州中医药大学、河北中医学院、成都医学院、成都大学的专家学者进行了撰写；成都中医药大学裴瑾、李芸霞、谢晓芳进行了统稿，英文稿由成都中医药大学王寒冰审稿，世界中医药学会联合会翻译中心进行润色和审校，在此一并表示感谢！

尽管我们在编写过程中竭尽所能，但由于作者较多、涉及交叉学科领域较广，系统中药学是我们开创的新学科，需要不断总结与发展，因此，本教材若存在不足或疏漏之处，恳请专家、同道和读者提出宝贵意见，以便再版时修订提高。

编　者
2021年6月

In the vast history of Chinese Nations, Chinese Medicine has been always blessing and protecting Chinese people. Despite countless disasters and plagues, the sons and daughters of China have been reborn, prosperous and endless. Countless TCM masters and ancestors as Shen Nong, Hua Tuo, Zhang Zhongjing and Li Shizhen, found the nature-given treasure Chinese Medicinals, which have been carrying out miraculous effects in the course of generations of Chinese people fighting against diseases. They can clear heat and detoxify, dispel wind and dissipate dampness, strengthen the body and dispel evils, as well as prolong lifespan. The effect is excellent both for many acute and chronic diseases. How does the above mysterious effect happen? What substances contained in Chinese medicinal and its formula or patent medicines? What kind of methods or techniques should be applied to explore their effect-related substance and active mechanism? Chinese and foreign scientists, medical scientists and people all over the world are looking forward to unraveling the mystery of Chinese medicine treasures.

Is one Chinese medicinal a system? Is the formula a complex system composed by multiple branch systems? Can Complex System Science (CSS) be applied to do research on Chinese medicinals and formulae? Taking the "large Chinese Materia Medica" as the theoretical basis, Systematic Chinese Material Medica (SCMM) Team introduced the CSS theory into Chinese Material Medica (CMM), and put forward a new theory that CMM is a complex system created by CMM ecological environment system interacting with human complex system, and propose there is a six - elemental co-acting system that affects this complex system and may reflect the magic mechanism of CMM and formulae.

SCMM is the wisdom crystals of generations of Chinese Medicinal masters and experts, and the inheritance and innovation of "Large Chinese Material Medica" thought of Professor Ling Yikui. With the guidance of the "Large Chinese Material Medica" thought, it has established the undergraduate major of CMM, cultivated numerous Chinese medicine talents and a series of Chinese medicinal textbooks have been published. Thus, it laid a thick foundation for the development of SCMM.

The generation of SCMM is to salute to all predecessors and scientists during the Chinese Medicine development. In order to better inherit and innovate "Large Chinese Material Medica" thought, constantly develop the achievements of predecessors, deeply explore the functioning mechanism of Chinese medicinals as well as the factors resulting in effects, since the year of 2000, Prof. Peng Cheng has led his team to launch a research on Fuzi (Aconiti Lateralis Radix Preparata) with the supports of National 973 Plan, and projects of the National Natural Science Funding. They inherited the "large Chinese Material Medica" thoughts, and fully combined the theory and methods of modern system science, to study its different sources, diverse processed products, various preparation processes, as well as spatial, ecological, quantitative, chemical, and biological characteristics from different chemical levels, so to endeavor illustrating the dynamic change process among time, dose and effect, and revealing the material basis, biological effect and application rules of Fuzi. Based on that, it forms three branch systems of SCMM, sublime its core as "Variety-Quality-Pharmacy-Proterty-Efficacy-Application" and the multiple evaluation technique. Hence, the theory and technology of SCMM tends to be maturing. In 2019, Prof. Peng Cheng gathered Chinese Medicine experts and Chinese Medicinal experts from 14 colleges and universities nationwide to organize a composing committee, and compiled the 13th Five-year Plan innovative Chinese Materia Medica textbook Systematic Chinese Materia Medica of National TCM higher Education.

Aiming to let more scientists and pharmacologists deeply know the mechanism of Chinese Medicinal exerting its efficacy, to widely exert the Chinese Medicinal values in drug development and innovation, trigger active academic arguments, promote international exchanges and cooperation in research and industry, let the world people share the fruits of 5000 year's development of Chinese Medicine, and finally do more contributions for the health care and medical career for worldwide human beings, based on the previous innovative textbook *Systematic Chinese Materia Medica*, through revising, translating, composing bilingually, this textbook will be published in both Chinese and English Language.

The book includes two parts as the pandect and monograph. The pandect mainly introduces the systematic Chinese materia medica as well as the scientific connotation, cognitive processes and modern research on the key elements of *systematic Chinese materia medica*. The monograph part is categorized according to efficacy of medicinals. In each part, it further elucidate each medicinal the basic characteristics including variety and quality, pharmacy, property and efficacy, as well as application. The compilation of this textbook strives for the following six requests. ① Systematicness: According to the knowledge and technology system of *Systematic Chinese Materia Medica*, the pandect is laid out in terms of seven aspects, namely overview, variety, quality, pharmacy, property, efficacy and application. The monograph part introduces Chinese medicinals from aspects of basic overview, variety and quality, pharmacy, property and efficacy, and application. Thereby comprehensively and systematically expound the knowledge and technology system of Systematic Chinese Materia Medica. ② Scientificalness: The theory, technology, and method of Chinese material medica are thoroughly researched and clarified to reflect the characteristics sufficiently. Presentation in writing seeks to be objective, fair and harmonious, avoiding ambiguity and controversy. *The Pharmacopoeia of the People's Republic of China (2020 Edition)* is chosen as the reference to write the origin, quality standard, property, efficacy and indication of each Chinese medicinal in the book. ③ Innovativeness: The book not only constructs the knowledge and technology system of SCMM, but also summarizes the latest achievements of systematic research of Chinese material medica, which reflects the update and progress on knowledge in textbook. ④ Practicability: Aiming at the current problem of too many, small, confused and repetitious knowledge particles, this book sticks to set knowledge points tightly reflecting "frontier of the subject, practical application, practicing need", for the purpose of "easy to teach, easy to learn, and easy to apply". ⑤ Foresight: This book not only keeps pace with the times by reflecting the update knowledge, technology and achievements of the discipline development, but also lays the foundation for the intersection and integration among Chinese Medicine, Chinese Materia Medica and Systematic Science etc.. ⑥ Accuracy: This book has a strong professional nature. The translations of ancient books, names of Chinese material medica, prescriptions and terms are in line with international standards, which mainly include the *WHO International Standard Terminologies on Traditional Medicine in the Western Pacific Region* (2007), *International Standard Chinese-English Basic Nomenclature of Chinese Medicine* (Li Zhenji, 2008), and the English version of *The Pharmacopoeia of the People's Republic of China*. It has attached five annexes for in the convenience of readers searching. The translation of ancient writings strives to meet "accuracy, smooth, and elegance".

Led by Chengdu University of TCM, this book is compiled in collaboration with experts from

Changchun University of Chinese Medicine, Anhui University of Chinese Medicine, Southern Medical University, Shaanxi University of Chinese Medicine, Yunnan University of Chinese Medicine, Guangdong Pharmaceutical University, Chinese Academy of Medical Sciences · Institute of Medicinal Plant Development, Henan University of Chinese Medicine, Guizhou University of TCM, Hebei University of Chinese Medicine, Chengdu Medical College and Chengdu University. Pei jin, Li Yunxia, and Xie Xiaofang from Chengdu University of TCM made the draft. For the English version, Wang Hanbing from Chengdu University of TCM, and experts from Translation Center of World Federation of Chinese Medicine Societies, they have done the editing, revision and polishing work. We would like to extend our sincere thanks to them all for their great contributions!

We have done our best in the process of compiling. However, due to the large number of authors, the wide range of interdisciplinary areas, the limited time, and the fact that Systematic Chinese Materia Medica is a completely new discipline we set, there are still some academic problems worthy of discussion and research, and need to be summarized and developed in the process of implementation. Therefore, we sincerely expect all experts, colleagues and readers' suggestions and finding of mistakes for revision and improvement in the second edition.

Editor

June, 2021

目录 | Contents

总　论
Overview

各　论
Monograph

总 论
Overview

第一章 概　　述
Chapter 1　Overview

当今自然科学呈现两极化发展的趋势，不断分化、综合。具有原创思维的中药学怎样合理分化、系统集成，是中药学必须面对和解决的问题。为了促进中药学科整合、学术创新、产业集成和提高中医药临床疗效，采用复杂系统科学的研究思路，阐释"系统中药学"的科学内涵、认知过程和现代研究进展，具有重要的历史、现实和未来意义。

Today, natural sciences present the trend of polarized and has been constantly differentiated and integrated. How to rationally differentiate and systematically integrate the Chinese Materia Medica with original thoughts is a problem that shall be confronted and solved. In order to promote the integration of Chinese Materia Medica disciplines, academic innovation, industrial integration, and improve the clinical efficacy of Chinese Materia Medica, the research ideas of the Complex Systems Science is applied to explain the scientific connotation, cognitive process and modern research progress of "Systematic Chinese Materia Medica", which will be of great significance in the history, reality and future.

第一节　系统中药学的科学内涵
Section 1　The Scientific Connotation of Systematic Chinese Materia Medica

复杂系统科学是 21 世纪的科学，它是研究系统复杂性规律的科学。自美籍奥地利生物学家贝塔朗菲（Ludwig Von, Bertalanffy）提出系统科学以来，系统科学的理论和方法不断演变和发展，系统论、信息论、控制论、协同论、突变论、耗散结构，以及相变论、混沌论、超循环论等新科学理论相继诞生。我国科学家钱学森首次提出了"开放的复杂巨系统"的概念和方向，认为所谓"复杂性"实际是开放的复杂巨系统的动力学特征。成思危认为，复杂科学有三个主要特点：研究对象是复杂系统；研究方法是定性判断与定量计算相结合、微观分析与宏观综合相结合、还原论与整体论相结合、科学推理与哲学思辨相结合的方法；研究深度不限于对客观事物的描述，而是更着重于揭示客观事物构成的原因及其演化的历程，并力图尽可能准确地推测其未来的发展。彭成认为，系统是若干要素组成的同外部环境相互作用的具有特定功能的有机整体；系统的要素是构成系统的元素，是系统发生、发展和变化的基础；系统的结构是系统的内部组织，是各要素在相互作用中形成的关系；系统的功能是系统在与环境相互作用中表现出来的特性、行为、效能和作用。而中药是一个复杂体系，中药的生态环境和中药作用的机体也是一个复杂体系，要认识和研究这三个复杂体系，就必须在复杂系统科学理论和方法的指导下，坚持"系统中药学"的特色，应用多维评价的方法，研究中药复杂系统的关键要素、结构与功能，即中药的品种、品质、制药、药性、功效、应用（简称"品、质、制、性、效、用"）。

Complex Systems Science is the science in the 21st century, which is a science that studies the law of system complexity. Since Austrian American biologist Ludwig Von Bertalanffy put forward the concept of systems science, its theories and methods have been constantly evolving and developing. New scientific theories such as Systematics, Informatics, Cybernetics, Synergetics, Catastrophe Theory, Dissipative Structure, Dissipative Structure, Phase Transformation Theory, Chaos Theory and Hypercycle Theory have been innovated one after another. Chinese scientist Qian Xuesen put forward the concept and direction of "Open Complex Giant System" for the first time. He insisted that the so-called "complexity" was actually the dynamic characteristics of Open Complex Giant System. Cheng Siwei believes that the complex science has three main characteristics, the research object is a complex system, the research method is the combinations of qualitative judgment and quantitative calculation, microscopic analysis and macroscopic analysis, reductionism and holism, scientific reasoning and philosophical speculation. The research depth is not limited to describe the objectives, but focuses more on revealing the causes of formation and progress of objective, and try to speculate their future development as accurately as possible. According to the thinking of Peng Cheng, the system is an organic whole with certain functions, which contains different essential factors interacting with the external environment with specific functions; the essential factors of the system are the elements of the system, and the basis of the occurrence, development and change of the system; the structure of the system is the internal organization of the system and the relationship formed by the interaction of various elements; the function of the system is the characteristic, behavior, efficiency and effect of the system in the interaction with the environment. Chinese Materia Medica is a complex system, so as the ecological environment it lives and the organism it works on. To study and understand these three complex systems, we must be under the guidance of the theories and methods in Complex Systems Science, adhere to the characteristics of "Systematic Chinese Materia Medica", use the multidimensional evaluation method and study the key elements, structure and function of Chinese herbal medicinal complex systems, including the variety, quality, processing, property, efficacy and application of Chinese medicinal.

一、品种
1 Variety

品种包括药材品种、炮制品种和中成药品种。①药材品种包括自然环境下野生的药用植物物种和药用动物物种，也包括人工栽培的药用植物品种和驯化家养的药用动物品种，还包括天然药用矿物及人工加工品。②炮制品种是中药临床应用的主要形式，即中药经加工炮制后的各种中药临床应用饮片，也包括临床应用的新型饮片，如单味中药浓缩颗粒（中药配方颗粒）、中药颗粒饮片、袋泡剂、煮散剂、超微粉等，其中配方颗粒应用较为广泛。③中成药品种是在中医药理论指导下，以中药饮片为原料，经过药学和临床研究，并经国家药品监督管理部门批准，按规定的生产工艺和质量标准制成的可直接供临床使用的制剂。

The varieties of Chinese Medicinal include that of the medicinal materials, the processed Chinese medicinal and the Chinese patent medicines. ① The varieties of medicinal materials include wild medicinal plant species and medicinal animal species in nature, as well as cultivated medicinal plant species, domesticated medicinal animal species, natural medicinal minerals and artificial products. ② Processed varieties are the main form of Chinese Medicine in clinical practice, including concentrated granules of single Chinese Materia Medica (traditional Chinese medicine formula granule), decoction granules, bagged drugs, cooked powder, superfine powder, etc. in which, the formula granules are more widely used. ③ The varieties of Chinese patent medicines are preparations, instructed by Chinese medicine theories, originated from decoction pieces, approved by the State Drug Administration after pharmaceutical and clinical research, and are produced with accepted production process and quality standard. They can be used directly in clinic.

我国现存最早的医学典籍《黄帝内经》收载成药9种，包括丸、散、膏、丹、药酒等剂型；《伤寒杂病论》收载成药60余种，剂型有丸剂、散剂、膏剂、栓剂、洗剂、灌肠剂等；北宋政府官办药局"惠民和剂局"，专司制药和售药，并编写了《太平惠民和剂局方》，该书是我国历史上第一部由国家刊行的中成药药典，收方788首，对后世影响极大。国家"十三五"重点图书《中国临床药物大辞典·中药成方制剂卷》收载中成药约6500种、中成药制剂8490种，剂型几十种。

In *Huang Di Nei Jing (Huangdi's Internal Classic)*, the earliest written work of Chinese medicine, 9 kinds of Chinese patent medicines were recorded such as Wan (Pill), San (Powder), Gao (Paste), Dan (Pellet), Yaojiu (medicinal liquor). The *Shanghan Zabing Lun (Treatise on Cold Damage and Miscellaneous Diseases)* recorded more than 60 kinds of Chinese patent medicines, in which pharmaceutical forms of Wan, San, Gao, Shuan (Suppository), Xi (Lotion), and Guanchang (Enema), etc. In Northern Song Dynasty, the government set up the Huimin Heji Bureau in charge of drug producing and sales and also published the classic *Taiping Huimin Heji Ju Fang (The Prescriptions of the Bureau of Taiping People's Welfare Pharmacy)*. It is the first national Chinese patent medicine pharmacopoeia,

collecting 788 prescriptions in it and has a great influence on later generations. In the 13th Five-Year Plan the State key books *Dictionary of Chinese Clinical Medicine · Volume of Traditional Chinese Medicine Prescriptions*, 6500 Chinese patent medicines and 8490 Chinese patent medicine prescriptions are collected, involving dozens of pharmaceutical forms.

二、品质
2 Quality

品质即指中药的质量，它反映的是中药种质、种苗、栽培、采收、产地加工、炮制、制剂等方面固有的整体特性的质量，包括外在品质和内在品质两部分。①外在品质主要指中药的性状质量，其质量评价内容包括以"辨状论质"为基础的形、色、气、味和以显微鉴别、理化测定为手段的质量评价。②内在品质主要包含遗传物质和药效物质。中药遗传物质主要是研究中药的遗传品质，即研究药材的生物遗传特性和优势，如优质品种的种质资源、遗传多样性、品种多样性、遗传分子标记，以及遗传物质与优质药材的生产、临床疗效的关系。中药药效物质是标定中药内在品质的主要方式，其研究主要应用化学和生物学的技术和方法，揭示基于临床疗效的中药有效部位、有效组分、有效成分，并达到可用分子式和结构式表示的具有一定物理常数的质量标志物。

The quality of Chinese Medicinal refers to the inherent overall characteristics of quality in germplasm, seedlings, cultivation, harvesting, processing, preparation and other aspects. The quality of Chinese Medicinal includes external quality and internal quality. ① External quality mainly refers to the character quality of Chinese Medicinal, and the quality evaluations include "character-based" assessment of shape, color, flavor, and taste, and quality evaluation based on microscopic identification and physicochemical determination. ② Intrinsic quality includes the genetic material and pharmacodynamic substances.

The genetic material refers to the study of the biological genetic characteristics, which refers to the advantages of Chinese Medicinal, such as the germplasm resources of high-quality varieties, genetic diversity, variety diversity, genetic molecular markers, as well as the relationship between genetic material and the production and clinical efficacy of high-quality medicinals. The pharmacodynamic substance is the main way to calibrate the intrinsic quality of Chinese Materia Medica. Chemical and biological techniques and methods are usually used to reveal the effective parts, active components and active ingredients of Chinese Materia Medica based on clinical efficacy, and achieve the mass markers with certain physical constants which can be expressed by molecular formula and structural formula.

三、制药
3 Pharmacy

制药主要包括药材产地加工、饮片炮制、中成药制药。①药材产地加工是指药用部位收获至形成商品药材而进行的初步处理和干燥等产地加工过程,主要包括采收、净制、干燥、规格分级、包装、贮藏等。其中,干燥的加工方法非常丰富,如阴干、烘干、熏硫、蒸、煮、烫、发汗等产地加工方法。传统形成的药材产地加工方法不仅具有区域药材生产、中医流派、医家用药习惯等特征,并蕴涵着丰富的科学道理,赋予了中药性状、规格、品质、药性等诸多内涵。②饮片炮制是中医药的一大特色,其历史悠久,技术独到,理论和技术体系完整,作用显著。饮片炮制的方法众多,临床上常用的传统炮制饮片多通过净制法、切制法、炒制法(加辅料或不加辅料炒)、炙法(加酒、醋、姜汁、蜂蜜等辅料)、煅法、蒸法、煮法、燀法、发酵法、发芽法、制霜法、烘焙法、水飞法等制备而成,而新型饮片,多采用现代制药技术制备而成。③中成药制药不仅是传统的膏、丹、丸、散,而更多的是现代中成药生产制剂,其剂型达50多种,包括固体剂型、半固体剂型、液体剂型、气体剂型等。

Pharmacy includes the processing in the production place of medicinal materials, the processing of decoction pieces and the pharmacy of Chinese patent medicines. ① The processing of medicinal materials in the production place refers to the preliminary processing and drying of the medicinal parts from harvested to commercial medicinal materials, which includes the harvesting, cleansing, drying, classification, packaging and storage. Drying methods are rich, such as drying in shade, baking, sulfuring, steaming, boiling, scalding, sweating and other methods. The traditional processing methods of medicinal material production place not only have characteristics of regional production of Chinese medicinal materials, schools of Chinese medicine, prescription habits and so on, but also contain abundant scientific principles, endowing Chinese Medicinal with such connotations as character, specification, quality and medicinal properties. ② The processing of decoction pieces is a major feature of Chinese Materia Medica, with a long history, unique technology, complete theory and technical system, and remarkable effects. The processing methods are numerous. For example, the traditional processed pieces commonly used in clinic are prepared with cleansing, cutting, stir-frying (with adjuvant or not), stir-frying with liquid adjuvants (with liquor, vinegar, ginger, honey or other adjuvants), calcining, steaming, decocting, blanching, fermenting, sprouting, crystallizing or powdering, baking, grinding with water, while the new types of decoction pieces are usually prepared with modern pharmaceutical techniques. ③ Pharmacy of Chinese patent medicines refers not only to the traditional forms such as paste, pellet, pills and powder, but also refers to more than 50 types of modern Chinese patent medicines, the pharmaceutical forms of which, including solid, semisolid, liquid, gas pharmaceutical form, and so on.

中药制药过程是广泛的，既包括药材加工、饮片炮制、中成药制药，也包括中药汤剂的煎煮、中药人工制品、中药曲类发酵和中药配方颗粒的制备、中药生物工程、中药制药设备等方面的内容。

The pharmacy of Chinese medicine is extensive, including the processing of medicinal materials, processing of decoction pieces, and pharmacy of Chinese patent medicine, as well as formula decocting, artificial products of Chinese medicine, fermentation of Chinese Medicinal, preparation of Chinese medicine dispensing granules, biological engineering of Chinese medicine, pharmaceutical equipment, and so on.

四、药性
4 Property

药性是中药作用于机体的基本性质和特征的高度概括，是中药基本理论的核心，是中药区别于植物药和天然药物的显著标志。药性的主要内容包括四气、五味、归经、升降浮沉、有毒无毒、补泻、润燥等。①四气即寒热温凉四种性质，是药物作用于机体后产生寒、热等不同效应的高度概括。②五味是指药物有酸、苦、甘、辛、咸不同的药味，因此具有不同的作用。③归经表示药物对人体作用的部位，归是作用的归属，经是脏腑经络的概称。④升降浮沉表示药物对人体作用的不同趋向性。⑤有毒无毒是指药物对机体是否有损害作用，并不是所有的中药都有毒性，有毒中药专门指那些药性强烈，对人体有毒性或副作用，安全剂量小，用之不当或药量超过常量，即对人体产生危害，甚至可致人死亡的中药。⑥药物虚实补泻是从药物作用于机体所发生的反应概括出来的，是与所治疾病的虚实性质相对应而确定的。⑦润燥是对药物祛除燥邪或湿邪，以及治疗燥证或湿证的作用性质的概括，是相对燥邪、湿邪，或燥证、湿证而言的，主要是反映药物对人体阴液变化的影响。

Property is the highly generalization of the primary properties and characteristics of Chinese medicinal acting on human body. It is the core of the basic theory of Chinese Medicinal and acts as a significant symbol of Chinese medicinal differing from botanic and natural medicinals. The main contents of the property of Chinese medicine include the four qi, the five flavors, meridian (channel) tropism, ascending, descending, floating and sinking, toxic and non-toxic, reinforcement and reduction, moistening and dryness and so on. ① Four qi refer to four properties like cold, hot, warm and cool. It is a generalization of the medicinal action on the body to produce cold, heat and other different effects. ② Five flavors refer to the medicine with different medicinal tastes including acid, bitter, sweet, spicy and salty, and therefore the medicine has different effects. ③ The meridian tropism ("Gui Jing" in Chinese) refers to the place where the medicinal acts on the human body. "Gui" means the attribution of the function; "Jing" is the general name of Zang-fu organs and channels. ④ Ascending, descending, floating and sinking indicate the different tendencies of Chinese materia medica effects on human body. ⑤ Toxic and non-toxic refer to whether the medicinal is harmful to the body or not. It doesn't mean all Chinese Medicinal are toxic. Toxic Chinese Medicinal specifically refers to those with strong properties, toxic effects or side effects on the human body, and with small safe doses. The improper use or overuse of these medicines can be harmful to the human body, and even cause death. ⑥ The deficiency and excess, reinforcement and reduction of medicines are summarized from the reaction of medicines on the body and correspond to the property of the disease being treated. ⑦ Moistening and drying are summaries of medicinals to remove dryness or dampness, as well as the treatment of corresponding syndromes related to dryness or dampness. It mainly reflects the influence of medicinals on the change of human body's Yin fluid.

除此之外，在历代文献中，药性还有走守、动静、刚柔、猛缓及敛散、滑涩、轻重等记载。

In addition, there are some other records of property in the ancient literature, including migratory and settled, dynamic and static, firm and soft, fierce and relaxative, convergent and emanative, slippery and dry, slight and heavy, etc.

五、功效
5 Efficacy

功效是系统中药学的核心和主体,是系统中药学区别于传统主流本草学、现代药理学的重要特征,是现代中药学的学科标志。中药功效是在中医药理论指导下,对中药治疗作用、保健作用的理性概况,主要分为治疗功效和保健功效。

Efficacy is the core and subject of Systematic Chinese materia medica, acting as the feature to make systematic Chinese materia medica different from traditional mainstream herbalism and modern pharmacology, thereby becoming the subject mark of modern Chinese materia medica. Efficacy is a rational overview of both the therapeutic effects and health care effects of Chinese materia medica under the guidance of Chinese medicine theory. It is mainly divided into therapeutic efficacy and health care efficacy.

治疗功效又可分为消除疾病发生的原因、发挥治本作用的对因治疗功效和改善疾病症状、发挥治标作用的对症治疗功效,以及对疾病直接发挥治疗作用的对病治疗功效。①对因治疗作用是祛除病邪,消除病因,恢复脏腑功能的协调,纠正阴阳偏盛偏衰的病理现象。简言之,即祛邪、扶正、调理脏腑功能。②对症治疗作用是指中药治疗功效中能消除或缓解患者自觉痛苦症状或临床体征的特殊效用。③对病治疗功效是针对中医的"病"发挥治疗作用的功效,如截疟、驱蛔虫等,分别针对疟疾、蛔虫病发挥治疗作用。

The therapeutic efficacy could be divided into etiology-targeted efficacy that has fundamental effect to eliminate the causes of disease, and symptom-targeted efficacy that has palliative effect to improve the symptoms, as well as disease-targeted efficacy. ① Etiology-targeted efficacy aims to remove pathogens, eliminate the cause of disease, restore the coordination of zang-fu organs functions, and correct the imbalance between yin and yang. ② Symptom-targeted efficacy refers to the special efficacy of Chinese medicine to relieve the symptoms or clinical signs and suffering. ③ Disease targeted on diseases is to exert the therapeutic efficacy directly on the "diseases" of Chinese medicine, such as effects of preventing malaria and dispelling ascarid are respectively suitable for treating malaria and ascariasis.

保健功效是在中医药理论指导下将中药对人体预防或养生、康复等作用进行概括和总结而形成的,包括预防功效和养生功效。①预防功效是指采用以药物为主的多种手段,如烟熏、洗浴、佩带或内服等,防止某些疾病的发生和发展。②养生功效是指采用中药以增强人体适应能力,强身健体,调理情志,养护脏腑,延缓衰老等方面的作用。

Health care efficacy, including preventive efficacy and health maintenance efficacy, refers to the prevention, health maintenance, and rehabilitation of Chinese Medicinal on human beings under the guidance of Chinese medicine theory. ① Preventive efficacy refers to using a variety of medicinal based means, such as smoking, bathing, wearing or oral administration, to prevent the occurrence and development of diseases. ② Health maintenance efficacy refers to the use of Chinese medicine to enhance adaptability, strengthen the body, regulate emotions, maintain the function of zang-fu organs, and delay aging

另外,随着现代研究的不断深入,中药新的功效不断被发现、认识和使用。如青皮、枳实升压、抗休克;泽泻、山楂降血脂;罗布麻降血压;砒霜抗癌治疗白血病等。

With the development of modern research, new effects of Chinese materia medica have been constantly discovered, recognized and used. For example, Qingpi (Citri Reticulatae Pericarpium Viride) and Zhishi (Aurantii Fructus Immaturus) have the effect of raising blood pressure and preventing shock; Zexie (Alismatis Rhizoma) and Shanzha (Crataegi Fructus) can lower blood fat; Luobuma (Apocyni Veneti Folium) can lower blood pressure; Pishuang (Arsenicum Sablimatum) can treat leukemia, and so on.

六、应用
6 Application

中药临床应用是医药结合的桥梁，反映中药临床合理应用的精髓和中医临床治病救人的根本，主要包括中药临床应用的形式、方法和规律。其应用形式主要有饮片和成药，应用方法与规律主要包括配伍、用法、用量、禁忌等方面的内容。

The clinical application of Chinese medicinal includes the forms, methods and rules of the clinical application, which is a bridge of the combining of clinical practice and medicinal pharmacy. It reflects the essence of the rational clinical application of Chinese medicinal and the foundation of curing diseases. The clinical application forms of Chinese medicinal include decoction piece and patent medicines, and the application methods and rules mainly include compatibility, administration, dosage, contraindication and other aspects.

配伍：指按照病情的不同需要和药物的不同特点，有选择地将两种或两种以上的药物配合在一起应用。古人将中药的配伍关系总结为七个方面，称为"七情"，即单行、相须、相使、相畏、相杀、相恶、相反。

Compatibility of Chinese medicinal refers to the selective application of two or more medicinals in combination based on needs of patient's condition as well as characteristics of medicinals. The ancient people summarized the compatibility of Chinese medicinal into seven aspects, known as the "Qiqing (seven emotions)", including

single application, mutual reinforcement, mutual assistance, mutual restraint, mutual suppression, mutual inhibition and antagonism.

中药饮片和中成药的用法：主要包括给药途径、不同剂型、服药方法等方面的内容。①中药饮片和中成药的给药途径，主要包括胃肠道给药和不经胃肠道给药两类。其中，不经胃肠道给药又包括注射给药、呼吸道给药、皮肤给药、黏膜给药等。②中药剂型包括汤剂、颗粒剂、丸剂、片剂、灌肠剂、栓剂、注射剂、气雾剂、洗剂、搽剂、软膏剂、膏药、涂膜剂、巴布剂、离子透入剂、滴眼剂、滴鼻剂、含漱剂等。③服药方法主要是根据病情需要和药物特性，选择适当的服药时间，也是合理用药的要求。

Administration of Chinese medicine decoction pieces and Chinese patent medicines includes routes of administration, pharmaceutical form and method of taking medicine. ① The routes of administration of Chinese medicine decoction pieces and Chinese patent medicines mainly include gastrointestinal administration and non-gastrointestinal administration. Non-gastrointestinal administration also includes injection administration, pulmonary administration, skin administration, and mucosal administration. ② The pharmaceutical forms of Chinese Medicinal include decoction, granule, pill, tablet, enema, suppository, injection, aerosol, lotion, liniment, ointment, plaster, cataplasm, ion penetration agent, eye drops, nose drops, gargle, etc. ③ The method of taking medicine is based on the treatment needs of disease and the characteristics of medicine, and then choose the appropriate time to take medicine, which is also the requirement of rational use of medicine.

中药的用量：不仅包括中药饮片单味药用于治疗的常用有效量、方剂中各药的相对用量、药物的实际利用量，也包括中成药应用的剂量。①单味药常用有效剂量的实质，是药物应用于机体后，能够产生特定生物效应的量；②方剂中的相对用量是指在方剂中，单味药与其他药物配合后产生共同效应的需要量；③实际利用量主要是指由于药材质量、炮制、剂型、制剂、服法等多种因素的影响，药物实际利用不同的量。因此，在中药饮片和中成药实际应用中应高度重视。

Dosage of Chinese Medicinal includes not only the common and effective dosage of a single medicinal, the relative dosage of each medicinal in prescriptions and the actual dosage of the medicine, but also the dosage of Chinese patent medicine. ① The substance of the commonly used effective dosage of a single medicinal is the amount of the medicinal applied to human body to produce specific biological effects. ② The relative dosage in the prescription refers to the amount of single medicinal required to produce a common effect when in the combination with other medicinals in the prescription. ③ The actual dosage mainly refers to different doses of the medicinal influenced by the quality, processing, pharmaceutical form, preparation, method of administration and other factors. Therefore, the actual dosage should be attached great importance in the application of Chinese medicine decoction pieces and Chinese patent medicine.

用药禁忌：主要包括证候禁忌、配伍禁忌、妊娠禁忌和饮食宜忌四个方面。①证候禁忌是指某些病证应当避免使用某种或者某类中药饮片或中成药。②配伍禁忌是指两药合用后使治疗效应下降，或使毒副作用增强，或产生新的毒副作用效应者，原则上都不宜合用。历来把这些视为配伍禁忌药，并概括为"十八反"和"十九畏"。③妊娠禁忌是指妇女在妊娠期间使用某些饮片或中成药会损害母体及胎元以致引起堕胎的药物，包括禁用药与慎用药两类。禁用药多为大毒的药物、引产堕胎药、破血消癥药、峻下逐水药；慎用药包括通经祛瘀、行气破滞、辛热燥烈、滑利通窍类药物。④饮食宜忌是指服用中药饮片及中成药期间禁忌进食某些食物，简称食忌，又称忌口，以免降低、破坏药效，或引发不良反应。

Medication contraindications include four aspects: syndrome contraindication, compatibility contraindication, pregnancy contraindication, and dietary contraindication. ① Syndrome contraindication refers to the fact that some diseases and syndromes should avoid using certain type of Chinese medicine decoction pieces or Chinese patent medicine. ② Compatibility contraindication refers to the fact that two medicinals used together can reduce treatment efficacy, enhance or create new toxic and side effect, so these medicinals in principle should not be used together. The compatibilities of these medicinals have been regarded as taboos, and summarized as "eighteen incompatible medicaments" and "nineteen medicaments of mutual restraint". ③ Pregnancy contraindication, including prohibited medicinals and medicinals given cautiously, refers to the use of certain decoction pieces or Chinese patent medicines during pregnancy which will damage the mother and fetus and cause abortion. Most of the prohibited medicinals are poisonous medicinals, induced abortion medicinals, medicinals for stasis-breaking and eliminating abdominal mass, medicinals for drastically purging water; medicinals given cautiously include medicinals of dredging meridians and removing blood stasis, promoting qi to break stagnation, pungent and hot, or dry and drastic, smoothing and dredging orifices. ④ Dietary contraindication refers that certain food should not be taken while taking some Chinese medicine decoction pieces and Chinese patent medicine, so as to prevent the reduction and destruction of the efficacy, or the occurrence of adverse reaction.

另外，儿童、老人由于生理、心理不同于成年人，药物在吸收、分布、代谢、排泄的过程与成人有差异，儿童应根据体重或年龄计算用药剂量和使用途径，尽量避免使用含有毒性成分的中成药，并根据中成药治疗效果，尽量缩短儿童用药疗程，及时减量或停药；老年人因机体组织器官衰老，对药物的吸收、代谢速度减慢，应避免使用对肝脏、肾脏等药物代谢器官有损害的药物，也应避免对心脏、血管等组织有损害的药物。运动员因其职业特殊性，对含有兴奋性成分的药物应避免使用；而中成药的服用则应按药品说明书的要求安全合理使用。

In addition, as the physiology, psychology of children and the elderly are different from that of the adults, it is different from adults in drug absorption, distribution, metabolism, and excretion. For children, the dosage and route of medication should be calculated along with their weight or age, and avoid the use of medicine containing toxic ingredients, shorten the course of medication according to the therapeutic effect, and timely reduce or stop taking medicine. For the old, due to the aging of the body tissues and organs, the absorption and metabolism of medicinals are slowed down. The elderly should avoid using

medicinals that damage the metabolic organs of drugs such as liver and kidney, and medicinals that damage the tissues such as heart and blood vessels. Athletes should avoid using medicines containing excitatory ingredients because of the particularity of their occupation. Chinese patent medicine should be reasonably and safely used according to the requirements of the package instruction.

由此可见，系统中药学是研究中药复杂系统品种、品质、制药、药性、功效、应用等关键要素发生、发展、变化规律的科学。

Thus, the systematic Chinese materia medica is a science of researching on occurrence, development and change of the key elements of the Chinese materia medicia complex system, including variety, quality, pharmacy, property, efficacy and application.

第二节　系统中药学的认知过程

Section 2　The Cognitive Process of Systematic Chinese Materia Medica

纵观本草的发展，尤其是主流本草的发展历史，我们可以清晰地看到，从古至今，中医药无不重视整体、系统、动态的变化过程，已经有"系统中药"的萌芽。而真正出现系统中药学的认知，是中国中药高等教育以来，逐渐认识、提出、形成和发展起来的科学体系。

Throughout the development of medicinals, especially the history of mainstream medicinals, we can clearly find that the Chinese medicine consistently has been attaching great importance to the overall, systematic and dynamic natural process in all ages, and "systematic TCM" had sprouted in ancient China. Since the higher education of Chinese medicine, the cognition of Systematic Chinese materia medica has authentically appeared, which is a scientific system

that has been gradually recognized, proposed, formed, and developed.

1956 年 8 月 6 日，国务院正式行文批准在北京、上海、成都、广州建立四所中医学院。1956 年 9 月 1 日招生，中药学仅是中医学专业的一门课程，涉及本草、方剂相关内容。1959 年 5 月 8 日，经原中华人民共和国卫生部（59）131 号文批准在原成都中医学院开办中药本科专业，招生 60 人。中药本科专业的创办，使传统中药人才培养进入国家高等教育系列，成为我国高等教育的重要组成部分，也是我国中医药高等教育史上的一个里程碑。但中药本科专业建设与教材无可借鉴。为此，凌一揆教授提出"大中药"的概念。"大中药"包括本草与方剂、中药栽培与鉴定、中药炮制与制剂、中草药化学、中药药理等方面的内容。为了创办中药本科专业，构建"大中药"体系,凌一揆、雷载权教授主编了《中药学讲义》《方剂学讲义》,徐楚江、冯向贤老师编写了《中药制剂学讲义》《中药炮炙学讲义》,贾敏如、李方尧教授编写了《中药鉴定学讲义》,曾万章、万德光教授编写了《药用植物学讲义》,万德光教授编写了《药用动物学讲义》,陈道森、邓先久老师编写了《中药栽培学讲义》,肖崇厚教授编写了《中草药化学》,沈映君教授参编了《中药药理学》。其后,原成都中医学院主编了第一版全国高等中医院校教材《中药学》《中药炮制学》《中药鉴定学》《中药化学》和规划教材《临床中药学》《中药药理学》《药用动物学》等中药专业主干课程。

On August 6th, 1956, the State Council officially approved the establishment of four Chinese medicine colleges in Beijing, Shanghai, Chengdu and Guangzhou. The enrollment work started on September 1st, 1956, Chinese materia medica is just a course of the specialty of Chinese medicine, involving contents of Bencao (materia medica) and prescriptions. On May 8th, 1959, approved by the NO. 131 document of former Ministry of health of the People's Republic of China (59), the undergraduate specialty of Chinese materia medica was set up in the former Chengdu college of TCM, enrolling 60 students. The establishment of the specialty brought the cultivation of Chinese materia medica talent into the national higher education series and turned it into a significant part of the higher education in China, which is also a milestone in the history of the higher education of Chinese medicine in China. However, there is no reference for the construction and the teaching materials of this specialty, for which, professor Ling Yikui put forward the conception of "large Chinese Materia Medica (Dazhongyao)", which includes the contents of medicinals and prescriptions, cultivation and identification of Chinese Medicinals, processing and preparation of Chinese Medicinal, chemistry of Chinese materia medica, pharmacology of Chinese medicine and so on.

In order to establish the undergraduate specialty of Chinese Materia Medica and construct the system of the "large Chinese Materia Medica", professor Ling Yikui and professor Lei Zaiquan edited the *Chinese Materia Medica Lecture Notes* and *Formula Lecture Notes;* teacher Xu Chujiang and teacher Feng Xiangxian compiled the *Preparation of Chinese Materia Medica Lecture Notes* and *Processing of Chinese Materia Medica Lecture Notes;* professor Jia Minru and professor Li Fangyao edited the *Identification of Chinese Materia Medica Lecture Notes;* professor Zeng Wanzhang and professor Wan Deguang compiled *Pharmaceutical Botany Lecture Notes;* professor Wan Deguang also compile the *Pharmaceutical Zoology Lecture Notes.* Moreover, teacher Chen Daosen and teacher Deng Xianjiu compiled *Cultivation of Chinese Herbal Medicine Lecture Notes;* professor Xiao Chonghou compiled *Chemistry of Chinese herbal medicine;* professor Shen Yingjun participated in the edition of *Pharmacology of Chinese Materia Medica.* Later, Chengdu college of traditional Chinese medicine (named Chengdu University of TCM today) compiled the first edition of textbooks for national Chinese medicine colleges and universities, including *Chinese Materia Medica, Science of Processing Chinese Materia Medica, Identification of Chinese Materia Medica, Chemistry of Chinese Materia Medica*, and the planning textbooks, such as *Clinical Chinese Medicine, Pharmacology of Chinese Materia medica, Pharmaceutical Zoology* and other main courses of specialty of *Chinese Materia Medica.*

"大中药"概念的提出和"大中药"课程体系的构建,是凌一揆教授"系统中药"思想的主要内容。为了揭示系统中药学的科学内涵和关键要素,彭成教授于2000年以来,在国家973计划、国家自然科学基金重点项目等国家级项目的支持下,针对中药品种的多样性、化学成分的复杂性、药效作用的多向性、临床应用的广泛性,选择常用中药附子作为研究对象,研究附子不同来源，不同炮制品种，不同制备工艺，不同化学层次的空间特征、生态特征、数量特征、化学特征和生物学特征，试图阐明附子空间、时间、剂量与效应之间的动态变化过程，揭示中药附子的物质基础、生物效应和应用规律；系统研究了参附注射液的品种、质量、安全性与有效性、临床和制药生产关键技术应用，实施全程自动化数字监控，进行品质控制。并首次提出中药"品质性效用"和中药注射剂"品质制性用"的多维评价研究模式，系统研究附子和参附注射液的品种、品质、制药、药性、功效、应用，取得了明显的社会和经济效益。其中，"附子的系统研究与开发应用"获得2010年度四川省科学技术进步一等奖，"参附注射液品质控制与产业化关键技术应用"获得2013年度国家科学技术进步二等奖。王永炎院士函评"附子的系统研究与开发应用"时写到："对附子进行'品、质、性、效、用'一体化的研究与开发当是首创，项目体现了科学性、前瞻性、创新性和实用性，是一种值得向国内外推广辐射的新模式，具有中医药的原创思维和原创优势。"肖培根院士在函评意见中写到"本项目构建的中药系统研究'多维评价'的理论、方法和实践体系，对中药资源的系统研究与应用，具有示范推广作用"。

The proposition of the conception of "large Chinese Materia Medica" and construction of relevant course system are the main contents of the "Systematic Chinese Materia Medica", which is a thought from professor Ling Yikui. Since the year of 2000, for revealing the scientific connotation and key elements of Systematic Chinese Materia Medica, supported by national projects such as the National 973 Program and the National Natural Science Foundation of China, with a focus on the diversity of Chinese Medicinal, the complexity of chemical components, the multi-directionality of pharmacodynamic effects as well as the universality of clinical applications, professor Peng Cheng had taken the widely used Chinese medicine Fuzi (Aconiti Lateralis Radix Praeparata) as the research object to study its different sources, diverse processed products, various preparation processes, as well as spatial, ecological, quantitative, chemical, and biological characteristics from different chemical levels, so to endeavor illustrating the dynamic change process among time, dose and effect, and revealing the material basis, biological effect and application rules of Fuzi. In addition, he systematically studied the variety, quality, safety and efficacy, and clinic application and pharmaceutical key technique application, and implemented automatic digital monitoring throughout the process to control the quality. For the first time, he proposed the multi-dimensional evaluation research modes of "variety, quality, property, efficacy, application" for Chinese Materia Medica and "variety, quality, pharmacy, property, application" for Chinese medicine injection. The systematical research on the variety, quality, pharmacy, property, efficacy and application of Fuzi and Shenfu Zhusheye (Injection), has acquired obvious social and economic benefits. Among them, the program "Systematic Research, Development and Application of Fuzi" was rewarded the first prize of Science and Technology Progress Award of Sichuan province in 2010, and "Quality Control and Industrialized Key Technology Application of Shenfu Zhusheye" won the Second prize of the National Science and Technology Progress Award in 2013. Academician Wang Yongyan evaluated by letter on "Systematic Research, Development and Application of Fuzi" as follows: the integrative research and development on "variety, quality, property, efficacy, application" of Fuzi is an initiative project, which embodies the scientificity, foresight, innovation and practicality of the study. For its original thinking and advantages of Chinese medicine, it is a novel mode worthy of spreading domestICly and overseas. Moreover, academician Xiao Peigen commented that the theory, method and practice system of "multi-dimensional evaluation" for the systematic study of Chinese medicine established in this project has a demonstration and popularization effect on the systematic research and application of Chinese medicine resources.

2006年，成都中医药大学本科教学评估时，彭成教授带领成都中医药大学药学院的专家，对成都中医药大学中药本科教育的理念进行了总结，即为"医药结合、系统中药、实践创新"，并对"系统中药学"进行了解释，即"系统中药学是指中药是一个系统，是研究中药认采种制用（品质性效用）等理论和技术的系统知识"。2010年，彭成教授在《中药与临床》杂志发表论文，详细阐述了"系统中药"产生的背景和科学内涵，并应用复杂系统科学研究的思路，结合系统中药学的特点，提出"多维评价"是"系统中药"研究的优选方法，还以中药附子为研究实例，系统阐释了"系统中药""品、质、性、效、用""多维评价"的实践方法。2012年，针对中药注射剂研制与生产过程中存在的关键科学和技术问题，彭成教授在《中药与临床》杂志发表论文，提出中药注射剂"品质制性用"的研究模式，并以参附注射液为例，解析中药注射剂研制与生产过程中"品种、质量、制药、性效、临床应用"几个关键问题的科学内涵，为中药注射剂的研制与生产提供了新的思路。2017年，彭成教授在《中药与临床》杂志发表论文，再论"品、质、制、性、效、用"的科学内涵，自此，系统中药学的理论技术体系和实践方法日渐成熟。

In 2006, during the undergraduate teaching evaluation of Chengdu University of TCM, with the leading of Professor Peng Cheng, the experts of Pharmacy School of Chengdu University of TCM summarized the concept of undergraduate education of TCM of Chengdu University as "combination of medicine and drug, Systematic Chinese Materia Medica, practice and innovation". They also gave explanation for "Systematic Chinese Materia Medica" which is "Chinese medicine is a system, which is a systematic knowledge of theories and technologies on the identification, harvest, cultivation, pharmacy, application (variety, quality, property, efficacy, application) of Chinese medicine". In 2010, professor Peng Cheng published a paper in *Pharmacy and Clinics of Chinese Materia Medica*, elaborating the background and scientific connotation of Systematic Chinese Materia Medica in details. Besides, being based on the thought of complex system scientific research and the characteristics of Systematic Chinese Materia Medica, he put forward that "multi-dimensional evaluation" is the preferred method for the study of "Systematic Chinese Materia Medica". In addition, this paper also took the Fuzi as a research example, systematically explaining the practical methods of "Systematic Chinese Materia Medica", "variety, quality, property, efficacy, application" and "multidimensional evaluation". In 2012, aiming at the key scientific and technical problems in the development and production of Chinese medicine injections, professor Peng Cheng published a paper in the journal of *Pharmacy and Clinics of Chinese Materia Medica,* in which he put forward the research mode of "variety, quality, pharmacy, property, application" of Chinese medicine injection and analyzed the scientific connotation of several key issues of "variety, quality, pharmacy, property and efficacy, clinical application" in the development and production of TCM injections by taking Shenfu Injection as an instance, which provided a novel idea for the development and production of Chinese medicine injections. In 2017, Professor Peng Cheng published another thesis in the *Pharmacy and Clinics of Chinese Materia Medica,* in which he discussed the scientific connotation of "variety, quality, pharmacy, property, application" again. Since then, the theoretical and technical system and practice methods of Systematic Chinese Materia Medica have gradually matured.

第三节　系统中药学的现代研究

Section 3　Modern Research on Systematic Chinese Materia Medica

一、品种的研究
1 The Research on Variety

（一）药材品种
1.1 Variety of Materia Medica

中药药材品种的研究，主要包括中药品种考证、中药品种调查、中药品种比较、中药品种鉴定和中药品种与生态环境、栽培养殖、采收加工、物质基础、药理毒理、功效应用等方面的内容。

The research on the variety of Chinese materia medica includes the verification, investigation, comparison and identification of the variety of Chinese medicine as well as the contents among variety of Chinese medicine and ecological environment, cultivation, harvest and processing, material basis, pharmacology and toxicology, application and efficacy.

目前，药材品种研究的热点领域主要有种质资源、新品种培育、规范化种养殖和道地药材研究等；药材品种研究的现代方法主要有DNA分子遗传标记技术、中药化学指纹图谱技术、组织形态三维定量分析等。

Presently, the hot areas of the research on variety of medicinal materials mainly include germplasm resources, new breed cultivation, cultivation standardization, and genuine regional medicinal and so on. The modern methods of the variety of medicinal material research cover DNA molecular genetic marker technology, Chinese medicine chemical fingerprinting technology, three-dimensional quantitative analysis of tissue morphology, etc.

1. DNA分子遗传标记技术　为从居群和分子水平上揭示中药材道地性的生物学实质提供了可能，同时可用于中药材鉴定与道地性研究的RFLP、RAPD、AFLP、测序技术、DNA barcoding技术等DNA分子遗传标记技术，又具有快速、微量、特异性强及不受生长发育阶段、供试部位、环境条件影响等特点。

1.1.1 DNA molecular genetic marker technology provides the possibility to reveal the biological essence of the genuine regional nature of Chinese materia medica from population and molecular level. Meanwhile, the technology can be used for identification and authentic research on Chinese materia medica, including RFLP, RAPD, AFLP, sequencing technology, DNA barcoding technology, which also has the characteristics of quickness, trace, high specificity and not affected by growth and development stage, test site and environmental conditions.

2. 中药化学指纹图谱技术　已广泛应用于中药药材品种质量标准研究，涉及薄层扫描（TLCS）、高效液相色谱（HPLC）、气相色谱（GC）、高效毛细管电泳（HPCE)等色谱法，紫外光谱（UV）、红外光谱（IR）、质谱(MS)、核磁共振（NMR）、X-射线衍射等光谱法以及各种色谱光谱联用分析技术。

1.1.2 Chinese medicine chemical fingerprinting technology has been widely applied to the study of quality standards of the variety of traditional Chinese medicinal materials, which involves chromatography, such as thin layer chromatography (TLCS), high-performance liquid chromatography (HPLC), gas chromatography (GC), high performance capillary electrophoresis (HPCE), and spectroscopy including ultraviolet spectrum (UV), infrared spectrum (IR), mass spectrometry (MS), nuclear magnetic resonance (NMR) and X-ray diffraction; as well as various

Chromatography-spectrum analysis techniques.

3. 组织形态三维定量分析　全面表征中药组织形态结构细胞的空间位置和结构与功能的关系，而且实现了中药组织鉴定三维定量与数字可视化。

1.1.3 Histomophological three-dimensional quantitative analysis can comprehensively characterize the relationship between the spatial position, structure and function of Chinese medicine tissue morphological structure cells, which realizes the three-dimensional quantitative and digital visualization of Chinese medicine tissue identification.

（二）炮制品种

1.2 Variety of Processing

近年来，中药炮制品种在炮制辅料、炮制技术、炮制规范、炮制原理、新型饮片等方面的研究取得了一系列的创新和发展。

Recently, a series of innovations and developments have been gained during the studies of processing adjuvants, processing technology, processing norms, processing principle, and new types of decoction pieces on Chinese medicinal materials.

1. 炮制辅料研究方面　先后建立了姜、蜜、酒、醋、盐等国家标准，对麦麸、蛤粉、滑石粉、河砂、酒、醋、盐、姜、蜂蜜、油等辅料的炮制作用进行了研究。

1.2.1 Research on Adjuvants in Processing Chinese Medicinal Materials

National standards for adjuvants as ginger, honey, liquor, vinegar, salt, etc. have been established, and then the processing effects of wheat bran, pulverized-clamshell, pulverized-talcum, river sand, liquor, vinegar, salt, ginger, honey, oil and other adjuvants have been studied.

2. 炮制技术和炮制规范研究方面　不仅将饮片炮制老药工的炮制经验数据化，建立了科学、实用的规范化的炮制工艺模式，为中药饮片生产的规范化、规模化创造了良好的条件，而且相继修订和增补了常用中药及藏、蒙、维等特色民族医药的饮片炮制规范。另外，饮片生产中

有诸多以主观判断为主的情况，如"火力"的控制仍然主要靠药工"以手试温"，"火候"的判断主要通过眼看、鼻嗅、口尝、手试等方法，对药材形状、颜色、大小、断面、气、味、质地等进行多方位判断，炒制过程中炒香、炒焦和蒸制中"黑如漆，甜如饴"，以及毒性中药半夏、川乌、附子等饮片"口尝微有麻舌感"等。

1.2.2 Research on Technology and Norms of Processing Chinese Medicinal Materials

Not only digitized the processing experience of seasoned pharmaceutical workers in the processing of decoction pieces and established the scientific and practical standardized processing mode to create a good condition for the standardization and scale-up of the production of decoction pieces, but also revised and supplemented the processing standard of Chinese medicine and characteristic ethnic medicines such as Tibetan, Mongolian and Uygur medicines successively. In addition, there exist quite number of conditions of subjective judgment in the production of decoction pieces. For instance, the Huoli (control of fire force) is still depended on the experienced pharmaceutical workers to "test the temperature by hand", and the "Huohou (control of time and temperature)" is mainly judged by the methods of seeing, sniffing, tasting, and hand-testing, as well as the multi-directional judgement on the shape, color, size, cross-section, gas, taste, and texture of medicinal materials, such as stir-heating the medicinals till fragrant, stir-frying to brown, and steaming, the characteristics of "black as lacquer, sweet as maltose" in steaming, and the state of "slightly tingling taste" of Banxia (Pinelliae Rhizoma), Chuanwu (Aconiti Radix), Fuzi and other poisonous decoction pieces.

3. 新型饮片研究方面　主要有单味中药浓缩颗粒（中药配方颗粒）、中药颗粒饮片、袋泡剂、煮散剂、超微粉等新型饮片。

1.2.3 Research on New Types of Decoction Pieces

There are single Chinese medicinal

concentrated granule (granule of Chinese medicinal formula), granular decoction pieces of Chinese medicine, teabag, medicinal powder for boiling, ultra-fine powder and other new types of decoction pieces.

中药浓缩颗粒是以中药饮片为原料，经提取、分离、浓缩、干燥、制粒、包装等工艺制成的产品，具有不用煎煮，调剂、服用方便，清洁卫生等优点；以成方颗粒为主、单味中药浓缩颗粒为辅的颗粒制剂，是一种兼顾随证调方和复方合煎两个特点的汤剂改革尝试。

Chinese medicinal concentrated granule is made from decoction pieces through extraction, separation, concentration, drying, granulation, packaging and other processes, which possesses the characteristics of free of frying or dispensing, conveniently taking, cleanliness, etc. It is mainly composed of granules of Chinese medicinal formula and supplemented by single Chinese medicinal concentrated granules, which belongs to an innovative attempt of decoction with two features, namely "adjusting formula as syndrome changes" and "boiling compound recipes together".

中药颗粒饮片是在传统饮片的基础上，根据每种药物发挥最大效益的原则，经加工制成一定颗粒状，干燥、灭菌，单味定量分装而成的一种统一规格、统一剂量、统一质量标准的新型饮片，颗粒饮片既保持了传统中药饮片的固有优点，又弥补了不足，是目前取代传统饮片的最佳新型饮片，是国际上竞相大力研究推广使用的饮片新剂型。

Granular decoction pieces of Chinese medicine, as a novel type of decoction pieces, is each medicinal to process into granular shape after drying, sterilizing, and single quantitative packaging on the basis of traditional decoction pieces according to the principle of maximizing the benefits of each medicine, then packed in unified specification, unified dose and unified quality standard. It not only maintains the inherent advantages of traditional decoction pieces, but also makes up for the shortcomings, which is the best and newest type to replace traditional decoction pieces, as well as the new form of decoction pieces that is currently being actively researched and promoted.

袋泡剂是将经过炮制后的药物研成粉末，用耐热水浸泡、通透性较好的滤纸机械包装成协定剂量，供配方使用。其有效成分易于渗出、服用方便，但因存在含淀粉、糖类药物容易虫蛀变质，熟地黄、黄精等少数药物不易粉碎，乳香、没药等树脂类药物细粉不易被水渗透等现象，不利于全面推广应用。当今中药饮片产业的发展主流是不再拘泥于传统中药饮片一种剂型，饮片产业正在向着多剂型、方便型、科学型方向发展，发展速度越来越快，产品的技术含量越来越高。

Teabag refers to powders prepared from processed medicinals, and mechanically packed into standard dose by the filter paper with hot water resistance and good permeability for the use of the formula. It is easy to take and the effective constituent inside can ooze quickly. However, due to the existence of several disadvantages, it is not conducive to the comprehensive application. For instance, the medicinals containings starch and sugar are easy to get worm-eaten spoilage and medicinals like prepared Shudihuang (Rehmanniae Radix Praeparata, prepared), Huangjing (Polygonati Rhizoma), etc. are difficult to smash, as well as the fine powder of resinous medicinals including Ruxiang (Olibanum) and Moyao (Myrrha), etc. is not easily permeable by water. Presently, the mainstream of the development of the Chinese medicine decoction pieces industry is no longer confined to one traditional decoction piece form, but develops towards a multiple-pharmaceutical form, convenient and scientific direction, with higher speed and higher technological content of products.

（三）中成药品种

1.3 Variety of Chinese Patent Medicines

中成药是中医临床应用的形式，中成药的

主要研究内容包括组方原理、给药剂型、制备工艺、质量控制、有效性、安全性和临床应用。

Chinese patent medicine is a form of clinical application of Chinese medicine, and its main research contents include prescription principle, pharmaceutical form, preparation procedure, quality control, efficacy, safety and clinical application.

处方是中成药研究的基础，中成药处方的来源主要有经方、验方、协定方和科研方。

Prescription is the basis of research on Chinese patent medicine, and the sources of their prescriptions mainly contain classical formula, experiential effective formula, hospital-verified formula and scientific research formula.

中成药的剂型和制备方法是中成药研究开发的核心内容，研究结果直接关系到中成药的安全性、有效性、稳定性、适用性和经济性。中成药剂型的选择应根据药物的性质和临床用药的需要而定，首先要考虑起效快慢、作用时间长短、给药途径与方式、作用部位；其次还要考虑生物利用度高低、用药剂量大小、质量是否稳定可控、使用是否安全方便等；再根据临床治疗和药物性质设计工艺，选择工业化生产路线。

The pharmaceutical form and preparation procedure are the core contents of Chinese patent medicine research and development, and the research results are directly related to its safety, efficacy, stability, applicability and economy. The choice of pharmaceutical form of Chinese patent medicine should be based on the property of the medicinal and the need of clinical use. The first consideration should be given to the speed of efficacy, the duration of action, the route and method of administration, and the place of action. Secondly, it is necessary to consider the level of bioavailability and the dosage, whether the quality is stable and controllable, whether the use is safe and convenient. Then, design process and choose the industrial production route according to the clinical treatment and medicinal properties.

中成药质量研究的关键在于建立适合中成

药品种自身特点的质量控制与评价科学方法，即制定科学的质量标准。中成药的质量控制与评价研究一般包括中药材原料质量控制和中药制剂质量控制两大部分。中药材质量控制标准的核心内容是鉴别和含量测定，鉴别方法要求专属、灵敏，含量测定方法要求能控制有效成分含量，且要进行方法学考察，以确保中成药产品质量的可控性。中成药制剂的质量控制的核心内容为制法、理化性质、鉴别、含量测定与稳定性的研究。

The key to study the quality of Chinese patent medicine is to establish a scientific method of quality control and evaluation suitable according with the characteristics of Chinese patent medicines, that is, to establish scientific quality standards. The quality control and evaluation of Chinese patent medicine generally includes two major parts as the quality control of raw materials and the quality control of traditional Chinese pharmaceutical preparation. And the core contents of the quality control standard for Chinese medicinal materials are identification and content determination. The identification method is required to be exclusive and sensitive, and the content determination method is required to be able to control the content of effective constituents, Hence, the vital contents of the quality control of Chinese patent medicine are the study of preparation, physical and chemical properties, identification, content determination and stability.

中成药的功能应用与作用机制研究，要从实验研究和临床研究两个方面揭示中成药的物质基础作用原理。尤其要在中医药理论指导下，应用制药新技术、新工艺、新设备和新辅料，以提高中成药的研究水平，创新药物或进行中成药大品种的二次开发。如在急救用药方面，已经研发了全国中医医院急症必备中成药50多个，其中参附注射液、参麦注射液、清开灵注射液、醒脑静注射液、灯盏花素注射液、双黄连注射液等已广泛应用。在重大疾病用药方面，复方丹参滴丸、地奥心血康、心可舒胶囊等是治疗冠心病心绞痛常用的有效之品；以薏苡仁油为主要成分的康莱特注射液对原发性非小细胞肺癌及原发性肝癌有良好的治疗效果；以蟾蜍、斑蝥、鸦胆子油、砒霜为主要原料制成的中成药品种对肿瘤的治疗有很好的疗效；清开灵注射液、板蓝根冲剂、新雪颗粒、金莲清热颗粒、灯盏细辛注射液、复方苦参注射液和香丹注射液等中成药防治呼吸道病毒感染有较好疗效。另外，中成药大品种的二次开发，成效显著。如复方丹参方、参附方、藿香正气方的二次开发，是中成药大品种二次开发成功的典范。

In order to study the functional application and mechanism of action of Chinese patent medicine, we should reveal the fundamental action principle of it from two aspects, namely experimental research and clinical research. In particular, with the guidance of Chinese medicine theory, new pharmaceutical techniques, new technologies, new equipment and new auxiliary materials should be applied to improve the research level of Chinese patent medicine, innovative medicinals or carry out the secondary development of large varieties of Chinese patent medicine. For example, in the field of emergency medicine, more than 50 essential Chinese patent medicines have been developed in Chinese medicine hospitals in China, among which Shenfu Zhusheye, Shenmai Zhusheye, Qingkailing Zhusheye, Xingnaojing Zhusheye, Dengzhanhua Zhusheye and Shuanghuanglian Zhusheye have been widely used. In addition, in terms of medication for serious diseases, Fufang Danshen Diwan (Dripping Pills), Di'ao Xinxuekang Jiaonang (Capsules), Xinkeshu Jiaonang, etc. are commonly used effective products for the treatment of coronary heart disease and angina pectoris; Kanglaite Zhusheye with Yiyiren (coix seed oil) as the main component has good therapeutic efficacy on primary non-small cell lung cancer and primary liver cancer; the Chinese patent medicine made of Chanchu (Bufo bufo gargarizans Cantor), Banmao (Mylabris), Yadanziyou (Bruceae Fructus oil) and Pishuang as the main raw materials has a good

efficacy on the treatment of tumor. Furthermore, Chinese patent medicine such as Qingkailing Zhusheye, Banlangen Keli, Xinxue Keli, Jinlian Qingre Keli, Dengzhanxixin Zhusheye, Fufang Kushen Zhusheye and Xiangdan Zhusheye have good therapeutic efficacy on respiratory virus infection. Besides, the secondary development of large variety of Chinese patent medicine has achieved remarkable progress. For example, the secondary development of Fufang Danshen Prescription, Shenfu Prescription and Huoxiang Zhengqi Prescription is a successful model for the secondary development of large variety of Chinese patent medicine.

二、品质的研究
2 The Research on Quality

中药品质研究的核心是中药的质量，主要包括遗传物质、有效成分、毒性成分与有害物质、全成分指纹图谱等研究内容。

The core of Chinese medicine quality research is quality, which includes the research contents of genetic material, effective constituents, toxic components and harmful substances, fingerprint of whole components, etc.

（一）中药遗传品质研究
2.1 Research on the Genetic Quality of Chinese Medicine

中药遗传品质研究主要是研究优质药材的生物遗传特性和优势，如优质品种的种质资源、遗传多样性、品种多样性、遗传分子标记，以及遗传物质与优质药材的生产、临床疗效的关系。

The research on genetic quality of Chinese medicine mainly focuses on the biological genetic characteristics and advantages of high-quality medicinal materials, such as germplasm resources, genetic diversity, variety diversity, genetic molecular markers of high-quality varieties, as well as the relationship between genetic materials and production, clinical efficacy of high-quality medicinal materials.

（二）中药有效成分研究

2.2 Research on the Effective Constituents of Chinese Medicine

中药有效成分是指具有一定生物活性，可以用分子式和结构式表示，并具有一定物理常数的单体化合物。如青蒿素是从青蒿（黄花蒿）Artemisa annua L. 中提取的一种抗疟有效成分，柴胡皂苷 A、柴胡皂苷 B₂、柴胡皂苷 C 和柴胡皂苷 D 是柴胡抗溃疡的有效成分；但至今大部分中药的有效成分仍未得以阐明，如《中国药典》一部收载的 2598 种中药材（包括部分饮片和提取物）及其制剂中，仅 60% 有化学成分研究报道，约 20% 进行过较系统的成分研究，其研究任务任重而道远。

The effective constituents of Chinese medicine refer to the monomer compounds with certain biological activity, which can be expressed by molecular formula and structural formula, and have certain physical constants. For example, artemisinin is an antimalarial effective constituent extracted from Qinghao (Artemisiae Annuae Herba), Artemisa annua L., saikosaponin A, saikosaponin B₂, saikosaponin C and saikosaponin D are effective constituents of Bupleurum chinense against ulcer. However, most of the effective constituents of Chinese medicinals have not been clarified so far. For instance, only 60% of the 2,598 kinds of traditional Chinese medicinal materials (including some decoction pieces and extracts) and their preparations included in *Volume I of Pharmacopoeia of the People's Republic of China* have been reported to have the studies of chemical components, and about 20% have been conducted systematic studies, which indicates (a long way to go for) the research on the effective constituents of Chinese medicine is far away.

（三）中药毒性成分与有害物质研究

2.3 Research on the Toxic Components and Harmful Substances of Chinese Medicine

分外源性的有害物质和内源性的毒性成分。①外源性有害物质主要来源于两个方面，一是重金属的污染，如砷、铅、汞、铜和镉等金属元素的污染与药用植物种植环境、土壤、水源、农药化肥使用、存储运输和炮制等多个因素相关，关系到中药产品质量；二是农药等残留，包括杀虫剂、杀菌剂、除草剂、生长调节剂等。其中，六六六、DDT 等化学性质稳定，在环境中降解缓慢，且脂溶性强，易于在生物体内富集，残留毒性大。②内源性有毒有害物质主要是指内源性毒性成分，如川乌、附子、草乌等含有的乌头碱，马钱子中的士的宁和关木通、广防己、青木香所含的马兜铃酸等。

The toxic components and harmful substances of Chinese medicine could be divided into exogenous harmful substances and endogenous toxic components. ① Exogenous harmful substances mainly come from two aspects, one is the pollution of heavy metals, such as arsenic, lead, mercury, copper and cadmium, which is related to the cultivation environment, soil, water, use of pesticides and fertilizers, storage, transportation and processing of medicinal plants, and they can influence the quality of Chinese Medicinal products. The other is pesticide residues, including pesticides, fungicides, herbicides, growth regulators. Among them, benzene hexachloride, DDT, etc. have properties of stable chemical, slow degradation in the environment, strong lipid solubility, easy accumulation in living organisms, and strong residual toxicity. ② Endogenous toxic and harmful substances mainly refer to endogenous toxic components, such as the aconitine in Chuanwu, Fuzi, and Caowu (Aconiti Kusnezoffii Radix), etc., and the strychnine in Maqianzi (Strychni Semen), as well as the aristolochic acid in Guanmutong (Aristolochiac Manshuriensis Caulis), Guangfangji (Aristolochiae Fangchi Radix) and Qingmuxiang (Aristolochiae Radix).

（四）中药全成分指纹图谱研究

2.4 Research on Fingerprint of Whole Components of Chinese Medicinal

中药化学成分的含量高低只是中药品质的化学表征，并不能完全代表中药的毒效关系。

因此，全成分指纹图谱研究成为目前中药品质研究的重要手段。近年来利用高效液相色谱（HPLC）、气相色谱 - 质谱联用技术（GC-MS）、高效液相色谱 - 质谱联用技术（HPLC-MS）等技术方法，建立中药指纹图谱，进行品质研究，为中药材的质量评价提供了更加可靠的依据。而中药品质的核心还是需要落实到中药的疗效，基于遗传物质、化学表征、生物活性评价的品质研究是未来的主要研究方向。

The content of chemical ingredients in Chinese Medicinal is only a chemical characterization of its quality, however, which cannot completely represent the relationship between toxicity and efficacy. Accordingly, research on fingerprint of whole components of Chinese Medicinal becomes a significant method for the quality research of Chinese Medicinal. Recent years, establishing the fingerprint of Chinese Medicinals by using the technologies including HPLC, GC-MS, HPLC-MS, etc. to study the quality of Chinese Medicinal provided a more reliable basis for the quality evaluation of traditional Chinese materia medica. The core of Chinese Medicinal quality is destined to the efficacy, and the quality research based on genetic material, chemical characterization and biological activity evaluation is the main research direction in the future.

三、制药的研究
3 The Research on Pharmacy

中药制药研究，主要包括药材产地加工、饮片炮制、提取工艺、制剂工艺、自动化生产等制药过程。以参附注射液为例，来阐述制药研究的主要环节。

The research on pharmacy of Chinese Medicinal includes the pharmaceutical process such as the origin processing of medicinal materials, processing of decoction pieces, extraction process, preparation process, and automatic production. Taking Shenfu Zhusheye

as an example, we will elaborate the main links of pharmaceutical research.

（一）产地加工与饮片炮制
3.1 Origin Processing and Decoction Pieces Processing

附子的产地加工是降低附子毒性的重要手段之一，其传统加工中强调胆巴浸泡，胆巴的质量直接影响附子药材的质量，因此先制定了胆巴的质量标准。参附注射液以黑顺片入药，因此对黑顺片的炮制工艺过程中胆巴浸泡、漂洗次数、蒸煮处理等每个工艺步骤的总生物碱、双酯型生物碱、单酯型生物碱、核苷类物质（尿苷、腺苷）、糖类物质（果糖、葡萄糖、蔗糖、麦芽糖）、无机盐离子、浸出物、灰分等指标的变化规律进行了研究，制订了黑顺片炮制工艺及工艺技术参数，既能保证附片的减毒存效，又能保证中药注射剂的质量。红参产地加工与炮制，即选好的参根剪去须根及支根，装入蒸笼中蒸 2 ~ 3 分钟，先武火后文火，蒸至参根呈半透明时熄火，冷后取出晒干或烘干，建立了鉴定红参药材的 TLC 法和近红外光谱法和人参皂苷、糖蛋白等成分含量测定方法，并建立了红参内控标准的指纹图谱。

Origin processing of Fuzi is one of the important methods to reduce its toxicity. Danba (a kind of bittern) immersion is emphasized in its traditional processing, and the quality of Danba directly affects the quality of Fuzi. Therefore, we have established quality standards for Danba. Shenfu Zhusheye is formulated with Heishunpian (a processed decoction piece of Fuzi), and we studied the change law of total alkaloids, diester-type alkaloids, monoester alkaloids, nucleosides (uridine, adenosine), carbohydrate (fructose, glucose, sucrose, maltose), inorganic salt ions, extracts, ash content, etc. during the processing steps of Heishunpian, such as Danba immersion, rinsing times, steaming, and so on. Finally, we set up the processing technology and technical datum of Heishunpian, which can not only reduce the toxicity and maintain the effect, but also guarantee the quality of the traditional Chinese medicine injection. Specifically, the origin processes and decoction pieces processing of Hongshen (Ginseng Radix et Rhizoma Rubra), refers to cut off the fibrous roots and branch roots from selected ginseng roots, and then steam them in a steamer for 2 to 3 minutes with mild heating fire after strong fire, then turn off the fire when the ginseng roots are translucent. Finally, after cooling down, dry them in sun or in a stove. Our project team has established TLC method, near-infrared spectroscopy method, and content determination methods of ginsenoside, glycoprotein as well as other component for the identification of Hongshen, and the fingerprint of the internal control standard.

（二）提取与制剂工艺研究

3.2 Research on Extraction Process and Preparation Process

黑顺片的提取工艺是关系到参附注射液安全有效的重要因素。采用 UV、HPLC、HPLC/MS、HPLC/ ELSD 等分析方法，深入研究黑顺片提取工艺中煎煮时间、煎煮次数、加水量等因素变化过程中水提液总生物碱、酯型生物碱和双酯型生物碱的量时曲线，在组分水平和分子水平上探讨煎煮时间、加水量与黑顺片化学成分谱（库）的生物碱成分及毒性关系，黑顺片成分与功效关系，揭示了传统水煎对黑顺片毒性成分的控制规律；通过黑顺片生物碱成分模拟水解分析，确定毒性成分的水解影响因素、水解产物和黑顺片提取的最佳时间。对红参提取时回流加醇时间、乙醇浓度、回流升温时间、冷却时间，各次回流液的醇度、体积，对浓缩时的蒸汽压力、真空度、浓缩时间、浓缩液的相对密度及温度，以及主要阶段的蛋白质、树脂、鞣质、草酸盐、钾离子、含量、热原、指纹图谱、微生物数及部分阶段的溶血、异常毒性进行研究，确定红参提取工艺。对参附注射液工艺中除淀粉、蛋白质、鞣质、树脂等高分子物质和除热原、灭菌工艺、内包材等进行研究，建立产品各阶段药物含量、指纹图谱等方面的质量控制方法。

The extraction process of Heishunpian is a vital factor affecting the safety and effectiveness of Shenfu Zhusheye. We used UV, HPLC, HPLC/MS, HPLC/ELSD and other analytical technologies to lucubrate the amount-time curves of total alkaloids, monoester alkaloids, diester-type alkaloids in aqueous extracts of Heishunpian with process of changes of decoction time, number of times of decoction and amount of water added. We discussed the relationship between decoction time and water amount and alkaloids and toxicity on the levels of component and ingredient, as well as relationship between constituents and efficacy, which revealed the control regulation of traditional decoction on toxic components in Heishunpian. Based on the simulated hydrolysis analysis of alkaloids in Heishunpian, the influencing factors of toxic components hydrolysis, the optimal time for extracting the hydrolysates and Heishunpian were determined. Alcohol time in reflux, ethanol concentration, heating time in reflux, cooling time, alcohol concentration and volume of each reflux liquid in the extraction of Hongshen, steam pressure, vacuum degree, concentration time, relative density and temperature of the concentrated liquid during concentration, and content of protein, resin, tannin, oxalate, potassium ion, pyrogen, fingerprint, number of microorganisms in the main stage, as well as hemolysis and abnormal toxicity in part of the stage were studied to determine the extraction process of Hongshen. Moreover, establish quality control methods for medicinal content, fingerprint and other aspects in each stage of the product by studying on the removal of starch, protein, tannin, resin and other high-molecular substances, pyrogen removal, sterilization process, inner packaging materials, etc.

（三）自动化生产与在线检测

3.3 Automatic Production and Online Testing

应用网络控制技术、中药指纹图谱质量控制和近红外在线检测等技术，对参附注射液的生产自动控制系统的主要设备和主要技术参数进行研究，对工艺参数进行实时在线存储、传输、备份和反馈，通过红外在线自动监测仪和软系统对参附注射液生产线的监控点实现远程在线控制。

With techniques of network control, quality control with Chinese Medicinal fingerprint and near infrared online detection, we studied the main equipment and technical parameters of the production automatic control system of Shenfu Zhusheye which realized the real-time online storage, transmission, backup and feedback for process parameters, and the remote online control of monitoring points for Shenfu Zhusheye production line through infrared online automatic monitor and soft system.

四、药性的研究
4 The Research on Property

(一) 四气
4.1 Four Qi

四气是指寒、热、温、凉四气，又称为四性，主要反映药物影响人体阴阳盛衰、寒热病理变化的作用性质，是中药最基本的药性。早在《神农本草经》序录就提出，药"有寒热温凉四气"。药物寒热温凉，是从药物作用于机体所发生的反应概括出来的，与所治疾病的寒热性质相对应。也就是说药物寒热温凉的性质是由用药后机体的反应和病证的寒热决定的。具体而言，能够减轻或消除热证的药物，一般为寒性或凉性；反之，能够减轻或消除寒证的药物，一般属热性或温性。四性之外，还有平性，指药物性质平和、作用较缓和，实际上仍略有微寒、微温的差异，其性平是相对而言，仍未超出四性的范围。

Four *qi,* also known as four properties, involves cold, hot, warm and cool. Four *qi* mainly reflect the effects of medicines on exuberance and debilitation of *yin* and *yang*, and the pathological changes of cold and heat in the human body, which are the most basic properties of Chinese Medicinal. As early as in the preamble of *Shennong Bencao Jing (Shennong's Classic of Materia Medica)*, it was proposed that medicines possess four properties, including cold, hot, warm and cool. The cold, hot, warm and cool properties of medicines are summarized from the reactions of medicinals on the body, which are correspond to the cold and hot properties of diseases. That is to say, the cold, hot, warm and cool properties of medicines are determined by the reaction of the body after treatments as well as the cold and hot properties of diseases. Specifically, medicines capable of reducing or eliminating heat syndrome are generally cold or cool. Conversely, medicines capable of reducing or eliminating cold syndrome are generally hot or warm. In addition to the four properties, there is also neutral property, which means that the properties of medicinals are gentle and possess a relative moderate efficacy. Actually, there are still slight differences between cold and warm of the neutral property, which is defined as a comparative term and still within the scope of four properties.

现代对中药四气的研究，通常将其分为寒凉及温热两大类进行，主要针对中医临床寒热病证的表现与机体各系统功能活动变化的关系，研究四性与中枢神经系统、自主神经系统、内分泌系统、能量代谢等有密切关系。①中枢神经系统方面，多数寒凉药对中枢神经系统呈现抑制性作用，如金银花、板蓝根、钩藤、羚羊角、黄芩等；多数温热药则具有中枢兴奋作用，例如麻黄、麝香、马钱子等。②自主神经系统方面，多数寒凉药能降低交感神经活性、抑制肾上腺皮质功能、升高细胞内 cGMP 水平，相反多数温热药能提高交感神经活性、增强肾上腺皮质功能、升高细胞内 cAMP 水平。③内分泌系统方面，主要是通过影响下丘脑 - 垂体 - 肾上腺皮质、下丘脑 - 垂体 - 甲状腺以及下丘脑 - 垂体 - 性腺内分泌轴发挥作用。如温热药人参、黄芪、白术、当归、鹿茸、肉苁蓉、刺五加、何首乌等可兴奋下丘脑 - 垂体 - 肾上腺皮质轴，使血液中 ACTH、皮质醇含量升高；附子、肉桂、紫河车、人参、黄芪、何首乌等具有兴奋下丘脑 - 垂体 - 甲状腺轴的作用，使血液中促甲状腺激素或 T_3、T_4 水平升高；人参、刺五加、淫羊藿、附子、肉桂、鹿茸、紫河车、补骨脂、冬虫夏草、蛇床子、仙茅、巴戟天等可以兴奋下丘脑 - 垂体 - 性腺内分泌轴。④能量代谢方面，不同药性的药物对能量代谢功能的作用与影响下丘脑 - 垂体 - 甲状腺轴功能、Na$^+$-K$^+$-ATP 酶活性有关，温热药能够促进机体的能量代谢，而寒凉药则表现为抑制机体的能量代谢。另外，还应用化学、生物热力学、系统生物学等对四气的物质基础、热力学过程、系统生物学变化进行了研究。

The modern research on four *qi* of Chinese Medicinal is usually divided into two categories: cold and cool, warm and hot. It mainly focuses on the relationship between the clinical manifestations of cold and hot syndromes of Chinese medicine and the changes of functional activities of various systems of the organism. The research on four *qi* is closely related to the central nervous system, autonomic nervous system, endocrine system and energy metabolism etc. ① In terms of the central nervous system, majority of the cold and cool medicinals have inhibitory effects on the central nervous system, such as Jinyinhua (Lonicerae Japonicae Flos), Banlangen (Isatidis Radix), Gouteng (Uncariae Ramulus Cum Uncis), Lingyangjiao (Saigae Tataricae Cornu) and Huangqin (Scutellariae Radix) etc. While most of the warm and hot medicinals have central excitatory effect, such as Mahuang (Ephedrae Herba), Shexiang (Moschus) and Maqianzi etc. ② In terms of autonomic nervous system, most of the cold and cool medicinals can reduce sympathetic nerve activity, inhibit adrenocortical function, and increase intracellular cGMP level; On the contrary, most warm and hot medicinals can improve sympathetic nerve activity, enhance adrenocortical function and increase intracellular cAMP level. ③ As for the endocrine system, medicinals mainly exert efficacy by affecting the hypothalamic-pituitary-adrenal axis, hypothalamic-pituitary-thyroid axis, and hypothalamic-pituitary-gonadal endocrine axis. Such as Renshen (Ginseng Radix et Rhizoma), Huangqi (Astragali Radix), Baizhu (Atractylodis Macrocephalae Rhizoma), Danggui (Angelicae Sinensis Radix), Lurong (Cervi Cornu Pantotrichum), Roucongrong (Cistanches Herba), Ciwujia (Acanthopanacis Senticosi Radix et Rhizoma Seu Caulis) and Heshouwu (Polygoni Multiflori Radix), which possess a warm property and can stimulate the hypothalamic-pituitary-adrenal axis and increase the ACTH and cortisol levels in blood. Medicines such as Fuzi, Rougui (Cinnamomi Cortex), Ziheche (Placenta Hominis), Renshen, Huangqi and Heshouwu can stimulate the hypothalamic-pituitary-thyroid axis and increase levels of thyrotropin or T_3 and T_4 in blood. Besides, Renshen, Ciwujia, Yinyanghuo (Epimedii Folium), Fuzi, Rougui, Lurong, Ziheche, Buguzhi (Psoraleae Fructus), Dongchongxiacao (Cordyceps), Shechuangzi (Cnidii Fructus), Xianmao (Curculiginis Rhizoma) and Bajitian (Morindae Officinalis Radix) can excite the hypothalamus-pituitary-gonadal endocrine axis. ④ In terms of energy metabolism, the effects of different medicinals on energy metabolism are related to the function of the hypothalamus-pituitary-thyroid axis and Na$^+$-K$^+$-ATPase activity. Medicines with warm and hot properties can promote energy metabolism in the body, while medicines with cold and cool properties can inhibit the body's energy metabolism. In addition, chemistry, biothermodynamics, and systems biology have also been applied to study the material basis, thermodynamic processes and system biological changes of four properties.

（二）五味

4.2 Five Flavors

五味本义是指辛、甘、酸、苦、咸五种口尝而直接感知的真实滋味，后来随着用药实践的发展，五味成了药物功效作用的概况。由此可知，确定味的主要依据一是药物的滋味，二是药物的作用。现代研究表明，五味的物质基础是不同类型的化学物质，而这不同类型的化学物质作用于机体，产生药理作用，从而调节人体阴阳，扶正祛邪，消除疾病。

The original meaning of five flavors refers to the true taste directly perceived by the five tastes of pungency, sweetness, sourness, bitterness and saltiness. Later, with the development of medication practice, the five flavors represent a general conception of medicinal efficacy. Therefore, the principal basis for determining the flavor is the taste and functions of medicinals, respectively. Modern research shows that the material basis of five flavors are based on different types of chemical substances, and these various chemical substances can act on the body to produce pharmacological effects, thereby regulating *yin* and *yang* of the body, reinforcing the healthy *qi* and eliminating the pathogenic factors and diseases.

①辛味药主要含挥发油，其次为生物碱、苷类等，辛能散、能行，具有发散、行气、行血等功效，主要与扩张血管、改善微循环、发汗、解热、抗炎、抗病原体、调整肠道平滑肌运动等作用相关。②甘味药多含糖类、苷类、蛋白质、氨基酸、维生素等成分，甘能补、能和、能缓，具有补虚、和中、调和药性、缓急止痛等功效，具有调节机体免疫系统功能、增强机体抗病能力以及缓和拘急疼痛，调和药性等方面的作用。③酸味药多含有机酸和鞣质，酸能收、能涩，具有收敛固涩等功效，主要表现在抗病原微生物、收敛、止泻、止血、消炎等方面的作用。④苦味药多含各种生物碱、苷类、挥发油、黄酮、鞣质等，苦能泄、能燥，具有清热、燥湿、泻下等功效，主要有抗菌、抗炎、杀虫、平喘止咳、致泻、止吐等作用。⑤咸味药主要含碘、钠、钙、钾、镁等无机盐成分，多为矿物类及动物类药材，咸能软，能下，具有软坚散结和泻下等功效，具有抗肿瘤、抗炎、抗菌、镇静、镇痛、解热、降血脂、降血压、降血糖、抗凝血、利尿等方面的作用。

① Pungent medicinal mainly contains volatile oil, followed by alkaloids and glycosides etc. The pungency of medicinal has functions of dispersing, promoting *qi* and blood, which is mainly related to the effects of dilating blood vessels, improving microcirculation, sweating, antipyretic, anti-inflammatory, anti-pathogen and regulating the movement of intestinal smooth muscle. ② Medicinal with sweet property mainly contains saccharides, glycosides, proteins, amino acids and vitamins etc. The sweetness of medicinal can tonify, harmonize and act slowly with the effect of tonifying deficiency, harmonizing the middle energizer, regulating the nature of medicinal and relieving spasm and pain, which could be used to regulate the immune system and enhance the disease resistance of the body, relieve pain and regulate the nature of medicinal. ③ Sour medicinal mainly contains organic acid and tannin with astringent action. It has the effects of securing and astriction, which are mainly manifested in functions of antiviral microorganism, astringency, antidiarrhea, hemostasis and antivomitting etc. ④ Bitter medicinal contains a variety of alkaloids, glycosides, volatile oil, flavonoids and tannins etc. The bitter property of medicinal can discharge and dry dampness with functions of clearing heat, drying dampness and purgation, which can exert effects of antibacterial, anti-inflammatory, relieving cough and asthma, diarrhea and preventing vomiting etc. ⑤ Salty medicinal mainly contains iodine, sodium, calcium, potassium, magnesium and other inorganic salt components, which are mostly mineral and animal medicinal. The saltiness of medicinal has functions of softening hardness and purging with the effects of softening hardness and dissipating binds and purgation, which are mainly related to the efficacy of antitumor, anti-inflammation, antibacterial, sedation, analgesia, antipyretic, lowering blood lipids, antihypertension, antihyperglycemia, anticoagulation and diuresis etc.

中药五味，不一定是用以表示药物的真实滋味，更主要是用以反映药物作用在补、泄、散、敛等方面的特征性，而研究五味与化学成分、药理作用之间的规律性，对探索中药五味学说的现代内涵，具有重要意义。

The five flavors of Chinese Medicinal are not necessarily used to mean the true taste of the medicinal, but mainly to reflect the action characteristics of medicinals in tonifying, purging, dispersing and astringing etc. It is of great significance to study the regularity among five flavors, chemical constituents and pharmacological actions to explore the modern connotation of five flavors theory of Chinese medicine.

（三）归经

4.3 Meridian Tropism

归经是中药药性理论的重要组成部分，"归"是指药物的归属，即指药物作用的部位，"经"是指经络及其所属脏腑；归经是药物对机体治疗作用及适应范围的归纳，是中药对机体脏腑经络选择性的作用。归经的现代研究，多从药物的药理作用、药物在体内的分布、受体结合等方面开展工作。

Meridian tropism (Guijing) is an important part of Chinese medicine theory. The "Gui" refers to the attributions of medicinals in the body, that is, the place where the medicinal acts. "jing" refers to the meridians and their viscera and bowels. Meridian tropism (Guijing) is the induction of the therapeutic effect of medicinals on the body and the scope of adaptation. It is the selective effect of viscera and bowels, meridians and collaterals of Chinese medicinal. The modern study of meridian tropism mainly focuses on the pharmacological effects, the distribution in vivo and the binding of receptors of medicinals.

1. 药理作用方面 李仪奎等对429种常用中药按药理活性分组，统计各组的归经频数，发现两者之间存在相关性。如具有抗惊厥作用的钩藤、天麻、全蝎、蜈蚣等22味中药均入肝经，入肝经率达100%，而与不具有抗惊厥作用中药的入肝经率仅为42.9%，有显著差异；具有泻下作用的大黄、芒硝、芦荟等18味中药入大肠经率亦达100%，明显高于其他411味中药10.5%的入大肠经率；具有止咳作用的杏仁、百部、贝母等18味药，具祛痰作用的桔梗、前胡、远志等

23味药，具平喘作用的麻黄、地龙、款冬花等13味药，入肺经率分别为100%、100%和95.5%，符合"肺主呼吸""肺为贮痰之器"的论述；鹿茸、淫羊藿、补骨脂等53味壮阳中药全部入肾经，符合中医认为肾主生殖的理论。

4.3.1 Pharmacological Effects

Li Yikui et al. divided 429 commonly used medicinal into groups according to their pharmacological activities and found that there was a correlation between meridian tropism and pharmacological effects via counting the frequency of the meridian tropism of each group. For example, 22 Chinese medicinal with anticonvulsant effects such as Gouteng, Tianma (Gastrodiae Rhizoma), Quanxie (Scorpio) and Wugong (Scolopendra) all enter into the liver meridian, that is, 100% anticonvulsants enter the liver meridian, while only 42.9% of medicines without anticonvulsant effects enter into the liver meridian, which show a significant difference. 100% of 18 Chinese medicinal with purgative effects such as Dahuang (Rhei Radix et Rhizoma), Mangxiao (Natrii Sulfas) and Luhui (Aloe) etc. enter the large intestine meridian, which is significantly higher than that of 10.5% of other 411 Chinese medicinal. The frequencies of 18 medicines with antitussive effects, such as Xingren (Armeniacae Semen Amarum), Baibu (Stemonae Radix) and Beimu (Bulbus Fritillaria), of 23 medicinal with expectorant effects, such as Jiegeng (Platycodonis Radix), Qianhu (Peucedani Radix) and Yuanzhi (Polygalae Radix), of 13 medicines with calm panting effects, such as Mahuang, Dilong (Pheretima) and Kuandonghua (Farfarae Flos) entering into the lung meridian are 100%, 100% and 95.5%, respectively, which are consistent with the discussions of "lung mainly manages respiration" and "lung is the container of phlegm". 53 Chinese medicinal with invigorating yang effects such as Lurong, Yinyanghuo, Buguzhi all enter into the kidney meridian, which are in line with the recognition that kidney is mainly responsible for reproduction.

2. 药物在体内分布方面 对23种中药的有效成分在体内的分布与中药归经之间的联系进行分析，发现其中20种中药归经所属的脏腑与其有效成分分布最多的脏腑基本一致（61%）和大致相符（26%），符合率高达87%。如鱼腥草（归肺经）所含鱼腥草素肺组织分布多，丹参（归心、肝经）所含隐丹参酮肝、肺分布最多；³H-川芎嗪的肝脏、胆囊摄取率最高，与川芎归肝、胆经相符，³H-麝香酮主要分布于心、脑、肺、肾等血液供应充足的组织和器官，并能迅速透过血脑屏障进入中枢神经系统，与麝香归心经、通关利窍、开窍醒脑的传统认识相符。采用同位素示踪，高效液相色谱分析和放射自显影等技术对32味中药归经及其在体内吸收、分布、代谢、排泄方面进行定性、定位和定量的动态观察，显示其与相应药物归经的脏腑基本相符；由此可以得出，中药有效成分在体内选择性分布是中药归经的物质基础。

4.3.2 Drug Distribution in the Body

It was found that the viscera and bowels of meridian entry of 20 Chinese medicinal and those of having the most active constituents were basically the same (61%) and roughly the same (26%) with a high compliance rate of 87% via analyzing the relationship between the distribution of the active ingredients of 23 Chinese medicinal in the body and their meridian entries. For example, the houttuynin of Yuxingcao (Houttuyniae Herba) is mainly distributed in lung tissue, and Yuxingcao entering the lung meridian. Cryptotanshinone of Danshen (Salviae Miltiorrhizae Radix et Rhizoma) is mostly distributed in liver and lung tissues, and Danshen enters into the heart and liver meridians. The uptake ratio of 3H-ligustrazine in liver and gallbladder is the highest, which is consistent with the liver and gallbladder meridian entries of Chuanxiong (Chuanxiong Rhizoma). 3H-muscone is mainly distributed in sufficient blood supplied tissues and organs such as heart, brain, lung and kidney etc., and can quickly enter the central nervous system through the blood-brain barrier, which is consistent with the traditional understanding of Shexiang that entering the heart meridian, tonifying joints and orifices and inducing resuscitation. The meridian entries of 32 Chinese medicinal and their absorption, distribution, metabolism, and excretion in the body are qualitatively, regionally, quantitatively and dynamically observed through isotopic tracing, HPLC analysis and autoradiography technologies. The results showed that the distributions of medicines are consistent with their corresponding viscera and bowels of meridian tropism. Thus, it can be concluded that the selective distribution of active ingredients in vivo is the material basis of meridian tropism of medicines.

3. 受体结合研究方面 受体具有明确定位的特点，与归经概念的特征极为相似，中药归经极有可能是与其作用于某种或某几种受体有关。以受体结合来研究归经，可以在更深层次上揭示归经的机制，避免中西医内脏概念不一致所导致的确定归经定位难的不足。如附子所含消旋去甲乌药碱具有兴奋心肌 α、β 受体的作用；去甲猪毛菜碱具有兴奋 β、α 受体的作用；氧化甲基多巴胺为 α-受体激动剂，具有强心、升压作用，与附子归心经相符；槟榔可作用于M胆碱能受体而引起腺体分泌增加，使消化液分泌旺盛、食欲增加，与中医药理论中的槟榔归胃、大肠经一致。

4.3.3 Binding of Receptors

The receptors possess a definite location, which is very similar to the characteristic of meridian tropism concept. The meridian tropism of Chinese medicine may be related to its function of working on some or several types of receptors. The mechanism of meridian tropism can be deeply revealed through receptor binding study, which can avoid the difficulty of determining the meridian tropism due to the inconsistency of visceral concepts between Chinese and Western medicine. For example, the higenamine in Fuzi can stimulate α and β receptor of cardiac muscle. Salsolinol has the function of exciting β, α receptor. Oxidized methyl dopamine is an α-receptor agonist with cardiotonic and pressure-increasing effects, which is consistent with Fuzi entering the heart meridian. Binglang (Arecae Semen) can act on M cholinergic receptors and cause glandular secretion of glandular, which result in the increased with glandular secretion ipeptic juice and appetite increasing and is consistent with Binglang entering the stomach and large intestine meridian according to Chinese medicine theory.

（四）升降浮沉

4.4 Ascending, Descending, Floating and Sinking

升降浮沉是药物作用在人体内呈现的一种走向和趋势，向上向外的作用称为升浮，向下向内的作用称为沉降。一般来说，具有解表、透疹、祛风湿、升阳举陷、开窍醒神、温阳补火、行气解郁及涌吐等功效的药物，其作用趋向主要是升浮；具有清热、泻火、利湿、安神、止呕、平抑肝阳、息风止痉、止咳平喘、收敛固涩及止血等功效的药物，其作用趋向主要是沉降。目前对中药升降沉浮理论的实验研究较少，主要是结合方药的药理作用进行辨析。如补中益气汤可以选择性地提高在体及离体动物子宫平滑肌的张力，加入升麻、柴胡的制剂作用明显；如果去掉升麻、柴胡则作用减弱且不持久，单用升麻、柴胡则无作用；说明升麻、柴胡具有升阳举陷之功。柿蒂提取物对大鼠膈肌标本的收缩呈现先增强后抑制的作用，并且随浓度增高，增强效应持续的时间越短，抑制效应出现的时间越早，抑制作用越强，体现了柿蒂降逆的功效。有些中药具有升浮和沉降的双向作用趋向，如麻黄发汗、解表具有升浮的特性，又能止咳平喘、利尿消肿而具有沉降的特性；白芍上行头目祛风止痛，具有升浮的特性，又能下行血海以活血通经，又具有沉降的特点；黄芪既能补气升阳、托毒生肌，具有升浮的特性，又能利水消肿、固表止汗，具有沉降的特点。

Ascending, descending, floating and sinking are the trend and tendency of medicines after acting on the human body. The upward and outward actions are called ascending and floating, while the downward and inward actions are called sinking and descending. In general, medicines with functions of releasing exterior, promoting eruption, expelling wind and dampness, elevating *yang* and raising the prolapsed organs, opening the orifices, tonifying fire and warming *yang*, moving *qi* to relieve depression and vomiting tend to be ascending and floating. Medicines with functions of clearing heat, discharging fire, draining dampness, tranquilizing, checking vomiting, calming liver *yang*, extinguishing wind to arrest convulsions, relieving cough and asthma, securing and astriction and arresting bleeding tend to be sinking and descending. At present, there are few experimental studies on the theory of ascending, descending, floating and sinking of Chinese Medicine, which are mainly differentiated and analyzed according to the pharmacological effects of formulas. For example, Buzhong Yiqi Tang (Decoction) can selectively increase the tension of uterine smooth muscle in vivo and in vitro, and this effect can be enhanced in the addition of Shengma (Cimicifugae Rhizoma) and Chaihu (Bupleuri Radix). The removal of Shengma and Chaihu can weaken and even destabilize this effect. However, it will not be effective when Shengma and Chaihu are used alone, which indicates that Shengma and Chaihu have the effects of elevating yang and raising the prolapsed organs. The effect of Shidi (Kaki Calyx) extraction on the contraction of diaphragmatic muscle in rat is firstly enhanced, then subsequently inhibited and along with the increasing of concentration, the shorter the duration of the enhancement effect lasted, the earlier the inhibition effect appeared, and the stronger the inhibition effect was, which reflect the descending counterflow effect of Shidi. Some Chinese medicinal show a two-way action tendency of ascending, floating and descending, sinking. For example, the effects of sweating and relieving exterior syndrome of Mahuang reflect the characteristics of ascending and floating, while the effects of relieving cough and asthma and inducing diuresis to reduce edema show the characteristics of descending and sinking. Baishao (Paeoniae Radix Alba) ascends to head and eyes and can dispel wind and relieve pain with the characteristics of ascending and floating. Besides, it can also go downward the sea of blood to activate blood and unblock the meridian, which show the characteristics of descending and sinking. Huangqin can not only tonify qi and raise yang, promote pus discharge and tissue regeneration with the characteristics of ascending and floating, but also drain water and disperse swelling and secure the exterior to check sweating with the characteristics of descending and sinking.

（五）有毒无毒
4.5 Toxicity and Non-toxicity

有毒无毒是通过中药对机体是否有毒性损害作用，而加以判别区分。绝大多数中药没有毒害作用，属无毒；只有那些药性强烈，对人体有毒性或副作用，安全剂量小，用之不当或药量超过常量，即对人体产生危害，甚至可致人死亡的中药有毒性，属有毒中药。我国古代医药学家，早在公元前《国语》中就有以含乌头的肉喂狗，以验其毒性记载，具有现代毒理实验的萌芽，而真正开始应用现代毒理学的理论、技术和方法来研究中药的毒性、毒作用机制及产生毒作用的物质基础，始于 20 世纪 20 年代，国内外学者才开始应用现代毒理学方法对中药的毒性进行系统研究。其研究主要包括三方面的内容，一是研究有毒中药对人体可能发生危害的剂量（浓度）、接触时间、接触途径等，以及危害的程度，就是研究有毒中药的毒性结果，为安全性评价和管理法规制订提供毒理学信息，包括有毒中药的急性毒性、长期毒性、遗传毒性、生殖毒性、致癌性等；二是研究有毒中药经皮肤、黏膜和各种生物膜进入靶部位，在体内分布，经生物转化成活性物质，与体内靶分子发生反应而引起生物体危害的过程，就是研究有毒中药对生物体毒作用的细胞、分子及生化机制；三是依据基础毒理学、机制毒理学提供的资料和临床应用的经验，研究有毒中药或有毒中药组成的药品，按规定使用，是否具有足够低的危险性，为临床安全合理用药提

供依据。

Toxicity and non-toxicity are distinguished by whether Chinese medicinal have toxic damage to the human body. Most of Chinese medicinal have no toxic effects and are non-toxic medicines. Only those medicines that possess strong medicinal properties, toxicity or side effects to the human body with a small range of safe dosage and do harm to human body or even cause death in an improper or overdosed medication are called toxic medicines. As early as in *Guoyu (Discourses of the States)* in BC, it was recorded that ancient Chinese medical scientists feed dogs with meat containing Wutou (Aconite Main Root) to test the toxicity, which showed the germination of modern toxicology experiments. In the 1920s, the toxicity, mechanism of toxic effects and the material basis of toxicity of Chinese medicinal were explored basing on the theory, technology and methods of modern toxicology. Researchers at home and abroad began to systematically study the toxicity of Chinese medicinal in the application of modern toxicological methods from then on. The research mainly includes three aspects: The first is to study the dosage (concentration), exposure time, route of exposure and the degree of damage of toxic medicines that may cause to the human body. Thus, to provide toxicological information for safety evaluation and formulation of management regulations, including acute toxicity, long-term toxicity, genetic toxicity, reproductive toxicity and carcinogenicity of toxic medicines. The second is to study the process that causing biological damage when toxic medicines are combined with the targets through the skin, mucous membranes and various biofilms to distribute in the body and converted into active substances to react with target molecules via biotransformation. That is, studying the cells, molecules and biochemical mechanisms of toxic Chinese medicinal on organisms. Thirdly, based on the data provided by basic toxicology and mechanism toxicology and clinical application experience, researches on the toxic medicines or medicinal containing toxic medicinals are conducted to determine whether medicines are of low risk and provide a basis for the safe and rational clinical use.

五、功效的研究
5 The Research on Efficacy

（一）治疗作用
5.1 Therapeutic Effect

中药最主要的用途是治病，其治疗作用是中药功效的主流；凡符合用药目的并能达到防治疾病的作用称为治疗作用。其治疗作用又可分为消除疾病发生的原因、发挥治本作用的对因治疗作用和改善疾病症状、发挥治标作用的对症治疗作用。

The main purpose of Chinese medicinal is to treat diseases and its therapeutic effect is the mainstream of Chinese medicinal efficacy. The effect that meets the purpose of medication and can prevent and treat diseases is defined as the therapeutic effect. The therapeutic effect can be divided as follows: Elimination of the cause of diseases, exerting the effect of treating the root of etiology, improving the symptoms of diseases and exerting the effect of treating the tip of symptoms.

1. **对因治疗作用**　不外是祛除病邪，消除病因，恢复脏腑功能的协调，纠正阴阳偏盛偏衰的病理现象。简言之，即祛邪、扶正、调理脏腑功能。如麻黄散寒，西瓜解暑，常山截疟等属祛邪去因作用；人参补气，附子助阳，当归补血等属扶正作用；而柴胡疏肝，丹参调经，杏仁止咳则属调理脏腑功能。

5.1.1 Etiological Treatment

It is to eliminate the evil and pathogeny, restore the coordination of viscera and bowels function, and correct the pathological exuberance or weakness phenomenon of *yin* and *yang*. In a word, it focuses on eliminating the pathogenic factors, reinforcing the healthy qi and regulating viscera and bowels function. For example, Mahuang dispels cold, Xigua (Aconitum carmichaelii Debx.) relieves summer-heat, and Changshan (Dichroae Radix) prevents recurrence of malaria, which is achieved by the treatment of removing pathogenic factors and expelling pathogeny. Renshen tonifies *qi*, Fuzi raises yang, and Danggui enriches blood, which show their effect of reinforcing the healthy *qi*. The liver soothing of Chaihu, the menstruation regulation of Danshen, and the suppression of cough of Xingren reflect the regulation effect on viscera and bowels function.

2. **对症治疗作用**　是指中药治疗功效中能消除或缓解患者自觉痛苦症状或临床体征的特殊效用，这一作用，无论是从古代医药文献的记载、古今临床应用实例，还是根据现代药理、药化研究结果，均可证明其客观存在。如麻黄平喘、生姜止呕、延胡索止痛、三七止血皆属"对症"功效。

5.1.2 Symptomatic Treatment

It refers to the special effect of Chinese medicinal to eliminate or relieve the conscious painful symptoms of patient or clinical signs. This effect can be proved objectively from the records of ancient medical literature, clinical examples from ancient and modern times, and the results of modern pharmacology and medicinal research. For example, Mahuang can calm panting, Shengjiang (Zingiberis Rhizoma recens) can check vomiting, Yanhusuo (Corydalis Rhizoma) can relieve pain and Sanqi (Notoginseng Radix et Rhizoma) can stop bleeding, which all reflect the symptomatic treatment efficacy of medicines.

中药治疗作用的现代研究，主要是根据中药的功能主治，首选符合中医理论、具有中医特色的试验方法及病证动物模型，直接证实其功效作用；其次可选用现代医学的疾病动物模型及实验方法，间接研究其功效作用。由于中药常具有多方面的功效或通过多种方式发挥作用等特点，应选择相应的技术方法加以研究。通过研究，首先应回答中药是否有效，有效的范围、作用的强度、起效的快慢与持续的时间；其次应明确中药的主要药效作用和次要药效作用是什么，与同类中药比较有什么优势和特色；最后应排除各种影响实验结果的干扰因素，全面分析、综合归纳实验结果，找出内在规律，上升到中药功效理论的高度，用以阐明中药药效作用的规律。

The modern research on the therapeutic effect of Chinese medicine is mainly based on the functions and indications of medicines. The efficacy of Chinese medicine is directly confirmed by selecting the optimum experimental method and animal model that are in accordance with the theory and characteristics of Chinese medicine. Secondly, the animal models and experimental methods of modern medicines can be applied to indirectly study its efficacy. Due to the characteristics of various functions and functioning in many ways of Chinese medicinal, the corresponding technical methods should be selected for research. The efficacy, effective range of dosage, intensity of the effect, speed and duration of functioning should be answered firstly through research. Secondly, the main and secondary efficacy of Chinese medicine should be clarified, and what are the advantages and characteristics compared with similar medicines. Finally, all kinds of interfering factors that affect the experimental results should be eliminated, and the experimental results should be comprehensively analyzed and summarized to find out the inherent regularity and even integrated with the theory of Chinese medicine to clarify the regularity of efficacy.

（二）保健作用

5.2 Health Care Effect

中药保健作用是在中医药理论指导下，对中药预防或养生保健作用的概况和总结。

The health care effect of Chinese medicine is an overview of the prevention or health care effects of Chinese medicinal under the guidance of Chinese medicine theory.

1. 中药预防作用 是治疗作用的延伸，但与治疗作用有本质的区别。治疗作用是针对疾病，而预防作用是应用中药治未病，是使"无病机体"保健健康。一般采用的方式是用一些中

药烟熏、洗浴、佩带以及内服而发挥防病作用。《本草纲目》记载，苍耳"为末水服，辟恶邪、不染疫疾"；茅香、兰草"并煎汤浴，辟疫气"；大蒜"立春元旦，作五辛盘食，辟温疫"；黄连"预解胎毒""小儿初生，以黄连煎汤浴之，不生疮及丹毒"。

5.2.1 Preventive Effect of Chinese Medicinal

It is an extension of the therapeutic effect, but it is fundamentally different from the therapeutic effect. The therapeutic effect is aimed at the disease, while the preventive effect is the application of Chinese medicine for the preventive treatment of diseases, which helps to keep the disease-free body healthy. The commonly used method to prevent diseases is the application of smudging, bathing, wearing and administration of Chinese medicinal. As recorded in *Bencao Gangmu (Compendium of Materia Medica)*, the evil and epidemic disease can be avoided when taking the powder of Canger (Xanthii Fructus); taking a bath with Maoxiang (Cymbopogon citratus (DC.) Stapf.) and Lancao (Orchida Herba) boiled is water can eliminate epidemic disease; eating Dasuan (Allii Sativi Bulbus) in the start of spring and New Year's day can avoid epidemic disease; children taking a bath with Huanglian (Coptidis Rhizoma) soup at birth can be prevented from congenital disease and sores.

2. 中药养生保健作用 中药养生源远流长，早在《神农本草经》就记载了大量养生延年的药物。如灵芝"久食，轻身不老，延年"。

5.2.2 Health Care Function of Chinese Medicinal

There is a long history of health preservation of Chinese medicinal. As early as recorded in *Shennong Bencao Jing*, a large number of medicines can be used for health promotion and prolonging life. For example, eating Lingzhi (Ganoderma) for a long time can keep body in a young state and lifespan can be extended.

中药养生保健作用的现代研究，主要是根据受试中药预防保健功用的特点，选用合格实验

动物及相关材料，在国家认证通过的实验室或基地，按照国家保健作用评价程序和检验方法，科学评价中药在免疫调节、延缓衰老、增智、促进生长发育、抗疲劳、减肥、保护心血管系统、抗辐射、抗癌、抗突变等保健作用。如中药免疫调节作用至少应完成细胞免疫、体液免疫和单核 - 巨噬细胞功能方面的试验；中药延缓衰老作用应进行生存试验、过氧化脂质含量测定和超氧化物歧化酶活性检测；中药促智作用需选用跳台试验、避暗试验、穿梭箱试验、水迷宫试验等，研究受试中药对记忆获得、巩固和再现的作用；中药抗疲劳作用必须进行负重游泳试验和爬杆试验；中药减肥作用需完成受试药物对大鼠肥胖模型的减肥试验；中药抗辐射作用首先应进行小鼠抗辐射 30 天存活试验，若结果为阳性，需继续进行外周血象、骨髓象、染色体畸变和精子畸形检查，以确定中药抗辐射的保健作用。

The modern research on the health care function of Chinese medicine is mainly based on the characteristics of the preventive and health care functions of the tested medicines. Qualified experimental animals and related materials are selected, and the functions of Chinese medicinal are scientifically evaluated in immune regulation, delay of aging, intelligence increase, promoting the development of growth, anti-fatigue, reducing weight, protection of cardiovascular system, anti-radiation, anti-cancer and anti-mutation etc. For example, the immunomodulatory effect of medicines, tests should be completed at least in the aspects of cellular immunity, humoral immunity and mononuclear macrophage function. Survival test, lipid peroxidation content and superoxide dismutase activity detection should be carried out for the anti-aging effect of medicines. To study the effect of medicine on memory acquisition, consolidation and reproduction of memory, the gangplank test, dark avoidance test, shuttle box test and water maze test should be applied. The anti-fatigue effect of medicines must be tested by weight-bearing swimming and pole climbing. The effect of medicines on reducing weight needs

to complete the experiment of the tested drug on the obesity model of rats. The anti-radiation effect of medicines should firstly be tested in mice for anti-radiation survival for 30 days. If the result is positive, peripheral blood imaging, bone marrow imaging, chromosome aberration and sperm malformation should be further examined to determine the anti-radiation healthy effect of medicines.

另外，随着现代研究的不断深入，中药新的功效不断被发现、认识和使用，如青皮、枳实升压抗休克，泽泻、山楂降血脂，罗布麻降血压，砒霜抗癌、治疗白血病等，有显著疗效。

Besides, with the constantly deepening of modern research, new functions of Chinese medicinal have been discovered, recognized and applied. For example, the boosting and anti-shock effect of Qingpi and Zhishi, hypolipidemic effect of Zexie and Shanzha, hypotensive effect of Luobuma, and anti-cancer and treatment for leukemia of Pishuang, all show significant therapeutic effects.

六、应用的研究
6 The Research on Application

（一）中药饮片
6.1 Chinese Decoction Pieces

中药饮片临床应用的现代研究，主要包括组方配伍、用法用量等方面的研究内容。

The modern research on the clinical application of Chinese decoction pieces mainly includes the compatibility of prescriptions, administration and dosage etc.

1. 组方配伍

饮片组方配伍应用，是中医药治疗疾病的显著特点，是反映中医临床用药特色的关键。饮片组方配伍应用主要围绕饮片的配伍层次、配伍关系、配伍环境、配伍比例等方面进行研究。

6.1.1 Compatibility of Prescriptions

The compatibility and application of decoction pieces are the remarkable characteristics of Chinese medicine in treating diseases and crucially reflect the characteristics of clinical medication of Chinese medicinal. The compatibility application of decoction pieces mainly focuses on the level and relationship of compatibility, as well as the environment and proportion of compatibility etc.

（1）配伍层次的研究：包括饮片配伍、组分配伍、成分配伍等三个方面。

6.1.1.1 It includes the compatibility of decoction pieces, components and ingredients, respectively.

①饮片配伍研究的主要内容是药效物质基础与作用机制，不论何种配伍关系，配伍后均将产生物质基础和生物效能的变化，达到增效减毒的作用；饮片配伍也可以根据药物的性质和临床的需求，通过不同的药物组合、不同的配伍环境、不同的炮制品种、不同的用量比例、不同的给药剂型、不同的煎服方法、不同的给药途径等，控制中药饮片发挥疗效的方向。

① The main contents of the research on the compatibility of decoction pieces are the pharmacodynamic material basis and mechanism of action. Regardless of the compatibility relationship, the material basis and biological efficacy can be changed after compatibility so as to increase efficacy and reduce toxicity. The compatibility of decoction pieces can also be based on the properties of medicinals and clinical needs via studying different medicinal combinations, various compatibility environments, different processed varieties, different dosage proportions and forms, different decocting methods and ways of administration to control the therapeutic approach of Chinese medicinal slices.

②组分配伍主要是以系统科学思想为指导，以药化、药理、药物信息学、计算科学和复杂性科学等多学科技术为手段，从临床出发，遵循传统配伍理论与原则，强化主效应，减轻或避免副效应，形成针对特定病证的组效关系明确的中药组分配伍形式。组分配伍研究主要包括组分的提取、分析、评价和作用机理研究几方面，其核心就是药效物质和作用原理研究。

② Component compatibility is mainly guided by systematic scientific idea and application of multi-disciplinary technologies such as pharmaco-chemistry, pharmacology, pharmaceutical informatics, computational science and complexity science etc. From the view of clinic application, the traditional compatibility theories and principles to strengthen the main effect and alleviate or avoid side effects should be followed so as to form the compatibility form of medicine components for specific disease with definite relationship of combination effect. The study of component compatibility mainly includes the aspects of component extraction, analysis, evaluation and mechanism research, and the core of which is the study of pharmacodynamic substances and action mechanism.

组分提取：根据中药的性质与功用，采用溶剂提取、溶剂分配、超临界萃取等技术方法，提取不同极性或不同类别的化学成分提取物，再用大规模工业色谱分离制备技术，对提取物进行纯化，获得组分。

Component extraction: According to the property and function of Chinese medicinal, different kinds of chemical components can be extracted by solvent extraction, solvent distribution and supercritical fluid extraction. Then large-scale industrial chromatography separation technology is conducted to purify the extraction to obtain components.

组分分析：组分样品是典型的复杂体系，包含种类众多、含量变化迥异的化合物。必须采用定性、定量的分析方法，如色谱、光谱、化学指纹图谱等技术手段，分析揭示中药组分的物质基础。

Component analysis: The component sample is a typical complex system that contains a wide variety of compounds with varying contents. It is necessary to use qualitative and quantitative analysis methods, such as chromatography, spectroscopy and chemical fingerprints to analyze and reveal the material basis of medicine components.

组分评价：在中医药功效理论指导下，主要选择反映拟治疗病证相对特异的动物模型或指标，以整体、器官药理水平评价样品组分的活性，必要时结合细胞和分子药理实验，阐明各种组分单独应用和配伍后各层次效应及分子网络调控通路，探索活性组分，揭示组效关系，并根据不同药物组分组合的活性综合评价结果，寻求组分间的最佳配伍配比关系。

Component evaluation: Under the guidance of the efficacy theory of Chinese medicine, animal models or indicators that are relatively specific for disease treatment are selected to evaluate the activity of component samples at the pharmacology level of whole and organ. If necessary, combining cell and molecular pharmacological experiments to clarify the various levels of effects and molecular network regulatory pathways after the individual application and compatibility of various components. The active components and the relationship between combination and effect are well studied to explore the optimum compatibility relationship among components according to the comprehensive evaluation results of the activity of different components.

组分作用机理研究：得到药效确切的中药组分后，从临床出发，以药化、药理、药物信息学、计算科学和复杂性科学等多学科技术为手段，进一步深化研究，阐明其治疗病证的药效物质和作用原理。

Study on the action mechanism of components: Once obtaining the components of Chinese medicinal, multi-disciplinary technologies such as pharmaco-chemistry, pharmacology, pharmaceutical informatics, computational science and complexity science should be applied in the view of clinical use to further deepen the research and clarify the medicinal substances and action mechanism in the treatment of diseases.

③成分配伍是在饮片配伍、组分配伍研究的基础上，进一步揭示各组分中化学成分之间的配伍配比关系，以期较清晰地说明其与组分配伍、饮片配伍的内在本质联系。如附子大黄属典型的寒热配伍，附子味辛甘大热，"能行、能补"，大黄味苦性寒，"能泄"；附子可温补心阳、肾阳、脾阳和去寒邪，大黄可通腑泻浊除积滞。附子大黄配伍源于《金匮要略·腹满寒疝宿食病脉证治第十》载大黄附子汤，方中以大黄苦寒攻下、通腑降浊，附子辛热散寒、温阳气，二药相合，寒热并用，温通并行，辛苦通降，相反相成，主治阳虚便秘证。为揭示附子大黄成分配伍对阳虚便秘的治疗作用及其作用机制，在附子大黄饮片配伍、组分配伍治疗阳虚便秘动物模型的基础上，采用乳鼠的结肠 Cajal 间质细胞（结肠 ICC）模型研究附子大黄成分配伍对结肠 ICC 的作用机制。结果表明附子大黄饮片配伍，对阳虚便秘模型动物的排便疗效优于单用附子或大黄，作用机制与其调节胃肠激素和肠神经递质的分泌有关；附子大黄组分附子总碱与大黄总蒽醌配伍，对阳虚便秘模型大鼠的作用最优，其发挥温阳通便功效的作用机制与调控肠运动相关胃肠肽的分泌有关，主要与调节 MTL、SS、AchE 的水平有关；附子大黄成分乌头碱大黄素配伍，1∶2配伍对结肠 ICC 具有减毒增效作用。

③ Composition compatibility: It is based on the study of the compatibility of decoction pieces and components and further reveals the compatibility relationship among various chemical compositions of components so as to clearly explain its intrinsic essential relationship with the compatibility of component and decoction pieces. For example, the compatibility of Fuzi and Dahuang is a typical hot-cold combination. The medicinal properties of Fuzi are pungent, sweet and hot, which can promote *qi* and tonify *yang*. The medicinal propertiy of Dahuang is bitter and cold, which can discharge fire. Fuzi can warm and tonify *yang* of heart, kidney and spleen and dispel cold evil, while Dahuang can free viscera and bowels, purge turbidity and remove stagnation. The compatibility of Fuzi and Dahuang originates from the Dahuang Fuzi Tang (Decoction) in *Jingui Yaolue (Synopsis of the Golden Chamber: the tenth chapter, the treatment of abdominal cold hernia*

and persistent food disease). In this prescription, Dahuang is bitter and cold and has the effects of purgation, clearing viscera and bowels and purging turbidity, Fuzi is pungent and hot and can expel cold and warm *yang*. The compatibility of these medicines indicates the combined use of the cold and hot, warming and clearing out, moving and descending with pungency and bitterness, in antagonism and complement, which can treat *yang* deficiency constipation. To reveal the therapeutic effect of Fuzi and Dahuang on the treatment of *yang* deficiency constipation and its mechanism of action, based on the decoction pieces and component compatibility of Fuzi and Dahuang in the treatment of *yang* deficiency constipation animals, a colon Cajal interstitial cells (colon ICC) model in KM suckling mice is used to study the mechanism of compositions compatibility of Fuzi and Dahuang in the treatment of colonic ICC. As a result, the combination of Fuzi and Dahuang decoction pieces had a better defecation effect on *yang* deficiency constipation model animals than the use of Fuzi or Dahuang alone. The mechanism of action is related to its regulation of the secretion of gastrointestinal hormones and intestinal neurotransmitters. The compatibility of total alkaloids in Fuzi and total anthraquinone in Dahuang has the optimum effect on *yang* deficiency constipation rats. Its mechanism of exerting the laxative effect of warming *yang* is related to the regulation of gastrointestinal peptides secretion that is associated with bowel movements, which mainly depends on the regulation of MTL, SS and AchE levels. The compatibility of aconitine in Fuzi and emodin in Dahuang (1 : 2) possesses the effect of reducing toxicity and enhancing efficacy on colonic ICC.

（2）配伍关系的研究 主要指中药七情配伍。现代主要采用化学分离分析技术和药理学实验方法，研究中药七情配伍关系中各药效物质（有效组分和有效成分）间增效、减毒和调节的内在联系。

6.1.1.2 Research on Compatibility Relationship

It mainly refers to the compatibility of seven emotions of Chinese medicinal. In modern times, chemical separation and analysis techniques and pharmacological experimental methods are mainly used to study the internal connection of synergism, detoxification and regulation among various medicinal substances (effective components and ingredients) in the compatibility of seven emotions of medicines.

①单行 即不用其他药物辅助，单独应用于临床。如独参汤，以一味人参补气固脱，用于气虚欲脱或阳虚欲脱者。

① Single application: That is to say, the medicinal is used alone in clinic without the aid of additional medicinals. Such as Dushen Tang (Decoction), which Renshen is used alone to invigorate *qi* for relieving desertion. It is used for the treatment of *qi* or *yang* deficiency with collapse.

②相须 指性能功效相类似的药物配合应用，增强其原有疗效。如大黄芒硝相须为用，治疗积滞便秘，尤以热结便秘为宜。现代研究表明生大黄能刺激肠道，增加蠕动而促进排便；芒硝的主要成分为硫酸钠，在肠中不易吸收，易形成高渗盐溶液，使肠道保持大量水分，容积增大，刺激肠黏膜感受器，反射性地引起肠蠕动亢进而致泻。二药伍用，泻下之力量更强。

② Mutual reinforcement: It refers to the application of medicinals with similar performance and effect to enhance their original efficacy. Such as Dahuang and Mangxiao, which are used together for the treatment of stagnant constipation, especially heat constipation. Modern research shows that Dahuang in raw material can stimulate the intestine, increase peristalsis and promote defecation. The main component of Mangxiao is sodium sulfate, which is not easily absorbed in the intestine and can form hypertonic salt solution so as to keep much water in the intestinal tract and increase its volume, stimulate the intestinal mucosa receptors and reflexively lead to the active intestinal peristalsis to cause diarrhea. The promotion effect of diarrhea could be enhanced in the combination of the two medicinals.

③相使　指性能功效相似的药物配合应用，以一种药物为主，另一种药物为辅，辅药能提高主药的疗效。如黄连木香配伍，治疗湿热下痢，黄连清热燥湿止痢，木香行气化滞止痛，相使为用。现代研究表明黄连体外对痢疾杆菌有抑制作用，体内对痢疾杆菌感染致死小鼠有保护作用；黄连木香配伍，木香能使黄连中盐酸小檗碱的达峰时间提前、血药浓度增加，对14种（株）能够引起感染性腹泻的病原菌有较强的抗菌活性，对在体或离体胃肠道运动有抑制作用，有一定的抗炎镇痛作用，其治疗感染性腹泻的范围和强度较优。

③ Mutual assistance: It refers to the application of medicinals with similar performance and efficacy and taking one medicinal as the main medicine and another as the adjuvant. The subsidiary medicinal can improve the efficacy of the main medicinal, such as the compatibility of Huanglian and Muxiang (Aucklandiae Radix) in the treatment of dampness-heat diarrhea. Huanglian can clear heat and dry dampness, and Muxiang can move qi and remove food stagnation to relieve pain. Modern studies show that Huanglian has an inhibitory effect on dysenteriae in vitro and a protective effect on mice caused by dysentery infection in vivo. In the compatibility of Huanglian and Muxiang, Muxiang can advance the peak time of berberine hydrochloride in Huanglian and increase blood concentration. It has strong antibacterial activity against 14 kinds of pathogenic bacteria that can cause infectious diarrhea. It also has an inhibitory effect on the gastrointestinal movement in vivo or in vitro as well as anti-inflammatory and analgesic effects, and the effective range and intensity are good in the treatment of infectious diarrhea.

④相畏、相杀　是同一配伍关系的两种提法。相畏，指一种药物的毒性反应或副作用，能被另一种药物减轻或消除；相杀，指一种药物能

减轻或消除另一种药物的毒性或副作用。如附子与甘草配伍，附子的毒性能被甘草减轻和消除，所以说附子畏甘草；甘草能减轻或消除附子的毒性或副作用，所以说甘草杀附子的毒。现代毒理学研究证明，附子的毒性主要是心脏毒、神经毒，毒性组分主要是酯性生物碱，毒性成分主要是乌头碱。甘草能明显降低附子的毒性，以乌头碱计，附子单煎液总生物碱含量为0.22%，附子甘草分煎后混合液为0.02%，附子甘草合煎液为0.01%；甘草皂苷、甘草黄酮、甘草多糖均能降低附子酯性生物碱的毒性，附子酯性生物碱LD_{50}为37.69 mg/kg，附子酯性生物碱与甘草皂苷、甘草黄酮、甘草多糖1∶2配伍，毒性明显下降，LD_{50}分别为110.58、104.78、83.59 mg/kg；甘草总黄酮能延长乌头碱诱发的小鼠心律失常的潜伏期，甘草类黄酮和异甘草素能使乌头碱诱发的动物心律失常持续时间明显减少；甘草酸在体内的水解产物葡萄糖醛酸能与乌头类生物碱的羟基结合，生成低毒或无毒的葡萄糖醛酸络合物而由尿排出，从而降低附子的毒性。

④ Mutual restraint and mutual suppression: These are two formulations of the same compatibility. Mutual restraint refers to the toxicity or side effects of one medicinal being reduced or eliminated by another medicinal. Mutual suppression refers to that one medicinal can reduce or eliminate the toxicity or side effects of another medicinal. For example, in the compatibility of Fuzi and Gancao (Glycyrrhizae Radix et Rhizoma), the toxicity of Fuzi could be reduced and eliminated by Gancao, thus, Fuzi is considered to be restraint of Gancao. Gancao could reduce or eliminate the toxicity or side effects of Fuzi, so Gancao could suppress the toxicity of Fuzi. Modern toxicology research has proved that the toxicity of Fuzi mainly lead to cardiotoxicity and neurotoxicity, and the toxic components and compositions are mainly ester alkaloids and aconitine, respectively. Gancao could markedly reduce the toxicity of Fuzi. According to the content of aconitine, the content of total alkaloids in Fuzi Danjianye

(Decoction) is 0.22%, the mixture of separately decocted Fuzi and Gancao is 0.02%, and the mixture of Fuzi and Gancao decocted together is 0.01%. Glycyrrhizin, glycyrrhiza flavonoids and Glycyrrhiza Polysaccharide could reduce the toxicity of ester alkaloids of Fuzi, of which the LD_{50} is 37.69mg/kg. The compatibilities of ester alkaloids in Fuzi with Glycyrrhizin, glycyrrhiza flavonoids, Glycyrrhiza Polysaccharides in 1 : 2 lead to significantly reduced toxicity and LD_{50} is increased to 110.58, 104.78 and 83.59mg/kg, respectively. Total flavonoids in Gancao could prolong the latency of arrhythmia induced by aconitine in mice. Flavonoids and isoliquiritigenin in Gancao could significantly reduce the duration of arrhythmia induced by aconitine in animals. Glyoxylic acid, the hydrolysis product of glycyrrhizic acid in the body, could combine with the hydroxyl group of aconitine alkaloids to form low-toxic or non-toxic glucuronic acid complexes and be excreted from the urine, thereby reducing the toxicity of Fuzi.

⑤相恶　指两种药物合用，一种药物与另一药物相互作用而致原有功效降低，甚至丧失药效。如丁香恶郁金，因郁金能削弱丁香的行气作用。现代研究证明，丁香配伍郁金能抑制动物胃肠的运动，桂郁金和绿丝郁金可减弱丁香对小鼠胃排空的促进作用，抑制呕吐家鸽的止吐作用。

⑤ Mutual inhibition: It refers to the combination of two medicinals that one medicinal can interact with another medicinal to reduce the original efficacy or even deprive its efficacy. For example, Dingxiang (Caryophylli Flos) inhibits the effects of Yujin (Curcumae Radix), because Yujin can weaken the effect of Dingxiang on moving *qi*. Modern research proves that Dingxiang and Yujin can inhibit gastrointestinal movement in animals. Guiyujin and Lvsiyujin can attenuate the effect of Dingxiang on gastric emptying in mice and inhibit the antiemetic effect of vomiting pigeons.

⑥相反　指两种药物合用，能产生毒性反应或副作用。如甘遂、大戟、海藻、芫花与甘草配伍，将产生毒副作用，属中药"十八反"。现代毒理学研究表明甘遂、大戟、海藻、芫花与甘草配伍，LD_{50}下降，毒性增强；连续给药7天，观察实验动物各系统症状指征，检测肝功、肾功、心肌酶谱，做心、肝、肾组织病理观察，发现配伍前后，药物对呼吸系统均无明显影响，但对实验大鼠循环、消化、神经系统有不同程度的损害，导致实验动物心率加快，ALT升高、心肌酶谱各项指标异常变化，心脏、肝脏、肾脏组织充血、出血，小灶性炎细胞浸润，细胞组织肿胀变性及空泡样改变；说明"十八反"药物不宜配伍使用。但不可一概而论，情况非常复杂。如附子与贝母配伍，也属"十八反"配伍。现代研究，附子与贝母合煎，没有新的化学成分的产生，但附子毒性成分乌头碱的溶出明显增多，乌头碱在血中的保留时间明显延长，毒性增加，附子强心作用减弱；乌头碱与贝母总碱配伍，明显延长室性心动过速和室颤时间，增加乌头碱的心脏毒性，降低去甲乌药碱提高心肌收缩力的作用；附子能剂量依赖性地增加LM_2细胞凋亡率，浙贝母也有增加LM_2细胞凋亡的作用，附子与浙贝母1 : 1配伍，能使LM_2细胞凋亡率显著降低，表明两药合用对LM_2肿瘤的抑制作用减弱。但附子与浙贝母单1 : 2配伍，对小鼠Lewis肺癌具抑瘤作用。

⑥ Antagonism: It refers to the combination of two medicinals that can produce toxic reactions or side effects. For example, the compatibilities of Gancao and Gansui (Kansui Radix), Daji (Euphorbiae Pekinensis Radix), Haizao (Sargassum), Yuanhua (Genkwa Flos) can be toxic and cause side effects, which belong to the "eighteen incompatible medicaments" of Chinese medicine. Modern toxicology studies show that the compatibilities of Gancao and Gansui, Daji, Haizao, Yuanhua can decrease the LD_{50} and increase the toxicity. For 7 days of continuous administration, the systemic symptoms of experimental animals are observed, liver function, renal function, and myocardial enzyme spectrum are detected and pathological observations on the heart, liver and kidney tissues are performed. It is found that the medicinal has no significant effect on the respiratory system before or after the compatibility. However, it has different degrees of damage on the circulation, digestion and nervous system of experimental rats, resulting in accelerated heart rate, increased ALT content, abnormal changes of myocardial enzymes, congestion and bleeding of heart, liver and kidney tissues, and small focal inflammation cells infiltration, swelling and degeneration of cellular tissue and vacuole-like changes, which indicates that medicinals of "eighteen incompatible medicaments" should not be used in combination. But it cannot be generalized due to the complicated situation. For example, the compatibility of Fuzi and Beimu also belongs to the "eighteen incompatible medicaments" compatibility. Modern research has shown that the compatibility of Fuzi and Beimu produce no new chemical ingredients. However, the dissolution of aconitine—the toxic component of Fuzi, is significantly increased and the retention time of aconitine in blood is significantly prolonged and toxicity is increased as well, which lead to an attenuated cardiotonic effect. The compatibility of aconitine with total fritillaria significantly prolongs ventricular tachycardia and ventricular fibrillation time, increases the cardiotoxicity of aconitine and reduces the effect of higenamine on myocardial contractility. Fuzi can increase the apoptosis rate of LM_2 cells in a dose-dependent manner, and Zhebeimu (Fritillariae Thunbergii Bulbus) also increases the apoptosis of LM_2 cells. The compatibility of Fuzi and Zhebeimu (1∶1) can significantly reduce the apoptosis rate of LM_2 cells, which indicates that the combination of the two medicinals can weaken the inhibition of apoptosis rate on LM_2 tumors. However, the compatibility of Fuzi with Zhebeimu (1∶2) has an antitumor effect on Lewis lung cancer in mice.

（3）配伍环境的研究：主要包括配伍外环境和配伍内环境的研究。外环境是指中药配伍前影响药效物质基础与作用机制的因素总和，包

括中药的品种、产地、炮制、制剂等影响配伍的因素。内环境是指配伍后影响药效物质基础与作用机制的因素总和，包括配伍的不同形式、不同条件、不同的配伍过程发生的物理、化学和生物效应的总和。如附子与甘草配伍，附子为单基原植物，不同产地毒性差异较大，毒性物质主要为双酯性生物碱，炮制后双酯性生物碱含量明显降低，久煎有利于双酯型生物碱水解，水解产物为苯甲酸，煎煮超过6小时后，双酯型生物碱基本全部水解，毒性基本消失；配伍甘草，酸性环境改变了毒性成分氮原子的正电效应和空间结构，有利于双酯型生物碱水解成单酯型生物碱；甘草皂苷具有对抗附子酯性生物碱的心脏毒性效应，和甘草酸铵通过酸性基团结合成盐，改变生物碱的存在形式，发挥协同抑制作用，达到降低双酯型生物碱毒性的目的。又如附子大黄配伍，附子总生物碱含量呈升高趋势，酯性生物碱的含量呈降低趋势，大黄主要成分含量影响较小；经人工胃液和人工肠液孵化后，总生物碱含量显著升高，双酯型生物碱含量降低；人工肠液对新乌头碱和次乌头碱的稳定性强于乌头碱，人工胃液对大黄主要成分的稳定性强于人工肠液。

6.1.1.3 Research on the Compatibility Environment

It mainly includes research on the external and internal environment of compatibility. The external environment refers to the sum of the factors that affect the basis of the substance and the mechanism of action before the compatibility of medicines, such as the variety, origin, processing and preparation of medicines. The internal environment refers to the sum of the factors that affect the substance base and mechanism of action after compatibility, including physical, chemical and biological effects of different forms, conditions and compatibility processes. For example, the compatibility of Fuzi and Gancao, Fuzi is a simple primitive plant and the toxicity of Fuzi varies greatly in different places. The toxic substance is mainly the diester alkaloids. After processing, the content of diester alkaloids is significantly reduced. Long time decoction of Fuzi is beneficial to the hydrolysis of diester alkaloids and the hydrolysis product is benzoic acid. Decoction for more than 6 hours can hydrolyze all the diester alkaloids and the toxicity is basically gone. The acidic environment in the compatibility of Fuzi and Gancao changes the positive charge effect and the spatial structure of the nitrogen atom of the toxic component, which is beneficial to the hydrolysis of the diester alkaloids to the monoester alkaloids. Glycyrrhizin has a cardiotoxic effect against aconite ester alkaloids, and can be combined with ammonium glycyrrhizinate to form salts via acidic groups so as to change the existing form of alkaloids and exert a synergistic inhibitory effect to reduce the toxicity of diester alkaloids. For another, the content of total alkaloids in Fuzi is increased in the compatibility of Fuzi and Dahuang, and the content of ester alkaloid is decreased and the content of the main components of Dahuang has little effect. After incubation with artificial gastric juice and artificial intestinal fluid, the contents of total alkaloids and the diester alkaloids are increased significantly and decreased, respectively. The artificial intestinal fluid is more stable to neoaconitine and hypoconitine than aconitine, and artificial gastric juice is more stable to the main components of Dahuang than artificial intestinal fluid.

（4）配伍比例的研究：中药剂量比例不同，药物配伍后发生药效、药性的变化不同，临床适应证就不同。如黄连与吴茱萸配伍，是典型的寒热配伍，配伍剂量比例不同，主治功效差异很大。黄连与吴茱萸6：1配伍为左金丸，黄连与吴茱萸1：6配伍为反左金丸。左金丸主治肝火犯胃之胁肋胀痛，呕吐吞酸，嘈杂嗳气，口苦咽干，舌红，脉弦数。反左金颠倒二药的用量比例，则药性偏温热，临床常用于脘痞嘈杂泛酸，又呕吐清水，畏寒，舌苔白滑，偏于胃寒甚者。现代研究表明，左金丸与反左金在相同模型上体现了不同的证治药效，左金丸能明显防治大鼠的热型（包括胃热Ⅰ°和胃热Ⅱ°模型）急性胃黏膜损伤，符合左金丸的临床证治；但在胃寒

模型中，由于证治不符，药效越来越差。反左金在胃热模型中几乎无效；但在胃寒模型中（包括胃寒Ⅰ°、胃寒Ⅱ°和胃寒Ⅲ°模型）则体现出显著的保护作用，且随着三个模型寒性程度的增强，其防治胃黏膜损伤的作用也随之增强；在胃寒Ⅱ°模型中病理检测反左金的疗效明显优于左金丸；而在胃寒Ⅲ°模型上，这种差距体现的更明显，反左金防治胃黏膜损伤的疗效从损伤指数和病理检测上都明显地优于左金丸，左金丸的作用较差。实验结果还表明单味黄连或吴茱萸的药效不如二者配伍使用好。

6.1.1.4 The Research on Compatibility Proportion

Different dosage ratios of medicines will lead to different clinical effects due to different efficacy and medicinal properties after the compatibility of medicines. For example, the compatibility of Huanglian and Wuzhuyu (Euodiae Fructus) is a typical combination of cold and hot. The indications vary in different dosage proportions. The compatibilities of Huanglian and Wuzhuyu in 6 : 1 and 1 : 6 called Zuojin Wan and Fanzuojin Wan, respectively. Zuojin Wan is mainly used to treat syndromes of liver fire invading the stomach, vomiting and swallowing acid, gastric upset and belching, bitter taste in the mouth and dry throat, red tongue and string-like pulse. Fanzuojin Wan reverses the dosage ratio of these two medicinals and is relative to the warm, which is often used in clinical applications of gastric stuffiness and upset and pantothenic acid, vomiting water, fearing of cold, white tongue fur, and with more cold affecting stomach. Modern research indicates that Zuojin Wan and Fanzuojinwan show different effects towards syndromes on the same model. Zuojin Wan can significantly prevent acute gastric mucosal injury in rats (including stomach heat Ⅰ° and stomach heat Ⅱ° models), which is consistent with the clinical diagnosis and treatment of Zuojin Wan. However, in the model of stomach cold, the efficacy is getting worse due to the inconsistency of therapeutic effects of Zuojin Wan and Fanzuojin

Wan which is almost ineffective in stomach heat models. Further more has significant protective effects in stomach cold models (including stomach cold Ⅰ°, stomach cold Ⅱ° and stomach cold Ⅲ° models), and as the increasing of coldness, its effect in preventing and treating gastric mucosal injury also increased. In the model of stomach cold Ⅱ°, pathological detection of Fanzuojin Wan is significantly better than that of Zuojin Wan. Inaddition, in the model of stomach cold Ⅲ°, this gap is more obvious. The efficacy of Fanzuojin Wan in preventing and treating the gastric mucosal injury is better than Zuojin Wan in terms of injury index while pathological examination, while the effect of Zuojin Wan is worse. The experimental results also show that the efficacy of Huanglian or Wuzhuyu when used alone is not as good as the compatibility.

2. 用法用量

包括用量与用法两个方面。（1）用量：是指为了达到一定治疗目的，中药饮片所应用的剂量，一般指日服药量，中药饮片的用量与药物自身性质，临床需要、患者情况以及地域、季节等因素有关，不能一概而论。汤剂一般为一日一剂，每剂分2次或3次服用；病情急重者，可每隔2~4小时左右服药1次，昼夜不停，使药力持续，利于顿挫病势；发汗药、泻下药，因药力较强，服药应中病即止，一般以得汗、得下为度，不必尽剂，以免汗、下太过，损伤正气；呕吐病人服药宜小量频服。剂量的现代研究主要应注意量效关系、时效关系。（2）用法：主要包括给药途径、服药方法等方面的内容。①给药途径，主要包括胃肠道给药和不经胃肠道给药两类。不经胃肠道给药包括注射给药、呼吸道给药、皮肤给药、黏膜给药等。②服药方法是根据病情需要和药物特性，选择适当的服药时间，也是合理用药的要求，包括晨起空服，饭前服，饭后服，睡前服，发作前服，热药凉服，凉药热服等方式。

6.1.2 Administration and Dosage of Chinese Medicinal

(1) Medicinal dosage: It refers to the dosage of Chinese decoction pieces in the application of certain therapeutic purposes, generally refers to the daily dose of medicine. The dosage of Chinese decoction pieces is related to the property of the medicinal, clinical needs, conditions of patients and regions and seasons etc., which cannot be treated as the same. Decoctions are usually taken once a day and is usually taken twice or three times a day. Patients with severe illness can take medicinal every 2 to 4 hours though day and night so as to enhance the durability of medicinal, which helps to alleviate the disease. The treatment of sweating medicinal and purgative medicinal should be stopped immediately once the symptoms are relieved due to the strong efficacy of these medicinal. Generally, moderate relief of sweating and diarrhea are enough. It is not necessary to take all the medicine to prevent excessive sweating and damage of healthy *qi*. Patients with vomiting should frequently take medicinal in a small amount. The relationship of dose-effect and time-effect should be studied with attention in the modern research of dosage. (2) Medicinal administration: It mainly includes the route of administration and the method of taking medicine. ① Routes of administration mainly include gastrointestinal administration and parenteral administration. Parenteral administration includes injection, respiratory administration, skin administration and mucosal administration etc. ② The method of taking medicine is to choose the appropriate time for taking medicine according to the needs of disease condition and characteristics of medicine, which is also a requirement for the reasonable use of medicinal. Taking medicinal in the morning, before meals, after meals, before sleeping, before the attack, hot medicine in cool condition and cold medicine in hot condition are all included in the methods of taking medicinal.

另外，中药饮片临床应用时，还要注意证候禁忌、配伍禁忌、妊娠禁忌，饮食宜忌和儿童、孕妇、老人的用药特点，密切关注药物在吸收、分布、代谢、排泄过程中的差异。

Besides, in clinical applications of Chinese decoction pieces, we should also pay attention to the syndrome contraindication, compatibility contraindication, pregnancy contraindication, diet contraindication, the characteristics of children, pregnant women, and the elderly, and the differences in the absorption, distribution, metabolism and excretion of medicinal.

（二）中成药

6.2 Chinese Patent Medicines

中成药是中医药的重要组成部分，其应用具有悠久的历史。我国现存最早的医学典籍《黄帝内经》，载方13首，其中就有9种成药，包括丸、散、膏、丹、药酒等剂型。医圣张仲景《伤寒杂病论》收载成药60余种，其中剂型有丸剂、散剂、膏剂，以及栓剂、洗剂、灌肠剂等。宋代政府高度重视中成药的研究、收集、制作和使用，尤其是北宋政府官办药局"惠民和剂局"，专司制药和售药，并编写了《太平惠民和剂局方》，该书是我国历史上第一部由国家刊行的中成药药典，收方788首，对后世影响极大；如纳气平喘黑锡丹，开创化学制剂的先例；又如清心开窍的至宝丹，疏肝解郁的逍遥散，解表化湿的藿香正气散等，至今沿用。

Chinese patent medicines are the important constitutes of Chinese medicine and has a long history in application. *Huang Di Nei Jing*, the earliest extant medical classic in China, contains 13 prescriptions, among which there are 9 patent medicines, including pill, powder, paste, pellet, medicinal liquor and other pharmaceutical forms. Zhang Zhongjing, the medical sage, collected more than 60 kinds of patent medicines in *Shanghan Zabing Lun*, among which the pharmaceutical forms includes pill, powder, paste, suppository, lotion and enema etc. The government in Song Dynasty attached great importance to the research, collection, production and application of Chinese patent medicine, especially the government-run pharmacy of the Bureau of People's Welfare Pharmacies in Northern Song Dynasty, which is specialized in pharmaceutical、preparing and

medicinal sales. It compiled *Taiping Huimin Heji Ju Fang* with 788 prescriptions, which was the first Chinese patent medicine pharmacopeia published by the state in the history of China and impacted greatly of generations. For example, *Heixi Dan (Pellet) creates a precedent for chemical agents with the effect of promoting inspiration to relieve asthma. Zhibao Dan (Pellet) with the effect of clearing and opening the mind, Xiaoyao San (Powder) with the effect of relieving the depressed liver and Huoxiang Zhengqi San (Powder) with the effect of relieving dampness and resolving dampness* are still in use up to now.

中华人民共和国成立以后，中成药的研发和应用得到很大发展。目前，中成药品种8000多种，中成药剂型达50余种，其中常用的中成药剂型有固体剂型、半固体剂型、液体剂型、气体剂型等。①固体剂型主要有散剂、颗粒剂、胶囊剂、丸剂、滴丸剂、片剂、浸膏剂、栓剂、丹剂等，以及锭剂、贴膏剂、茶剂、膜剂、海绵剂、糕剂、熨剂、条剂、钉剂、线剂、曲剂、灸剂、烟剂等。②半固体剂型主要有煎膏剂、流浸膏剂、软膏剂、凝胶剂等剂型。③液体剂型主要有合剂（含口服液）、酒剂（亦称药酒）、酊剂、糖浆剂等，以及注射剂、乳剂、露剂、搽剂、洗剂、油剂等。④气体剂型主要有气雾剂、喷雾剂；气体剂型可用于呼吸道吸入、皮肤、黏膜和腔道给药。

After the founding of the People's Republic of China, the research and application of Chinese patent medicines have been greatly developed. At present, there are tens of thousands of Chinese patent medicines and there are more than 50 pharmaceutical forms of Chinese patent medicines. The commonly used forms of Chinese patent medicines include solid, semi-solid, liquid and gas form etc. ① Solid preparation forms mainly include powder, granules, capsule, pill, dropping pills, tablet, extract, suppository and pellet etc., as well as pastille, emplastrum, medicated tea, film agent, sponges, medicinal cake, medicated ironing, medicinal roll, nail preparations, medicated thread, fermented medicine, moxa-preparation and fumicants etc. ② Semi-solid preparation forms mainly include soft extract, fluid extract, ointment and gel-forming agent etc. ③ Liquid preparation forms mainly include mixture (including oral liquid), vinum (also known as medicated liquor), tincture and syrup etc., and injection, emulsions, distillate medicinal water, liniments, lotions and oiling agent etc. ④ Gas pharmaceutical forms mainly include aerosol and spray. The pharmaceutical form of gas can be used for respiratory tract inhalation, skin, mucous membrane and cavity administration.

中成药的研究主要包括创新药物研发和中成药大品种二次开发。中成药的创新研究包括创新药物的发现、处方组成原理、成药制备、质量标准、稳定性控制、药理毒理研究、临床试验等方面的内容。中成药大品种二次开发，主要包括质量提升，有效性、安全性和经济性再评价等方面的内容。概言之，主要包括三方面的研究内容：①处方组成与制药方法研究。处方是中成药研究的基础，中成药处方主要来源于经方、验方、医院制剂和科研协定方，其组成应遵循三方面的原则，一是理法方药一致性原则，二是君臣佐使的配伍原则，三是突出临床应用的原则。制药方法的研究是中成药研究开发的核心内容，研究结果直接关系到中成药的安全性、有效性、稳定性、适用性和经济性。应根据临床的需要、药物的性质和工业化的程度选择适宜的剂型、设计制备工艺及工业化生产。②中成药的功能主治与作用机制研究。中成药的功效和主治病证的确定，要求全面、准确，突出主要作用和临床定位。研究中应以药效学的实验研究和客观标准化的临床研究为主，同时多学科结合，从而阐明其发挥疗效的物质基础和作用机制，指导临床安全合理应用。③成药的质量控制与评价方法研究。中成药的质量好坏直接影响其疗效发挥，建立适合中成药品种自身特点的质量控制与评价方法至关重要。中成药的质量控制与评价研究一般包括中药材原料质量控制和中药制剂质量控制两大部分，部分中成药以中药提取物、有效部位或有效成分为中间体原料的，还要进行中间体原料

的质量控制研究。

The research of Chinese patent medicines mainly includes the research and development of innovative medicinals and the secondary development of large varieties of Chinese patent medicines. The innovation research of Chinese patent medicines includes the discovery of innovative medicines, the principle of prescription composition, the preparation of Chinese patent medicines, quality standards, stability control, pharmacology and toxicology research and clinical trials etc. The secondary development of large varieties of Chinese patent medicines mainly includes quality improvement, effectiveness, safety and economic re-evaluation. In summary, it mainly includes three aspects as follows: ① Research on prescription composition and pharmaceutical methods. Prescriptions are the basis for the research of Chinese patent medicines. Prescriptions of Chinese patent medicine mainly come from classical prescriptions, proved recipes, hospital preparations and scientific research parties. Its composition should follow three principles, the first is the principle of the consistency of regularity and medicine, the second is the principle of compatibility of the sovereign, minister, assistant and guide, and the third is the principle of clinical applications. The research of pharmaceutical methods is the core content of the development of Chinese patent medicines. The research results are directly related to the safety, effectiveness, stability, applicability and economics of Chinese patent medicines. According to the clinical requirements, the property of medicine and the degree of industrialization, the appropriate preparation forms, the preparation process and industrial production should be selected properly. ② Study on the function indications and mechanism of action of Chinese patent medicine. The efficacy and indications for diseases of Chinese patent medicines should be comprehensive and accurate, which highlight the main role and clinical location of medicines. The research should be based on pharmacodynamic experimental research and objective standardized clinical research, and multi-disciplinary integration so as to clarify the material basis and mechanism of action and guide the safe and rational application in clinic. ③ Research on quality control and evaluation methods of Chinese patent medicines. The quality of Chinese patent medicines directly affects its efficacy. It is of vital importance to establish quality control and evaluation methods for the characteristics of Chinese patent medicines. The research on quality control and evaluation of Chinese patent medicines generally includes two parts: quality controls of raw materials of Chinese medicinals and Chinese pharmaceutical preparations. Some Chinese patent medicines are made from extracts, effective parts or active ingredients of medicines as intermediate raw materials, thus quality control of these intermediate raw materials is also required.

中成药的合理应用主要包括依法用药、辨证用药、安全用药几方面。①依法用药：首先应按照中华人民共和国《药品管理法》的要求，依法合理应用中成药；其次，应按照国家基本药物制度和医疗工伤保险药物目录，做好合理用药；再者，按照处方药与非处方药分类管理，合理用药；最后，根据《药品管理法》和《医疗机构制剂注册管理办法》的相关规定，合理使用医疗机构的中药制剂，满足人民群众的需求。②辨证用药：辨证使用中成药，主要是根据患者的临床表现，辨析确立疾病的证候属性，进而立法、处方、用药，即"法随证立，方从法出"；但在应用过程中应注意，同一疾病由于发病的时间、地区以及患者体质的不同，或是处于不同的发展阶段，可以见到不同的证；不同的疾病在发展过程中，可以出现相同的证，因而中成药在应用时，可采用"同病异治"或"异病同治"的方法。中医临床实践中，常碰到一些疾病，病因病机单一，证候属性区分度不强，可直接按照西医的病名、病理状态和理化检查结果来使用中成

药，即辨病论治；如高脂血症，属中医"痰浊""瘀血"的范畴，可选用血脂康胶囊、绞股蓝总苷胶囊等中成药。临床实践中，常将中医的辨证与西医的辨病结合起来，辨证辨病结合使用中成药；如冠心病心绞痛是西医病名，中医辨证属胸痹气滞气瘀、瘀血阻络、寒凝心脉、心气不足、气阴两虚等证候类型，分别选用速效救心丸、复方丹参滴丸等治气滞血瘀证，选用地奥心血康、血塞通颗粒等治瘀血阻络证，选用冠心苏合滴丸、宽胸气雾剂等治寒凝心脉证，选用通心络胶囊、补心口服液等治心气不足证，选用黄芪生脉饮、滋心剂型，已成为中医药临床治疗危重病症的独特武器。③安全用药：由于历史原因，一些早期的注射剂品种审批不严格，安全试验和临床试验不够完善，以及由于中药材原料品种混乱、成分复杂、制剂工艺不规范、质量标准不完善、联合用药不合理、给药途径不恰当，以及患者体质等因素，造成中药注射剂频频出现不良反应，甚至出现死亡病例。因此，中药注射剂的使用，一要辨证用药，严格按照药品说明书的功能主治使用，禁止超范围用药；二要严格按照药品说明书推荐剂量、调配要求、给药速度、疗程使用药品；三要根据适应证，合理选择给药途径；四是中药注射剂亦单独使用，谨慎联合用药，如确需联合使用其他药品时，应谨慎考虑与中药注射剂的间隔时间以及药物相互作用等问题；五是对老人、儿童、肝肾功能异常患者等特殊人群应慎重使用，加强监测；六要加强用药监护，用药前要认真检查药物，用药过程中应密切观察用药反应，发现异常，立即停药，采用积极救治措施，救治患者。

The rational application of Chinese patent medicines includes using the medicine legally, syndrome differentiation and its medication and using medicines safely. ① Using medicines legally: Firstly, Chinese patent medicines should be reasonably applied following the requirements of the *Pharmaceutical Management Law* of the People's Republic of China; Secondly, the rational use of medicinals should follow the national essential medicinal system and list of medical medicinals of medical injury insurance; Also, medicines should be used rationally according to the classified management of prescription drugs and over-the-counter drugs. Finally, following the relevant provisions of the *Pharmaceutical Management Law* and the *Measures for the Administration of Preparation Registration of Medical Institutions*, the Chinese pharmaceutical preparations of medical institutions are reasonably used to meet the needs of patients. ② Syndrome differentiation and its medication: The dialectical use of Chinese patent medicines is mainly based on the clinical manifestations of patients to identify and establish the syndrome attributes of the disease, and then establish treatment methods, determine prescriptions and use drugs in the disease. That is, "the methods of treatment are the basis for formulating prescriptions, and prescriptions are the embodiment of treatment methods". However, in the process of application, it should be noted that different syndromes can be seen in the same disease due to the attack time, region and constitution of patients or different development stages of diseases. Accordingly, the same syndrome can appear in the development of different diseases. Therefore, in the application of Chinese patent medicine, the method of "different treatments for the same disease" or "the same treatment for different diseases" can be adopted. In the clinical practice of Chinese medicine, some diseases with single etiology and pathogenesis and inapparent differentiation of syndrome attributes are often encountered. Chinese patent medicines can be used directly according to the disease, pathological status, and physical and chemical examination results of western medicine, which is known as "disease identification and treatment". Such as hyperlipidemia, which belongs to the category of "phlegm turbidity" and "stasis blood" in Chinese medicine, Chinese patent medicines such as Xuezhikang Jiaonang and Jiaogulanzonggan Jiaonang (total glycocide) can

be selected. In clinical practice, Chinese patent medicines are often used in combination of the syndrome differentiation of Chinese medicinal and the disease differentiation of Western medicines. For example, coronary heart disease and angina pectoris are of Western diseases. Meanwhile The syndrome differentiation of Chinese medicine is chest impediment, qi stagnation and blood stasis, blood stasis in the collateral, cold coagulation of heart pulse, deficiency of heart *qi*, and deficiency of *qi* and *yin*. Suxiaojiuxin Wan and Fufang Danshen Diwan are selected to treat the syndrome of *qi* stagnation and blood stasis; Diaoxinxuekang and Xuesaitong Keli are selected to treat the syndrome of blood stasis in the collateral; Guanxinsuhe Diwan and Kuanxiong Qiwuji (Aerosol) are selected to treat the syndrome of cold coagulation of heart pulse; Tongxinluo Jiaonang and Buxin Koufuye (Mixture) are selected to treat the syndrome of heart *qi* deficiency; The use of Huangqi Shengmai Yin (Decoction) and Zixin Jixing (Preparation forms) have become an unique weapon in the clinical treatment of critical disease syndrome. ③ Use medicines safely: Due to some historical reasons, such as the undemanding approval of some early injections, insufficient trials of safety and clinical test, the confused variety of raw materials of Chinese medicinal, the complex composition, the irregular preparation technology, the incomplete quality standards, the unreasonable combination of drugs, the inappropriate route of administration and difference of patients' constitution, there are frequent adverse reactions and even deaths event in the injections of Chinese medicinal. Therefore, the use of injections must be differentiated and used strictly in accordance with the functions of the drug instructions. It is forbidden to use drugs beyond the range of medication. Secondly, the drugs should be used strictly in accordance with the recommended dosage, formulation requirements, speed of administration and treatment course of instructions. Thirdly, the route of administration must be rationally determined by the indications. Fourthly, injections of Chinese medicinal should be used alone and carefully combined. If it is necessary to use injections with other drugs, the interval time and drug interaction with the injection should be carefully considered. Fifthly, the elderly, children and patients with abnormal liver and kidney function should be used with caution and monitored. Sixthly, we must strengthen the monitoring of medication, carefully check the medication before taking medicines, closely observe the medication reaction, and the medication should be stopped immediately in case of abnormal reactions and adopt active treatment measures to rescue patients.

第二章　中药的品种
Chapter 2　Variety of Chinese Medicinals

中药具有独特的理论体系和多基原、多品种、多产地、多功效、多用途等系统性特点。中药品种是一个含义较广且独具特色的概念，中药品种主要包括中药材品种、炮制品种（饮片品种）和中成药品种。

Chinese medicinal (CM) has a unique theoretical system and systematic characteristics of multiorigins, multivariety, multifunctions, multiuse, etc. The variety of CM is a broad and special concept; it mainly includes the variety of Chinese materia medica, processed Chinese medicinal products (traditional Chinese medicine decoction pieces) and Chinese patent medicines.

第一节　中药品种的含义
Section 1　The Meaning of Chinese Medicinal Variety

在本草典籍中，中药"品"和"种"的含义有区别，但有时亦通用。如《本草经集注》中说："以神农本经三品，合三百六十五为主"，这里的"品"，指上中下三品，即药物分类的类型；"又进名医副品，亦三百六十五，合七百三十种"，这里的"种"是指个药，即药味。又如《本草纲目》中说，"每品具气味、产采、治疗、方法"，所说的"品"则是指个药，都与现在所说的"品种"存在差别。中药品种主要包括中药材品种、炮制品种（饮片品种）和中成药品种；与生物学的"品种"含义不同。生物学上"种"指"物种"，是生物分类的基本单位，又可分为变种、亚种、变型和品种。现行的"品种"概念[2]，一般是指栽培上的经济植物类别，是人类通过驯化野生的不同种、变种或类型得到的，而野生植物没有品种之分。

In the material medica classic, the means of "pin" and "zhong" in Chinese medicines are different, but sometimes they are same. Sometimes "pin" refers to the type of Chinese Medicine classification, and "zhong" refers to a certain Chinese Medicine, for example: *Bencaojing Jizhu (Collective Commentaries on Classics of Materia Medica)* wrote that: *Shennong Bencao Jing* recorded 365 kinds of TM and which were divided into 3 'pin'. On the basis of this book, 365 other TM are recorded, and a total of 730 'zhong' of TM were recorded", but sometimes "Pin" refers to a TM, for instance, *Bencao Gangmu* said "Every 'pin' TM were recorded their smell, place of production, harvest, treatment and usage ". So, there are differences between modern "pinzhong" and ancient "pinzhong". TM variety is mainly composed of three parts: Chinese materia medica variety processed Chinese medicinal product (Chinese medicinal decoction pieces) variety, and Chinese patent medicines variety, which is different from biological "variety". Biological "zhong" refers to "species", is the basic unit of taxonomy, which can be divided into variants, subspecies, varieties. Modern "pinzhong" means "variety", generally refers to cultivated economic plants, and there is no concept of "pinzhong" in wild species.

一、中药材品种
1 Variety of Chinese Materia Medica

中药材品种通常是指中药所有来源的生物物种或矿物化合物，中药材基原则一般是指某一中药所有来源的生物物种或矿物化合物，可分为单基原、双基原和多基原。单基原品种中药材常常来源于单一的物种，例如中药材丹参来源于唇形科植物丹参 *Salvia miltiorhiza* Bge.；多基原品种中药材往往较为复杂，其来源常不止于一个物种，如中药材远志来源于远志科植物远志 *Polygala temuifolia* Willd. 或卵叶远志 *Polygala sibirica* L. 的干燥根；此外，即便是同一个物种来源的中药，也会由于入药部位等的不同而形成两个或两个以上的中药材品种。如植物紫苏 *Perilla frutescem* （L.）Britt. 的不同部位均各成一药，分别为紫苏子（干燥成熟果实）、紫苏叶（干燥叶）、紫苏梗（干燥茎）。根据中药材品种的真、伪、优、劣，还可分为正品、地区习用品、代用品、伪品。

Variety of Chinese materia medica refers to all the biological species or mineral compounds which could be used as Chinese medicinal. Chinese medicinal origin principles refer to biological species or a mineral compound which is/are the source of a Chinese medicinal, and can be divided into single-origin, double-origin and multi-origin. Single-origin means Chinese medicinal derive from a single species, for example, Danshen is derived from Salvia miltiorhiza Bge., Multi-origin variety is more complex, it means Chinese medicinal derives from more than one species, such as Yuanzhi, its original plants are Polygala temuifolia Willd. or Polygala sibirica L., in addition, even deriving from the same plant, it may produce more than

one variety due to the difference in application, etc., for instance, the different part of Zisu Perilla frutescem (L.) Britt. can make into Zisuzi (Perillae Fructus, dry ripe fruit), Zisuye (Perillae Folium, dry leaf) and Zisugeng (Perillae Caulis, dry stem). According to the authenticity, hypocrisy, superiority and inferiority, Chinese medicinal is divided into, the authentic, the regional folk medicine, the substitute and the fake.

正品： 中药正品是经本草考证的、名实相符的，并经临床验证的优良中药材品种。"名实相符"是指药，名、基原、采集、产地加工、炮制、贮藏各项，以及药材的性状、功能、主治各项，都符合标准并与文献记载的相一致。中药正品允许在全国范围内作商品药材流通和向国外出口销售。凡是现行《中国药典》和地方标准收载的品种，和道地药材品种都属于正品。

The authentic: the authentic is the genuine, excellent, verified clinically Chinese Medicine that is recorded in materia medica classic. "The genuine" refers to that the medicine, the name, source origin, collection methods, origin processing, processing of materia medica, storage, as well as the properties, functions, and indications are consistent with standards and documents. The authentic is allowed to circulate nationwide and export as merchandise. All the varieties included in the current *Chinese Pharmacopoeia* and local standards, as well as genuine regional materia medica are genuine.

地区习用品： 我国卫生部于1987年颁布的《地区性民间习用药材管理办法》，对"地区习用品"的定义为"地区性民间习用药材系指国家药品标准未载，而在局部地区有多年生产、使用习惯（其他地区没有使用习惯）的药材品种"，且审核批准的地区性民间习用药材，只准在本地区内销售使用。

The regional folk medicine: The *Regional Folk Medicines Management Measures*, promulgated by the Ministry of Health of China in 1987, defines "regional folk medicine" as "Chinese Medicine is not recorded in national standards, but produced and has been used in local areas for decades". And the approved regional folk medicine can only be sold in the local area.

代用品: 中药代用品是伴随着正品出现的,由来已久。汉代,张仲景的药方中即有"无猪胆,以羊胆代之"的先例。中药代用品出现的原因是商品药材短缺。代用品可分用同属近缘品种代替正品、用栽培品代替野生正品、用非药用部位代替药用部位、用人工合成(培育)品代替正品、用性效相近的中药代替短缺的正品中药五类。

The substitute: The appearance of the substitute is accompanied by the authentic and has a long history. In the Han Dynasty, Zhang Zhongjing had a precedent of sheep gallbladder replacing pig gallbladder. The reason for the emergence of substitutes is the shortage of commercial medicinal. Genuine products can be replaced by related species, wild varieties can be parts replaced by cultivated products, medicinal parts can be replaced by non-medicinal parts. artificially synthesized (cultivated) products and Chinese medicinal with similar properties and efficacy are used to replace genuine products.

伪品: 中药材伪品可分为两种情况,一种情况是,"以非药品冒充药品"者,如用面粉、玉米粉、石膏经模压加工制成假冬虫夏草,用淀粉或植物果实包以黄土冒充牛黄等,这种作伪情况较少见,对于从事相关专业者来说不难鉴别;另一种情况是,"以他种药品冒充此种药品",由于不少中药材品种存在多基原和异物同名的情况,此类冒充现象比较常见,也比较复杂和严重。

The fake: The fake can be divided into two types. One is impersonating medicine with non-medicine, for example, flour, corn flour and aquamarine are shaped with molds to make fake Donchongxiacao, wrapping starch or fruit of some plants with loess in order to impersonate Niuhuang (Bovis Calculus), this kind of circumstance is rare, and it is not difficult to identify for those engaged in related professions. Another is that one medicine is impersonated by other. Because different Chinese medicinal may have the same name,

and the same Chinese medicinal may come from different plants. This kind of impersonation is more common, complicated and serious.

二、炮制品种
2 Variety of Traditional Processing of Chinese Medicinal

炮制品种是指在中医药理论的指导下,依据辨证施治用药需要和药物自身性质,以及调剂、制剂的不同要求,采用传统制药技术将中药材炮制成不同规格的饮片形式而形成的品种。如中药材半夏在临床上常用的饮片品种有半夏、法半夏、清半夏、姜半夏等。

Under the guidance of the theory of Chinese medicine, according to the needs of syndrome differentiation and treatment, the property of the medicine, as well as the different requirements of preparation and dispensing, treated with traditional Chinese pharmaceutical technology, Chinese materia medica is processed into diverse traditional Chinese medicine decoction pieces, and then forms multiple varieties. Taking Banxia as an example, its processing varieties include Banxia, Fabanxia (prepared), Qingbanxia (prepared with alum) and Jiangbanxia (prepared with ginger).

中药炮制涉及的方法和使用的辅料众多,其对应的不同炮制品种也十分丰富。目前,常用的中药炮制方法有炒制法(加辅料或不加辅料炒)、炙法、发酵法、发芽法、制霜法等。临床上常使用的品种大多数为炮制品种。

There are many methods and pharmaceutic adjuvant used in the processing of Chinese medicinal, and the corresponding varieties are very plentiful. At present, the commonly used methods of processing include stir-frying (with or without adjuvants), stir-baking method, fermentation, sprouting, frost like powdering, etc. Most of the varieties used in clinic are Traditional Chinese medicine processed products.

但是,目前有的炮制品种已经濒临绝境,这些炮制品种或因工艺复杂,如"仙半夏";或因辅料不易得，如"鳖血柴胡"；或因炮制时间过长，如"九转南星"等原因而渐渐消失。

However, some processed products due to the complex craftsmanship, such as "Xian Banxia", some because of rare pharmaceutic adjuvant, such as "Biexue Chaihu", and some on account of taking too long time, such as "Jiuzhuan Nanxing", a part of traditional Chinese medicine processed products are on the verge of extinction.

三、中成药品种
3 Variety of Chinese Patent Medicines

中成药为中药成药的简称，中成药品种是在中医药理论指导下，以中药饮片为原料，经过药学和临床研究，并经国家药品监督管理部门批准，按规定的生产工艺和质量标准制成的可直接供临床使用的制剂。制剂方法的不同，可形成不同的中成药品种。

Chinese patent medicines are the abbreviation of complete preparation of Chinese patent medicines. The varieties of Chinese patent medicines are prepared directly for clinical use under the guidance of Chinese medicine theory, using Chinese materia medica as raw materials, after pharmacy and clinical research, and approved by the State Drug Administration, based on the prescribed production process and quality standards. Different preparation methods can form different Chinese patent medicine varieties.

第二节 中药品种的发展
Section 2 Development of Chinese Medicinal Variety

中医药学著作历千百年之嬗递传承，关于中药品种的一些经典论述是对其的认识过程的反映，其发展史的相关记载，对我们继承传统的中药品种经验和研究发展中药品种的理论与实践均有重要的意义。

Traditional Chinese medicine Classics have been inherited for hundreds and thousands of years, and the contents in the books reflect the understand process of Chinese medicinal variety. These records on the development history of Chinese medicinal variety, have a great significance for us to inherit the experience and develop the theory in the later period.

一、中药材品种的发展
1 The Development of Chinese Materia Medica

中药的发现和应用，经历了极其漫长的实践过程。中药材品种的丰富发展，是我国劳动人民长期的实践和经验的升华，"神农尝百草"的传说，就反映了我国劳动人民发现及应用药物、积累临床经验的艰苦实践过程。

The discovery and application of CM is an extremely long practical process. The booming development of Chinese materia medica variety is the result of the long-term practice and cumulative experience of people's hard-working. The legend of "Shen Nong tasted hundreds of medicinals" reflects the tough process of discovering and applying medicinals, as well as accumulating clinical experience.

（一）古代本草论药材品种
1.1 The Development of Ancient Chinese Medicinal Variety

《诗经》可以说是我国现存文献中最早记载药用生物的书籍，书中收录100多种药用动植物名称，如苍耳、芍药、枸杞等。与《诗经》类似的还有《山海经》。

Shi Jing (The Book of Songs) can be deemed to be the earliest book recording Chinese medicinal in the existing literature in China. In this book, more than 100 names of CM are contained, such as Cang'er, Shaoyao (Paeonia lactiflora Pall.), Gouqi (Lycium barbarum L.), etc. Shanhai Jing (The Book of Mountains and Seas) is similar to Shi Jing in this aspect.

《神农本草经》被认为是现存最早的药学著作，全书载药 365 种，按药物功效将中药分为上、中、下三品，上品如人参、甘草、地黄等，中品如干姜、葛根、当归等，下品如附子、大黄、巴豆等。

Shennong Bencao Jing, is the earliest book on materia medica in China. 365 medicines are recorded in this book, and are divided into three grades according to their efficacy and properties. The upper grade includes Renshen, Gancao, Dihuang (Rehmanniae Radix), etc., middle grade includes Ganjiang (Zingiberis Rhizoma), Gegen (Puerariae Lobatae Radix), Danggui, etc., and the lower grade includes Fuzi, Dahuang, Badou (Crotonis Fructus).

东汉时期，张仲景著《伤寒杂病论》，总结了"麻黄配桂枝"等经典配伍药对，被后世誉为"成方之祖"，为药材品种的临床应用树立了典范。

At the end of Eastern Han Dynasty, Zhang Zhongjing, known as "the ancestor of prescription", wrote Shanghan Zabing Lun and summarized some Classic compatibility of medicinal, such as Mahuang with Guizhi (Mahuang Guizhi Tang, Decoction). He set a model for the clinical application of Chinese medicinal.

魏晋南北朝时期，陶弘景总结汉魏以来名医的用药经验，撰成《本草经集注》，载药 730 种，对药材的形态、性味、产地、采制、真伪鉴别等都做了较为详尽的论述。

During the Wei Jin Southern and Northern Dynasties, Tao Hongjing summarized the experience of famous doctors since the Han and Wei Dynasties, and wrote Bencaojing Jizhu. 730 kinds of Chinese materia medica and their form, property, original place, identification are recorded in this book.

唐朝时期出现了我国第一部官修药学专著——《新修本草》（又名《唐本草》）。全书载药 844 种，不仅开创了世界药学著作图文并茂方法的先例，还收集了安息香、血竭等外来药，并增加了水蓼、葎草等民间经验用药。《海药本草》《本草拾遗》《蜀本草》等本草典籍也记载不少当时新兴的中药材品种和外来药品种。

During the Tang Dynasty, China owned the first pharmacopeia sponsored officially--Xinxiu Bencao (Newly Revised Materia Medica), also known as Tang Bencao (Tang Materia Medica). The book sets a precedent for the world's pharmaceutical works. It contains 844 kinds of Chinese materia medica; these medicinals not only came from some typical folk medicinals, such as Shuiliao (Polygonum hydropiper L.) and Lvcao (Humulus Scandens), but also come from foreign countries, such as Anxixiang (Benzoinum) and Xuejie (Draconis Sanguis). Besides, Haiyao Bencao (Oversea Materia Medica), Bencao Shiyi (Supplement to Materia Medica) and Shu Bencao (Shu Materia Medica) all contain the content about emerging medicinals and abroad medicinals

宋代药物学发展迅速，中药材品种继续增加。该时期出现了《开宝重定本草》、《嘉佑补注神农本草》《本草图经》等著作。其中唐慎微的《经史证类备急本草》（简称《证类本草》），全书共载药 1740 多种，方药兼收，图文并重，且保存了民间用药的丰富经验。

In the Song Dynasty, pharmacology developed rapidly, and the varieties of Chinese materia increased continuously. During this period, Kaibao Chongding Bencao (Revised Materia Medica by Song Kaibao), Jiayou Buzhu Shennong Bencao (Remarks on Shennong's Classic of Materia Medica in Jiayou Year), Bencao Tujing (Illustration of Meteria Medica), etc., were created. Among them, Jingshi Zhenglei

Beiji Bencao (Classified Materia Medica from Historical Classics for Emergency), wrote by Tang Shenwei, records more than 1740 kinds of medicinals prescriptions rich in the pictures of medicinals and folk medication experience.

明朝医药学家李时珍经过长期的考查、研究和临床实践，撰成了《本草纲目》。该书载药1892种，其中新增药物374种，按自然属性分为16部60类，收载了多种民间药物，如紫花地丁、西红花、曼陀罗等中药材品种。

In the Ming Dynasty, after a long period of investigation, research and clinical practice, Li Shizhen, one of the greatest medical physician and pharmacologist in China, wrote *Bencao Gangmu*. The book contains 1892 kinds of medicines, among which 374 medicines are new at that time. The book also contains some folk medicines, such as Zihuadiding (Violae Herba), Fanhonghua (Croci Stigma) and Mantuoluo (*Datura stramonium Linn.*).

清朝时期，药物学家赵学敏著成《本草纲目拾遗》，共载药921种，补充了太子参、金钱草、西洋参等疗效确切的民间药及外来药。

In the Qing Dynasty, pharmacologist Zhao Xuemin wrote *Bencao Gangmu Shiyi (Supplement to Compendium of Materia Medica)*. There are 921 medicines recorded in the book, some folk and foreign medicines with definite effect, such as Taizishen (Pseudostellariae Radix), Xiyangshen (Panacis Quinquefolii Radix) and Jinqiancao (Lysimachiae Herba), are also compiled in this book.

（二）药材品种近现代发展

1.2 The Development of Modern Chinese Medicinal Variety

中药材品种随着中医药的发展不断增加，尤以近现代最为迅速。1935年编写《中国药学大辞典》，中药辞书的产生和发展是该时期中药学发展的一项重要成就。同期，随着中医药院校的出现，涌现出了第一批适应教学和临床需要的中药学讲义。至1959年，《中药志》对中药质量进行鉴别和比较，并增加了本草考证的内容。分别于1975年

和1986年出版的《全国中草药汇编》共收载中药材品种4000余种，系统全面地整理了关于中药材认、采、种、养、制、用等经验和国内外科研技术资料。90年代年出版的《中华本草》载药8980种，涵盖了当今中药学的许多内容，并增加了化学成分、药物制剂、药材鉴定和临床报道等内容，是一部反映20世纪中药学科发展水平的综合性本草巨著。此外，中药材品种的理论研究方面亦有发展。

With the development of Chinese medicine, the variety of Chinese materia medica continues to increase, especially in modern times. *Zhongguo Yaoxue Dacidian (Chinese Pharmaceutical Dictionary)*, written in 1935, was an important achievement in the development of science of Chinese Materia medica (SCMM) during that period. During the same period, with the emergence of Chinese medicine schools, the first batch of lecture notes on (SCMM) appeared. By 1959, the book *Zhongyao Zhi (Chinese Medicinal Herbal)* not only recorded the content of quality identification of Chinese medicine, but also added the content of textual research. *Quanguo Zhongcaoyao Huibian (National Collection of Chinese Herbal Medicine)* published in 1975 and 1986 respectively, collects more than 4,000 varieties of Chinese materia medica. The experience and the scientific and technological information in the recognition, acquisition, seeding, breeding, production, use, etc. of Chinese materia medica are comprehensively included in these two books. *Zhonghua Bencao* published in the 1990s, contains 8980 kinds of medicines, covering almost all the information of Chinese materia medica today, and includes the new content about chemical ingredients, pharmacological preparations, medicinal materials identification and clinical reports, etc. *Zhonghua Bencao* is a reflection of the development of Chinese medicine in the 20th century. In addition, the theoretical research on the variety of CM has also developed.

二、炮制品种的发展

2 The Development of Processed Chinese Medicinal

中药材经炮制能达到方便调剂、制剂以及减毒增效等目的，同时通过不同的炮制处理，产生了具有不同功用的中药炮制品种。我国中药炮制的起源很早，积累了非常丰富的经验。

Chinese medicinal can achieve the effects of easy-adjustment, convenient preparation, less toxicity and better medicinal effect by processing. At the same time, through different processing methods, different kinds of Traditional Chinese medicine processed products were produced. The origin of processing of materia medica is very early, and it has accumulated much experience.

（一）古代本草论炮制品种

2.1 The Development of Ancient Processed Chinese Medicinal

汉以前的古文献中所记载的都是比较简单的炮制内容和炮制原则。战国时期《黄帝内经》的《灵枢·邪客》篇中有"治半夏"的记载；《素问·缪刺论》中最早记载了炭药。

Before the Han Dynasty, ancient classics only recorded simple processing methods and principles. In the period of the Warring States period, *Huang Di Nei Jing* has the chapter about processing of Banxia.

汉代出现了大量的炮制方法和炮制品。东汉时期《神农本草经》中的 13 种炮制品种，包括发芽的大豆黄卷、鹿角胶、阿胶等；《伤寒杂病论》对方剂中使用的炮制品种做出脚注；东晋葛洪在《肘后备急方》中记载了 80 多种药物炮制方法，以及姜半夏等中药炮制品。

In the Han Dynasty, a large number of processing methods and products booming out, 13 traditional Chinese medicine processed products are written in *Shennong Bencao Jing*, including Dadouhuangjuan (Sojae Semen Germinatum), Lujiaojiao (Cervi Cornus Colla), E'jiao (Asini Corii Colla), and so on. The formula in *Shanghan Zabing Lun* contains footnote for

variety of processed Chinese medicine applied in prescriptions. In the Eastern Jin Dynasty, Ge Hong recorded more than 80 medicine processing methods in *Zhouhou Beiji Fang (Handbook of Prescriptions for Emergency)*, such as the processed products of Jiangbanxia prepared with ginger and other Chinese medicinals.

南北朝时期，我国有了中医药史上的第一部炮制学专著《雷公炮炙论》。书中记载了各种炮制中药材的方法，广泛地应用辅料炮制药物，制备不同的炮制品。

During the Northern and Southern Dynasties, China had the first monograph on processing technology in the history: *Leigong Paozhi Lun (Leigong Treatise on the Preparation)*. This book describes various processing methods, and widely describes the use of various pharmaceutic adjuvants to prepare different processed products.

唐代在炮制原则系统化和炮制新方法方面有较详细的记载。孙思邈的《备急千金要方》提出了类似于现今中国药典的炮制通则；《千金翼方》《仙授理伤续断秘方》等书中新增了炮制品种，如姜天南星、姜草乌、醋草乌等；《新修本草》《食疗本草》《外台秘要》等本草典籍中新增了许多炮制方法和炮制辅料。

In the Tang Dynasty, there were systematic and detailed records of processing principles and new processing methods. *Beiji Qianjin Yaofang* Essential prescriptions worth a Thousand Gold for Emergencies, completed by Sun Simiao, proposes general processing rules that similar to those of today's Chinese Pharmacopoeia. *Qianjin Yifang (Supplement to the Essential Prescriptions Worth a Thousand Gold)*, *Xianshou Lishang Xuduun Mifang (Monograph on Orthopedics and Traumatology of colestial Chinese)* and other books record new processing products, such as Jiang Tiannanxing prepared with ginger, Jiang Caowu prepared with ginger, Cu Caowu prepared with vinegar. Some classics, such as *Xinxiu Bencao, Shiliao Bencao (Materia Medica for Dietotherapy), Waitai Miyao (Arcane Essentials*

from the Imperial Library) and etc., record the new processing methods and accessories at that time.

宋代从注重汤剂的饮片炮制品种发展到同时重视成药中饮片炮制品种。王怀隐编著的大型方书《太平圣惠方》始载"乳制法"和巴豆霜；宋代的《太平惠民和剂局方》，书中特设专章讨论炮制技术，收录了185种中药的炮制方法和要求。

In the Song Dynasty, Chinese medicine scientists not only paid attention to the variety of decoction pieces in soups, but also began to value the variety of decoction pieces in Chinese Patent medicine medicines. *Taiping Shenghui Fang (Taiping Holy Prescriptions for Universal Relief)*, a large-scale formula book written by Wang Huaiyin, records the method of preparing with milk and Badoushuang firstly. *Taiping Huimin Heji Ju Fang* in Song Dynasty, compiled by Chen Shiwen and others, sets a special chapter to discuss the processing technology and contains processing methods and requirements of 185 kinds of Chinese medicinals.

元代王好古在《汤液本草》记载了同一种中药材的不同炮制品种；张元素在《珍珠囊》中记载了酒白芍和煨木香等炮制饮片。

In the Yuan Dynasty, Wang Haogu showed different processing products which come from same Chinese materia medica in the book of *Tangye Bencao (Materia Medica for Decoctions)*. Zhang Yuansu recorded diverse decoction pieces such as Jiubaishao *(prepared with Liguor)* and Weimuxiang *(Roasted)* in *Zhenzhunang (Pouch of Pearls)*.

明代，《本草发挥》和《本草蒙荃》中都记载了当时的炮制准则。《本草纲目》中记载了半夏、天南星、胆南星等炮制品种，记载的炮制方法近20大类，其中许多方法沿用至今。

In the Ming Dynasty, both *Bencao Fahui (Elaboration of Materia Medica)* and *Bencao Mengquan (Enlightening Primer of Materia Medica)* record the processing guidelines. *Bencao Gangmu* records processing products of Banxia,

Tiannanxing (Arisaematis Rhizoma), Dannanxing and other processed products, it also records nearly 20 processing methods, many of which are still used today.

清代，中药的炮制技术和品种不断增加。《本草述》收载300多种炮制品种；《本草述钩元》增加了中药黄芪蜜制、盐水制的炮制品；《修事指南》分论232种中药具体的炮炙方法；《本草纲目拾遗》特别收录了近70种的炭药。

In the Qing Dynasty, the processing technology and variety of Chinese medicines continued to increase. In the book of *Bencao Shu (Description of Materia Medica)*, more than 300 kinds of processed products are contained. The Mizhi Huangqi (honey) and Yanshui Zhi Huangqi (processing with saline) are includes in *Bencao Shu Gouyuan (Delving into the Description of Materia Medica)*. *Xiushi Zhinan (Bibliography on Medicinal Processing)* discusses 232 specific processing methods of Chinese medicine. Nearly 70 kinds of charcoal medicines are contained in *Bencao Gangmu Shiyi (Supplement to the Compendium of Materia Medica)*.

（二）炮制品种现代发展

2.2 The Development of Modern Processed Chinese Medicinal

1988年，出版了我国第一部《全国中药炮制规范》，共收载了554种常用中药炮制品种，既体现了全国统一制法，又兼顾到地方特点。2009年饮片首次列入《国家基本药物目录》，2010年版《中国药典》对饮片给予明确定义，解决了中医配方和中成药生产投料界定不清晰的问题。《中国药典》作为我国药品检验的最高标准，历版药典一部所载的绝大部分中药材在继承传统的基础上均经过了简单的净制、切制等炮制过程，亦均收载有中药炮制通则和单味中药的炮制项。

In 1988, China's first edition of *National Standards for Processing Chinese Traditional Medicine* was published, which includs 554 traditional Chinese medicine processing products used commonly. This book not only embodies the unified national manufacturing method, but also takes local characteristics into account. In 2009, traditional Chinese medicine decoction pieces were listed in the *National Essential Medicines List* for the first time. The 2010 edition of *Chinese Pharmacopoeia* clearly defined the definition of traditional Chinese medicine decoction pieces. *Chinese Pharmacopoeia,* as the highest standard for drug inspection in China. Most of the Chinese medicinal materials contained in the first volume of *Chinese Pharmacopoeia*, have undergone a simple process of preparation, cutting and other processing on the basis of inheritance. The general rules of processing and the processing of single traditional Chinese medicine are also contained.

三、中成药品种的发展
3 Development of Chinese Patent Medicines Variety

我国医药学家根据中药四气、五味、升降浮沉、归经、毒性等性能特点和临床医疗需要，在中医理论指导下和理、法、方、药的基础上，遵循君、臣、佐、使的遣方规律，将中药进行配伍加工制备得到中成药。

Under the basic theory of Chinese medicine and the principles of reason, law, formula, and medicine, following the characteristic of four *qi*, five flavors, ascending, descending, floating and sinking, meridian tropism, toxicity and clinical needs, and then according to the hierarchy of sovereign, minister, assistant and guide, Chinese medicinals are prepared and combined to get Chinese patent medicines.

（一）古代本草论中成药品种
3.1 The Development of Ancient Chinese Patent Medicines Variety

中药制剂的起源可追溯至夏朝，这个时期出现多种药物浸制而成的药酒，随后又发现了曲（即酵母，一种早期应用的复合酶制剂）。殷商时期，伊尹首创汤剂，总结出《汤液经》，标志着汤剂在中药制剂品种中的形成。《五十二病方》的用药记载有丸、散、膏、丹、药浴剂、药

熏剂、药熨剂、饼剂等10余种剂型。

The origin of Chinese pharmaceutical preparation can be traced back to the Xia Dynasty. A variety of medicinal liquors made during this period, and Qu (yeast, a compound enzyme preparation for early application) was discovered at that time. During the Yin and Shang dynasties, Yi Yin, the pioneer of decoction, wrote *Tangye Jing (The Classicals on Decoction)*, which marked the formation of decoction in the variety of Chinese patent medicine. Moreover, there are more than 10 types of dose forms, including pills, powder, paste, pellet, medicinal bath, Chinese medicinal fumigation, traditional Chinese medicine ironing, medicinal cake and so forth, are recorded in *Wushier Bingfang (Prescriptions for Fifty-two Diseases)*.

春秋战国时期，《黄帝内经》，收载成方13首，其中汤剂4首，除具有多种剂型外还提出了"君臣佐使"的制方之法，是春秋战国以前医疗成就和治疗经验的总结。《神农本草经》也论及了中成药制药理论和制备法则。

During the Spring and Autumn Period and Warring States Period, *Huang Di Nei Jing* a summary of the medical achievements and treatment experience before that period, contains 13 prescriptions, including 4 soups, and proposed the hierachy methods of prescription forming by sovereign, minister assistant and guide. Pharmaceutical theory and preparation rules of Chinese patent medicine are also mentioned in *Shennong Bencao Jing*.

东汉末年，张仲景的《伤寒杂病论》，首次记载用动物胶汁、炼蜜、和淀粉糊做丸的赋形剂等，一些著名的中成药如五苓散、理中丸、四逆散等一直沿用至今，并传扬海外，日本的汉方制剂也有许多是遵循张仲景的名方所研制出来的。

In the late Eastern Han Dynasty, using animal glue, honey, starch paste and etc. as excipient is firstly recorded in *Shanghan Zabing Lun*. Some well-known Chinese patent medicines such as Wuling San (Powder), Lizhong Wan, Sini San, etc. have been used today, and some of them were spread overseas. A portion of Japanese medicinal preparations are developed in accordance with famous prescriptions in this book.

晋代的《肘后备急方》，首次提出了"成药剂"的概念，并最先把成药列为专卷，该书收载成药数十种，对传统剂型的制备有较为详细的描述。

In the Jin Dynasty, *Zhouhou Beiji Fang*, wrote by Ge Hong, proposes the concept and lists a special volume of "patent medicine" for the first time. Dozens of patent medicine and details in preparation are contained in the book.

唐代孙思邈所著《千金药方》和《千金翼方》，共载方6500余首，既有唐以前著名医家用方，也有民间验方，同时自创了用于治疟的太乙神精丹（氧化砷）等多种成药方，磁朱丸、独活寄生汤（现为丸剂）等有效方剂被制成成药剂型流传至今。

In the Tang Dynasty, Sun Simiao compiled *Beiji Qianjin Yaofang (Essential Recipes for Emergent Use Worth A Thousand Gold)* and *Qianjin Yifang*, which contain more than 6,500 formulae, including famous medical prescriptions before Tang, folk prescriptions, and prescriptions created by himself. The effective prescriptions such as Cizhu Wan and Duhuo Jisheng Tang (Decoction) (changed into pills now) are made into patent medicine and spread widely nowadays.

宋朝时期，《太平惠民和剂局方》，共收载中药制剂788种，卷首有"和剂局方指南总论"，文中对"处方""合药"和"药石炮制"等均有作专章讨论。

During the Song Dynasty, *Taiping Huimin Heji Ju Fang* contains 788 Chinese patent medicines totally, At the beginning of the volume, there is a general introduction to the guidelines for Heji administration. In this paper, the "prescription", "the combination of medicinals" and "the processing of medicinal stones" are discussed in special chapters.

金元时期，各个中医流派创制了具有自己特色的成药，如攻下派创制的木香槟榔丸，滋阴派的大补阴丸，寒凉派的防风通圣散、益元散，以及补土派的补中益气丸等著名成药。

During the Jin and Yuan Dynasties, there have various medical schools creating diverse Chinese patent medicine with their own characteristics, such as Muxiang Binglang Wan created by the School of Purgation, Dabuyin Wan derived from School of Nourishing Yin, Fangfeng Tongsheng San and Yiyuan San of the School of Cold and Cool, and Buzhong Yiqi Wan (Dripping Pills) initiated by the School of the Reinforcing the Earth.

清代《温病条辨》，创制了不少治疗温病的有效方剂，为后世此方面药物的研制奠定了基础，如现代的中成药银翘解毒丸即是在银翘散的基础上研制而成。

In the Qing Dynasty, *Wenbing Tiaobian (Detailed Analysis of Warm Diseases)* records numerous effective prescriptions used to treat warm diseases, which laid the foundation for the development of medicines in this respect for later generations. For example, Yinqiao Jiedu Wan was developed on the basis of Yinqiao San.

（二）中成药品种近现代发展

3.2 The Modern Development of Chinese Patent Medicines Variety

新中国成立以后，1963年版的《中国药典》首次收载中成药197种，标志着中成药的发展开始走上了标准化、规范化、法制化的道路。历2010年版《中华人民共和国药典 临床用药须知·中药成方制剂卷》用中医术语规范了所载中成药的功能主治，全面规范了常用中成药的临床标准，结束了药典配套丛书中成药临床用药须知长期阙如的历史。药典收载的中成药品种数目在不断增加，最新的2020版《中国药典》收录了1607个中成药品种，与2015版的《中国药典》相比，新增了116个品种。

After the founding of the People's Republic of China, the *Chinese Pharmacopoeia*, published in 1953 and 1963, included 197 Chinese patent medicines for the first time, declaring that the development of Chinese patent medicine was on the road to standardization, specification and legalization. *Pharmacopoeia of the People's Republic of China Clinical Medication Instructions · Traditional Chinese Medicine Preparation Volume*, in 2010 edition, uses Chinese medicine terms to describe the function of Chinese patent medicine, fully standardizes the clinical standards of commonly used Chinese patent medicine, and fills in the blank history in this aspect of Pharmacopoeia supporting series. The number of Chinese patent medicine included in *Chinese Pharmacopoeia* is constantly increasing. The 2020 edition of the *Chinese Pharmacopoeia* contains 1,607 varieties of Chinese patent medicine. Compared with the 2015 edition of the Chinese Pharmacopoeia, 116 new varieties were added.

第三节 中药品种的现代研究
Section 3 Modern Research on Chinese Medicinal Variety

现代科学技术的不断进步发展，药用植物学、中药鉴定学、中药化学、药用植物栽培学、植物化学分类学等多学科之间的相互渗透，饮片剂型、炮制规范化、质量控制体系等方面的优化发展，制药新技术、新工艺、新设备和新辅料等的创新应用，都极大地促进了对中药的种质资源、品种及道地性的研究。

The continuous advancement of modern science and technology, the interpenetration of multiple disciplines such as medicinal botany, Chinese medicine identification, Chinese medicine chemistry, medicinal plant cultivation and phytochemical taxonomy, the optimization and development of tablet type, standardized processing and quality control system as well as the innovative application of new pharmaceutical technologies, new processes methods, new equipment and application of new pharmaceutic adjuvants, they all have greatly promoted the modern research on the germplasm resources, variety study and genuineness of Chinese medicine.

一、中药材品种的现代研究
1 Modern Research on Chinese Materia Medica Variety

目前，药材品种研究的主要领域有中药品种调查、道地药材研究、中药品种的栽培养殖、中药品种的比较等；药材品种的研究方式和手段也随着科学技术的发展在进步，如多光谱成像技术、化学指纹图谱技术、人工种子技术等都是品种研究中常涉及到的。

At present, the research of Chinese medicinal variety focus on the investigation of Chinese materia medica variety, the research on genuine regional materia medica, the cultivation of medicines and the comparison of medicine varieties, etc. The research methods of Chinese materia medica variety are also closely related to the development of science and technology, such as multi-spearal imaging technology, chemical fingerprint, artificial seed technology.

（一）中药品种调查
1.1 The Investigation of Chinese Materia Medica Variety

进行中药材品种的现代研究，需先了解目前中药材品种的概况，一般会进行中药材品种调查。中药材品种调查主要以传统野外调查方法为基础，并结合先进适用的现代技术和方法，如影像、全球卫星定位系统、遥感、地理信息系统、计算机网络等，以确保数据的准确性和客观性，提高中药资源品种调查的效率和质量。

Before conducting modern research on varieties, it is necessary to understand the circumstance of verities, so, survey of Chinese materia medica varieties would be carried out. The survey mainly bases on traditional field investigation methods and take advanced modern technologies and methods, such as imaging, global satellite positioning system, remote sensing, geographic information system, computer network, etc., to ensure the accuracy and objectivity of the data as well as to improve the efficiency and quality of the investigation of Chinese medicine resources varieties.

建国以来，我国于20世纪60、70、80年代共完成了三次大规模中药材资源普查。其中始于1983年的第三次中药资源普查结果显示，我国中药资源种类达12807种。这上万种中药品种中重要的中药材品种大约有1000多种，最常用的品种只有500种左右。近年来，一些生长环境苛刻或资源量有限，或再生困难的品种，被大量盲目采挖导致其资源的急速减少以致枯竭，新的珍稀濒危种类因此逐渐产生。30多年后，为了进一步了解我国中药资源的生长分布情况，2018年，第四次全国中药资源普查全面展开，如今仍在如火如荼的进行。

Since 1949, China conducted three large-scale censuses of Chinese medicinal resources in 1960s, 1970s and 1980s. The third census, which began in 1983, shows that there are 12,807 kinds of Chinese medicinals. Among them, there are more than 1,000 kinds of important medicines varieties, and only about 500 kinds are the most commonly used. In recent years, due to the harsh growth environment, or limited resources, or difficulty in regeneration, some varieties decrease rapidly after blindly excavating. Thus, there have more and more endangered species. 30 years later, in order to further grasp the growth and distribution of Chinese medicinal resources in our country, in 2018, the fourth national general census of Chinese medicinal resources has been launched, and is still in its full swing.

（二）道地药材品种的研究

1.2 Research on the Genuine Regional Medicinal Variety

道地药材是具有中国特色、根植于中医药理论体系、来源于生产和用药实践、世所公认的特定产区的名优正品药材的代名词。从生物学角度出发，"道地性"是遗传、环境及药材表型三者在长期协同进化过程中，在某个特定时空上的一个反映，基原研究、性状研究、显微特征研究和理化研究是道地药材品种研究的常用的方法。近年来，DNA分子遗传标记技术、中药化学指纹图谱技术、组织形态三维定量分析、生物效价检测等一些新的鉴定方法，也作为道地药材品种研究的辅助手段之一。

Genuine regional medicinal refers to famous and genuine Chinese Medicinal with Chinese characteristics, rooted in the theoretical system of Chinese medicine, derived from production and clinical practice, growth in specific areas and recognized by the world. From the biological view, "Genuine regional" is a reflection of genetic, environmental and medicinal phenotypes in a specific time and space during the long-term co-evolution process. which is related to the background of genetic, environment and phenotype. Researches in origin, traits, and microscopic characteristics, physical and chemical researches are commonly used genuine regional medicinal methods. In recent years, some new identification methods such as DNA molecular genetic marker technology, chemical fingerprint and biological potency detection have also been used as one of the auxiliary methods.

（三）中药材品种的人工培育

1.3 The Artificial Cultivation of Chinese Materia Medica Variety

目前人参、西洋参、三七等大宗常用中药材商品几乎全部来源于栽培。然而，面对中药野生资源的日渐减少甚至衰竭以及中药材需求日增的巨大压力，只进行中药材的大规模栽培是远远不够的，必须选育高产优质品种，同时保证中药材质量和产量。

Currently, many commonly used medicines such as Renshen, Xiyangshen, Sanqi are almost derived from cultivation. However, facing the huge pressure of declining or even exhausting of wild medicine resources and increasing demand, large-scale cultivation is far from enough. Thus, it is necessary to breed high-yield and high-quality varieties and ensure their quality and yield simultaneously.

中药栽培品种日益增多，但属于真正中药品种的屈指可数。其原因是药用植物育种不仅注重产量更要注重质量，多年生植物的选育周期长，药用植物有多个药用部位、独特的生态生物学特性、浓厚的地域性等。因此中药材品种培育需要构建中药资源的核心种质库，把握品种选育目标，重视道地药材及野生品；重视数量性状研究，建立健全品种选育机制等。

Cultivated varieties are increasing day by day, but only a few varieties meet the requirements. The reason is that medicinal plant breeding not only focuses on yield but also on quality, the breeding cycle of perennial medicines is long, and medicinal plants have multiple medicinal parts, unique ecological and biological characteristics, and strong regional characteristics. Therefore, the breeding needs to construct a core germplasm bank of traditional Chinese medicinal resources, grasp the target of variety selection, attach importance to genuine regional materia medica and wild medicines, emphasize the study of quantitative traits and establish a sound variety selection mechanism.

（四）药材品种比较研究

1.4 The Comparative Research on Chinese Materia Medica Variety

该研究主要在相似中药品种中进行。品种比较研究可用于确定中药材品种的基源。如通过功效等的比较研究，多版《中国药典》对中药品种做出了改变，1995 年版《中国药典》将植物禹州漏芦（蓝刺头）*Echinops latifolius* Tausch. 从中药材漏芦的基源中分出，而与华东蓝刺头 *Echinops grijisii* Hance. 合称中药材禹州漏芦；2000 年版将华中五味子 *Schisandra sphenanthera* Rehd. et Wils. 从五味子中分出自成南五味子，2005 年版将黄柏 *Phellodendron chinense* Schneid. 与关黄柏 *Phellodendron amurense* Rupr.、葛根 *Pueraria lobate* (Willd.) Ohwi 与粉葛 *Pueraria thomsonii* Benth. 区分成不同的中药材；2010 年版将铁皮石斛 *Dendrobium officinale* Kimura et Migo 从中药材石斛中分列出，巫山淫羊藿 *Epimedium wushanense* T. S. Ying 从中药材淫羊藿中分列出等。比较研究还可以用于扩大药源等。

The research was mainly conducted on similar medicine varieties. This research can be used to determine the origin of Chinese materia medica. For example, by comparing the efficacy, *Chinese Pharmacopoeia* made adjustments to the original varieties of medicines, in the 1995 edition of *Chinese Pharmacopoeia*, the plant, Lancitou (*Echinops latifolius* Tausch.) was separated from origin plants of Loulu (Rhapontici Radix), and called Yuzhou Loulu (Echinopsis Radix) together with the Huadonglancitou (*Echinops grijisii Hance*); in the 2000 edition of the Chinese Pharmacopoeia, the Huazhongwuweizi (Schisandra sphenanthera Rehd. et Wils.) was separated from origin plants of Wuweizi (Schisandrae Chinensis Fructus), and became Nanwuweizi (Schisandrae Sphenantherae Fructus); in the 2005 edition, the Huangbai Phellodendron chinense Schneid was separated from Guanhuangbo (Phellodendri Amurensis Cortex), and the Gegen Puerariae lobatae Radix was separated from Fenge (Puerariathomsonii Benth.). In the 2010 edition, the Tiepishihu Dendrobium officinale Kimura et Migo was separated from Chinese medicinal Shihu Epimedium wushanense T.S.Ying was separated from medicinal plants of Yinyanghuo. Comparative studies can also be used to expand medicines source and ect.

二、炮制品种的现代研究
2 Modern Research on Processed Chinese Medicinal Variety

中药炮制作为传统的制药技术，具有悠久的历史和丰富的内容，现代科学技术的应用使传统炮制品种研究进入了一个新研究领域。现代炮制品种研究需要正确地运用现代科学知识和技术，传承并创新炮制方法与理论；只有阐明中药炮制理论和炮制方法的科学内涵，探索新的炮制工艺和辅料，才能丰富炮制品种。

Processing of materia medica is a traditional pharmaceutical technology with a long history and plenty knowledge. The application of modern science and technology has upgraded the study of processed Chinese materia medica variety into a new era. The research of modern processing medicinal products requires the correct use of modern scientific knowledge and technology, and need inheritance and innovation of processing methods and theories. Only by clarifying the scientific connotation of processing theory and methods, and exploring new processing techniques and pharmaceutic adjuvant, can we enrich the variety of processed products.

（一）炮制辅料研究
2.1 Study on Pharmaceutic Adjuvants

炮制方法中利用辅料炮制中药是具有特色的一类方法。中药炮制辅料按照形态分为液体辅料和固体辅料。有些辅料，如酒、醋、盐、姜、蜜等，在食品行业中的性质、应用、作用等都比较清晰，但作为炮制辅料，现今的认识大多仍停留在其传统功效、经验鉴别等方面。近年来，随着中药现代化的不断深入，国家非常重视中药的继承和创新问题，中药炮制辅料的规范化、标准化正是中药炮制的规范化、现代化、标准化关键问题之一。

Using pharmaceutics adjuvant is aunique method of processing of materia medica. According to the morphology, it could be divided into liquid pharmaceutic adjuvant and solid pharmaceutic adjuvant. Some pharmaceutic adjuvant such as liquor, vinegar, salt, ginger, honey, etc. are clear in the food industry in terms of their properties, applications, functions, etc., but as pharmaceutic adjuvants, knowledge of them still stays in their traditional efficacy, empirical identification methods, etc. .

In recent years, with the continuous deepening of the modernization of Chinese medicinal, China has attached great importance to its inheritance and innovation, and the pharmaceutic adjuvant is one of the key issues of the standardization, modernization and standardization of Chinese medicinal.

（二）炮制规范研究
2.2 Study on Processing Specifications

《中国药典》和地方标准，对多种中药进行了现代炮制技术、辅料等的要求，相继修订和增补了常用中药及藏、蒙、维等特色民族医药的饮片炮制规范。同时，针对中药饮片产业生产不规范等普遍问题，国家先后多次立项，将饮片生产一线技术人员的炮制经验数据化，建立了科学、实用的规范化炮制工艺研究模式，为中药饮片生产的规范化、规模化创造了良好的条件。

Chinese Pharmacopoeia and Chinese local standards have conducted researches on modern processing technology and pharmaceutic adjuvants, and the processing regulations for decoction pieces of traditional Chinese medicine, as well as Tibetan medicine, Mongolian medicine and Uighur medicine have successively revised and supplemented. At the same time, in response to the common problems of nonstandardization in the traditional Chinese medicine decoction industry, the state established multiple projects, to make processing experience of the prestigious technicians was digitized, and set up a scientific and practical research model for standardized processing techniques, which has created good conditions for standardized and scaled production of traditional Chinese medicine decoction.

饮片炮制过程中所用到的辅料缺乏符合自身特色的质量标准，辅料的操作规范亦不完善，譬如炮制用酒，药典规定一般使用黄酒，而在实际生产中又有白酒，且酒的质量及浓度也各有差异；辅料的标准及使用，长期困扰着企业生产，因此建立中药饮片辅料标准及规范使用势在必行。

The pharmaceutic adjuvant lacks quality standards that meet their own characteristics, and the operation specifications are not complete. For instance, Chinese Pharmalopoeia stipulates the wine for processing use should be yellow rice wine, yet the white wine existing in actual production. The standards of pharmaceutic adjuvant have been plaguing scientific research experiments and enterprise production, so it is imperative to establish standards and promote the standardized use of pharmaceutic adjuvant.

（三）炮制方法的研究

2.3 Study on Processing Methods

传统的炮制方法都是依靠手工或简单的加工设备，随着饮片生产规模的扩大，许多专用的机械设备应运而生。如风选机、洗药机、润药机、炒药机、切药机、蒸药箱、粉碎机等等，提高中药饮片生产的机械化、自动化、现代化水平。为了验证中药炮制理论的科学性、可行性和实用性，在中医药理论指导下，应用现代科学技术，采用多学科、多指标进行系统研究，并通过中医临床验证或模拟临床用药等形式进行了验证。

Traditional processing is primarily dependent on handwork or simple equipment. With the expansion of the production scale of traditional Chinese medicine decoction pieces, many special mechanical apparatuses came into being. Air sorting machine, medicine washing machine, medicine spraying machine, medicine cooking machine, medicine cutting machine, steaming medicine box, pulverizer, etc., these machines improve the level of mechanization, automation and modernization of traditional Chinese medicine decoction industry. In order to verify the scientificity, feasibility and practicability of Chinese medicine processing theory, under the basic theory of Chinese medicine, modern science and technology, multi-disciplinary and multi-index

systemic research, and through traditional Chinese medicine clinical verification (or simulated clinical medicine) were applied in further study.

（四）炮制新型饮片研究

2.4 Study on New Chinese Medicine Decoction Pieces

为满足大众多样化需求和提升医药行业服务质量，当今中药饮片产业正在朝着多样、方便、科学的方向快速发展。传统"饮片入药，临用煎汤"的用药方式，已渐渐不适应现代人的生活节奏。因此，从1993年始，经过20余年的改革尝试，我国研发出了多种新型饮片，主要有中药配方颗粒、中药颗粒饮片、粉末型饮片三大类。这些新兴饮片都符合中医药理论，保持了原中药饮片的药性药效，又具有不需煎煮、易于调剂、方便使用、质量可控等优点。

To meet the diverse needs of the public and improve the service quality, the traditional Chinese medicine decoction industry is rapidly developing in the direction of multi-form, being convenient and scientific. The traditional way of taking medicine, drinking the soup boiled from traditional Chinese medicine decoction pieces, has gradually become unfit for the rhythm of modern lifestyle. Therefore, since 1993, after more than 20 years of reform attempts, China has developed some new types of decoction pieces, mainly including traditional Chinese medicine formula granules, decoction pieces of coarse particles of Chinese medicine, Chinese medicine powdery decoction. These emerging decoction pieces conform to the theory of Chinese medicine, not only maintain the medicinal efficacy of the original decoction pieces, but also have the advantages of decoction-free, easy adjustment, convenient use, and controllable quality.

三、中成药品种的现代研究
3 Modern Research on Chinese Patent Medicines Variety

中成药的临床应用越来越广泛，且不断有新

的中成药品种出现。近年来，在中医药理论指导下，通过应用和推广制药新技术、新工艺、新设备和新辅料，改进传统剂型，推动了既具有中国传统医药特色又符合现代科学发展的中成药新品种的创制，使得中成药品种在重大疾病防治、品种的二次开发和新剂型等方面均取得了成果，极大地丰富了中成药的品种。

The clinical applications of Chinese patent medicine are becoming more and more extensive, and new varieties of Chinese patent medicine are constantly appearing. In recent decades, under the guidance of basic theory of Chinese medicine, Chinese patent medicine varieties makes visible achievement in new variety research for. prevention and control of major diseases, the secondary development of varieties and new pharmaceutical forms by the application and popularizing of new pharmaceutical technologies, processes, equipment and excipients, improving the research level and pharmaceutical forms and promoting the creation of new varieties that have both the characteristics of Chinese medicine and the modern science.

（一）新剂型研究
3.1 Research on New Pharmaceutical Form

现代科学的发展给中成药新剂型研究提供了更加宽广的空间，产生了许多新剂型，如注射液、胶囊、颗粒剂、滴丸等。许多对重大疾病有良好治疗效果的中成药被开发成注射液，对一些危亡重症的抢救施治有明显作用，如治疗心血管疾病的参附注射剂、参麦注射剂、生脉注射剂，治疗脑血管疾病的清开灵注射液、醒脑静注射液、灯盏花素注射液等。胶囊亦是新剂型研究的重点，如治疗冠心病心绞痛地奥心血康、心可舒胶囊，治疗肿瘤的安替可胶囊治疗糖尿病的参芪降糖胶囊等。此外一些新中成药品种，如复方丹参滴丸、速效救心丸、金芪降糖片、消渴丸等在防治重大疾病上有着重要地位。现在还出现了一大批全新的中成药品种，主要有缓释制剂、控释制剂、靶向制剂。

Modern science provides a broader space for the research of new formulations of Chinese patent

medicines, resulting in many new pharmaceutical forms, such as injections, capsules, granules, and pills. Many Chinese patent medicines that have good therapeutic effects have been developed into injections, which have obvious effects on the rescue of some critically illness. Such as Shenfu Zhusheye, Shenmai Zhusheye, Shengmai Zhusheye used to treat cardiovascular disease, Qingkailing Zhusheye, Xingnaojing Zhusheye, Dengzhanhuasu Zhusheye for treating cerebrovascular disease, etc. Capsules are also a focus, such as Di'aoxinxuekang and Xinkeshu Jiaonang for coronary heart disease and angina pectoris, Antike Jiaonang for treating tumors and Shenqi Jiangtang Jiaonang for diabetes. In addition, some new varieties, such as Fufang Danshen Diwan, Suxiao Jiuxin Wan, Jinqi Jiangtang Pian (Tablets), Xiaoke Wan, etc., play an important role in preventing and treating major diseases. There are also a large number of newly brand Chinese patent medicines mainly including sustained-release preparations, controlled-release preparations and targeted preparations.

（二）制备工艺的研究
3.2 Research on Preparation Technique

中成药的制备较为复杂，对制备技术，设备和辅料要求较高。现在已经有许多技术、新设备和新辅料应用在中成药制备工艺上，如超低温粉碎、超临界流体萃取、冷冻干燥、薄膜包衣、环糊精包合、固体分散等新技术，提取、浓缩、纯化、干燥、灭菌、制剂成型等中成药生产过程中组装式的自动流水线等新设备，以及纤维素衍生物、淀粉衍生物、合成半合成油脂、磷脂、合成表面活性剂、乙烯聚合物等新辅料。

The preparation of Chinese patent medicine is complicated, and the requirements on the preparation technology, equipment and pharmaceutic adjuvant are strict. Now, new technologies, such as ultra-low temperature crushing, supercritical fluid extraction, freeze drying, film coating, cyclodextrin inclusion, solid dispersion, etc., new equipments in automatic assenably line, such as extraction, concentration, purification, drying, sterilization, formulation forming, etc. And cellulose derivatives, starch derivatives, synthetic semi-synthetic fats, phospholipids, synthetic surfactants, ethylene polymers, etc., these new pharmaceutic adjuvants are used in preparation of Chinese patent medicine.

（三）中成药大品种二次开发研究

3.3 Research on the Secondary Development of Large Varieties of Chinese Patent Medicines

中成药二次开发应体现中医药的特色和优势，基于"临床 - 生产 - 市场"三维导向模式，注重产品的临床需求与设计、生产过程的现实化以及市场要求的灵活性和药品生产的经济成本。结合现代新方法新技术等，使传统中成药转变成安全、有效、稳定、方便、精密、可控的现代中成药新品种。

The secondary development of Chinese patent medicine is based on the three-dimensional guidance model of clinical-production-market, it also focus on the clinical needs, practical issues in the design and production process, the flexibility required and the economic cost. Combined with modern new methods and new technologies, Chinese patent medicine has been transformed into new modern varieties, which are safe, effective, stable, convenient, precise and controllable.

以参附汤的二次开发为例，参附汤是临床常用的经典名方，功能益气、回阳、救脱，主治阳气暴脱证。但需临时煎煮，且服用量大，不适于急重症抢救。通过对参附汤的二次开发，在其原方基础上将汤剂改制成参附注射液，既保留了原方的功能主治，又去杂存精减少剂量、临床应用更加方便，疗效亦大为提高，为中医急救良药，可用于心源性休克、感染性休克、中毒性休克、创伤性休克等。

Take Shenfu Tang (Decoction) as an example. The Shenfu Tang (Decoction) is a classic prescription. It has the functions of benefiting *qi*, restoring yang to save from collapse. However, it needs to be decocted temporarily in a large dose, which is not suitable for emergency treatment. Through the secondary development, the decoction was transformed into injection, which not only retained the original function, but also reduced the dose. Its clinical application becomes more convenient and the efficacy is also greatly improved, which used for cardiogenic shock, septic shock, toxic shock, traumatic shock and so on.

第三章 中药的品质
Chapter 3　Quality of Chinese Medicinals

中药品质是中药的生命，是中药质量的核心，受到中药种质、种苗、生长环境、栽培、采收、产地加工、炮制、制剂、储存、用法等多方面的影响。中药品质的内容主要包括中药材品质、中药饮片品质和中成药品质三部分。

The quality is the life and the core of Chinese medicinals. It is, affected by germplasm, seedlings, growing environment, cultivation, harvesting, origin processing, processing method, preparation, storage, usage and so on. Chinese medicinal quality mainly consists of three parts, the quality of Chinese raw medicinals, the quality of Chinese medicine decoction pieces and the quality of Chinese patent medicines.

第一节　中药品质含义
Section 1　The Meaning of Chinese Medicinal Quality

"中药品质"是指中药的质量，强调"合乎标准"或"规格品"的概念[5]，反映了中药种质、种苗、栽培、采收、产地加工、炮制、制剂等方面固有的整体特性的质量，包括内在品质和外在品质两部分。中药内在质量系指药材内含有效成分的种类与数量，对药材品质起决定性作用；而外在品质主要指药材的形状、大小、质地、色泽等，突出和反映药材的内在质量。

The "Chinese medicinal quality" refers to the quality of Chinese Medicinals, emphasizing the concept of "complying with the standards" or "specification". It reflects the quality of the inherent integral characteristics in germplasm, seedlings, cultivation, harvesting, processing, preparation, etc., for both intrinsic and extrinsic quality. The intrinsic quality refers to the type and quantity of active ingredients in the medicinals, which plays a decisive role in the quality of Chinese materia medica. The extrinsic quality mainly refers to the shape, size, texture, color, etc. of the medicinal materials, highlighting and reflecting the intrinsic quality.

传统方法主要从药物的"形、色、气、味"评价中药质量，以眼观、手摸、鼻闻、口尝等简便的方法来鉴别药材的形状、大小、色泽、表面特征等特征，这种传统的评价方法能快速有效的鉴别中药的品质优劣。如人参以"马牙芦""枣核艼""铁线纹""皮条须""珍珠点"为鉴别要点，天麻习称"鹦哥嘴""红小瓣""肚脐眼"。这些鉴定术语简洁、形象、便于记忆，至今也常用于中药品质鉴定。

Chinese medicinals are observed from their "shape, color, smell and taste" by traditional methods to access their quality by simply sight-seeing, hand-touching, nose-smelling, and mouth-tasting for differentiating medicinals from shape, size, color, appearance, etc. This method can quickly and effectively identify the quality of

Chinese medicinals. For example, Renshen, or ginseng can be differentiated by horse-teeth-print rhizome, Juju be seed root iron wire lines, thong fiber, and pearl point. Tianma is characterized by

"parrot beak", "red pigtail" and "belly button". These concise and visual identification terms are easy to remember and still commonly used to identify the quality of Chinese medicinals now.

第二节　中药品质的发展
Section 2　Development of Chinese Medicinal Quality

在对中药的认识初期即产生了中药品质评价的概念，中药品质随着中药品种的发展，其内涵渐渐丰富，古人逐渐认识到饮片大小、用药方式、药物剂型等因素都能影响中药的品质。中药品质包含中药材品质、中药饮片品质和中成药品质。饮片包括了部分经产地加工的中药切片（包括切段、块、瓣）、原药材饮片以及经过炮制的药材饮片。仅经过净制和切制形成的中药饮片，其品质与原药材一致，而经过醋炙、酒炙、麸炒、蛤粉炒等炮制手段得到的饮片，其品质与炮制条件密切相关，因此中药饮片品质的发展伴随中药材品质和炮制技术而发展。

The concept of quality evaluation of Chinese medicinals came into being at the early stage when people get knowledge of Chinese medicine. With the development of Chinese medicine species, the connotation of quality of Chinese medicinal gradually enriched. Ancient people gradually realized that the size of decoction pieces, the way of medication, the pharmaceutical form and other factors can affect the quality. The quality of Chinese medicinal includes the quality of raw material of Chinese medicinal, that of Chinese medicine decoction pieces and that of Chinese patent medicine. Chinese medicine decoction pieces include a part of Chinese medicinal only pre-processed in the production site (pieces, tubers or flaps), genuine medicinal pieces and processed Chinese medicine processing products. The qualities of Chinese medicine decoction pieces only cleaned, cut and selected are consistent with the original Chinese medicinalse, while the qualities of Chinese medicine decoction pieces processed by vinegar, liquor, and wheat bran or clam meal powder are closely related to the processing conditions. Therefore, the development of Chinese medicine decoction pieces quality is accompanied by the development of genuine Chinese medicine quality and processing techniques.

一、中药材及饮片品质的发展
1 The Development of Chinese Materia Medica Quality and Chinese Medicine Decoction Pieces Quality

东汉《神农本草经》中记载的"土地所出，真伪陈新""有毒、无毒"和"性、效、用"的论述，就是原始的中药品质观的体现；书中还提到产地、采收、加工、真伪等因素能影响中药品质。张仲景的《金匮玉函经》中记载"凡咀药，欲如豆大，粗则药力不尽"，阐明饮片粒度能影响药效从而影响品质。

In the Eastern Han Dynasty, statements as "land production、authentic or false、old or new"、"toxin or non-toxin""nature, efficacy, application", recorded in *Shennong Bencao Jing*, are the embodiment of the initiate concept in the quality of Chinese raw medicinal and Chinese medicine decoction pieces. It also mentioned that the origin, collection processing and authenticity could affect the clinical efficaly of Chinese medicine. *Jingui*

Yuhan Jing (Golden Chamber Yuhan Classic), written by Zhang Zhongjing, also mentioned that "the medicines you take it by chewing should be as big as beans. If the medicines are too big, its effect will not work well". It indicates that the size of decoction pieces can affect the efficacy and then the quality.

魏晋南北朝时期，梁陶弘景在《本草经集注》中，根据中药材的产地与性状，把中药的品质分四个层次表述：优良品质用"最佳""最好""最胜"等；良好品质用"为良""为好""为佳"等；一般品质用"可用""亦入药""少用"等；劣等品质用"不好""不佳""不堪用"等，奠定了中药"辨状论质"的品质观念；同时，还将"㕮咀"改为切制，对药物提出了"细切"要求，并指出了饮片品质影响疗效。

During the Wei, Jin, Southern and Northern Dynasties, Tao Hongjing divided the quality of Chinese medicine into four grades, which are the best, the good, the general and the inferior, according to the origin and traits in his book, *Bencaojing Jizhu*. It established the idea of distinguishing the shape and nature of Chinese medicinal for the quality. In this book, it also developed requirements on cutting that the medicine shall be cut into small pieces, and points out that the qualities of decoction pieces could affect the efficacy.

唐朝《新修本草》即开创了图文鉴定的方法鉴别中药材的真伪。南朝刘宋时期《雷公炮炙论》记载了药物的炮炙、熬煮、修事之法等，随后经过历代医药学家不断充实、完善。

In the Tang Dynasty, *Xinxiu Bencao* created a method to identify the authenticity of Chinese medicinal by graphic identification. *Leigong Paozhi Lun* in the Liu and Song Period of Southern Dynasties recorded the methods for processing medicinal, including stir-baking, decocting-boiling carving, and etc., and these methods were enriched and perfected by later medical practitioners.

宋代炮制方法有很大改进，炮制目的从减低

药物的毒副作用到增强和改变疗效等方向，极大地提高了中药饮片的品质。如《太平圣惠方》记载巴豆要去皮膜、加热压去油制霜，降低其峻烈之性，就是强调炮制对饮片品质影响的重要性。

In the Song Dynasty, the processing methods improved constantly. The processing purposes were developed from reducing the toxins and side effects to enhancing and changing the medicinal efficacy, which greatly improved the quality of Chinese medicine decoction pieces. For example, *Taiping Shenghui Fang* recorded the processing methods for Badoushuang by peeling the skin and membrane, heating and pressing the medicinal to remove oil to make frost for reducing its drastic nature and this emphasized the importance of processing on the quality of the decoction pieces.

元代，《汤液本草》中记载了黄芩、黄连、黄柏、大黄等中药材不同炮制品的临床应用和疗效，表明古人对炮制影响药物的性能有了更加深刻的认识。张元素在《珍珠囊》中也记载了炮制的中药饮片的临床应用，以及提升饮片品质的炮制方法。

In the Yuan Dynasty, it recorded the applications and efficacy of different processing products of various Chinese materia medica such as Huangqin, Huanglian, Huangbo, and Dahuang in *Tangye Bencao*, showing that the ancients had a deeper understanding on influence of processing on property of Chinese medicinals, Zhang Yuansu also recorded the clinical application of Chinese medicine decoction pieces and the processing methods for improving the quality in the *Zhenzhunang*.

明代李时珍撰写的《本草纲目》，对中药基源、产地、采收加工、炮炙、性、效、用均有记述或评价，系统地说明了的中药材和中药饮片的品质观[10]。官修本草《本草品汇精要》中，记载了各个中药材和中药饮片的质（质地和形态）、色（药材颜色）、味（药材气味）、代（代用品种）、赝（伪品和真、伪品的鉴别方法）等。

In the Ming Dynasty, *Bencao Gangmu* written by Li Shizhen thoroughly described or evaluated the origin, place of origin, harvest, processing, properties, effects and use of Chinese medicinals and systematically explained the quality concept of Chinese raw medicinals and Chinese medicine decoction pieces. *Bencao Pinhui Jingyao* (*Concise Herbal Foundation Compllication*), an official medicinal book, recorded the texture, morphology, color, odor, substitution, and identification methods, etc. of Chinese raw medicinals and Chinese medicine decoction pieces.

清代赵学敏的《本草纲目拾遗》除了将《本草纲目》收载的中药和炮制品、炮制技术进行拾遗补缺外，还特别收录了近70种的炭药，并将张仲景提出的"烧炭存性"的理论拓展到"炒炭存性"，亦是古人对炮制方法提升中药品质的思考。

In the Qing Dynasty, in addition to supplementing the processed products and processing methods contained in the *Bencao Gangmu*, Zhao Xueming also compiled nearly 70 kinds of carbonized medicines into *Bencao Gangmu Shiyi* (*Supplement to the Compendium of Materia Medica*). Besides, he developed the theory that "Chinese medicinals are carbonized, to preserve its properties", created by Zhang Zhongjing, into that "Chinese medicinals are parched to be carbon, to remain functions", which demonstrated the ancestors' thinking on improving the quality of Chinese medicine by processing methods.

二、中成药品质的发展
2 The Development of Chinese Patent Medicine Quality

古代医家在大量药剂实践中积累了宝贵经验，在此基础上总结、提炼了剂型、制药、施药三个主要因素对中成药品质的影响。

The ancient physicians accumulated precious experience from a great amount of pharmaceutical practices. On this basis, the effects of pharmaceutical form, pharmacy and application

on the quality of Chinese patent medicine were summarized and refined.

（一）古代本草论中成药品质
2.1 The Development of Chinese Patent Medicine Quality in Ancient Times

中成药的出现较早，在夏禹时代（公元前2000多年）就有了利用酒制药的实践；汤剂也是最早应用的剂型之一，在商代就得到了应用，伊尹还在《汤液经》中总结了汤剂应用的经验；战国时期的《黄帝内经》记载了汤、丸、散、药酒等剂型，其《素问》篇写到："治温以清，冷而行之；治清以温，热而行之。"表明了古人对用药方式影响中成药的品质和药物疗效的认识。

Chinese patent medicines appeared quite early. In the Xia Yu era (more than 2000 BC), there was the practice of using liquor to make medicine. The decoction, applied in the Shang Dynasty, was one of the earliest application forms as well. Yi Yin summarized the experience in the application of decoction in *Tangye Jing*. During the warring states period, *Huang Di Nei Jing* recorded decoction, pill, powder, tincture and other pharmaceutical forms. It was written in *Suwen (plain question)* chapter that "treating hot diesease by clearing, cool down and move it; treating cold disease by warming, heat up to move it", showing the ancients understood that the medication methods can affect the quality and the efficacy of Chinese patent medicine.

秦汉时期，我国中成药制备的理论与技术有了显著的发展。炼丹术兴起，开启化学药物使用的先河；《神农本草经》书中提出："药性有宜丸者、宜散者、宜水煎者、宜酒渍者、宜煎膏者"，表明了古人对剂型影响中成药品质的认识；东汉时期张仲景所著的《伤寒论》《金匮要略》在药物组方、配伍、剂量、剂型、制法、应用等方面有独特的见解。

During the Qin and Han Dynasties, the theory and technology of Chinese pharmaceutical preparations in China developed rapidly. The rise of alchemy opened the way of using chemical drugs. *Shennong Bencao Jing* put forward that "depending on medicinal properties, some medicines are suitable for pill, some for powder, some for decoction, some for tincture and some for fluid extract", it means that Chinese patent medicine quality affected by pharmaceutical form was recognized. In the Eastern Han Dynasty, Zhangzhongjing had an unique view on the formulation, combination of medicines, dosage, pharmaceutical form, preparation methods, and application, which were wrote down in *Shanghan Lun* (*Treatise on Cold Damage Diseases*) and *Jingui Yaolue*.

唐代孙思邈所著的《备急千金要方》《千金翼方》中，收载了各科应用方剂，载有方论 5000 余首，如天王补心丹、小青龙汤、四逆散等，并设有制药总论专章，极大地促进了中成药的发展。

In the Tang Dynasty, Sun Simiao's *Beiji Qianjin Yaofang*（*Essential Prescriptions Worth a Thousand Gold for Emergencies*）and *Qianjin Yifang* collected prescriptions for various applications, containing over 5000 prescriptions and their explanations, such as Tianwang Buxin Dan (Pills), Xiaoqinglong Tang (Decoction), Sini San (Powder) etc.. These books also had a special chapter and general theory. This greatly promotes the development of Chinese patent medicine.

宋代统治者设立了太医局卖药所（即太平惠民药局），制备成药出售；公元 1103 年，制药部从卖药所分出，成立了修合药所，专制备成药以供惠民药局出售，这是我国最早的官营制药厂。《太平惠民和剂局方》中收载方剂 300 多个，该书既有配方手册的作用，又有推广成药的用途，使中成药的处方、制法与应用有了较统一的规范和准则。

In the Song Dynasty, the royal medicine store (Taiping people's welfare bureau) was established to sell ready-made medicines. The Ministry of Pharmacy was separated from the royal patent medicine store in 1103 AD and established the Xiuhe Medicine Office specializing in preparing medicines for Huimin Medicine Bureau to sell, and this is the earliest official pharmaceutical factory in China. In 1151 AD, more than 300 formulas were contained in *Taiping Huimin Heji Ju Fang*,

written by Chen Shiwen et al. This book was not simply a formula manual, but also promoted the use of patent medicines, so that the prescriptions, preparation methods and applications of Chinese patent medicines have relatively unified specifications and guidelines.

明代李时珍的《本草纲目》，总结了 16 世纪以前我国的用药经验，药物剂型近 40 种，书云："水火不良，火候失度，则药亦无功。"阐述了汤剂煎煮方法对中成药品质的影响。

In the Ming Dynasty, the medication experience in China before the 16th century and nearly 40 kinds of pharmaceutical forms were summarized in *Bencao Gangmu*. This book saying unqualified water and improperfire described that the way to make a decoction could affect the quality of some Chinese patent medicines.

（二）中药品质的现代发展

2.2 The Development of Chinese Patent Medicine Quality in Modern Times

新中国成立以后，为了加强中成药品质的管理，颁布了《中华人民共和国药典》《中华人民共和国药品管理法》《新药审批办法》等，还在全国各地相继建立了各级药品监督管理部门及检验机构。药品管理法规的实施，从法律意义上对中药的生产、经营和使用进行规范，最大限度地确保中药的质量。

After the founding of new China, in order to strengthen the management of Chinese patent medicines, *Pharmacopoeia of the People's Republic of China, Drug Administration Law of the People's Republic of China, Provisions for New Drugs Approval*, etc. were issued; supervision and management departments and inspection institution at various levels were established all over the country. The implementation of drug management regulations regulates the production, operation and application of Chinese medicinal, and ensures its quality to the greatest extent.

20 世纪 80 年代以来，遗传学、植物学、植物化学、分析化学、中药化学、药理学和药效学等学科的分析方法和手段相继被引入，对于中药质量的控制研究也逐步进入以化学评价为主的研究模式。

Since the 1980s, analytical methods and techniques in genetics, botany, phytochemistry, analytical chemistry, Chinese medicine chemistry, pharmacology, and pharmacodynamics have been introduced one after another. The researches on the control of Chinese medicinal quality have also gradually evolved into a model based on chemical evaluation.

现代中药品质主要从本草考证、原植物与资源调查、种质遗传特征、产地、栽培技术、性状、显微特性、炮制、化学成分、制剂和药理药效等方面进行了研究，并对一些品种进行了化学成分的分离和鉴定，针对中药材中一个或几个成分建立了定性或定量分析方法。现代分析技术的应用逐渐减少人为的主观误差，大大提高工作效率及分析结果的精密度和准确度。中药品质标准从过去的一般性要求，逐步发展到有定性、定量、检查及稳定性等控制项目，含量测定从单一成分发展到多成分，指纹图谱等新技术的使用更是让中成药品质评价变得更加全面和完善。

The modern researches on Chinese medicinal quality are mainly studied from Chinese materia medica researches, original plants and resource investigation, germplasm, cultivation techniques, microscopic characteristics, processing of Chinese materia medica, chemical composition, preparations and pharmacological effects; and the chemical components of some varieties were separated and identified, and qualitative or quantitative analysis is established for one or several components in some medicines. The applications of modern techniques reduce subjective errors, greatly improving the efficiency, precision and accuracy of results. The quality standards of Chinese medicinal have gradually evolved from the general requirements to qualitative, quantitative, inspection and stability control items. The content determination was developed from a single component to multiple components. The use of new technologies such as fingerprints let the quality evaluation system become more comprehensive and complete.

第三节　中药品质的现代研究
Section 3　Modern Research on Chinese Medicinal Quality

现代科技进步为中药品质研究补充了许多空白，中药品质评价不再仅仅依赖人为经验的判断，而是有具体、可靠的数据支撑。中药品质评价的方法，不再限于眼观，口尝等方法，分子生物学、植物学、药物化学等学科，以及化学指纹图谱、多光谱、基因测序等方法都为中药品质的现代研究的进步做出了贡献。

The advancement of modern science has filled many blanks in quality research of Chinese medicinals. The evaluation of Chinese materia medica quality no longer merely relies on the judgment of human experience, but is supported by concrete and reliable data. The methods for the evaluation of Chinese materia medica quality are no longer limited to primitive methods, such as visual observation and oral taste. Subjects such as molecular biology, botany, medicinal chemistry, and methods, for example, chemical fingerprinting, multispectral, gene sequencing, all contribute to modern researches on Chinese medicinal quality.

一、中药材及饮片品质的现代研究
1 Modern Research on Chinese Materia Medica Quality and Chinese Medicine Decoction Pieces Quality

影响中药材和中药饮片品质的因素有很多，

如中药材的种质种苗、产地、采收时间、炮制手段、药用部位、产地加工等因素均可对中成药品质产生影响。

There are many factors that affect the quality of Chinese material medica and Chinese medicine decoction pieces, such as germplasm and seedlings, place of origin site, harvest time, processing methods, medicinal parts, processing on the origin site and so forth.

（一）种质种苗对中药材品质的影响

1.1 The Effects of Germplasm and Seedlings on Chinese Meteria Medica Quality

种质种苗是从源头上影响中药品质的因素，是中药材生产的物质基础。对于多基源的中药，种质种苗的不同能显著影响中药的有效成分，如同一条件生长 4 年的甘草属 5 个种的甘草酸含量存在显著差异，其中以乌拉尔甘草含量最高，其次是胀果甘草、光果甘草，而刺毛甘草和刺果甘草含量甚微；对于单基原的中药，种质种苗亦有区别，如选育的青蒿新品种不仅比野生青蒿中青蒿素质量分数提高 0.2% 以上，且产量较野生青蒿增产 10% 以上。中药种质种苗的选育不仅仅能影响中药的品质，还能促进中药资源的可持续利用，满足日益增长的临床需求。

Germplasm and seedlings are the source factors, and are the material basis of Chinese materia medica production. For multi-origin Chinese materia medica, the differences in germplasm and seedlings may have a significantly effect on active ingredients. For example, the contents of glycyrrhizic acid in five species of Gancao grown under the same condition for 4 years are significantly different, among which the content in *Glycyrrhiza uralensis* is the highest , followed by *G. inflate* and *G. glabra*, while *G. echinta* and *G. pailidifora* have little. For single-origin medicines, germplasm and seedlings could affect the qualities as well. For example, compared with wild varieties, the selected new varieties of Qinghao (Artemisiae Annuae Herba) have an increased amount of artemisinin by more than 0.2%

and its production increases by more than 10% The germplasm and seedlings can not only affect the quality of Chinese materia medica, but also promote the sustainable use of medicinal resources to meet the growing clinical needs.

（二）中药炮制对饮片品质的影响

1.2 The Effects of Processing Methods on Chinese Decoction Pieces Quality

在加工炮制的过程中，受加热、水浸及辅料等因素的影响，中药材中所含成分的质和量往往会发生变化，导致成分、制剂、药理作用和临床疗效也随之发生变化，从而影响到中成药的品质。如"手拈散"中延胡索经醋炙后，止痛的功效成分生物碱的含量大大增加，"小金丸"中草乌经炮制后，乌头碱含量可降低至万分之四以下。

During the processing procedures, due to the influence of heating, water immersion, auxiliary materials, etc., the quality and quantity of ingredients contained in Chinese materia medica may be changed, resulting in differences in the pharmacological effects and clinical efficacy, which affect the quality of Chinese patent medicines. For example, after Yanhusuo is processed with vinegar, its content of alkaloids with the function of pain-relieving increased greatly; the content of aconitine in Caowu can be reduced to less than four ten thousandths after processing in "Xiao Jin Wan".

（三）中药材及饮片品质评价指标

1.3 Quality Evaluation Index of Chinese Materia Medica and Chinese Medicine Decoction Pieces

中药中有效成分通常是指具有一定生物活性和治疗作用，可以用分子式和结构式表示，并具有一定物理常数（如熔点、沸点、旋光度、溶解度等）的单体化合物，比如从中药黄花蒿中提取的青蒿素。在半个世纪前，绝大多数控制中药品质的方法基本上都是通过测定其单一成分含量进行控制的，借以判断药品是否"合格"，这种方法具有划时代的贡献，使中药材及其产品从没有化学成分控制到有化学成分控制，如

2020版《中国药典》中苦杏仁以苦杏仁苷为检测指标，川芎以阿魏酸为检测指标。

The active ingredients in Chinese materia medica refer to monomer compounds that have certain biological activities, therapeutic effects, and can be explained in molecular formula and structural formula, and have certain physical constants (melting point, boiling point, optical rotation, solubility, etc.), for example, the artemisinin extracted from the Huanghuahao. Half a century ago, the main methods used to determine whether a medicinal was "qualified" are to measure the content of a single ingredient. This method has an epochmaking contribution, transferring Chinese materia medicas and their products from no chemical composition control to chemical composition control. For example, 2020 edition of *Chinese Pharmacopoeia* records that Kuxingren (Armeniacae Semen Amarum) uses bitter amygdalin as its detection index, and Chuanxiong uses ferulic acid as its detection index.

如今，质量控制中药品质不再局限于某一个单一的有效成分，而是朝着多指标，多个有效组分的方向发展。例如2020版《中国药典》中将红花的质量控制指标定为羟基红花黄色素 A 和山奈酚两种指标性成分；附子以新乌头碱、次乌头碱和乌头碱作为指标成分。

Nowadays, the quality control of Chinese medicinal is no longer limited to a single active ingredient, but is developing towards multiple indicators and multiple components. For instance, 2020 edition of *Chinese Pharmacopoeia*, Honghua (Carthami Flos) uses hydroxysafflor yellow A and kaempferol as quality control indicators; Fuzi uses neo-aconitine, hypoaconitine and aconitine as indicators.

有效组分控制中药品质：单一成分控制中药质量的观点将药材本身内部各种成分的综合作用割裂开来，未考虑到中药的组分是一个复杂系统。有效组分是指能够直接或间接影响中药或方剂疗效的化学成分群。不管是单味药还是复方，

针对其功能主治，均有与之对应的药效物质，有效组分是其中所含的针对某一病症的有效成分的最佳组合。通过对中药或复方中的有效组分加以分析研究，可有效地控制其质量标准，能较为全面地反映出某种中药或复方的品质。

Effective components control the quality: The view of single ingredient control of the quality breaks down the internal comprehensive actions of all the ingredients, and does not take into account that the compositions in Chinese medicinal are a complex system, and the interaction between various ingredients. Effective component refers to a group of chemical compositions that can directly or indirectly affect the efficacy of Chinese medicinal or formula. no metter single Chinese medicinal or formula contain medicinal substances targeting at its indications and efficacy, and the effective component is the best combination contained in it for a certain disease. By analyzing and researching the effective components in Chinese medicinal or formula, its quality standards can be effectively controlled and comprehensively reflected.

全成分指纹图谱控制中药品质：中药所含物质基础与药效是密切相关的，是特定的药效组分有序的组合，各成分之间具有量和比例的关系。为了全面了解中药化学成分的量和比，多成分结合指纹图谱的综合评价被广泛的应用。近年来，利用气相色谱 - 质谱联用技术（GC-MS）、高效液相色谱（HPLC）、高效液相色谱 - 质谱联用技术（HPLC-MS）等方法对中药中的多组分进行分析，建立指纹图谱进行质量鉴定的方法被广泛采用。中药指纹图谱还可以用于药材真伪的鉴别。如 HPLC-MS 技术能区别阿胶和其他皮类的特征峰，使假阿胶原形毕露。当单纯的一类指纹图谱的研究不足以反映中药的复杂性和整体性时，可结合遗传学进行品质评价。

Full-component fingerprint to control the quality: The containing of medicinal material basis is closely related to the medicinal efficaly, that is orderly combination of specific pharmacodynamic components. There is a quantity and ratio between the ingredients in Chinese medicine. In order to fully understand the quantity and ratio of the chemical components in Chinese medicinal, the fingerprint is used widely. In recent years, gas chromatography-mass spectrometry (GC-MS), HPLC, high performance liquid chromatography-mass spectrometry (HPLC-MS) and other technical methods were used extensively to establish fingerprints of Chinese medicinals for quality control. These methods could be used in identification of authenticity of Chinese material as well. For instance, HPLC-MS can be used to distinguish Ejiao from the fake, because of the characteristic peaks. When single fingerprint is not enough to reflect the complexity and integrity of Chinese medicinals, it would be combined with genetics to carry out quality evaluation.

（四）有害物质影响中药材及中药饮片品质
1.4 Harmful Substances Affect the Quality

除有效成分外，中药材、中药饮片的毒副作用也是影响中药材、中药饮片品质的重要因素之一。中药的毒副作用主要来源于两个方面，一是外源性的污染物，如重金属、农药残留等；二是内源性的代谢产物。

In addition to active ingredients, substances that can produce toxic and side effects are also one of the important factors that affect the quality of Chinese materia medica and traditional Chinese medicine decoction pieces. These substances mainly divided into two types, one is exogenous pollutants, such as heavy metals, pesticide residues, etc.; the other is endogenous metabolites.

中药的外源性有害物质：主要是重金属和农药残留，目前中药材重金属、农残检测也加入中药品质评价项目中。国内外的中医药工作者对中药材的质量控制做了很多重金属的研究，大部分西方国家和日本均制定了严格的重金属含量标准。为了规范我国进出口药用植物质量和市场流通中药材及其饮片的质量，在《药用植物及制剂进出口绿色行业标准》和《中国药典》对重金属含量均进行了相关的规定，其中砷、铅、汞、铜和镉是中药材及其饮片重金属常规分析指标。在中药材的种植过程中，往往要使用一些农药，包括杀虫剂、杀菌剂、除草剂、生长调节剂等。但有些农药如六六六，DDT 等，由于其化学性质稳定，在环境中降解缓慢，易于在生物体内富集，具有惊人的残留毒性。

Exogenous harmful substances: it mainly refers to heavy metals and pesticide residues. At present, the detection of heavy metals and pesticide residues has been added to the quality evaluation project of Chinese medicinal. A lot of research on heavy metal content has been done in the quality control. Most western countries and Japan have established strict standards for heavy metal content. In order to ensure the quality, relevant regulations on heavy metal content was stipulated in the *Green Industry Standard for the Import and Export of Medicinal Plants and Preparations* and *Chinese Pharmacopoeia*. Arsenic, lead, mercury, copper and cadmium are routine analysis indexes. In the cultivation process, some pesticides are often used, including insecticides, fungicides, herbicides, growth regulators, etc. However, some pesticides such as hexadecimal, DDT, etc., because of their stable chemical properties, degrade slowly in the environment, are prone to accumulate in organisms, and have alarming residual toxicity.

内源性有害物质：这类有害物质可分为两类，一类既是毒性成分，又是有效成分，如川乌、附子、草乌等中的乌头碱，马钱子中的士的宁等。对于这类物质，目前中国规定大部分实行限量检查或规定其含量范围，这一类有害物质可以经过炮制而大大减少，且按照规定用量一般不会损害人体。另一类是仅为有毒成分，如千里光中的吡咯里西啶类生物碱等，对于这些毒性成分，特别是慢性毒性成分，是中药毒理学的研究重点。

Endogenous harmful substances: They can be divided into two types. One type is both toxic and effective ingredients, such as aconitine in Chuanwu, Fuzi, Caowu, and the Shidining in Maqianzi. For these substances, the Ministry of Health of China stipulates that most of them are carried out limit inspection or ltoimit their content range. This kind of harmful substances can be greatly reduced by processing, and do not damage the human body generally within the prescribed dosage. Another type is only toxic ingredients, such as the pyrrolizidine alkaloids in Qianliguang (Senecionis Scandentis Hebra). These toxic ingredients, especially those with chronic toxic ingredients, are research focus of Chinese medicine toxicology.

二、中成药品质的现代研究

2 Modern Research on Chinese Patent Medicine Quality

中成药品质研究的主要内容包括了建立中成药品质标准体系、控制中成药的安全性、提高中成药品质可控性和有效性几个方面。目前已经建立和完善不同剂型的常规检验标准；探索了新的检验方法，如液相色谱 - 质谱联用、DNA 分子鉴定、薄层 - 生物自显影技术等；优化了控制中成药安全性的标准；实行 GMP 帮助企业规范生产工艺等。除此之外，影响中成药品质最主要的三个因素，即中成药的制备工艺、辅料和剂型是现代研究的重点。

The main research aspects in Chinese patent medicine quality modern research includes: establishing a quality standard system, controlling the safety as well as improving the controllability and effectiveness. At present, routine inspection standards for different pharmaceutical forms have been established and perfected, new testing methods were introduced, such as liquid chromatography-mass spectrometry (LC-MS), DNA molecular identification, thin layer-biological self-imaging technology, etc.; and the safety control standards has been optimized; GMP has been implemented to help companies improve production techmics and etc.. In addition, the preparation technology, auxiliary materials and pharmaceutical forms are what the research focus on.

（一）制备工艺对中成药品质的影响

2.1 Effect of Preparation Technology on Quality

中成药的制备工艺各环节对品质均有影响，包括提取、分离、纯化、浓缩与干燥工艺、制剂成型工艺等，都可能造成中成药药效成分的挥发、氧化、降解、沉淀，甚至消失，从而影响质量。应用现代科学技术对工艺技术条件进行筛选，使制备工艺科学、合理、先进、可行，使中成药达到安全、有效、可控、稳定的效果。如复方夏枯草膏中夏枯草的有效成分为齐墩果酸，该成分难溶于水，易溶于醇，故采用 90% 的乙醇提取。

All aspects of the preparation process, including extraction, separation, purification, concentration and drying, preparation, etc., have impact on quality, for which may cause the volatilization, oxidation, degradation, precipitation, or even disappearance of the effective components. Using modern technologies to select the technological conditions of the process makes the preparation process become scientific, reasonable, advanced and feasible, also makes Chinese patent medicine can achieve a safe, effective, controllable and stable effect. For example, Oleanolic acid, the effective ingredient of Xiakucao (Prunellae Spica) in Fufang Xiakucao Gao (Paste), is insoluble in water but soluble in alcohol, so it can be extracted with 90% ethanol.

（二）辅料对中成药品质的影响

2.2 Effect of Auxiliary Materials on Quality

在药物加工成各种类型的制剂时，通常都要加入一些有助于制剂成型、稳定，并能使制剂成品具有某些必要的理化特征和生理特性的辅助物质，即辅料。辅料选用是否得当直接影响药物的生物利用度、毒副作用以及临床功效的发挥。如 β - 环糊精包合后能掩盖药物的不良气味，渗油、挥发等问题也能得到解决；益母草膏的制备过程中，常加入高浓度的炼蜜，抑制微生物的繁殖，达到增加煎膏剂稳定性的目的。

When medicinals are processed into various pharmaceutical forms, auxiliary materials called adjuvants or exciponts are usually added. These adjuvants help preparation take shape, stay stability, and can make the finished product have certain necessary physical, chemical and physiological characteristics. Auxiliary materials can directly affect the bioavailability, toxic and side effects, and clinical effects of medicinals. For example, package with β-cyclodextrin can cover the bad smell of the medicinals, and solve the problems of oil leakage and volatilization, in the preparation process of Yimucao Gao (Paste), high concentration of refined honey is often added to inhibit the reproduction of microorganisms and achieve the purpose of increasing the stability of the decoction.

（三）剂型对中成药品质的影响

2.3 Effect of Pharmaceutical Forms on Quality

剂型与中成药品质直接相关，相同的中药成方，由于剂型不同，服后产生的功效、持续时间、作用特点都可能出现较大的差异。因剂型不同，其给药方式也不相同，可影响体内药物的吸收和功效。如口服制剂中，液体剂型的释药性能高于片剂、丸剂等固体剂型。不同剂型中成药的品质控制标准差异比较大，而相同剂型中成药有许多共同的特征。历版药典中，均将常见剂型的常规检测内容单独列出，放在药典附录，方便查询。

Pharmaceutical forms are directly related to the quality of Chinese patent medicine. For the same recipe, due to the different pharmaceutical forms, the efficacy, duration, and characteristics of the effects may be different significantly. Different pharmaceutical forms have different medication ways, which can affect the absorption and efficacy of medicinals in the body. For example, in oral preparations, the release performance of liquid pharmaceutical forms is better than that of solid pharmaceutical forms such as tablets or pills. The quality control standards of Chinese patent medicines in different pharmaceutical forms are quite different, while Chinese patent medicines in the same pharmaceutical form have many common characteristics. In every edition of *Chinese Pharmacopoeia*, the routine tests of common pharmaceutical forms are listed separately and placed in the appendix of the pharmacopoeia, which is not only for convenient inquirly, but also reflects the emphasis on medicinal quality control in China.

第四章　中药的制药
Chapter 4　Pharmacy of Chinese Medicinals

第一节　中药制药的含义
Section 1　The Meaning of Chinese Medicinal Pharmacy

中药的制药是指将原生药材制备成临床可使用的中药制剂形式的过程和方法，包括药材的产地加工、饮片炮制和中药制剂三方面。历代医家以中药材田间采收和产地加工为源头，经历"燔鹿角""治蚕卵"等传统原始炮制方法，形成膏、丹、丸、散、汤等成药制剂形式，逐渐完善中药制药理论和实践依据。中药的制药贯通药物形成的整个环节，是决定药物质量优劣的关键技术，也是药物能发挥良好临床疗效的重要保障。

Chinese medicinal pharmacy refer to the process and methods of preparing raw medicinal materials into the clinically usable forms of Chinese medicinal preparation, including the processing of medicinal materials in producing area, the processing of medicinal decoction pieces or medicinal slices, and the preparations of Chinese medicinals. Chinese medicine masters of past dynasties took collecting in the field and processing in producing area as original methods. The processing methods have gone through traditional primitive methods such as "Fanlujiao (broiling deerhorn)" and "Zhicanluan (treating silkworm eggs)", and formed preparation forms such as Gao (paste), Dan (pellet), Wan, San, Tang (decoction), etc., gradually improving the theoretical and practical basis of traditional Chinese medicinal processing. Chinese medicinal pharmacy is applied to the whole process of medicinal formation, which is the key technology of determining the quality of medicinals, and also an important guarantee of good clinical efficacy for medicinals.

中药材产地加工又称初加工，是指中药材在采收后，为形成合格的商品药材所进行的初步加工或一般修制处理。

Processing of medicinal materials in producing area, also known as primary or primitive processing, refers to the preliminary processing or general treatment processing of medicinal materials in order to get qualified commercial medicinals.

中药炮制是以中医药理论为指导，根据药物自身性质，以及调剂、制剂和临床应用的不同要求，将中药材制成中药饮片所采取的一项制药技术。

Processing of Chinese medicinals is the pharmaceutical technology which is used to make medicinal materials into prepared medicinal slices based on Chinese medicine theory, and medicinal characters, as well as the different requirements of dispensing, preparations and clinical applications, and it is adopted to make Chinese medicinals into Chinese materia medica pieces.

中药制剂系指以中药饮片为原料，在中医药理论指导下，根据《中华人民共和国药典》等标准规定的处方，将药物加工制成具有特有名称，并标明功能主治、用法用量和规格，可直接用于临床的药品。

Under the guidance of Chinese medicine theory, taking the prescriptions listed in *Chinese Pharmacopoeia* and other standards as the references, Chinese medicinal preparations are bound to use medicinal slices as materials to be made into clinical medications, which should have specific names, be marked with functions and indications, administration and dosage, and specifications.

第二节　中药制药的基本任务
Section 2　Basic Tasks of Chinese Medicinal Pharmacy

一、中药材产地加工
1 Processing of Chinese Medicinal Materials in Producing Area

中药材产地加工又称初加工，是根据医疗、调剂、制剂的需要对采收后的药材进行加工处理的技术。中药材的质量除了与品种、产地、采收季节等因素密切相关外，产地加工也对其有重要影响。

Processing of medicinal materials in producing area, also known as primary processing, is the technology for processing collected medicinal materials according to the requirement of medical treatment, dispensing and preparations. The quality of Chinese medicinal materials is not only closely related to factors such as variety, producing area, harvest season, etc., but also to the processing in producing area, which has an important impact on it.

常用的产地加工方法有除杂、分离或清除非药用部位、碾捣、揉搓、发汗、干燥等，应根据药材药用部位和性质的不同选用不同加工技术。规范化的产地加工是保障中药质量的源头环节，产地加工与中药质量的相关性主要体现在：

The common processing methods in producing area include removing impurities, separating or removing non-medicinal parts, grinding, kneading, sweating, drying, etc. Different processing techniques should be adopted according to different medicinal parts and properties. Standardized processing in producing area is the source to ensure the quality of Chinese medicinal. The correlation between origin processing and Chinese medicinal quality is mainly reflected in:

（一）清除杂质及非药用部位，保证药材纯净度
1.1 Removing Impurities and Non-medicinal Parts to Ensure the Purity of Medicinal Materials

药材采收后，经过挑选、筛选、风选和水选等方法可清除夹带的杂质，如筛选延胡索中的砂石、风选苏子、水选乌梅等；经过去根、去茎、去皮、去壳、去核等方法可剔除或分离非药用部位，如荆芥去根、龙胆除去残茎、厚朴在产地刮去栓皮、苔藓等、山楂去核等，以提高药材质量。

After the medicinal materials are harvested, the impurities can be removed through the processing techniques of selecting, screening, wind and water selection, such as, screening sand and stones in Yanhusuo, selecting Suzi (Perillae Fructus) by wind, and selecting Wumei (Mume Fructus) by water. The non-medicinal parts can be removed or separated by removing roots, stems, peel, shells and kernels to improve the quality of medicinal materials. For example, removing the root of Jingjie (Schizonepetae Herba), removing the residual stem of Longdan (Gentianae Radix et Rhizoma), peeling Houpo (Magnoliae Officinalis Cortex) and removing moss, coring Shanzha, etc. improve the quality of medicinals.

（二）保持药效，防止霉变，利于贮运

1.2 Keeping Efficacy, Preventing Mildew, Facilitating Storage and Transportation

新鲜药材体内含有大量水分和营养物质，直接堆放或包装贮藏，可造成堆内湿度、温度增高，利于微生物传播萌发和侵入，造成药材发热、霉烂；新鲜药材体积大，不易贮运。药材采收后，进行干燥处理、钝化酶类，缩小体积，以达到保持药效，防止霉变，便于贮运的目的。传统的干燥方法有晒干、阴干、烘干等。现代有冷冻干燥、微波干燥、远红外加热干燥。

The fresh medicinal material contains plenty of water and nutrients. If they are directly stacked or packaged in storage, it will bring about the increase of humidity and temperature, contributing to the transmission, germination and invasion of microorganism, causing heat emission and rot of medicinal materials. Fresh medicinal materials are large in size, and thus difficult to store and transport. The medicinal material should be dried after it is collected, the enzymes in it should be inactivated, and the volume has to be reduced so as to keep efficacy, prevent mildew, and facilitate storage and transportation. The traditional drying methods include sun drying, shade drying, and drying. Modern methods include freeze drying, microwave drying, and far infrared heating and drying.

（三）产生新的活性成分

1.3 Generating New Active Ingredients

有些药材在采收后常需"发汗"处理，使药材干燥后油润、光泽或香气更浓烈，还可使某些化学成分含量增加或产生新的活性成分。如地黄发汗过程中梓醇发生水解，使其分子结构中具有的烯醚和缩醛活泼基团被打开失去糖基并进行重排，或者发生亲核反应生成稳定的呈色物质。

Some medicinal materials often need the processing of "sweating" after being collected

to make them oily, lustrous or more fragrant. The processing can also increase the content of some chemical ingredients or produce new active ingredients. For example, in the sweating processing of Dihuang, catalpol is hydrolyzed, causing that the active groups of ene ether and acetal in the molecular structure are opened to lose glycosyl group and rearranged, or a nucleophilic reaction occurs to generate stable chromogenic substances.

（四）降低或消除药物的毒性、刺激性或副作用

1.4 Reducing or Eliminating Toxicity, Irritation or Side Effects of Medicinals

枇杷叶、狗脊等药材表面有毛状物，服用时可能黏附或刺激咽喉的黏膜，发痒引起咳嗽，产地加工时需清除表面绒毛；泥附子经胆巴溶液、浸盐等过程制成盐附子，或进一步经浸泡、煮沸、切制等工艺制成黑顺片或白附片可降低毒性。

There are trichomes on the surface of some medicinal materials such as Pipaye (Eriobotryae Folium) and Gouji (Cibotii Rhizoma), which may stick to or irritate the mucous membrane of the throat, causing cough because of itching when they are taken. The surface fluff should be removed during processing in producing area. And the toxicity of Nifuzi can be reduced when it is processed into Yanfuzi by Danba solution and salt soaking, or by further processing of soaking, boiling and slicing, thus made into Heishunpian or Baifupian.

二、中药炮制

2 Processing of Chinese Medicinals

中药炮制是根据中医药理论，依照临床辨证施治用药的需要和药物的自身性质，以及调剂、制剂的不同要求，将中药材制成中药饮片所采取的一项制药技术。中药炮制技术历史悠久，中药炮制方法、技术、炮制品的应用散在于历代中医药文献中，并形成了炮制专著，如《雷公炮炙论》《炮制大法》《修事指南》等。中

药炮制历经两千多年的发展，在中医临床上被医家充分认可并得到广泛应用。

Based on the theory of Chinese medicine, processing of Chinese medicinals is the pharmaceutical technology which is adopted to make medicinal materials into prepared medicinal slices to meet the requirements of clinical syndrome differentiation, the nature of the medicinal, as well as the different requirements of dispensing and preparations. The processing technology of Chinese medicinal has a long history, its methods, techniques and applications of the processed products recorded in the traditional Chinese medicine literature in previous dynasties, and the monographs on processing have been formed, such as *Leigong Paozhi Lun, Paozhidafa (Main Solution of Processing), Xiushi Zhinan*. Processing of Chinese medicinal has been fully recognized and widely used in clinical practice after more than 2000 years of development.

中药材经净制、切制、炮炙（炒、炙、煅、蒸、煮、𤃩、复制、发酵发芽、制霜、烘焙、煨等）处理后成为饮片，是中医临床预防和治疗疾病的物质基础，炮制使中药的效应物质基础产生不同程度的变化，其性味、归经、升降浮沉及毒性等有所改变或调整，故炮制与中药质量密切相关。

Medicinal materials, after a series of treatment such as purifying, cutting and processing (stir-frying, broiling, calcining, steaming, boiling, blanching, complex producing, fermentation and germination, making frost-like powder, baking, simmering, etc.), are made into prepared medicinal slices, thus providing the material bases for clinical applications of prevention and treatment of diseases. The methods of processing can alter some effective material bases, further resulting in changes or adjustments in the medicinal nature, flavor, meridian entry, ascending and descending, floating and sinking, toxicity, etc. Therefore, processing is closely related to the quality of Chinese medicinals.

（一）增强药物疗效

2.1 Enhancing the Therapeutic Effects of the Medicinals

药物经炮制后可从多方面增强疗效。中药材切制过程中细胞破损、表面积增大等，药效成分易于溶出。炒、蒸、煮、煅等热处理可增加药效成分的溶出率；炮制辅料的助溶、脱吸附等作用，使难溶于水的成分水溶性增加。又如"逢子必炒"，多数种子外有硬壳，经热炒后种皮爆裂，便于成分煎出。款冬花、紫菀等化痰止咳药经蜜炙后，增强润肺止咳作用。

The therapeutic effects of medicinals can be enhanced in many ways after being processed. In the process of medicinal slicing, cells are damaged and the surface areas enlarged, which makes the medicinal ingredients dissolve easily. The dissolution rate of medicinal ingredients is increased by heating procedures like stir-frying, steaming, boiling, and calcining. The functions of solubilization and desorption of processed excipients can assist the solubility of water-insoluble components. Another example goes to the principle that when it comes to seeds, stir-frying is the essential procedure in processing, since most seeds have hard shells outside, and the seed shell bursts after being stir-fried, making it easier to let the useful ingredients out. After being processed with honey, the expectorant and anti-tussive medicinals such as Kuandonghua and Ziwan (Asteris Radix et Rhizoma) can enhance the effectiveness of moistening the lung for arresting cough.

（二）降低或消除毒副作用

2.2 Reducing or Eliminating the Toxicity and Side Effects

《中国药典》收载毒性中药品种72种，其中大毒者10种，有毒者42种，有小毒者30种，炮制可降低或消除药物的毒性或副作用。炮制解毒的方法包括浸渍、漂洗、砂烫、醋炙，蒸，煮、制霜等。如乌头经煮制后毒性降低且作用保留，朱砂经"水飞"后降低毒性，巴豆制霜后，缓和刺激性。中药成分复杂，作用多样，如果某作用不为具体病情所需，即为副作用，通过炮制使之符合病情需要。如麻黄既能平喘，又能发汗散寒，宜于风寒外束，无汗气喘者。对于肺热喘急而有汗者，将麻黄蜜炙，削弱其发汗作用而增强其平喘之功。

72 kinds of toxic Chinese medicinals are listed in *Chinese Pharmacopoeia*, including 10 kinds with severe toxicity, 42 kinds with medium toxicity and 30 kinds with mild toxicity. Processing can help to reduce or eliminate the toxicity and side effects of Chinese medicinal. There are many methods of detoxification, such as soaking, rinsing, scalding with sand, vinegar broiling, steaming, boiling, making frost-like powder and so on. For example, boiling can reduce the toxicity of Wutou and remain its effect; Shuifei (levigating) can decrease the toxicity of Zhusha (Cinnabaris), and making frost-like powder of Badou can alleviate its irritation. Chinese medicinal has complex ingredients and various effects, and it may bring about side effects if certain effect is unwanted in the specific condition. Hence it should be processed to meet the requirement of treatment. Mahuang, for example, can not only relieve asthma, but can release cold through perspiration, which is preferable for the treatment of non-sweating patients with asthma triggered by wind-cold. But for people sweating and coughing due to lung heat, Mahuang processed with honey can weaken its sweating effect to enhance its antiasthmatic effect.

（三）改变药物性味归经，满足临床辨证施治需要

2.3 Changing the Properties, Flavors and the Meridian Tropism to Meet the Requirement of Clinical Syndrome Differentiation and Treatment

炮制可改变中药的四气五味、作用趋向（升降浮沉）及归经。如生地黄，性寒，具清热、凉血、生津之功，经蒸制成熟地黄后，性由凉变温，功由清变补，滋阴补血、养肝益气。莱菔子，生用涌吐风痰，升多于降；炒莱菔子，降多于升，用于降气化痰，消食除胀。干姜，生品归脾、胃、肺经，温中散寒，回阳通脉，燥湿消痰；砂烫后长于温中散寒，温经止血，主归脾、胃经；炒炭后固涩止血，主归脾、肝经。

Processing can change the four *qi* and five flavors, function trends (ascending and descending, floating and sinking) and meridian entries. For example, Shengdihuang (raw), cold in nature, has the functions of clearing heat, cooling blood and engendering fluid. The nature of Shengdihuang (raw) changes from being cool to warm after being steamed, and its function changes from clearing to tonifying, thus Shudihuang (prepared) nourishing *yin*, tonifying blood, and nourishing liver and *qi*. The unprocessed Laifuzi (Raphani Semen), with more functions in ascending, can be adopted to induce vomiting, wind sputum and in contrast, the Chaolaifuzi (stir-fried), with more functions in descending, is used to reduce *qi*, resolve phlegm, and eliminate distension. The unprocessed dried ginger enters meridians of lung and stomach, and has the effect of warming interior for dispersing cold, rescuing Yang and promoting blood circulation and drying dampness to eliminate phlegm; while the processed one by scalding with hot sand enters the meridians of spleen and stomach and has the effect of warming interior for dispersing cold, and warming channel for arresting bleeding; when stir-fried to scorch, it enters meridians of the spleen and Liver, and has the effect of astringing for hemostasis.

（四）便于调剂和制剂，保证药效

2.4 Facilitating Dispensing and Preparations to Ensure Efficacy

中药材经净制、切制成一定规格的片、丝、段、块等，便于分剂量和配药方，保证调剂、制剂的剂量准确，也利于调配煎煮。质地坚硬的矿物药、甲壳类及动物化石类药材，难粉碎，不易煎出，通过炒、煅等加热处理，使质地酥脆而便于粉碎，如砂烫醋淬穿山甲、龟甲等。

Medicinal materials are cleaned and cut into certain specifications of slices, filaments, segments, blocks, etc., making them convenient for adjusting doses and prescriptions to ensure accurate dosages and preparations, and also conducive to decocting. When it is difficult to grind the hard medicinals like mineral medicines, crustaceans and animal fossils, process them by means of heat treatment such as stir-frying and calcining in order to make the crisp texture easy to be pulverized. For example, Chuanshanjia (Squama Manitis) and Guijia (Testudinis Carapax et Plastrum) are processed products by using the stir-baking in sand with hot vinegar quenched.

（五）洁净药物，利于贮藏保管
2.5 Cleaning the Medicinals for Storage

中药在采收、贮存、运输过程中常混有泥沙杂质及残留的非药用部位和霉败品，因此必须经过严格的分离和洗净，使其达到所规定的净度要求，保证贮存过程不发生虫蛀和霉变。如桑螵蛸必须经过蒸制，杀死虫卵后再干燥贮存。

Medicinal materials are often mixed with impurities, residual non-medicinal parts and moldy products in the process of collection, storage and transportation. Therefore, they must be strictly separated and cleansed in order to meet the requirement for cleanliness and to ensure that no moth and mildew grows during storage. For example, Sangpiaoxiao (Mantidis Oötheca) must be steamed to kill the eggs before being dried and kept in storage.

（六）矫臭矫味，利于服用
2.6 Removing Unpleasant Odor for Oral Administration

某些动物类、树脂类或其他有特殊不良气味的中药，服用后易出现恶心、呕吐、心烦等不良反应。常用酒制、蜜制、水漂、麸炒等方法炮制，矫臭矫味利于患者服用。

After taking some animal medicinals, resin herbs or other medicinals with undesirable flavors, people are prone to have adverse reactions such as nausea, vomiting and vexation. Methods like processing with liquor, stir-frying with honey, rinsing with water, stir-frying with bran are commonly used to remove the unpleasant odor, thus being acceptable for patients to take.

三、中药制剂
3 Preparation of Chinese Medicinals

中药制剂系指以中药饮片为原料，在中医药理论指导下，根据处方将药物加工制成具有特有名称并标明功能主治、用法用量和规格，可直接用于临床的药品。中药制剂应根据药物性质、剂型特点、临床要求、给药途径等筛选适宜的辅料，并确定制剂处方，利用先进的设备和技术等制成中药制剂，达到安全、有效、稳定、方便、可控的制剂标准，满足"速效、高效、长效""剂量小、副作用小、毒性小""服用、携带、生产、运输、贮存方便"的要求。

Under the guidance of Chinese medicine theory and according to prescriptions, traditional Chinese medicinal preparations use medicinal slices as materials to process medicinal materials into clinical medications, which should have specific names, be marked with indications, functions, usage and dosage, and specifications. Specifically, by selecting the appropriate excipients according to the medicinal properties, preparation forms, clinical requirements, routes of administration and so on, determining the prescription of preparation, and using advanced equipment and technology, the traditional Chinese medicinal preparations must reach the standard of clinical medications for safety, effectiveness, stabilization, convenience and controllability, meeting the requirements of "fast efficiency, high efficiency and long-term effect", "low dosage, less side effects and minor toxicity", and "be easy to take, carry, produce, transport and store".

中药制剂是将中医临床有效方药，按照中医药理论，采用现代科技加工制成具有特殊形态和质量特性的中药制剂，以满足临床需要。中药制剂过程是对方药与疗效关系认识、对有效物质研究与富集的过程，是通过特殊技术控制给药方法使药效发挥的过程。制剂技术是对合适剂型、工艺路线、适宜辅料和科学包装进行统一的有效手段，是中药制剂研究工作的核心。

Under the guidance of Chinese medicine theory and adopting modern science and technology, Chinese medicinal preparations are to make effective clinical prescriptions into Chinese medicinal preparations with specific forms and properties to meet clinical requirements. So the preparation of Chinese medicinal is the process of correlating the prescription and the curative effect, researching and enriching its effective substances, and it is also the process of exerting efficacy by controlling administration methods with special techniques. Preparation technology is an effective means of unifying appropriate preparation forms, process routes, appropriate auxiliary materials and scientific packaging, and it is the core of the research work of traditional Chinese medicinal preparation.

（一）中药制剂技术与中药质量的相关性

3.1 Correlation between Preparation Techniques and Medicinal Quality

中药制剂技术常从剂型选择、制备工艺、配伍作用等多角度保证制剂质量，实现中药制剂安全有效。①选择合适剂型。通过将有毒中药制成蜜丸、蜡丸、糊丸等剂型延缓其峻猛之性。②根据药性选择适宜提取方式。根据药性不同，将药物采用粉碎、水提、醇提等工艺处理以减毒。③利用中药复方"组分合和"作用，达到增效减毒。汤剂常通过合煎、先煎、久煎等方式，使有效成分尽可能完全溶出，使有毒成分与其他成分发生反应而降低，保证安全有效。④在保证传统制剂特色的基础上，吸纳现代制剂的工艺技术优势，通过缓控释、纳米化等制剂新技术制备得到缓控释制剂、靶向纳米制剂、定位释药制剂等新剂型，以改善药物溶解度、影响体内吸收代谢、实现组织靶向性等，达到减毒增效的目的。

Chinese medicinal preparation techniques often determine the quality of the preparation from the diverse aspects such as pharmaceutical form selection, preparation techniques, and compatibility functions to realize safety and effectiveness.

① Choosing appropriate pharmaceutical forms. By making the medicinals with toxicity into honey pills, wax pills, paste pills and other forms, the ferocity of medicine can be weakened.

② Selecting proper extraction methods according to the medicinal nature. To reduce the toxicity, medicinals should be processed by crushing, water extraction, alcohol extraction, etc. according to their nature.

③ Making the advantage of the components interaction of Chinese medicinal compounds to increase efficacy and reduce toxicity. Effective ingredients in decoction can be completely dissolved if it is processed through such ways as combined decocting, decocting first and long-time decocting so that the toxic ingredients react with other ones to reduce toxicity and ensure safety and effectiveness.

④ On the basis of ensuring the characteristics of traditional preparations and absorbing the technological advantages of modern preparations, new preparation forms such as sustained-controlled release preparations, targeted nano-preparations and localized drug release preparations are obtained through sustained-controlled release and nano-preparation technologies, so as to improve drug solubility, affect metabolism of absorption, and realize histo-targeting, so as to achieve the purpose of reducing toxicity and increasing efficiency.

（二）中药制剂技术的传承与发展

3.2 Inheritance and Development of Chinese Medicinal Preparation Technology

1. 中药传统制剂技术

中药的传统剂型包括膏、丹、丸、散、汤等。

3.2.1 Traditional Chinese Medicinal Preparation Techniques

Traditional preparation forms of Chinese medicinals include Gao (paste), Dan (pellet), Wan (pill), San (powder), Tang (decoction), etc.

在战国秦汉时期《黄帝内经》《神农本草经》《难经》等著作中关于膏药已有记载，为猪脂膏之类的软膏与中药混合后涂在狗皮上供外敷，称为狗皮膏药。魏晋时期炼丹术盛行，出现黑膏药。近代随着现代工艺的发展，膏药逐渐被橡胶膏剂、巴布膏、凝胶膏剂等现代贴膏剂代替。

Plasters have been recorded in *Huang Di Nei Jing, Shennong Bencao Jing, Nanjing (Classic of Questioning),* etc. since the Warring States period, Qin and Han dynasties. The plaster of the past was the combination of herbs and ointment made of pig fat, and such mixed components pasted on the dog skin for external application, so it was called Goupi Gaoyao (Plaster). Hei Gaoyao appeared in the Wei and Jin dynasties when alchemy was prevalent. With the development of modern technology, plasters are gradually replaced by rubber plasters, Babu plaster, gel paste and so on.

散剂为中药传统制剂的常用剂型之一，在《黄帝内经》中有记载，《伤寒论》《金匮要略》中达五十余方。除常用粉碎法外，还有灰化、取烟、制霜、澄粉、风化及一些特殊的制法。①含有毒中药饮片的散剂：常将除有毒中药之外的中药细粉混合，以等量递增法与有毒中药粉末混匀，过筛即得。②含低共熔混合物的散剂：冰片、薄荷脑等药物混合时会出现润湿或液化现象，称为低共熔现象。此类散剂的制备，若形成低共熔物后，药效增强，宜先形成低共熔物，再与其他药物混合；若形成低共熔物后，药效无明显变化，视情况灵活运用；若形成低共熔物后，药效减弱，则用其他组分分别稀释低共熔组分后轻轻混合，避免出现低共熔现象。③含液体药物的散剂：复方散剂中含挥发油、非挥发性液体药物、酊剂、流浸膏等液体一般可利用处方中其他固体组分吸收后研匀；若液体组分多，可加适量辅料吸收；若液体组分为非挥发性有效成分，可适当加热浓缩后再用其他固体粉末吸收，或加入固体粉末或辅料，低温干燥后研匀。

Powder, one of the commonly used traditional preparation forms, is recorded in *Huang Di Nei Jing*. Besides, *Shanghan Lun* and *Jingui Yaolue*

record more than 50 prescriptions of it. In addition to the commonly used methods of grinding, there are also methods such as cineration, smoke extraction, making frost-like powder, milling into powder, weathering and other special preparation methods.

① Powder containing Chinese medicine decoction pieces with toxicity

Generally, mix the different powders of non-toxic medicinal materials, then blend them into the toxicity-contained powder, increase the amount with equal increment progressively, and finally the processed powder is made after being sifted.

② Powder containing low eutectic mixture

The phenomenon of wetting or liquefaction occurs when medicinal materials like Bingpian (Borneolum Syntheticum) and Bohenao (l-menthol) are mixed, which is called eutectic phenomenon. If the formation of low eutectic occurs in the preparation, the efficacy of the medicinal will be enhanced, so the low eutectic should be first formed before being mixed with other medicinals. If there is no significant change in the efficacy of the eutectic after the formation of the eutectic, it can be used flexibly according to the situation; if the efficacy is weakened after the formation of the eutectic, the eutectic components should be diluted with other components and mixed gently to avoid Eutectic phenomenon.

③ Powder containing liquid medicinals

Some compound powders contain volatile oils, non-volatile liquid medicinals, tinctures, liquid extracts and etc., so grinding is adopted after they are absorbed by other solid components in the prescription. If there are excessive liquid components, the appropriate amount of excipients can be added to help absorb the liquid. If the liquid is composed of non-volatile active components, it can be heated and concentrated properly and then be absorbed by other solid powders, either solid powders or excipients can be added, and grinding is adopted after the mixture is dried at low temperature.

丸剂早在《五十二病方》中就有记述，《太平惠民和剂局方》记载方剂788个，其中丸剂284个。《伤寒杂病论》《金匮要略》中有用蜂蜜、糖、淀粉糊、动物药汁作黏合剂的记载。金元时代始有丸剂包衣，明代有朱砂包衣，清代用川蜡为衣料，作为肠溶衣的雏形。传统丸剂内服后胃肠道中溶散缓慢，药效迟缓，作用持久，多用于慢性病治疗，即"水丸取其易化、蜜丸取其缓化、糊丸取其迟化，蜡丸取其难化"，满足不同治疗需求。传统丸剂大多取其"缓"，但也有以药汁等水性基质制丸，以获得较快速的疗效。如乌梅丸以水泛丸，张仲景认为"一遇急症，即令其速服之"。现代制备水溶性基质的滴丸，如复方丹参滴丸、速效救心丸，拓展了丸剂治疗急性疾病的功用。传统丸剂一般采用泛制法和塑制法制备。前者系指在转动的适宜设备中，将饮片细粉与赋形剂交替润湿、撒布、不断翻滚、粘结成粒，逐渐增大的制丸方法，主要用于水丸、水蜜丸、糊丸、浓缩丸的制备。后者系指饮片细粉加适宜的黏合剂或润湿剂，混合均匀，制成软硬适宜、可塑性好的丸块，再依次制成丸条、分粒、搓圆而制成丸粒的制备方法，多用于蜜丸、水蜜丸、浓缩丸、糊丸和蜡丸的制备。随着中药制药机械发展，丸剂制备逐渐摆脱手工制作，发展成为工业化批量生产。

Pill preparations are early recorded in *Wushier Bingfang*, and 788 prescriptions including 284 pill preparations are recorded in *Taiping Huimin Heji Ju Fang*. It has been recorded that honey, sugar, starch paste and animal medicinal decoction have been used as pill adhesives in *Shanghan Zabing Lun* and *Jingui Yaolue*. Pill coating began in the Jin and Yuan dynasties, and cinnabar coating appeared in the Ming Dynasty, Chuanla (Sichuan wax), the prototype of enteric coating was used as the material of coating in the Qing Dynasty. The traditional pills, after oral administration, are slow in dissolving and dispersing in the gastrointestinal tract. Due to the slow but long-lasting effect, they are mostly used for the treatment of chronic diseases. Pills have different forms to meet the requirements of different treatment. For example, choose water pills when they are needed to melt quickly; choose honey pills when they are needed to melt slow; choose paste pills when they are needed to melt tardily; choose wax pills when they are needed to melt hardly. Mostly, traditional pills take the advantage of their "slow effects", but there are also some pills made with water-based matrix (eg. medicinal juice) to have a faster curative effect. For example, Wumei Pill can be dissolved with water, and Zhang Zhongjing believed that "In case of an emergency, it should be quickly taken." Modern preparation of water-soluble matrix dripping pills, such as Fufang Danshen Diwan and Suxiao Jiuxin Wan, has increased the functions of pills for treating acute diseases. Traditional pills are generally prepared by the "Fanzhi method (the universal making processing)" and "Suzhi method (the moulding processing)". The former refers to the method of gradually increasing the size of pills by wetting, spreading, rolling and bonding with excipients and fine powder of medicinal slices in a suitable rotating device. It is mainly used for the preparations of water pills, honey pills, paste pills and concentrated pills. The latter refers to the preparation method in which the fine powder of prepared slices and the appropriate adhesive or wetting agents are mixed evenly to form pill masses with proper hardness and plasticity, sequentially making them into pieces, granules and pills. This method is mostly used in the preparations of honeyed pills, water-honeyed pills, concentrated pills, paste pills and wax pills. With the development of pharmaceutical machinery, the preparation of pills has gradually got rid of manual production and developed into industrial mass production.

2. 中药现代制剂技术

随着社会进步和技术的发展，传统剂型和制剂工艺等方面显出诸多不足，逐渐形成了中药现代剂型。按给药途径和方法分类，经胃肠道给药的剂型有合剂、颗粒剂、片剂、胶囊剂等，经直肠给药的剂型有灌肠剂、栓剂等，注射用药有注射剂，经皮肤给药有软膏剂、橡胶贴膏、涂膜剂等，经黏膜给药有滴眼剂、滴鼻剂等，经呼吸道给药有气雾剂等。近四十年来，我国在对传统剂型的改进及优化方面进行了许多卓有成效的研究，如汤剂改制为颗粒剂（如正柴胡饮颗粒）、合剂（如四物合剂）、糖浆剂（如健脾糖浆）、注射剂（如参附注射剂）等；丸剂改制为片剂（如银翘解毒片）、口服液（如杞菊地黄口服液）、酊剂（如藿香正气水）、滴丸剂（如丹参滴丸）等。

3.2.2 Modern Preparation Techniques of Chinese Medicinals

With the progress of society and the development of technology, many deficiencies in traditional preparation forms and preparation techniques have emerged, and modern preparation forms of Chinese medicinals have gradually formed. The preparation forms are different in line with the different routes and methods of administration. For example, the preparation forms for gastrointestinal administration include mixtures, granules, tablets, capsules, etc., the preparation forms for rectal administration include enemas, suppositories, etc., the preparation form for injection includes injections, the preparation forms for percutaneous administration include ointments, rubber patches, coating agents, etc., the preparation forms for administration through mucous membrane include eye drops, nasal drops, etc., and the preparation form for respiratory administration includes aerosols, etc. In the past 40 years, China has carried out many fruitful studies on the improvement and optimization of traditional preparation forms, for example, the conversion of decoctions into granules (eg. Zhengchaihu Yin Keli), mixtures (eg. Siwu Heji), syrups (eg. Jianpi Tangjiang), and injections (eg. Shenfu Zhusheye); the conversion of pills into tablets (eg. Yinqiaojiedu Pian), mixture (eg. Qijudihuang Kofuye), tincture (eg. Huoxiangzhengqi Shui), pills (eg. Danshen Diwan) etc.

中药现代剂型研究依赖于中药制剂前处理、提取分离纯化、浓缩干燥、成型工艺等技术的发展。①粉碎是中药前处理过程的必要环节。超声粉碎、超低温粉碎等现代超微细粉化技术能够使细胞内活性成分等直接暴露，提高药物溶解速率。②中药成分复杂，提取和精制是提高提取有效成分并最大限度的除去杂质的首要环节。目前广泛采用的水提醇沉法消耗大、成本高，且生产周期长、提取效率低，对该工艺的改进和优化日益增多，如半仿生提取法、超临界流体萃取法、超声波提取法、絮凝沉淀法、膜分离技术、超滤技术、大孔吸附树脂技术。③中药提取液的浓缩是中成药制剂的首要环节。目前夹层式浓缩锅设备简单，清洗方便，但传热系数低。节能高效的新型干燥技术及设备如喷雾干燥、旋转闪蒸干燥等被广泛应用。④以颗粒剂为例，成型工艺是制备中的核心技术，选择优良的辅料和合理的工艺条件，可改变传统工艺干燥时间长、药材中对热不稳定的成分损失较多等情况。中药颗粒剂的发展应加强对新型辅料的开发研制，并不断将新工艺、新设备合理应用于制备中。

The research on modern preparation forms of Chinese medicinal depends on the technology development of pre-treatment, extraction, separation and purification, concentration and drying, and molding.

① Pulverization is a necessary step in the pre-treatment of Chinese medicinals. Modern ultra-fine pulverization technologies such as ultrasonic pulverization and ultra-low temperature pulverization can directly expose the active components in cells and improve the dissolution rate of medicinals.

② Due to the complex components of Chinese medicinal, extraction and refining is the primary step to improve the extraction of effective components and remove impurities to the maximum extent. At present, the widely used method of water extraction and alcohol precipitation has the characteristics of high consumption, high cost, long production cycle and low extraction efficiency, so the improvement and optimization of the process are increasing, such as semi-bionic extraction, supercritical fluid extraction, ultrasonic extraction, flocculation precipitation, membrane separation technology, ultrafiltration technology and macroporous absorption resin technology.

③ The concentration of Chinese medicinal extract is the first step of Chinese patent medicinal preparation. At present, the sandwich-type concentrator is simple in operation and easy to clean, but its heat transfer coefficient is low. Novel drying techniques and facilities with energy saving and high efficiency are widely used. For example, spray drying and rotary flash drying etc.

④ Taking granules as an example, the molding processing is the core technology in the preparation. The selection of excellent excipients and reasonable processing conditions can shorten the drying time and reduce the loss of thermal unstable ingredients of medicinal materials. Thus, for the development of Chinese medicinal granule preparations, in the development of Chinese medicine granules, we should strengthen the research and development of new excipients, and constantly apply new technology and equipment to the preparations.

第三节　中药制药的现代研究

Section 3　Modern Research on Chinese Medicinal Pharmacy

中药材的产地加工与炮制作为中药产业链中密切相连的两个环节，是影响中药饮片质量的关键。目前，中药饮片的生产正由加工与炮制分段化模式向一体化模式转变。随着现代制药技术的发展，中药制剂进入了药材种植、产地加工规范化、饮片炮制规范化、制剂工艺规范化、剂型现代化、质控现代化的新阶段。

The processing in producing area and processing of Chinese medicinal materials, as two links in the Chinese medicine industry chain, are the key factors affecting the quality of traditional Chinese Medicine decoction pieces. At present, the production of traditional Chinese medicine decoction pieces is changing the processing in producing area and preparation of Chinese medicinal materials from piecewise mode to integrated mode. With the development of modern pharmaceutical technology, Chinese medicinal pharmacy has entered a new stage of the standardization of planting, production area processing, decoction piece processing, preparation technology, and modernization of

pharmaceutical form and quality control.

一、特色产地加工方法
1 Characteristic Processing Methods in Producing Area

（一）发汗
1.1 Fahan (Sweating)

有些药材在加工过程中晒或微火烘至半干或微蒸煮后堆积发热，使内部水分向外渗透，当药材内部的水汽达到饱和，遇堆外低温，水气凝结成水珠附于药材表面，称为"发汗"。

In processing, after being dried in the sun, slightly heated to half dry, or slightly steamed, some medicinal materials accumulate heat, making the internal water release outwards. When the vapor inside the medicinal materials reaches saturation, and meets the low temperature outside, the vapor will be condensed into droplets attached to the surface of the medicinal materials, and this process is called "sweating".

"发汗"会引起药材外观形状及内在质量的

变化，从而赋予药材独特的品质。传统认为药材"发汗"后的性状和质量较未"发汗"更好，如厚朴"紫色多润"，玄参"色黑微有光泽"，续断"断面墨绿色"，秦艽"色棕黄"以及杜仲"内皮暗紫色"等都是药材"发汗"后质量上乘的表现。

The processing of "sweating" will cause changes in the appearance and quality of medicinal materials, thus endowing medicinal materials with unique qualities. It is traditionally believed that the properties and quality of medicinal materials after "sweating" are better than those without this processing. For example, Houpo becomes "purple and moist", Xuanshen (Scrophulariae Radix) becomes "black and slightly glossy", Xuduan (Dipsaci Radix) has "dark green section", Qinjiao (Gentianae Macrophyllae Radix) has "the color in brown yellow" and Duzhong (Eucommiae Cortex) has "dark purple bast" after the processing in "sweating", and the above medicinal properties are signs of high quality.

（二）熏制
1.2 Xunzhi (Fumigation)

有些药材为使色泽洁白，防止腐烂，常在干燥前后用硫磺熏制。如白芷、山药、川贝母等，硫磺熏制产生的二氧化硫是较强的还原剂，能漂白或阻止某些变色反应，使药材色泽明艳；二氧化硫还能杀死药材上残留病菌、害虫及虫卵，并与药材里的水分结合成亚硫酸，既可抑制微生物生长，又使植物组织细胞膜透水性增加，加快水分蒸发，易于干燥。

Some medicinal materials, such as Baizhi (Angelicae Dahuricae Radix), Shanyao (Dioscoreae Rhizoma), Chuanbeimu (Fritillariae Cirrhosae Bulbus), are often fumigated with sulfur before and after the processing of drying, making the color white and preventing rot. Sulfur dioxide produced by sulfur fumigation is a strong reducing agent, which can bleach or prevent some discoloration reactions and make medicinal materials bright in color. Sulfur dioxide can also kill residual bacteria, pests and eggs on medicinal materials, and combined with water in medicinal materials to form sulfurous acid, it can inhibit the growth of microorganisms, increase water permeability of cell membranes of plant tissues, and accelerate water evaporation to make the medicinal material dry easily.

硫熏是一种传统加工药材方法，但硫熏后，药材中硫化物残留增加，对人体组织器官会产生危害，还会使有效成分下降，同时污染环境。故国家限制使用硫磺熏制药材。《中国药典》2015版规定，中药材及饮片（矿物类除外）中二氧化硫残留量不得过 150mg/kg，山药、牛膝、粉葛、天冬、天麻、天花粉、白及、白芍、白术、党参等 10 种中药材及其饮片中二氧化硫残留量不得过 400mg/kg。

Sulfur fumigation is a traditional method for processing medicinal materials, but after sulfur fumigation, sulfide residues in medicinal materials increase, thus posing harm to human tissues and organs, reducing the effective ingredients, polluting the environment. Therefore, China restricts the use of sulfur fumigating medicinals. According to the 2015 edition of *Chinese Pharmacopoeia*, sulfur dioxide residues in medicinal materials and slices (except for minerals) shall not exceed 150 mg/kg, and sulfur dioxide residues in 10 kinds of medicinal materials including Shanyao, Niuxi (Achyranthis Bidentatae Radix), Fenge, Tiandong (Asparagi Radix), Tianma, Tianhuafen (Trichosanthis Radix), Baiji (Bletillae Rhizoma), Baishao, Baizhu and Dangshen (Codonopsis Radix) shall not exceed 400mg/kg.

（三）打靛
1.3 Dadian (Making Indigo)

青黛打靛是特色的产地加工方法，各个产地凭借历史传承和个人经验进行加工，其传统工艺一般需经过"浸泡发酵 - 搅拌打靛 - 淘花阴干"等几个关键步骤。其具方法为：鲜苗割回，放于木桶或大缸中，再放入清水，以叶腐烂、茎脱皮、枝脱节为度，将枝茎捞出，立即加入先用浸液淘洗并去掉砂质的石灰，充分搅拌，以乌绿色转为深紫红色为度，捞起液面泡沫，于烈日下晒干，即为"青黛"，其水下沉淀，即为"青淀"。

Making indigo is a characteristic processing method in producing area. The way of processing is based on historical inheritance and personal experience in each producing area. The traditional processing generally has several key steps of "soaking and fermentation, stirring, washing and drying" etc. The procedures are as follows: cut back fresh seedlings, put them in buckets or vats, and add clean water; keep them until the leaves rotten, the stems peeled, and the branches apart; take out the branches and stems; add the lime from which sand is removed, and fully stir the mixture until the mixture turns dark green to deep purplish red; then take away the foams on surface and dry the stuff under the sun, which is called "Qingdai (Indigo Naturalis)", and the sediments underwater are called "Qingdian (Indigo Naturalis)".

二、特色炮制方法
2 Characteristic Processing Methods

（一）酒制升提
2.1 Processing with Liquor for Ascending

酒，性大热，味甘辛，气味芳香。行药势，杀百邪，可引药上行。元王好古《汤液本草》"黄芩、黄连、黄檗、知母，病在头面及皮肤者，须用酒炒之，借酒以上腾也。咽之下、脐之上须用酒洗之，在下生用"。明陈嘉谟总结前人用酒制经验，提出"酒制升提"理论。指药物酒制后，增加或增强其上行、行散的作用，药物借酒之力走窜，向上、向外而达头目巅顶与肌肤四肢，以宣药势，活血通络。如黄连生用长于泻火解毒，清热燥湿。适于胃肠湿热所致的腹泻痢疾等，酒炙后引药上行，善清头目之火。

Liquor is sweet and spicy, hot in nature, fragrant in flavor, with certain property of guiding medicinal trend and the function of sterilization, it can guide the medicine ascending. Wang Haogu, a traditional Chinese medicine practitioner in the Yuan dynasty, proposed in his medical book named *Tangye Bencao (Materia Medica for Decoctions)* "When the disease goes to the head, face and skin, medicinals such as Huangqin, Huanglian, Huangbo and Zhimu (Anemarrhe Naerhizoma) should be stir-fried with liquor to exert its efficacy, and the sick parts under the throat and above the navel should be washed with liquor." Chen Jiamo in the Ming Dynasty summed up the previous experience in liquor making and put forward the theory of "the method of processing with liquor is conducive to the effects for ascending", which means medicinals processed with liquor will increase the ascending and dispersing effect, thus exert is actions upward and outward to reach head, skin, and limbs, making use of the advantage of liquor so as promote blood circulation and dredging collaterals. For example, the raw material of Huanglian, good at fire-downbearing and detoxification, clearing heat and dampness, is used for the treatment of dysentery caused by the dampness and heat in the gastrointestinal tract. After being processed with liquor, the medicinal is promoted for ascending to clear the fire in the head and eyes.

（二）醋制入肝
2.2 Processing with Vinegar for Entering the Liver Meridian

醋，性温，味酸苦，入肝经血分。《素问至真要大论》"醋先入肝"；明陈嘉谟提出"用醋注肝经且资住痛"，醋制能够引药入肝，增强活血疏肝止痛的作用。如生柴胡升散作用较强，多用于解表退热，醋制后缓和升散作用，疏肝止痛增强。

Vinegar is mild in nature, sour and bitter in flavor, and it enters the meridian of liver and blood level. In *Suwen Zhizhen Yaodalun (Treatise on Major Essentials of Plain Questions)*, it was recorded "vinegar enters the meridian of liver first". Chen Jiamo in the Ming dynasty put forward "vinegar flowing to liver meridian can relieve the pain". Vinegar can conduce to the drug effect on liver; enhance the effect of activating blood and relieving the pain in the liver. For example, the Shengchaihu (raw) has a strong ascending and dispersing effect, is often used for relieving exterior heat, and in contrast, Chaihu processed with vinegar weakens the ascending and dispersing effect, and strengthens the effect of relieving pain in the liver.

（三）炭炒止血
2.3 Charcoal Processing for Hemostasis

中药炭药使用已有二千多年的历史，早在《五十二病方》中就有"止血者燔发"的记载，唐代炭药止血的记载开始增多，金元时期炭药品种丰富，医家开始总结炭药与止血之间的关系。元代葛可九的《十药神书》明确提出炒炭止血的炮制理论。"大抵血热则行，血冷则凝……见黑则止"；"夫血者，心之色也，血见黑则止者，由肾水能止心火，故也"。

The use of carbonized medicinals in Chinese medicinal has a history of more than 2,000 years. There is a record of "burning one's hair to stop bleeding" in *Wushier Bingfang*. The records of carbonized medicinals for hemostasis began to increase in the Tang Dynasty, and the variety was rich in the Jin and Yuan Dynasties. Ancient doctors began to summarize the relationship between carbonized medicinals and hemostasis. The Book of *Shiyao Shenshu (Miraculous Book of Ten Recipes)*, written by Ge Kejiu in the Yuan Dynasty, clearly put forward the theory of charcoal processing to stop bleeding, that is "generally, the blood flows when it is warm, but the blood coagulates when it is cold, and the blood stops bleeding when it meets charcoal". Another saying goes that "blood is the color of the heart, and blood stops when meeting charcoal, that is why kidney fluid can stop heart fire".

炒炭止血是实践经验的总结，由于历史条件限制，古人只能用五行生克的朴素唯物主义观点来认识炭药的作用，具有片面性。现代研究表明：炭药止血与鞣质增加、可溶性钙增加、炭素吸附作用、本身存在止血成分炒炭后增加、产生新的止血成分等因素有关。

Charcoal processing for hemostasis is a summary of practical experience. Due to the limitations of historical conditions, the ancients can only use the simple materialism of the five elements to fragmentarily understand the role of carbonized medicinals, which is one-sided. Modern studies have shown that the function of carbonized medicinals used for hemostasis is related to the increase of tannin, the increase of soluble calcium, the adsorption of carbon, the increase of hemostatic components after charcoal processing, and the generation of new hemostatic ingredients.

三、中药新型制剂技术
3 New Preparation Techniques of Chinese Medicinals

随着国家制药工业发展，先后开发出透皮给药制剂、缓控释制剂、靶向制剂、智能化给药制剂等，实现了药物定时、定位、定量的传递。缓控释制剂使药物治疗作用持久、用药次数显著减少；迟释制剂在规定的部位或条件下释药，使药物更有针对性；靶向制剂使药物浓集于靶组织、靶器官、靶细胞，提高疗效，减少对正常细胞的毒性。

With the development of national pharmaceutical industry, some new forms of preparations such as transdermal drug delivery preparations, sustained and controlled release preparations, targeting preparations, intelligent drug delivery preparations,etc. have been successively developed, realizing the timing, positioning and quantitative delivery of drugs. The sustained and controlled release preparation makes the therapeutic effect of the drug last and reduce the frequency of medication obviously. The sustained and controlled one can release the drug in the regulated position or condition, which makes the drug acting more targeted. The targeting preparation makes the drug concentrate in the target tissue, target organ and target cell, improves the curative effect and reduces the toxicity of the normal cells.

中药制剂现代技术通常包括包合技术、固体分散技术、微囊与微球制备技术、纳米乳与亚微球制备技术、纳米粒制备技术、脂质体制备技术等。中药制剂现代技术推动了传统剂型向药物传递系统的发展，激光技术的出现促进了渗透泵释药系统的发展，环糊精包合技术、微型包囊技术、固体分散技术使缓控释给药更加成熟，脉冲技术使智能化给药成为可能。

The modern techniques of Chinese medicinal preparations usually includes inclusion technique, solid dispersion technique, microcapsule and microsphere preparation technique, nano-emulsion and sub-microsphere preparation technique, nano-particle preparation technique, liposome preparation technique and so on. The modern technology of Chinese medicinal preparations has promoted traditional preparation forms toward the development of drug delivery system, and the emergence of laser technique has promoted the development of osmotic drug delivery system. Cyclodextrin inclusion technique, micro capsule technique and solid dispersion technique make the administration of the sustained and controlled release preparation more mature, and pulse technique makes intelligent administration possible.

除制剂技术外，药用辅料也是推动新剂型发展的中药动力，特别是高分子辅料成为药物在渗透、释放、传递以及智能化给药过程中的重要组成部分，为中药缓释、控释、靶向制剂等研究提供了必备的物质基础。

Except for the preparation technology, medicinal excipients are also the important driving force for the development of new preparation forms. In particular, polymer excipients, an important part of medicinals in the process of penetration, release, transfer, and intelligent administration, provide a necessary material basis for researches on sustained release preparations, controlled release preparations and targeted preparations of Chinese medicinal.

随着中药制剂新技术理论实践、新设备革新、新辅料推广的逐渐成熟，中药的剂型不断发展，中药的制药也在不断改进，未来中药制剂的研究必将在充分运用制剂技术和现代药剂学的研究成果，不断研制发展中药制剂的药物递送系统。我们应该探究传统制药方法的科学内涵，传承和发展传统中科学的制药方法，利用新技术和新设备，不断开拓创新，使中药制剂更加科学有效，为人类健康事业保驾护航。

With the ongoing maturity of the theory and practice of new technology of Chinese medicinal preparations, innovation of new equipment, and promotion of new excipients, Chinese medicinal pharmacy continues to develop, and the processing of Chinese medicinal has improved as well. The future research of Chinese medicinal preparations will surely make full use of the preparation technology and research results of modern Pharmaceutics, and continuously develop the drug delivery system of Chinese medicinal preparations. We should explore the scientific connotation of traditional pharmaceutical methods, inherit and develop traditional Chinese and scientific pharmaceutical methods, use new technologies and new equipment, continue to innovate, make Chinese pharmaceutical preparations more scientific and effective so as to escort human health.

第五章 中药的药性
Chapter 5 Property of Chinese Medicinals

中药的药性是从不同的角度概括中药作用的特性，是反映学术特色的必备内容，也是学好中药的重要环节。

The property of Chinese medicinals is the characteristics of Chinese medicinals from different angles, the necessary contents to reflect the academic characteristics, and also an important part of learning Chinese medicinals.

第一节 中药药性的含义
Section 1 The Meaning of Chinese Medicinal Property

药性是中医药理论对中药作用性质或属性的高度概括，或称性能，是中药基本理论的核心。

Medicinal property, or performance, is a high generalization of the nature or attribute of Chinese medicine theory, and is the core of the basic theory of Chinese medicine.

"药性"一词最早见于《神农本草经》序例："药性有宜丸者、宜散者、宜水煮者、宜酒渍者、宜膏煎者，亦有一物兼宜者，亦有不可入汤酒者，并随药性，不得违越"。现代《中药学》教材将药性主要集中在四气、五味、归经、升降浮沉、毒性以及补泻、润燥、走守、猛缓、动静、刚柔等方面，称为"性能"，是中药学的主要特色，也是中药区别于植物药和天然药物的显著标志。

The word "medicinal property" was first found in the preface of Shennong Bencao Jing: "The medicinal property is varying and making for the appropriate pill, the appropriate powder, the appropriate water boil, the appropriate liquor stains, the appropriate ointment decoction, there also one thing, but also something not into the decoction liquor, it proper for making all forms, follow the medicine nature, do not violate". Modern Chinese Medicine textbook mainly focuses on the four *qi*, five flavors, meridian tropism, ascending, descending, floating and sinking, toxicity and reinforcement and reduction, moistening and dryness, walking, and staying slow and dynamic, rigid and soft, called "performance", is the main characteristics of Chinese medicinal, but also a significant symbol of the difference between Chinese medicinals and herba medicine or natural drugs.

第二节 中药药性的主要内容

Section 2 The Main Contents of Chinese Medicinal Property

中药的药性主要包括：四气、五味、归经、升降浮沉及毒性。其中四气、五味、归经和升降浮沉是中医借以认识药物性能与作用的基本依据，源于人们对于药物及其进入人体后作用的直观感受；而毒性有广义和狭义之分，体现了药物对疾病的治疗作用和对人体的伤害性，两者是一种辩证的关系。此外，还有补泻和润燥等，亦是中药的基本性能。

The medicinal properties of Chinese medicinals mainly include: four *qi*, five flavors, meridian tropism, ascending, descending, floating, sinking and toxic. Among them, four *qi*, five flavors, meridian tropism, ascending, descending, floating and sinking are the basis for Chinese medicine to understand the performance and effect of medicines, which originate from people's intuitive feelings about medicinals and their effects after entering the human body, while toxicity is divided into broad sense and narrow sense, which embodies the therapeutic effect of medicinals on diseases and its harm to human body. The two are dialectical relations. In addition, there are reinforcement (tonifying) and reduction (purging) and moistening and dryness as well, which are also the basic properties of Chinese medicinals.

一、四气
1 Four Qi

（一）四气的含义
1.1 The Meaning of Four Qi

四气，是指药物的寒热温凉四种药性，又称为"四性"。主要反映药物影响人体阴阳盛衰、寒热病理变化的作用性质，是中药最主要的性能。

Four *qi*, refers to the four properties of cold, hot, warm and cool medicines, also known as the "four properties natures". It mainly reflects the nature of the medicinal's effects on the ups and downs of yin and yang of the human body, and the pathological changes of cold and heat. They are the key properties (natures) of the Chinese medicines.

（二）四气的确定
1.2 Determination of four Qi

1. 根据药物所治疾病的寒热属性来确定 能够针对寒性病理状态，能减轻或消除寒证表现的药物，称为温热药，如附子、干姜、麻黄等，能改善畏寒、冷痛等寒象，发挥温热治疗效应，故标温热性，其祛寒力强者标为大热或热性，力稍次者标为温性，再次者标为微温。能够针对热性病理状态，能减轻或纠正热证表现的药物，称为寒凉药，如石膏、知母、黄连等，能改善或消除其发热、烦躁口渴、咽痛、疮痈肿毒热痛等热象，故标寒凉性，其清热力强者标为大寒或寒性，力稍弱者标为微寒或凉性。此外尚有性平药，指药性寒、热之性不显著，作用和缓的药物。

1.2.1 The determination of four *qi* is based on the cold and heat properties of the disease treated by the medicinal. Medicines for cold pathological state, can alleviate or eliminate cold syndrome performance of medicinals, are called warm medicines. For example, Fuzi, Ganjiang, Mahuang, can improve aversion cold, to cold pain and other cold symptoms, and play the effect of warming heating treatment, so they are warm and hot medicines, and the strongest cold-removing power is marked as big hot or hot nature medium; the is marked as warm; the third is marked as micro-temperature-mildwarm. Medicines for hot pathological state, can lighten or adjust heat syndrome, are called cold-cool medicines. such as Shigao (Gypsum Fibrosum), Zhimu (Anemarrhe Naerhizoma), and Huanglian, etc., which can improve or eliminate heat syptoms, such as fever, irritability, thirst, sore throat, sore carbuncle, swelling, toxins and heat pain. the medicinals with gentle effects of cold, heat not significantly.

2. **根据药物作用于机体的反应来确定** 药物作用于人体后，会直接或间接导致机体呈现类似于寒、热证的病理表现，即可确定药物的寒热属性。如大黄、黄芩、栀子等药，对正常动物可引起体温降低，竖毛等寒象反应，故多标为寒性；鹿茸、淫羊藿、蛤蚧等壮阳药，均能提高肾的功能活动，发挥壮阳、温煦等效应，多标为热性。故《神农本草经百种录》指出"入腹则知其性"。

1.2.2 Four *qi* is determined by the reaction of the medicinal acting on the body. After the medicinal acts on the human body, it will directly or indirectly cause the body to present pathological manifestations similar to cold and heat syndrome, which can determine the cold and heat properties of the medicinal. Such as Dahuang, Huangqin, Zhizi (Gardeniae Fructus) and other medicinals, to normal animals can cause hypothermia, vertical hair and other cold reactions, so more marked as cold; Lurong, Yinyanghuo, Gejie (Gecko) and other aphrodisiac, can improve the functional activities of the kidney and play the effects of Yang, warm and so on, more marked as heat. Therefore, *Shennong Bencaojing Baizhonglu* (*Shennong Herbal Classic 100 Kinds of Records*) pointed out that" when medicines go into the abdomen the natures could be known".

值得注意的是由于标定药物寒热属性的依据并不唯一，对同一药物标定的寒热属性就可能有多样性。如冰片，根据临床可治疗咽喉肿痛等病证，标为寒性，根据芳香之气，又有标为温性；又如薄荷根据其气芳香，质轻，可标为"温"，根据其"疏风热""利咽喉"，又多标为"凉"。

It is worth noting that because the basis for calibrating the cold and heat attributes of medicinals is not unique, the cold and heat attributes of the same medicinal may be diverse. Such as Bingpian, according to clinical treatment of sore throat and other diseases, marked as

cold, according to aromatic gas, but also marked as warm; such as mint according to its aroma, light, can be marked as "warm", according to its "dispersing wind and heat" "benefiting pharynx throat", and more marked as "cool".

（三）四性的临床意义

1.3 Clinical Significance of the Four Qi

分清疾病的寒热属性，是临床"八纲"辨证的一大纲领。"寒者热之，热者寒之"则是针对寒热证型的基本治则。掌握药性寒热，方可实现中医之理法，有效指导临床处方用药。具体而言，四性的临床意义主要有三个方面。

Distinguishing the cold and heat attribute of disease is a major program of clinical "eight principles" syndrome differentiation. "for cold, heating it, for heat giving cold" is the basic treatment for the cold and heat syndrome. Mastering the cold and heat of medicine can realize the principle of Chinese medicine and effectively guide clinical prescription. Specifically, the clinical significance of the four qi mainly has three aspects.

1. **祛除寒热病邪** 六淫外邪之中，寒邪、暑邪、火邪侵袭人体，是造成人体产生寒证、热证（或暑热证）的重要原因。有针对性地选择温热药以祛寒、寒凉药以清热或解暑，如寒邪在表，以辛温之麻黄、桂枝等散寒解表；表热之证，则以寒凉之薄荷、菊花等治疗表热。

1.3.1 Dispelling cold and heat disease evil. Six external evil, cold evil, heat evil, fire evil invading the human body, are the important factors why result in cold syndrome, heat syndrome (or heat syndrome). We can select the warm medicines to remove cold, and the cold medicine to clear heat targetedly. For example, cold evil is in the exterior, so warm medicine like Mahuang and Guizhi (Cinnamomi Ramulus) can disperse cold and relieve exterior; the syndrome of exterior heat, cold Bohe (Menthae Haplocalycis Herba), Juhua (Cinnamomi Ramulus) can treat the exterior heat.

2. **调整脏腑阴阳失调** 人体阴阳失调，往往导致机体出现偏寒或偏热的病理变化，寒凉药常能扶阴抑阳以制热，温热药常能扶阳消阴以除寒，如杨仁斋《直指方》说："温以调阳，寒以调阴，盖使阴阳调而得其正"。

1.3.2 Adjust the viscera yin and yang imbalance. The imbalance of yin and yang often leads to the pathological changes of cold or heat in the body. Cold medicine can often help yin and suppress yang to make heat; warm medicine can often help yang eliminate yin to remove cold, such as Yang Renzhai's *Zhizhi Fang (Zhizhi Prescription)*.

3. 消除典型的寒热症状　在寒热病证中，因为寒热邪气内盛，往往继发一些典型的寒热症状，如发热、心烦、口渴、红赤热肿及畏寒、冷痛等。利用相应的热性或寒性药物，可以消除这些典型的寒热症状。

1.3.3 Eliminate typical cold and heat symptoms. In the cold and heat disease syndrome, because of the cold and heat evil *qi*, often secondary to some typical cold and heat symptoms, such as fever, upset, thirst, red and red hot swelling and chills, cold pain. These typical cold or heat symptoms can be eliminated by the application of relevant hot or cold medicines.

此外，利用寒性药与热性药配伍，还用来治疗寒热错杂之证；或纠其一药的药性之偏，增强疗效；或采用"反佐"的配伍方式，防止不良反应。

In addition, the compatibility of cold medicines and heat medicines is also used to treat the syndrome of mixed cold and heat; or to correct the medicinal bias of one of its medicinals to enhance the curative effects; or to use the compatibility of "anti-zuo" to prevent the adverse reactions.

二、五味
2 Five Flavors

（一）五味的含义
2.1 The Meaning of the Five Flavors

五味，是指中药的辛、甘、酸、苦、咸五种味，有些中药还标有淡味或涩味，但涩附属于酸，淡附属于甘。早期的五味理论，来源于药物的真实滋味，后来五味作为中药的一种性能，主要用以反映部分药物散、敛、补、泻等作用的性质和特征。

Five flavors refer to the Chinese medicines with pungent, sweet, sour, bitter and salty five flavors. Some Chinese medicines are also marked with light flavor or astringent flavor, but astringent attachment belongs to sour flavor, light attachment belongs to sweet flavor. The early theory of five flavors came from the true flavor of medicines. Later, as a kind of performance of Chinese medicinals, five flavors were mainly used to reflect the properties and characteristics of some medicinals, such as dispersing, converging, supplementing and purging.

辛能行、能散，辛味药物多具有发散外邪、行气、行血等作用特点。如治疗表证的解表药，治疗气滞血瘀证的行气药或活血化瘀药多见辛味。祛风湿药、温里祛寒药也有外散的特点，化湿药、开窍药多为芳香之品，也往往标以辛味。

Pungent medicinals can promote moving and expelling, pungent medicines have the characteristics of spreading the external the evil, promoting the flow of *qi*, blood and other properties. For example, for the treatment of the exterior syndromes and the treatment of *qi* stagnation and blood stasis syndrome, we use the medicines with promoting *qi* and blood circulation and removing blood stasis, which are the pungent medicines. The wind-dampness expelling medicinals and interior-warming the inside of the medicines often have the characteristics of dispelling cold. The medicines removing dampness and resuscitation are mostly aromatic products, and are also considered as pungent medicines.

甘能补、能缓、能和，甘味表示药物具有补虚、缓急止痛、和中、调和药性或调和药味等作用特点。故补虚药、治疗挛急疼痛的缓急止痛药、健胃消食和中药等，多具有甘味。

Medicines in sweet flavor can tonify allievate and harmonize. Sweet flavor indicates those medicines have the function of tonifying deficiency, relieving pain in a hurry, and easing the medicine's effects or blending medicine flavor. Therefore, the medicines tonifying deficiency, relieving acute pain chronic pain, benefiting the stomach are mostly tasted sweet.

苦能泄、能燥、能坚，降逆止咳平喘药、止呕逆药多能降泄，分别治疗肺气壅遏与胃失和降；泻下药可，通泄，治疗大便秘结，清热泻火药可清泄，多见苦味。苦温燥湿药，如苍术、陈皮、厚朴，治疗寒湿证；苦寒燥湿药，如黄连、苦参、龙胆草，治疗湿热证，亦属苦味。此外，"苦能坚"，是指苦寒药通过清热泻火作用，消除热邪，以利于阴津的保存，故苦寒清泻是直接作用，存阴（或坚阴）是间接效果，如知母、黄柏等药治疗肾阴亏虚，相火亢旺。

Bitter medicines can release, dry, be firm reduce reverse cough and asthma medicine. Anti-nausea medicine can reduce the discharge, respectively, the treatment of lung *qi* repress and stomach disharmony; diarrhea-inducing medicines can be catharsis, for treatment of binding constipation, heat-clearing and purging gunpowder can clear, more bitter flavor. Bitter and warm dampness medicine, such as Cangzhu (Atractylodis Rhizoma), Jupi (Citri Reticulatae Pericarpium), Houpo, can treat cold and dampness syndrome, bitter cold dryness; dampness medicine, such as Huanglian, Kushen (Sophorae Flavescentis Radix), Longdancao can treat dampness and heat syndrome. It is also bitter. In addition, "bitter can firm" refers to the bitter cold medicine through clearing heat and reducing fire, eliminating heat evil, in order to facilitate the preservation of yin and jin, so bitter cold clear diarrhea is a direct effect, Cun Yin (or Jian Yin) is an indirect effect, such as Zhimu, Huangbo and other medicinals to treat kidney yin deficiency and ministerial fire hyperactivity.

酸与涩均能收、能涩，酸味与涩味表示药物具有收敛固涩的作用特点。习惯上将滋味为酸味的收涩药标定为酸，其滋味不酸者标定为涩味，但也往往酸涩并列。治疗自汗盗汗、久咳虚喘、久泻久痢、遗精滑精、尿频遗尿、崩漏不止、白带过多等滑脱不禁证候的敛肺、涩肠、止泻、固精、缩尿、止带药，多有酸味或涩味。

The sour and acerbity can collect, can astringent. The sour and astringent flavor indicates that the medicinal has the function of astringency. Habitually, the sour flavor of astringent medicine is calibrated as acid, and non-sour one as astringent, but is often sour and astringent. Treatment of self-sweating night sweat, long cough asthmatic, long diarrhea, spermatozoa, frequent enuresis, leakage, and leucorrhea with in contenance syndrome together convergence lung, astringent intestines, diarrhea, essence, urine, and stop belt medicine, with sour or astringent flavor.

咸能软、能下，咸味药多具有软坚散结、泻下通便的作用特点。如治疗癥瘕、瘰疬、瘿瘤、痰核的软坚散结药，多标以咸味。芒硝之软坚泻下，亦属咸味。此外，"咸能凉血""咸能入肾"，若干清热凉血药和滋肾补肾药，往往也标以咸味。

Salty can soften other things, relieve constipation by purgation. Salty medicines have the characteristics of resolving hard lump and relieving constipation by purgation. Such as the medicines for the treatment of scrofula, gall tumor, phlegm nucleus of resolving hard lump medicines are more standard with salty flavor. The soft firm diarrhea of Mangxiao, also belong to salty flavor. In addition, "salty can cool blood", "salty can enter the kidney", a number of clearing heat and cooling the blood medicines and kidney tonifying medicines are often marked with salty flavor.

淡能渗、能利，淡味表示药物，如茯苓、泽泻、薏苡仁，具有利水渗湿的作用特点。

Light can seep, can benefit. Medicines with light flavor such as Fuling (Poria), Zexie, Yiyiren (Coicis Semen), which indicate that they have the effects of the characteristics of clearing the dampness and promoting diuresis.

（二）五味的确定

2.2 Determination of the Five Flavors

中药的五味，主要是根据若干功效的作用特点，并结合其滋味而确定的。其中绝大多数是同时兼顾作用和滋味两方面特点的，只有少部分药物或只反映其作用特点，或只反映其真实滋味。由于在用药实践中，人们首先认识了药物的真实滋味。随着用药知识的积累，发现辛味与发散、甘味与补虚、酸味与收涩之间存在相关性，便逐渐以药物滋味来表示这些相关的作用特点，并形成了早期的五味理论。后来由于药物品种的增多，药物功用的拓展，有的药物具有某种滋味，却并无其相应的作用特点；而有的药物具有某些作用特点，却没有相应的滋味。如麻黄，虽有较强的发散作用，但在滋味上却无明显的辛味；山楂虽有浓烈的酸味，却不具有明显的收涩作用特点。因此，麻黄的"味"中，增加辛味以反映其能散的作用特点；保留山楂的酸味，只用以反映其实际滋味。

The five flavors of Chinese medicinals are mainly determined based on the characteristics of several functions and their taste. The vast majority of them take into account the characteristics of both effect and taste, whereas only a small number of medicinals only reflect their functional characteristics or their true taste. Because of the practice of medicinal use, people first understand the true taste of medicinals with the accumulation of knowledge of medicinal use. It is found that there is a correlation between the pungent and divergence; sweet is corresponding with tonifying deficiency, so as the sour taste and acerbity. Later, due to the increase of medicinal varieties and the expansion of medicinal function, some medicinals have certain taste, but there are no corresponding action characteristics, while some medicinals have some action characteristics, but there is no corresponding taste. Such as Mahuang, which has a strong divergent effect but is in the taste of no obvious pungent flavor; Shanzha has a strong sour taste, but does not have obvious characteristics of astringent effect. Therefore, in the "flavor" of

Mahuang, the symplectic flavor is added to reflect the function characteristics of its dispersing, and the sour taste of Shanzha is retained to reflect its actual taste only.

需要指出的是，对中药五味的标示尚存在一定分歧，一方面是由于确定药物五味的主要依据有滋味和作用两种，有少部分药物真实滋味和显示出的功效特点不一致；另一方面，由于中药的功效大多不止一种，其相应的作用特点也是多方面的，因而在确定某药的药味时，一般只列出一至两种主要或较为主要的味，不同文献对于同一药物之味的记述，存在较大的分歧。此外，由于中药功效存在复杂性，而五味理论所能表示的药物作用特性相对较为局限，有的功效，如杀虫、截疟、回阳救逆、升阳举陷等，尚不能用五味理论来加以概括和反映。

It should be pointed out that there are still some differences in the marking of the five flavors of Chinese medicinals, on the one hand, for the reason that the main basis for determining the five flavors of medicinals is taste and effect, there are a few medicinals with its true taste different form its efficacy characteristics. In addition, the complexity of the efficacy of Chinese medicine displays multipleact characterist Hence, when determining medical taste. one to main flavors liseed; and different documents record the same medica tase different oppearing divergence and the characteristics of medicinal action expressed by the theory of five flavors are relatively limited. Some efficacy, such as insecticidal, malaria interception, back-yang rescue, Yang lift depression and so on, can not be summarized and reflected by the theory of five flavors.

（三）五味的临床意义

2.3 Clinical Significance of the Five Flavors

五味是临床选药处方的依据之一，可以增强临床用药的准确性。如《神农本草经》记载主治"咳逆上气"的药物有 20 余种，而结合其五味的认识，则味辛散者宜治疗外邪郁闭引起的咳逆上气，味甘者宜治疗肺虚引起的咳逆上气，味酸者宜治疗肺气不敛引起的咳逆上气等等，从而避免了用药的盲目性。

Five flavors are one of the bases of clinical medicinal selection prescriptions, which can enhance the accuracy of clinical medicinal use. For example, *Shennong Bencao Jing* records that there are more than 20 kinds of medicinals for treating cough with *qi* reverse, Combined with the understanding of its five flavors, the drugs with the pungent flavor could be used to treat cough and *qi* reverse caused by external evil suppression, and the medicinals with sweet flavor could treat cough and *qi* reverse caused by the lung *qi* deficiency.

五味是中药性状鉴定的重要内容。如有无苦味，是鉴别苦杏仁与甜杏仁的主要依据；牛黄先苦而后微甜及入口的清凉感，对于判别其真伪十分重要。又如，乌梅、木瓜、山楂以酸味浓者质佳；黄连、黄柏、龙胆草以苦味重者质佳。

The five flavors are the important contents of the character identification of Chinese medicines. If there is any bitter flavor, it is the main basis for identifying Kuxingren (Armeniacae Semen Amarum, bitter Xingren) and Tianxingren (sweet almond); Niuhuang first is bitter and then become slightly sweet and has the cool feeling of entrance, that is very important to distinguish its authenticity, For example, Wumei, Mugua (Chaenomelis Fructus), Shanzha with strong sour is at good quality; Huanglian, Huangbo, Longdan with bitter taste is good.

三、归经
3 Meridian Tropism (Guijing)

（一）归经的含义
3.1 The Meaning of Meridian Tropism (Guijing)

归经是药物作用对人体部位的选择性，是药物作用的定位概念。"归"是指药物作用的归属，"经"是中医学脏腑经络及其相关组织的概称，寓有药物对机体不同部位具有识别、选择和定位走向的意思。比如清热药有清肝热、清胃热、清肺热、清心热之不同；补虚药有补肺、补脾、补

肾、补肝之异。

Guijing (meridian tropism) is the selectivity of medicinal action to human body and the concept of medicinal action position. "Gui" refers to the attribution of the action of medicinals."Jing "is the general term of the zang-fu channels and their related tissues in Chinese medicine. It means that the medicine has the meaning of identifying, selecting and positioning the different parts of the body. For example, clearing heat medicines have the differences of clearing the liver heat, clearing the stomach heat, clearing the lungs heat and clearing the heart heat; tonifying deficiency medicines have the difference of tonifying the lungs, tonifying the spleen, tonifying the kidney and tonifying the liver.

值得注意的是，在归经理论中，前人认为一些药对机体的某一部分具有特殊作用，其选择性特别强，因此在配伍中可以引他药达于病所而提高疗效，因而将这些药物称为引经药。

It is worth noting that in the theory of meridian tropism, predecessors think that some medicinals have a special effect on a certain part of the body, and their selectivity is particularly strong, so they can be used in compatibility to improve the efficacy of other medicinals. Therefore, these medicinals are called meridian medicinals.

（二）归经的确定
3.2 Determination of Meridian Tropism

中药归经是以脏腑学说和经络学说为理论基础，以药物所治病证的病位为依据而确定。由于历代医药家使用的辨证方法不同，所采用的确定药物归经的依据也有所不同，归经的标示也存在一定差异。

Meridian tropism of Chinese medicinal is based on the theory of viscera and meridian, and the disease position of the medicine. Because of the different syndrome differentiation methods used by medical physicians in the past dynasties, the basis of determining the meridian tropism of medicinals is also different, and there are some differences in the marking of the meridian tropism.

1. 以脏腑辨证理论确定药物归经　脏腑不但是认识人体生理功能的核心，同时也是辨别疾病的重要依据。明清以来，药物的治疗作用主要是通过对脏腑的生理功能与病理变化的影响而为人们所认识，因此，药物的归经也就直接归于某脏、某腑或在脏腑之后再加上经字，如心经、肾经等，如，杏仁、百部治疗咳嗽气喘则归肺经，山楂、神曲治疗食欲不振则归脾胃经，鹿茸、淫羊藿治疗阳痿、遗精则归肾经等。

3.2.1　By the theory of zang-fu syndrome differentiation to determine the meridian tropism of medicinals. The viscus is not only the core of understanding the physiological function of human body, but also an important basis for distinguishing diseases. Since the Ming and Qing dynasties, the therapeutic effect of medicinals is mainly recognized by the influence on the physiological function and pathological changes of the viscera. Therefore, the tropism of medicine is directly attributed to the viscera, the Zang or the Fu and their meridians, such as the heart meridian, the kidney meridian, etc. For example, Xingren and Baibu are used to treat cough and wheezing, entering the lung meridian; Shanzha (hawthorn) and Shenqu (Massa Medicata Fermentata) to treat loss of appetite entering the spleen and stomach meridian; Lurong and Yinyanghuo are used to treat impotence and nocturnal emission entering the kidney meridian.

2. 以经络辨证理论确定药物归经　经络内属于脏腑，外络肢节，五官九窍、四肢百骸，全身上下无处不到；体表发生病变，通过经络可影响到脏腑，脏腑发生病变，亦可通过经络反映至体表。经络既是辨认疾病部位的所在，也是药物作用的归宿。因此经络系统也成了药物归经的重要依据之一。如经络学说认为，足阳明胃经起于鼻旁……下行沿鼻外入上齿中，还出，环口绕唇……沿发际至于前额，白芷长于治前额疼痛、齿痛、鼻疾，则归胃经；肝经起于足大趾甲后丛毛处……沿股内侧中线进入阴毛中，绕阴器，至小腹，向外上方行至十一肋端入腹……上贯膈，

分胁肋，乌药、荔枝核长于治乳房胀痛、胸胁疼痛、疝气疼痛，则归肝经。

3.2.2　By the meridian differentiation theory to determine the medicinal entering the meridian. The meridian belongs to the viscera, externally connecting with collaterals and limbs, the five senses nine orifices, the limbs, the whole body everywhere; the body surface disease, through the meridian can affect the viscera, the viscera disease, can also be reflected to the body surface through the meridian. Meridian is not only the location of disease identification, but also the end-result of medicinal action. Therefore, the meridian system has become one of the important bases for the tropism of medicinals. Such as meridian theory that foot Yangming stomach meridian originar from the nose... Down along the nose into the upper teeth, but also out, around the lip... Along the hair line as for the forehead; Baizhi is good at treating forehead pain, tooth pain, nose disease, then belong to the stomach meridian; liver meridian originates from the foot after the big toenail plexus hair...Along the medial femoral line into the pubic hair, around the *yin* device to the lower abdomen, outward up to the top of the 11 ribs into the abdomen... Upper through diaphragm, divided into ribs, Wuyao (Linderae Radix), and Llizhihe (Litchi Semen) is good at treating breast pain, chest pain, hernia pain, and then enters the liver meridian.

由于所采用的辨证方法不同，故确定药物归经的依据也有所不同，同一药物标示的归经可存在差异。如麻黄发汗解表，按经络辨证理论则归膀胱经，按脏腑辨证理论则归肺经。

Because of the different syndrome differentiation used, the basis of determining the medicinal entering the meridian is also different, and the same medicinal can be warked different tropism. Such as Mahuang can sweat and release exterior, according to meridian syndrome differentiation theory, it enters bladder meridian, according to zang-fu syndrome differentiation theory, it entering lung meridian.

（三）归经的临床意义

3.3 Clinical Significance of Meridian Tropism

1. 丰富和完善了中药学的基本理论　归经同中药的四气、五味、升降浮沉、补泻等理论结合起来，构成了对药物性能较为全面的认识，药物的性味表示药物的作用性质，药物的升降浮沉表示药物的作用趋势，而药物的归经则说明了药物作用对机体部位的选择性，它揭示了药物作用的又一必不可少的特征。如同属辛温的药物，麻黄归肺经，能发散风寒；木香归脾胃经，能行气止痛；青皮归肝经，能疏肝破气；麝香归心经，能开窍醒神等。

3.3.1 Enriched and perfected the basic theory of Chinese medicine. Combined with the theory of four *qi*, five flavors, ascending, descending, floating and sinking, reinforcement and reduction of Chinese medicine, meridian tropism forms a more comprehensive understanding of medicinal performance. The meridian tropism of medicinals indicates the selectivity of medicinal action on body parts, which reveals another essential feature of medicinal action. As a pungent and warm medicine, Mahuang entering to the lung meridian, can spread wind-cold; Muxiang entering the spleen and stomach meridian, can move *qi* to relieve pain; Qingpi entering the liver meridian, can soothe the liver to break *qi*; Shexiang entering the heart meridian, can open the orifices and induce resuscitation.

2. 提高用药的准确性，增强临床疗效　按照归经原则选择用药，有助于提高"论治"的准确性。如同是风寒头痛，但因其疼痛的部位不同，所选药物也有所不同。如太阳头痛宜用藁本、羌活；阳明头痛宜用白芷、葛根；少阴头痛宜用细辛；厥阴头痛宜用吴茱萸。同时，在运用归经理论时，还可根据脏腑经络间的关系，按照中医五行学说相生相克规律来确定治疗原则，如滋水涵木法、益火补土法、培土生金法等。

3.3.2 Improve the accuracy of medicinal use, enhance clinical efficacy. The choice of medication according to the principle of meridian tropism is helpful to improve the accuracy of treatment. Like wind-cold headache, the choices of medicinals are varying according to the different pain location. Such as Taiyang headache should use Gaoben (Ligustici Rhizoma), Qianghuo (Notopterygii Rhizoma Et Radix); Yangming headache should use Baizhi, Gegen; Shaoyin headache should use Xixin (Asari Radix Et Rhizoma); Jueyin headache should use Wuzhuyu. At the same time, in the application of the theory of meridian tropism, we can also determine the treatment principles according to the relationship between the viscera and meridians, according to the mutually generating and restricting law of the five elements of Chinese medicine, such as the method of nourishing water to foster wood; the method of nourishing fire to strengthen earth, and the method of cultivating earth and producing metal (like strengthening spleen to tonify lung *qi)*.

四、升降浮沉
4 Ascending and Descending, Floating and Sinking

（一）升降浮沉的含义

4.1 The Meaning of Ascending and Descending, Floating and Sinking

中药的升降浮沉是用以表示中药对人体作用趋向的一种性能，升表示上升，降表示下降，浮表示向外发散，沉表示向内闭藏。

The ascending and descending, floating and sinking of Chinese medicinal is a kind of performance used to express the tendency of Chinese medicinal to act on human body. Ascending means rising, descending means falling, floating means diverging outward, and sinking means closing inward.

（二）升降浮沉的确定

4.2 Determination of Ascending and Descending, Floating and Sinking

药物升降浮沉的作用趋向，是与疾病的病势趋向相对而言的。根据升降出入的理论，对于各种病证，往往可以辨出不同的病势趋向，相对来说，药物便分别具有升降浮沉的作用趋向。如薄荷能解表、透疹，其性浮；枇杷叶能止呕吐，其性降；柴胡升阳举陷，其性升；五倍子，能敛汗、止血，其性沉。

The effect trend of medicinal rise and fall, floating and sinking is relative to the disease trend. According to the theory of ascending and descending, entering and exiting for all kinds of diseases, wc can often distinguish different trends of disease potential correspondingly, the medicinals also have the different acting trends as ascending, descending, floating and sinking. Such as Bohe can relieve exterior syndrome, promoting rash relieving, with the nature of floating; Pipaye can stop vomiting, with the nature of descending; Chaihu ascends Yang and lifts depression, with the nature rising; Wubeizi (Galla Chinensis), can astringe sweat, stop bleeding, with the nature of sinking.

（三）影响药物升降浮沉的因素

4.3 Factors Affecting the Ascending and Descending, Floating and Sinking of Medicinals

中药的升降浮沉不是一成不变的，可以通过炮制和配伍等措施，在一定程度上控制和改变，此即李时珍所谓"升降在物，亦在人也"。

The ascending and descending, floating and sinking of Chinese medicinals is not fixed. It can be controlled and changed to a certain extent through processing and compatibility measures, which is what Li Shizhen calls "ascending and descending in things, but also in people ".

1. 炮制　李时珍《本草纲目》认为"升者引之以咸寒，则沉而直达下焦；沉者引之以酒，则浮而上至巅顶，此非窥天地之奥而达造化之权者，不能至此"。一般来说，酒制、姜汁制可使药物升浮之性增强，而醋制、盐水制可使药物沉降之性增强。但这也不是绝对的，不同的药物运用相应的辅料进行炮制，或增强某一功效，或使归经更加专一，或降低毒副作用，或改变寒热之性，或矫味矫臭，或便于制剂。如姜汁炙竹茹，不是为了升散，而是增强止呕功效；酒制常山，不是为了增强升提之性，而是为了降低其涌吐之力。

4.3.1 Processing: Li Shizhen's *Bencao Gangmu* believes that "the ascending leads by the salty cold, then sinks and goes down to the coke; the sinking leads by the liquor, then floats up to the top of the top, this is not a glimpse of the world and the power of creation, can not come to this ". Generally speaking, liquor and ginger juice can enhance the rise of medicinals, while vinegar and brine can enhance the sedimentation of medicinals. But this is not absolute. Different medicinals are processed with corresponding excipients, either to enhance a certain effect, or to make the meridian more specific, or to reduce the side effects, or to change the nature of cold and heat, or to correct the smell, or to facilitate the preparation. Such as ginger prepared Zhuru (Bambusae Caulis In Taenias), not for the sake of dispersing, but to enhance the antiemetic effect; Changshan processed with liquor, is not for enhancing the nature of lifting, but its floating property relieving its vomiting.

2. 配伍　在复方中，药性升浮的药物在同较多药性沉降之药配伍时，其升浮之性可以受到制约；反之，药性沉降的药物在同较多药性升浮之药配伍时，其沉降之性亦可受到制约，使全方表现出多数药物的作用趋向。如麻黄与石膏或白术同用，其功效重在平喘、利尿，麻黄因发汗作用而表现出来的升浮之性受到抑制；若与桂枝同用，则功效重在发汗解表、外散风寒，其升浮之性更为强烈。

4.3.2 Compatibility: In compound, when the floating medicinal is compatible with more sinking medicinals, its floating property will be restricted; vice versa, the sinking medicinals is compatible with more floating medicinals,the sinking property can be restricted, That is to say settling property can be restricted, the whole prescription show the action trend of most medicinals. For example, when Mahuang and Shigao or Baizhu are used together, their function focuses on treating asthma, diuretic, its because the effect of Mahuang sweating the performance of the rising and floating is inhibited; if used with Guizhi, the effect is focused on sweating exterior, dispersing the wind cold, and its rising and floating functions are more strongly.

（四）药物升降浮沉的临床意义
4.4 The Clinical Significance of the Ascending and Descending, Floating and Sinking of Medicinals

1. 纠正机体气机失调　针对脏腑气机失调而不能自我调节恢复而引起的向上、向下、向外、向内的病势趋向，可利用药物的升降浮沉性质，逆其病势趋向，使之复常。如呕吐一证，因中焦虚寒，胃失和降而上逆作吐者，须用生姜、砂仁等降胃和中之药，逆其病势，以复胃气和降之常。

4.4.1 Improve the *qi* imbalance of the body. As to the upward, downward, outward and inward tendency caused by the imbalance of the viscera and *qi* movement, it can be hormalized by using the tendency of the medicinal properties. Such as the syndrome in vomiting, because of the deficiency of cold of the middle energizer, the stomach disharmony causes reverse vomiting, medicinals like Shengjiang (Fresh) and Sharen (Amomi Fructus) could be used to lower the stomach *qi* and harmonize the middle energizer, to treat the disease, to restore the stomach *qi* back to normal..

2. 因势利导，祛邪外出，顾护正气　人体病证表现出向上、向下、向外、向内的病势趋向有时是为了祛邪外出做出的保护性反应，治疗则应顺其病势趋向，以利于祛邪，如因饮食过多，胃腑拒纳而作呕者，应顺其上逆，因势利导，须以助吐之药，迅速吐出宿食，祛出邪气，以避免脾胃受伤。这也为"通因通用""塞因塞因"等治疗原则提供了药理学的理论依据。

4.4.2 Following the situation, dispelling evil out, protect the vital *qi*. Human body disease syndrome showing upward, downward, outward, inward trend is sometimes to dispel evil out of the protective response, and the treatment should be in line with the trend of disease, in order to help dispel evil. Such as people who eat too much and their stomach organs refused to accept and vomit. In order to follow the reverse trend vomitting-

inculced medicines should be given to quickly romitting、dispelling to avoid the dange of slecn & stomach. This also provides a theoretical basis for pharmacological treatment principles such as general purpose of Tongyin (unobstructed) and Sein (unobstructed) with different treatment methods.

五、毒性
5 Toxicity

（一）毒性的含义
5.1 Meaning of Toxicity

中药的毒性是药物对机体所产生的严重不良影响及损害性，是用以反映药物安全性的一种性能。对于中药毒性的认识，历来有广义和狭义之分。广义的毒性就是指药物的偏性。狭义的毒性，专指药物对人体的伤害性，毒药就是容易引起毒性反应的药。

The toxicity of Chinese medicinal is a serious adverse effect and damage caused by medicinals on the body, and it is a performance to reflect the safety of medicinals. The understanding of the toxicity of Chinese medicinal has always been broad and narrow. Generalized toxicity refers to the bias of medicinals. Narrow sense of toxicity, specifically refers to the harm of medicinals to the human body, and the poison is the medicinals easy to cause toxic reactions.

（二）影响毒性的因素
5.2 Factors Affecting Toxicity

毒性具有普遍性，并不意味着任何药物在任何情况下都会对人体造成伤害，引起毒性反应。药物使用后，是否对人体造成伤害以及毒性反应的大小，与多种因素有关。

The universality of toxicity does not mean that any medicinal in any case will cause harm and toxic reactions to the human body. After the use of medicinals, whether to cause harm to the human body and the size of toxic reactions, related to a variety of factors.

1. 剂量大小　药物毒性的大小主要取决于用药剂量的大小。在规定的毒性药品管理品种中，即使是毒性最强的砒霜，如果用量合理，也不会导致中毒。相反，通常认为无毒的药物，如果用量过大，也会导致中毒，甚至造成死亡。

5.2.1 Dosage: The toxicity of medicinals mainly depends on the dosage of medicinals. In the prescribed toxic medicinal management varieties, even the most toxic arsenic, if the dosage is reasonable, it will not lead to poisoning. On the contrary, medicinals are generally considered nontoxic, but if used too much, it can also lead to poisoning and even death.

2. **用药是否对证** 用药对证，能产生治疗效果，对人体有益；药不对证，即会导致新的病理偏向，对人体造成伤害，表现出毒性。如健康人或非适应证人服羊踯躅花，出现心动过缓，是中毒反应；但临床用治室上性心动过速，使心率减慢，恢复正常，即是治疗效果。

5.2.2 Medication based on the syndromes: Medication can produce therapeutic effect and benefit human body. Healthy people or non-adaptive witnesses take Yangzhizhuhua (Rhododendri Flos). Bradycardia is a toxic reaction; but clinical treatment of supraventricular tachycardia causes heart rate slowing down, returning to normal. That is, the therapeutic effect.

3. **药材品种** 不同品种的药材其毒性强弱是存在差异的。如白附子，有来源于毛茛科黄花乌头的块根的关白附和来源于天南星科独角莲的块茎的禹白附，前者的毒性比后者大。

5.2.3 Varieties of medicinal materials: The toxicity of different varieties of medicinal materials is different. For example, Baifuzi (Typhonii Rhizoma) has Guanbaifu (Aconiti Radix) from the root of Polygonaceae yellow aconitum and Yubaifu (Typhonii Rhizoma) from the tuber of Rhizoma Sinaceae, the former is more toxic than the latter.

4. **药材质量** 同种药材因产地、采集、贮存及入药部位等因素不同而存在质量差异，因而毒性强弱也可能不同。如桑寄生的宿主为无毒植物者，使用比较安全，寄生于有毒植物上者，其药材也含相应毒性成分，误服可能中毒。

5.2.4 Quality of medicinal materials: The quality of the same kind of medicinal materials is different because of the origin, collection, storage and medicating parts, so the toxicity may be different. If the host of sangjisheng mulberry parasitism is a nontoxic plant, it is safe to use; if parasitic on toxic plants, its medicinal materials also contain the corresponding toxic components, and it may cause poisoning by misuse.

5. **炮制** 合理的炮制可以降低药物的毒性，而不合理的炮制又可能导致药物的毒性增强。如附子内服多用炮制品，炮制目的主要是减毒，若炮制不规范，其炮制品容易造成中毒反应。又如雄黄入药只需研细或水飞，忌用火煅，火煅后会生成三氧化二砷（即砒霜），毒性大大增强。

5.2.5 Processing: Reasonable processing can reduce the toxicity of medicinals, and unreasonable processing may lead to increased toxicity of medicinals. For example, internally taking Fuzi are commonly processed products. As processing is to reduce toxicity, non-standardized processing may easily cause poisoning. If Xionghuang(realgar), is used as medicine, it only needs to be grinded in water, and avoid using fire calcining, because it will produce arsenic trioxide (Pishuang). As a result, the toxicity greatly enhanced.

6. **给药途径** 不同的途径给药，由于药物的吸收、分布与排泄可能存在差异，不仅会影响药物的治疗效果，也会影响药物的毒性。一般而言，按照毒性反应出现的早晚，其排列次序为：静脉注射，呼吸吸入，腹腔注射，肌内注射，皮下注射，口服，直肠灌注。

5.2.6 Route of administration: Different routes of medicinal administration, due to the possible differences in medicinal absorption, distribution and excretion, which will not only affect the therapeutic effect of medicinals, but also affect the toxicity of medicinals. Generally speaking, according to the soonevor later of toxic reaction, it is ordered as: intravenous injection, respiratory inhalation, intraperitoneal injection, intramuscular injection, subcutaneous injection, oral, rectal perfusion.

7. **配伍** 合理配伍，可使其毒性减轻，如配伍不当会使毒性增强，甚至产生新的毒性。如朱砂与昆布配伍，不仅两者的有效成分硫化汞和碘的含量明显下降，且会生成碘化汞，有汞离子游离，容易导致汞中毒。

5.2.7 **Compatibility**: Reasonable compatibility can reduce its toxicity. Improper compatibility will enhance the toxicity, or even produce new toxicity. If Zhusha is compatible with Kunbu (Laminariae Thallus Eckloniae Thallus), not only the contents of mercury sulfide and iodine obviously decreased, but also mercury iodide formed, and mercury ions are free, which can easily lead to mercury poisoning.

此外，不同的剂型、服药方法以及患者的个体差异等都是影响中药毒性的因素。

In addition, different pharmaceutical forms, medication methods and individual differences are all the factors affecting the toxicity of Chinese medicinals.

（三）正确对待中药的毒性

5.3 Treating the Toxicity of Chinese Medicinals Correctly

1. **避免两种片面性** 一是使用所谓无毒药时，毫无顾忌，盲目加大剂量以求高效，忽视安全，以致中毒，甚至造成死亡。二是使用有毒药特别是大毒药时，畏首畏尾，随意降低剂量以求安全，忽视疗效，以致疗效不佳或毫无疗效，控制不住病势，导致病情恶化，甚至死亡。

5.3.1 **Avoid two one-sidedness.** First, the use of so-called non-toxic medicinals, without scruples, blindly increases the dose in order to achieve efficiency and ignore safety, resulting in poisoning, and even cause death. Second, when using toxic medicinals, especially large poisons, some people are afraid of their heads and tails, so they reduce the dosage at will for safety and ignore the curative effect, resulting in poor or no curative effect, uncontrollable disease situation, and even death.

2. **有毒观念，无毒用药** 即在认识上要充分重视毒性的普遍性，明确药物都具有毒物的性质，如使用不当会对机体造成伤害；在具体用药

时，应做到合理用药，通过炮制、配伍等各种合理措施消除或降低药物的毒性反应，在充分保证用药安全的前提下追求最佳疗效。

5.3.2 **Toxic concepts, non-toxic medication.** That is to say, we should pay full attention to the universality of toxicity, making it clear that medicinals have the properties of poisons, such as improper use will cause harm to the body, and we should use medicinals rationally. Eliminate or reduce the toxic reaction of medicinals through processing, compatibility and other reasonable measures, and pursue the best curative effect on the premise of fully ensuring the safety of medicinal use.

3. **加强对药物毒性的研究和再次评价** 古代文献中有关药物毒性的记载，由于历史条件和个人认识的局限性，其中也存在若干错误。如《神农本草经》将丹砂（即朱砂）列在上品药之首位，视其为"无毒，多服久服不伤人"之药，而素称有毒的白花蛇及雷丸，其安全性远远大于若干"无毒"之品。还应当注意，本草文献中记载的毒性，一般是在口服情况下的急性中毒反应，而对中药的慢性毒性却知之甚少。应当借助现代的临床研究和毒理学研究，对中药的毒性加深认识或再次评价。

5.3.3 **Strengthen the study and re-evaluation of medicinal toxicity.** There are also some errors in the records of medicinal toxicity in ancient literature due to the limitations of historical conditions and personal understanding. For example, *Shennong Bencao Jing* listed Dansha (Zhusha) in the top of the medicinal, as "non-toxic, long-term take in bigger dose do not hurt people" medicine, and known as toxic Baihuashe (Bungarus Parvus) and Leiwan (Omphalia), its safety is far greater than a number of "non-toxic" products. It should also be noted that the toxicity recorded in the literature of medicinals is generally an acute toxic reaction under oral administration, but little is known about the chronic toxicity of Chinese medicine. Modern clinical and toxicological studies should be used to deepen the understanding or re-evaluation of the toxicity of Chinese medicine.

六、其他
6 Other

（一）补泻
6.1 Reinforcing and Reducing

药性的补泻，即通常所称的虚实补泻，是从药物所治虚实病证的疗效中总结概括出来的，它反映了药物在影响人体正邪消长、病证虚实变化方面的作用倾向，是说明药物作用性质的重要概念之一。

The reinforcing and reducing manipulation of medicinals, commonly known as excess and deficiency reinforcing-reducing, is summed up from the efficacy of the syndrome of deficiency and deficiency treated by medicinals. It reflects the tendency of medicinals influencing on waxing and waning changes, of body's healthy Qi and pathogeic evils and the deficiency and excess of disease syndrome, one of the essential conceptions indicating medicinal action property.

药物虚实补泻是从药物作用于机体所发生的反应概括出来的，与所治疾病的虚实性质相对应。凡能扶助正气，改善患者衰弱状态者为补，如人参、党参可用于脾气虚的倦怠乏力、食少便溏等虚证；反之，凡能祛除病邪，平其亢盛者为泻，如大黄可用于热结肠道、便秘、高热、神昏谵语等实证，有泻下攻积、清热泻火等作用。

Medicinals for the excess-deficiency and reinforcing-reducing are summarized from the reaction of medicinals on the body, corresponding to the excess and deficiency nature of the disease. Those who can support the right qi and improve the debilitating state of the patients are for reinforcing, such as Renshen and Dangshen, which can be used for deficiency syndrome such as burnout and fatigue, poor appetite and loose stool due to spleen and qi deficiency. Conversely, those who can get rid of the pathogenic disease and smooth the hyperactivity are for reducing. For example, Dahuang can be used for the intestinal excessive heat accumulation excess intestinal heat accumulation accompanied by constipation,

high fever, delirium, etc., and has the effects of purgation and invading accumulation, clearing heat and purging fire.

掌握药性的虚实补泻是合理运用中药的重要依据。若疾病属虚证时，当用具"补"性的药物以补之；若疾病属实证时，当用具"泻"性药物以攻之，此时不可再用"补"药；若证属虚实夹杂，则又当"补""泻"并用，攻补兼施。

It is an important basis for rational use of Chinese medicinal to master excess-deficiency and reinforcing-reducing of medicine. If the disease is a deficiency syndrome, "reinforcement (supplement)" medicinals should be used to supply it; if the disease is excess syndrome, "reduction" medicinals should be used to attack; at this time "tonifying" medicinals should not be used; if the syndrome is a mixture of deficiency and excess, the reinforcing and one reducing, and the attacking and the supplementing should be used together.

（二）润燥
6.2 Moistening and Dryness

药性的润燥，是对药物祛除燥邪或湿邪，以及治疗燥证或湿证的作用性质的概括，并用以反映药物对人体阴液变化的影响。

The moistening and dryness of medicinal properties is a summary of the effect of medicinals for removing dryness pathogen or dampness pathogen and treating dryness syndrome or dampness syndrome, and is used to reflect the influence of medicine on the change of yin fluid of human body.

药物的性润或性燥，是相对于燥邪、湿邪或燥证、湿证而言的。对此性能的确定，自然应以中医辨证理论为基础，以药物相应的功用为依据。一般说来，具有生津止渴，养阴润燥，润肺化痰止咳，润肠通便，滋补精血等功效，用以治疗津伤口渴，阴虚内燥，燥咳痰黏，肠燥便秘，精血亏耗等病证的药物，均具有濡润之性。反之，具有燥湿，化湿，利湿，化湿痰，祛风散寒，行气健脾，祛风湿等功效，用以治疗水湿内盛之病证者，多具有燥性。

The nature of the medicinal moist or dry, is the corresponding summary of medicinals dispelling dryness pathogen, dampness pathogen or the treatment of dryness and dampness syndrome. The determination of this property (performance) should be based on the theory of Chinese medicine syndrome differentiation and the corresponding function of medicinals. Generally speaking, medicinals has the functions of promoting fluid production, relieving thirst, nourishing yin and moistening dryness, moistening lung, resolving phlegm and relieving cough, moistening intestines and defecating, nourishing essence and blood, etc.

They can be used for the treatment of fluid injury and thirst, yin deficiency and internal dryness, dry cough and sputum stickiness, dry intestines, constipation, and blood depletion. All of them have the nature of moistening. On the contrary, the medicinals have the effects of drying dampness, dispelling dampness, eliminating dampness, dispelling dampness and phlegm, dispelling wind and cold, promoting qi and invigorating the spleen, and dispelling rheumatism. They are used to treat patients with the symptoms of dampness, which are mostly dry.

第三节　中药药性的现代研究

Section 3　Modern Research on Chinese Medicinal Property

对传统中药药性进行现代研究，主要是研究其相关化学成分、发掘其现代病理生理学机制和药理作用规律等，以期对药性进行客观解释，指导临床有效用药。

The modern study of Chinese medicine medicinal nature mainly focuses on its related chemical components, exploring its modern pathophysiological mechanism and pharmacological action law, in order to make an objective explanation of medicinal properties and guide clinical effective medicinal use.

一、四性的现代研究
1 Modern Research on the Four Qi

现代对寒热药性的认识，多以寒、热证所表现出的特定病理生理反应及生物化学变化为基础，观察中药对其是否产生热性或寒性效应，进而探究其作用机制。

Based on the specific pathophysiological reactions and biochemical changes of cold and heat syndrome, the modern understanding on the medicinal properties of cold and heat is mostly based on the observation of whether Chinese medicine has thermal or cold effects on it, and then to explore its mechanism of action.

中医热证的症状表现，多以机体能量代谢亢进，心率快、呼吸快、口腔温度升高、唾液分泌减少等交感神经 - 肾上腺系统功能活动增强，中枢神经兴奋等功能异常活跃的病理生理学变化为主；许多寒凉性质的中药，如大黄、黄连、黄芩等，能使热证病理反应及生化变化得以消除。中医寒证的症状表现则多以机体能量代谢低下，心率缓慢、呼吸缓慢、口腔温度低、血压偏低等交感神经 - 肾上腺系统功能活动低下，中枢抑制占优势等功能活动异常低下的病理生理学变化为主；许多温热性的中药如附子、干姜、肉桂等，能改善或纠正寒证病理反应及生物化学变化，使机体恢复正常。

The symptoms of Chinese medicine heat syndrome are characterized by hyperactive energy metabolism, rapid heart rate, rapid respiration, increased oral temperature, decreased saliva secretion and other pathophysiological hyperactivities related to sympathetic-adrenergic system and the central nervous system excitability. Many traditional Chinese medicines of cold nature, such as Dahuang, Huanglian, Huangqin, etc., can eliminate the pathological reaction and biochemical changes of the heat syndrome. The symptoms of cold syndrome of Chinese medicine are mainly characterized by low energy metabolism, slow heart rate, slow breathing, low oral temperature, low blood pressure, such pathophysiological hypoactirities related to low sympathetic-adrenergic system function, central nervous system inhibition. Many warm Chinese medicines, such as Fuzi, Ganjiang, Rougui, etc., can improve or correct the pathological reaction and biochemical changes of the cold syndrome and restore the body to normal.

一些现代研究还认为，本草中食物药的寒热偏性，与其热价的高低有关；或认为药性寒热与所含化学成分有关；也有学者认为药性与中药品种有关，而品种相同，在药用部位、采收时间、生态环境、加工炮制等条件影响下，寒热药性也可以发生变化。还有学者认为，中药药性只有在证的基础上才能得到充分表征，提出证候 - 药效 - 药性关系的研究模式。

Some modern studies also believe that the cold and heat deviation of food medicine in medicinals is related to its heat value; or that the cold and heat of medicine is related to the chemical composition contained; some scholars also think that medicinal nature is related to the Chinese medicine variety, For the same variety, its heat or cold natures can be varied along with the influence of the medicinal parts collecting time, ecotope processing. Some scholars believed that the medicinal properties of Chinese medicine can only be fully characterized on the basis of syndrome, and put forward the research model of the relationship between syndrome, pharmacodynamics and medicinal properties.

二、五味的现代研究
2 Modern Research on the Five Flavors

五味的现代实验研究主要是进行五味的有关化学成分与药理作用之间规律性的探讨。研究表明，滋味与药物的化学成分之间有密切的关系，

如酸（涩）味药多含有机酸和鞣质，当鞣质与胃肠黏膜或烧烫伤皮肤表面、局部出血组织、溃疡面接触后，在局部形成保护层，有助于创面免受刺激、制止出血和组织修复，故有止泻、止血和生肌等作用。辛味药一般含有芳香性挥发油，为解表药、化湿药、温里药、行气药、活血化瘀药和开窍药的主要有效成分。甘味药多含有糖类、蛋白质、氨基酸、苷类等人体代谢所需的营养成分，具有补充营养、强壮机体、增强或调节免疫功能、提高抗病能力等作用。寒性的苦味药多含生物碱和苷类，是其抗菌、抗炎、解热或利胆、泻下、止血等药效作用的主要有效成分。

The modern experimental study of five flavors is mainly to explore the regularity between chemical components and pharmacological effects of five flavors. Studies have shown that there is a close relationship between taste and chemical components of medicinals, such as acid (astringent) flavor medicinals containing organic acids and tannins. When Tannins and gastrointestinal mucosa or burn skin surface, local bleeding tissue, ulcer surface contacing, it will form a protective layer in the local and help the wound avoid irritation, stop bleeding and tissue repair, so it has the effects of stoping diarrhea, hemostasis and myogenesis etc. Pungent (Xinwei) medicines generally contain aromatic volatile oil, which is the main active component of exterior-relieving medicine, dehumidification medicine, interior warming medicine, qi movement medicine, promoting blood circulation for removing blood stasis medicine and resuscitation medicine. Sweet (Ganwei) medicines contain carbohydrate, protein, amino acid, glycosides and other nutrients needed for human metabolism, with the functions of supplementing nutrition, strenthening body, enhancing immune function, enhancing or regulating immune and improving disease resistance etc. Cold bitter medicines contain alkaloids and glycosides, which are the main active components of the antibacterial, anti-inflammatory, antipyretic or gallbladder, diarrhea, hemostasis and other medicinals.

三、归经的现代研究
3 Modern Research on Meridian Tropism

实验研究对归经与药理作用的关系研究较多，结果表明祛痰药大多归肺经，止血药大多归肝经，抗惊厥药大多归肝经，一般能与传统认识相吻合。有人通过部分中药在体内过程发现，无论是药动学的总体情况，还是药物成分吸收、分布与排泄，均与各药的归经密切相关。如用 ^{14}C 鱼腥草素给小鼠静脉注射后，大部分由呼吸道排出，为鱼腥草主要归肺经提供了依据。此外，还有人从微量元素含量、环核苷酸水平及受体学说与归经的关系，进行了一些研究，发现肝脏是 Fe、Cu、Mn、Zn 等微量元素富集的器官，而不少归肝经的药物，则富含这些元素。一些药物对动物不同脏器中环核苷酸水平的影响，与其相应的归经相关。受体学说与归经理论亦有相似之处，一些归心经的药物有效成分都明显兴奋心肌的 β_1 受体。

There are many experimental studies on the relationship between the meridian and pharmacological effects. The experimental results show that most of the expectorant medicinals belong to the lung meridian, most of the hemostatic medicinals belong to the liver meridian, and most of the anticonvulsants belong to the liver meridian, which is generally consistent with the traditional understanding. It has been found that whether it is the overall situation of pharmacokinetics, or the absorption, distribution and excretion of medicinal components are all closely related to the meridian entry of each medicinal. For example after intravenous injection of Yuxingcao ^{14}C, most of the houttuynia cordata was discharged from the respiratory tract, which provided the basis for the main lung meridian of Yuxingcao entering. Furthermore, some people have conducted some research on the relationship between trace element content, cyclic nucleotide level as well as receptor theory and entry of meridian, and it was found that the liver is an organ full of elements such as Fe、Cu、Mn、Zn, while many medicinals belonging to the liver meridian are rich in these elements. The effect of some medicinals on the levels of cyclic nucleotides in different organs of animals is related to their meridian entry. And there are similarities between the receptor theory and the theory of entry meridian. Some of the active components belonging to the heart meridian can obviously excite myocardial β_1 Receptor.

值得注意的是，中药归经中的部位是功能和脏腑组织的综合概念，并不能与现代解剖组织学中的内脏和器官完全等同起来。例如，归心经的药物如朱砂、黄连则未必就直接作用于解剖学的心脏，它除了能恢复正常的心律以外，还能改善人的精神、意识、思维活动等多个方面的病理状态，能够消除心烦、急躁、失眠、多梦、健忘等症状。

It is worth noting that the part of Chinese medicine entering the meridian is a comprehensive concept of function and viscera tissue, and can not be completely equivalent to the viscera and organs in modern anatomical histology. For example, medicinals such as Zhusha and Huanglian, which belong to heart meridian, do not necessarily act directly on the anatomical heart. In addition to restoring normal heart rhythm, it can also improve the pathological state of people's spirit, consciousness, thinking activity etc. and eliminate the symptoms of upset, impatience, insomnia, dreams, amnesia etc.

四、升降浮沉的现代研究
4 Modern Research on Ascending and Descending, Floating and Sinking

现代对升降浮沉理论的研究不多。如有人通过实验发现，能选择性地提高兔、犬在体或离体子宫平滑肌张力的方剂在加入柴胡、升麻后，其作用更为明显，而去掉此二药后，其作用减弱且不持久，从而肯定了兴奋子宫平滑肌是柴胡、升麻升浮药性的药理学基础之一。

Modern research on the theory of ascending and descending, floating and sinking is not much. Some people have found that the prescription that can selectively improve the tension of rabbit and dog uterine smooth muscle in body or in vitro is more obvious after adding Chaihu and Shengma, and the function is more obvious. After removing these two medicinals, its effect is weakened and not lasting, thus confirming that the excited uterine smooth muscle is one of the pharmacological bases of Chaihu and Shengma.

五、毒性的现代研究
5 Modern Research on the Toxicity

中药毒性的研究，历来受到国内外学者的高度重视，研究内容包括有毒中药物质基础、毒作用机制、解毒机理等。研究模式主要有：①"系统中药"指导下的多维评价与整合分析。对有毒中药的"品、质、性、效、用"进行多维评价，对有毒中药的"毒—效"物质基础—"毒—效"机制—增效减毒原理进行整合分析，从而揭示有毒中药"毒""效"的物质基础。②系统生物学与化学生物学指导下的毒性研究。以植物药毒性成分或动物药毒素作为小分子探针，研究有毒中药的化学生物学机制，揭示药性峻猛的"毒效物质"与靶分子之间的相互作用方式以及信息传递的过程。③网络药理学指导下的中药"毒与效"机制研究。通过创建疾病基因、药物靶标预测等一系列网络靶标分析方法，为中药毒效机制研究和整合分析提供了新的研究思路与方法。④基于代谢动力学的中药毒性研究。对有毒中药和含毒性成分的中药进行毒代动力学和药代动力学研究，揭示其体内过程等等。

Study on toxicity of Chinese medicines, has always been highly valued by scholars at home and abroad. The contents of the research include the basis of toxic Chinese medicine, the mechanism of toxic action, the mechanism of detoxification etc.. The main research models are as follows: ① Multi-dimensional evaluation and integrated analysis under the guidance of "Systematic Chinese Medicine". To carry on the multi-dimensional appraisal to the toxic Chinese medicinal as from the variety, the quality, the property, the efficacy, and the application. To integrate and analyze the principle of "toxic-effect" substance basis," toxic-effect "mechanism, increasing efficiency and reducing toxicity principle, so as to reveal the poisoning and being effective material basis of the toxic Chinese medicinals. ② Toxicological studies guided by systematic biology and chemical biology. Using phytotoxic components or animal toxins as small molecular probes study the chemical biological mechanism of toxic Chinese medicine and reveal the interaction mode and the process of information transmission between the drastic toxic substance and the target molecule. ③ Study on the mechanism of "toxicity and efficacy" of Chinese medicinal under the guidance of network pharmacology. Through the creation of disease genes, medicinal target prediction and a series of network target analysis methods, it provides a new research idea and method for the study and integration analysis of toxic effect mechanism of Chinese medicines. ④ Research on the toxicity of Chinese medicines based on metabolic kinetics. Toxicokinetics and pharmacokinetic studies on toxic Chinese medicines and Chinese medicines containing toxic ingredients are conducted to reveal their internal processes, etc.

此外，对配伍禁忌的研究也有一定进展，如甘草分别与大戟、芫花、甘遂配伍时，随着甘草相对剂量的增大，对小鼠的毒性也随之增强。对有毒中药的开发利用研究也逐渐引起重视，如利用乌头碱的麻醉止痛作用治疗风湿等疼痛性疾病、以眼镜蛇毒制剂镇痛或治疗小儿麻痹症后遗症等。

In addition, some progress has been made in the study of compatibility taboos. For example, when Gancao compatible with Daji, Yuanhua or Gansui. The toxicity to mice is also enhanced with the increase of relative dose of Gancao. The research on the development and utilization of toxic Chinese medicines has gradually attracted attention, such as the use of aconitine anesthesia and analgesic effect in the treatment of rheumatism and other painful diseases, with cobra venom preparation analgesia or treatment of poliomyelitis sequelae and so on.

第六章 中药功效
Chapter 6　Efficacy of Chinese Medicinals

中药的功效，是中药作用的最基本，最重要部分。中医正是通过运用中药的功效来防治疾病。中药的作用是指中药对机体的影响，主要包括治疗作用、保健作用和毒副作用。在中药学中功效是纽带，将药物的性能与其临床应用有机联系起来。中药功效是临床中药学的核心和主体，系统中"品质制性"均须体现"效"，也是学科发展最活跃的部分。

The efficacy of Chinese materia medica (CMM) is the basic and the most important part of the function of Chinese materia medica. In Chinese medicine, it is through the application of the medicinal efficacy to prevent and treat diseases. The efficacy of Chinese medicines refers to the influence on the body, mainly including therapeutic effects, health care effects and toxic and side effects. In Chinese medicine, efficacy is the link, which organically relating the characteristics of medicines with their clinical application. Efficacy of Chinese medicines is the core and main body of clinical CMM. In the systematic Chinese materia medica, the variety, quality, pharmacy, and nature are also must reflect the efficacy which is the most active part in the discipline development.

第一节　中药功效的含义
Section 1　The Meaning of Chinese Medicinal Efficacy

中药功效的形成经历了漫长的历史时期，从最初功效与主治混杂表述，且以主治为主，逐渐发展到出现对中药功效的表述。

The formation of efficacy of Chinese medicines has experienced a long historical period, from initially mixed expression of efficacy and indications as main contents, and taking indications as the majority, to the special expression of the efficacy.

中药功效的最初表述是对药物治疗疾病的客观直白的描述，如《神农本草经》谓五味子"主益气，……补不足，强阴，益男子精"。随着中药学的发展，逐渐形成较为成熟规范的功效术语，常与病因病机、治则治法结合，如与外感六淫邪气相对应的功效祛风、散寒、燥湿、润燥、清热等。

The initial expression of efficacy of Chinese medicines is an objective and straightforward description of the treatment of the medicinals on diseases, for example in the book of *Shennong Bencao Jing*, Wuweizi was recorded in charge of the main and beneficial replenishing qi supplementing deficiency, strengthening yin and benefiting men's essence. With the development of CMM, more mature and standardized terms of efficacy have been gradually formed, which are often combined with etiology, pathogenesis, treatment principles and methods, such as the efficacy corresponding to exogenous six evils, like dispelling wind, dissipating cold, drying dampness, moistening dryness, clearing heat, etc..

一、功效的认识及概念
1 Knowledge and Concepts of Efficacy

古代本草在论述药物时，一般是功效与主治不分，以主治为主，将功效混列其中。魏晋南北朝至唐宋，本草对药物功效与主治的表述基本与前朝本草相似，对功效的认识较为模糊，滞后于主治。随着中医病因、病机及防治学的发展，金元时期的本草开始进行药物功效的总结。明清时期的本草着力于药物功效的归纳。尤其清代《本草备要》《本草求真》诸书或将功效单列于药名之下，或作为眉批处理，这是中药功效专项分列的开始，也为近代中药学设立功效专项的体例的出现奠定了基础。此后中药功效得到快速发展。目前，中药功效已成为中药学的核心，功效作为纽带，将中药的性能、主治、配伍应用等知识得以有机地联系在一起。中药的功效亦是中药进行现代研究的中心点，围绕功效进行全方位的研究，进一步促进对功效的认识、理解，进而指导临床运用。

When discussing medicinal in herbal classics in Tang and Song Dynasties and before, the efficacy was often not separated from the indication, and indication was the main content. The understanding of efficacy is vague and lags behind that of indication. With the development of etiology, pathogenesis and prevention of Chinese medicine, herbal classics in Jin and Yuan dynasties tried to summarize the efficacy. In the Ming and Qing dynasties, herbal classics focused on induction of efficacy. In particular, in the classics of Qing Dynasty, such as *Bencao Beiyao (Compendium of Materia Medica)*, *Bencao Qiuzhen (Seeking Truth from the Grass)*, etc., efficacy was either separated listed under the name of the medicinal, or treated as note in the paper header. This is the beginning of the special separation of the efficacy of Chinese medicine, and also laid the foundation for the emergence of special style of efficacy in modern Chinese

medicine. Since then, the efficacy of Chinese medicine has developed rapidly. At present, the efficacy of Chinese medicine has become the core of Chinese medicine. As a link, the efficacy organically links the characteristics, indication, compatibility and application of Chinese medicine. The efficacy of Chinese medicine is also the central point of modern research of Chinese medicine. based on which the overall studies should be carried out to promote the recognition, understanding of medicinal efficacy than further guide clinical application.

目前对中药功效的含义研究较少，成都中医药大学张廷模教授首先提出中药功效的含义，指出中药功效是在中医理论指导下对于药物治疗和保健作用的高度概括，是药物对于人体医疗作用在中医学范畴内的特殊表述形式。其在理论上、内容上和形式上都有别于其他医药学对药物作用的认识和表述，具有明显的中医药特色。

At present, there is a little research on the meaning of efficacy of Chinese medicines. Professor Zhang Ting-mo of Chengdu University of Traditional Chinese Medicine, first proposed the concept for it as following, the efficacy of Chinese medicine is a high-level summary of the therapeutic and health care functions of medicinals under the guidance of Chinese medicine theory, and it is a special expression form of the medical effects of medicinals on human body in the scope of Chinese medicine. It has obvious characteristics of Chinese medicine in theory, content and form.

二、功效与性能的关系
2 Relationship of Efficacy and Property

中药的性能主要包括四气、五味、归经、升降浮沉、毒性等内容。中药的各种性能，都是以中医药理论为基础，从不同角度，对于中药功效性质和特征的高度概括，也是在中医药理论指导下认识和使用中药，并用以阐明其药效机理的依据。性能理论产生较早，《神农本草经·序例》

中已有四气、五味及有毒无毒的记载，金元时期本草对药物的归经、升降浮沉等理论进行了整理和完善。中药性能的认识和论定，以阴阳、五行、脏腑、经络中医药理论为依据，根据药物的临床主治作用，在长期用药实践中不断总结归纳出来，如药物能主治风热表证、脏腑实热证、血热出血证、湿热下注证等，从八纲辨证的寒热辨证来看，上述的主治证都是"热证"，而药物能纠正"热"的病理偏盛，因此都具有寒、凉的药性。四气、五味、归经、升降浮沉、毒性等每一种性能，从不同角度反映具体中药的不同个性，同时也可以表明某一类药物作用的某种共性。掌握了这些药物作用的性质和特征，对于临床根据不同证候的需要，准确精选相宜的药物，趋利避害，以达到预期防治疾病的目的，保证用药安全有效起到重要作用；或用以阐释药物功效的作用机理，也具有重要指导价值。因此，性能理论的产生很好的指导了临床医家的用药，使临床药物的使用方式从经验的重现变化为有理论指导的药物选择，在中药学的发展中，以中药性能作为核心的中药理论受到历代医家重视。

The property characteristics of Chinese medicines mainly contain the four-qi theory, the five-flavor theory, meridian tropism, the four-direction theory (ascending, descending, floating, sinking), toxicity, and so on. All the properties are based on the theory of Chinese medicine, and highly generalize the nature and features of efficacy from different perspectives. It is also the basis for understanding and applying Chinese medicine under guidance of theory of Chinese Medicine, and for clarifying the efficacy mechanism. The theory of Chinese medicine property was came into being early, In the preface of *Shennong Bencao Jing* , four qi, five flavors, toxicity and non-toxicity were recorded in the preface. The herbal books written during the Jin and Yuan Dynasties sorted out and improved the theories of meridian tropism, the four-direction theory, etc.. The property of Chinese medicine is recognized and determined based on the Chinese medicine theories such as yin-yang theory, five phase theory,

viscera organs theory, meridian and collateral theory, and clinieal indications, and summarized from the clinical practice. For example, if the indications of the medicinals contain exterior syndrome of wind-heat, excess heat in viscera and bowels, bleeding caused by blood heat, dampness-heat invading downward, etc., where all belong to the heat syndrome according to the eight principle syndrome differentiation. These medicinals can correct the 'heat' pathological symptoms, thus they all have the nature of cool or cold. The characteristics of four qi, five flavors, meridian tropism, ascending-descending-floating-sinking theory and toxicity,each of them reflect the property of different Chinese medicine from different perspective. Meanwhite, they also can iddicate some similarity of some kind of medicinal Mastering the properties and characteristics of the functions of Chinese medicine, plays an important role in the accurate medicinal selection along with clinical syndromes, seeking benefits and avoiding disadvantages, so as to reach the anticipated prevention and treatment purpose, and to ensure the safety and effectiveness of medicinal use. It is also important for explaining the principle of medicinal efficacy. Therefore, the characteristics theory can well guide the clinical doctors to use medicinals well, and make the use of medicinals gradually change from the recurrence of experience to the choice of medicinals with theoretical guidance.

由于在中药学的发展中，对功效的认识滞后于性能理论，因此，在临床用药中需要在药物性能理论指导下选择用药来弥补功效的不足。虽然目前对中药功效的认识日益完善，但是中药性能仍有其存在价值，就二者之间的关系需要进一步明确。

In the development of Chinese medicines, as the understanding of efficacy lags behind the theory of characteristics, it is necessary to choose medicinals according to the medicinal's characteristics theory in clinical medication to make up for the deficiency of efficacy. Although the understanding of the efficacy is toward perfect, the characteristics of Chinese medicines are still valuable. The relationship between the two needs to be further clarified.

中药的性能是对于具体中药功效性质和特征的高度概括，因此，性能具有"抽象"的特性，而药物功效是药物具体的防病治病作用，具有"具体"的特性。因此在指导药物临床运用时，性能与功效比较更"粗""泛""浅"，而功效与性能比较更"精""专""深"。两者具有层次上的差异。如药物的寒、热药性与清热解毒、温中止痛等功效比较，寒、热药性只反映这类药物作用的共同倾向，并不涉及具体功效与病证，属较高层次的概念，而清热解毒、温中止痛等功效是药物对机体的医疗作用，与具体证候热毒证，中焦寒证等一一对应，属较低层次的概念。因此，药性与功效是抽象与具体、共性与个性的关系。

The characteristics of Chinese medicines are highly generalization of the feature of the efficacy of Chinese medicines, which is "abstract", while the efficacy of Chinese medicines refers to the specific role of medicinals in the prevention and treatment of diseases, which is concrete. They are at different levels. Compared with effecacy, property is more rough, wide and specificial, and the efficacy is more accurate, specific and deeper. For instance, the cold and heat nature compared with the efficacy such as clearing away heat and detoxifying, warming the middle to relieve pain, the cold and heat natures only reflect the common tendency of this kind of medicinal, and do not involve specific efficacy and syndrome, which is at a higher level of concept. While the efficacy such as clearing away heat and detoxifying, warming the middle to relieve pain are the specific therapeutic effects of medicinals on the body, which correspond to the syndromes of heat toxin, deficiency cold one by one, which belongs to a lower level concept. Consequently, the relationship between characteristics and efficacy is the same as that of abstract and concrete, commonness and individuality.

功效是药物具体的防病治病作用，而性能是抽象的作用特性，并不代表具体作用，离开了具

体的药物和功效，性能就很难具有确定的意义。如徐灵胎《医学源流论·药石性同用异论》指出："同一热药，而附子之热，与干姜之热，迥乎不同；同一寒药，而石膏之寒，与黄连之寒，迥乎不同"，明确指出了药性寒、热药性与具体药物功效的是不同的。在临床用药中，应该把性能理论与具有药物功效结合起来，才能很好的指导临床用药。

Effecacy is the specific prevention and therapeutic functions of medicinals, property is the abstractive function characteristics which doesn't represent concrete functions. Without specific medicinals and efficacy, characteristics hardly have definite significance. For instance, Xu Lintai pointed out in Section *Yaoshi Xingtong Yongyi Lun of Yixue Yuanliu (On the Origin and Development of Medicine)* that as hot medicinal, the heat of Fuzi is absolutely different from the heat of Ganjiang; so as the cold medicinal, the cold of Shigao is entirely different from that of Huanglian's, which clearly indicates that the cold and hot nature of medicines is different from the specific efficacies. In clinic, we should combine the theory of property with the efficacy of property to guide clinical medication.

三、功效与主治的关系
3 Relationship of Efficacy and Indications

古代本草对中药效应最直接的认识和表述就是其所治病证即主治，从《神农本草经》开始对药物的记载以其所治病证为主，如白芷（即白芷）"主女人漏下赤白，血闭，阴肿，寒热，风头侵目泪出，长肌肤，润泽可作面脂"。中药的主治是用药后直接能观察到，因此其出现较早，随后主治和功效常混杂表述，至明朝出现功效专项表述后二者才逐渐分开。至近代中药学中中药功效与主治分项更为完善。

In the ancient herbal books, the direct understanding and expression of efficacy of Chinese medicines are embodied the syndromes it treats, or called indications of the medicinal. Since the book of *Shengnong Bencao Jing (Shennong's Classic of Materia Medica)*, the records of medicinals are mainly based on syndromes and symptoms they treat. For example, Baichai (named Baizhi today) was recorded as mainly for treating metrostaxis with red and white leucorrhea, amenorrhea, *raginal* swelling, cold and hot, tears caused by the wind invading the eyes, helping skin growth, moistening and can be used as facial fat'. The main indications of Chinese medicine can be observed directly after use, so it appears earlier、later, the efficacy and indication are used in mixture for expression. The two aspects were gradually separated when the special expression of efficacy appeared in Ming Dynasty. In modern times, the separation between efficacy and indication of Chinese medicine was more complete.

主治是药物在临床的主要适应病证，包括疾病、证候及症状。

Indication is the main clinical syndromes that the medicinal treats, including diseases, syndromes and symptoms.

功效与主治是中药的重要内容，二者关系密切，相互依存，相互促进。主功效是对主治病证核心病机治法的抽象和提炼，主治为具体的病证或症状。如《本草纲目》载蝉蜕："治头风眩晕，皮肤风热，痘疹作痒。"随着中医病因病机理论的发展，逐步认识到这些不同的主治病证或症状，却有着相同的病理基础，都是由于风热外邪侵袭而引起。因此将其治疗这些病症或症状的功效总结为"发散风热"或"疏散风热"。

As key contents of Chinese medicine, efficacy and indication are closely related, interdependent and mutually promoting. Main efficacy is the abstraction and refinement of treatments aiming at the core pathogenesis, and indication refers to specific syndromes or symptoms. For example, Chantui (Cicadae Periostacum) was recorded in *Bencao Gangmu* as 'mainly in indicated for headache and dizziness due to wind, heat-wind in skin, and itchy acne'. With the development of the theory of Chinese medicine etiology and pathogenesis, it is gradually recognized that these different syndromes or symptoms have the same pathological basis, that is to say, they are caused by the invasion of external wind-heat into body. Hence, the efficacy of treating these diseases or symptoms is summarized as 'dispelling wind heat' or 'dispersing wind heat'.

就临床运用而言功效又对主治的范围加以限定，如柴胡功效为"解表退热，疏肝解郁，升举阳气"，其临床常用于表证发热及少阳证，肝郁气滞证，中气下陷证等相应的病证，但是临床运用是灵活多变的，柴胡并不仅仅用于以上病证。

The efficacy in turn also limits the scope of indication, such as the efficacy of Chaihu is to "release the exterior evil and relieve fever, raise *yang* to lift visceral prolapse", and is usually used to treat exterior syndrome with fever, *less yang* meridian syndrome, syndrome of liver depression and qi stagnation, qi sinking of middle energizer, and other corresponding syndromes. However, the clinical application is flexible, and chaihu is not only used for the above diseases.

目前对药物功效有一定的认识，中药功效是临床中药学研究的核心。学习时先认识药物的功效，通过功效确定药物的主治病证。

At present, there is a certain understanding of the efficacy of medicinals, the efficacy of Chinese medicine is the core of clinical CMM research. When we are learning, first understand the efficacy of the medicinal, through the efficacy of the medicinal to determine the main symptoms.

四、功效的分类
4 Classification of Efficacy

中药的功效主要分为两大类，即治疗功效和保健功效。治疗功效包括对证、对病和对症功效，保健功效包括预防和养生功效。治疗功效是针对疾病，为常用作用，而保健功效针对"无病"状态，因而相对被忽视。但是治未病是中医的特色所在，强调未病先防，因此在今后的研究和临床应用中保健功效值得更多的关注。

The efficacy of Chinese medicines mainly

divided into two categories: therapeutic efficacy and health care efficacy. The therapeutic efficacy includes effects on syndrome, disease and symptom; and the health care efficacy includes functions of preventive effect and health preserving effect. The therapeutic efficacy is aimed at the disease, which is a common function, while the health care efficacy is aimed at the "disease free" state, so it is relatively ignored. But 'preventive treatment of disease' is the characteristic of Chinese medicine, which emphasizes prevention before disease. So, the health care efficacy deserves more attention in future research and clinical application.

（一）治疗功效

4.1 Therapeutic Efficacy

治疗功效分为对证治疗功效和对病治疗功效。在中医理论指导下，具体中药功效逐步被认识和总结出来，而中医认识疾病和治疗疾病的基本原则是辨证施治，中药功效最重要的是针对"证"的治疗，功效在认识上将中药治疗作用与中医"证"有机地联系起来是其成熟的标志，进而使中医的理、法、方药成为真正统一的整体。因此，治疗功效中绝大部分功效实际上是直接针对中医所特有的"证"而总结形成的。

The therapeutic efficacy contains therapeutic effect on syndrome and therapeutic effect on disease. Under the guidance of Chinese medicine theory, the specific efficacies of Chinese medicine are gradually recognized and summarized, and the basic principle of Chinese medicine to recognize and treat diseases is treatment based on syndrome differentiation. The most important efficacy of Chinese medicine is to target "syndrome". Thus, the efficacy of Chinese medicine organically links the therapeutic effect with the "syndrome" of Chinese medicine is its mature sign, and then makes the principle, method、prescription and medicinal actually unified as a whole. Therefore, most of therapeutic effects in efficacy are actually summarized directly target at "syndrome" of Chinese medicine.

1. **对证治疗功效**　"证"是对疾病所处一定阶段的病因、病性、病位等作出的综合性概括，是病情本质的概括。对证功效是针对中医所特有的"证"发挥治疗作用的功效。对证功效与"证"紧密相联，多数药物的功效是对证治疗功效。如发散风寒，主要针对"风寒表证"发挥治疗作用；清热解毒，主要针对"热毒证"发挥治疗作用。通过对证治疗功效使中医辨证论治，理、法、方、药成为一个有机的整体。对证功效既是性能理论产生的基础，又是临床用药的主要依据。例如薄荷疏散风热，既可推测其性能为辛凉，归肺经，又可推测其主治为风热表证。因此对证功效是联系性能理论与临床应用纽带，既能直接指导药物的临床应用，又具有重大的理论价值。

4.1.1 The Efficacy of the Therapeutic Effect of Syndrome

"Syndrome" is a comprehensive summary of the cause, property and location of the disease at a certain stage, so it is also a summary of the nature of the disease. The therapeutic effect on syndrome is the special function aimed at the unique "syndrome" of Chinese medicine. This therapeutic effect on syndrome is closely related to the 'syndrome', and the efficacy of most medicinals is the therapeutic effect on syndrome. For example, dispersing wind cold mainly plays a therapeutic role in "wind cold exterior syndrome"; clearing heat and detoxifying mainly plays a therapeutic role in "heat toxin syndrome". Through the effect of syndrome differentiation and treatment, the theory, method, prescription and medicinals of Chinese medicine become an organic whole. The therapeutic effect on syndrome is not only the basis of property theory, but also the main basis of clinical medication. For example, Bohe has the therapeutic effect of dispelling wind-heat, it can be inferred not only that it is pungent in flavor, cool in nature, meridian entry of lung, but also the indication of Bohe is for exterior wind-heat syndrome. Therefore, the therapeutic effect on syndrome is the link between property theory and clinical application, and it can not only direct the clinical application of medicinals, but also has great theoretical value.

2. 对病治疗功效　"病"是对某种特定疾病全过程的特点与规律的概括。对病功效就是针对中医的"病"发挥治疗作用的功效。如截疟、驱蛔虫等，分别针对疟疾、蛔虫病发挥治疗作用。中医不仅有辨证论治的特点，同时也有辨病治疗的特色。临床治病时，如果在"辨证论治"的基础上结合不同病的特点给药，即辨证与辨病有机结合，可以大大提高临床疗效。

4.1.2 The Efficacy of the Therapeutic Effect on Disease

'Disease' is the summarization of the characteristics and laws of the whole process of a specific disease. The therapeutic effect on disease is the effect of the medicinal on treating diseases. For example, the effects of preventing the attack of malaria, and expelling ascaris respectively play a therapeutic role in malaria and ascariasis. Chinese medicine not only has the characteristics of treatment based on syndrome differentiation, but also has that of treatment based on disease differentiation. In clinic, if the medicine is given on the basis of 'treatment based on syndrome differentiation' in combination with different diseases, that is the organic combination of syndrome differentiation and disease differentiation, the clinical efficacy may be greatly improved.

3. 对症治疗功效　症是对症状和体征的总称，是疾病过程中表现出来的个别、孤立的现象。对症治疗功效指消除或缓解患者某一自觉的症状或临床体征的治疗功效。如麻黄之平喘，生姜之止呕，柿蒂之止呃逆等皆属"对症"之功效。中医在治疗上强调"急则治标"，对症治疗功效正是体现了这一治则。

4.1.3 The Efficacy of the Therapeutic Effect on Symptoms

'Symptom' is a general term for symptoms and signs, which is the individual or isolated phenomenon in the process of disease. The

therapeutic efficacy on symptom refers to the therapeutic efficacy of eliminating or alleviating the conscious symptoms or clinical signs for patients. For instance, the antiasthmatic effect of Mahuang, the antiemetic effect of Shengjiang and the stopping hiccup effect of Shidi, etc. are all belong to therapeutic efficacy on symptom. In Chinese medicine, it is emphasized to "treat the tip in emergency", and this kind of effect just embodies the principle.

（二）保健功效
4.2 Health Care Efficacy

保健功效是在中医药理论指导下将中药对人体预防、养生、康复等作用进行概括和总结而形成的，包括预防功效和养生功效。

Health care efficacy is formed by summarizing the functions of prevention, health preservation and rehabilitation under the guidance of Chinese medicine theory, including preventive effect and health preserving effect.

1. 预防功效　预防功效是指采用以药物为主的多种手段，如烟熏、洗浴、佩带或内服等，防止某些疾病的发生和发展。中医学十分强调"治未病"，注意防病于未然。如《本草纲目》认为佩兰等药煎汤沐浴，可"辟疫气"。"小儿初生，以黄连煎汤浴之，不生疮及丹毒。"

4.2.1 Preventive Effect

Preventive effect refers to the use of a variety of means mainly with medicinals, such as smoking, bathing, wearing, oral administration, etc., to prevent the occurrence and development of certain diseases. Chinese medicine attaches great importance to 'preventive treatment of disease', which is to prevent disease in advance. For example, according to the book of *Bencao Gangmu*, the method of bathing with decoction extracted from Peilan (Eupatorii Herba) combined with other medicinals can 'ward off pestilental disease'; 'When children are born and bathed in decoction of Huanglian, without sores or erysipelas can be ward off'.

2. 养生功效　养生功效指中药增强人体适

应能力，强身健体，调理情志，养护脏腑，延缓衰老等方面的作用，在本草中常记载为"延年、轻身不老、悦颜色、黑须发"等。

4.2.2 Health Preserving Effect

Health preserving efficacy refers to the functions of Chinese medicine in enhancing the adaptability of human body, strengthening the body, regulating emotions, maintaining the viscera, delaying aging, etc. it is often recorded in herbal classic as "prolonging the life, lightening the body but not aging, pleasing complexion, blacking hair", etc..

现代社会人们更加重视自身的健康，因此养生功效的发展具有重要的实用价值。目前，我国实行药品和保健食品分类注册的管理方式，确定可作为保健品原料的中药按保健功能进行划分其养生保健作用。

In modern society, people pay more attention to their own health, so the development of health preserving effect has important practical value. At present, China implements the classified registration and management of medicinals and health-care food, and Chinese medicine that are approved by the state as raw materials for health care products are classified according to the functions of health care.

除以上功效分类方法外，还有其他的分类，如按不同辨证方法有针对八纲辨证的功效、针对病因辨证的功效等；按中医治疗学进行分类有对因功效、对症功效、对病证功效；按主治现代病症进行功效分类如降血压、降血糖、降血脂等。

In addition to the above classification methods for efficacy, there are other classifications. For example, according to different syndrome differentiation methods, there is efficacy for eight principle identification, efficacy for etiological identification, etc.; according to Chinese medicine therapeutics, there are different efficacies for the etiology, symptoms and signs, disease, respectively; according to the main indications of modern diseases, there are efficacies of lowering blood pressure, reducing blood sugar, lowering blood fat, etc.

第二节　中药功效的发展

Section 2　Development of Chinese Medicinal Efficacy

中药功效的发展经历了漫长的历史时期，随着医药学家对中药认识的深入，进而出现了中药功效，并对中药功效进行了深入的研究。

The development of the efficacy of Chinese medicines has gone through a long historical period. With the further understanding of Chinese medicinals by pharmacists, the efficacy of Chinese medicines emerged and has been studied deeply.

一、古代本草论功效
1 Efficacy of Chinese Medicinals in Herbal Classics

汉及汉以前，"功效"一词在《汉书》中已有广泛的使用，但在本草中未使用，功效多与主治混淆不分。

Before and at Han Dynasty, the word "efficacy" had been widely used in the classic *Hanshu (History of the Han Dynasty)*, but not used in herbal classics. The efficacy was often confused with the indication then.

唐、宋金元时期本草对药物的描述中提到功效一词，多用以表示药物的效应。如唐·苏颂《新修本草》曰："白菀即女菀，……无紫菀时亦用之，功效相似也。"宋·唐慎微《证类本草》曰："热酒调服之，大有功效也。"元·李东垣《珍珠囊补遗药性赋》曰："又有曾青铜，……与空青功效不相上下。"

During the Tang, song, and JinYuan Dynasties, the term "efficacy" was mentioned in the description of herbs, which was mostly used to express the effect of medicinals. For example, Su Song of Tang Dynasty said in *Xinxiu Bencao (Newly Revised Materia Medica)*, 'Baiwan (Aster ericoides) also named Nuwan... is also used when there is no Ziwan, as their efficacies are similar.' *Zhenglei Bencao (Materia Medica Arranged According to Pattern)* written by Tang Shenwei of Song Dynasty recorded that 'it has great effect when medicine being mixed with hot liquor'. Li Dongyuan of the Yuan Dynasty said in his book *Zhenzhunang Buyi Yaoxingfu (The Supplement of the Pearl Capsule and the rhythm of Medicine property)* that' there is also Zengqingtong (Azurite)... efficacy of which is the same as that of Kongqing (Azurite)'.

明清时期的本草着力于药物功效的归纳，药物功效极大发展。如明·龚廷贤《药性歌》录药性歌 240 首，多是对药物功效归纳，如人参"大补元气"，甘草"调和诸药"。且这一时期重视对相似药物功用异同的比较。明·贾所学撰、李延昰补订的《药品化义》对药物阐释按体、色、气、味、形、性、能、力八款进行，其"力"项，即为药物主要功效。

In Ming and Qing Dynasties, herbal classics devoted to summarizing efficacy, which contributed to great development of efficacy. For example, in the book of *Yaoxing Ge (Verse of Medicinal Properties)* in Ming Dynasty written by Gongtingxian, 240 songs of medicinal characteristics were collected, most of which summarized the efficacy of medicinals, such as Renshen 'strongly tonifying essential qi, and Gancao 'harmonizing the actions of medicinals'. In this period, more attention was paid to the comparison of the functions of similar medicinals. In the book of *Yaopin Huayi (Meaning of Medicine)* in Ming Dynasty, which was wrote by Jia Suoxue and supplemented by Liyanshi, medicinals were expounded in eight items as body, color, smell, taste, shape, property, energy and power, in which the item 'power' referred to the main efficacy of medicinals.

清代《本草备要》《本草求真》诸书或将功效单列于药名之下，或作为眉批处理。这是中药功效专项分列的开始，也为近代中药学设立功效专项的体例奠定了基础。清·黄宫绣《本草求真》是现存古代本草药物功效分类较为完善的临床中药专著。其于凡例开宗明义："是编开列药品总以气味相类共为一处，如补火等药，则以补火为类，滋补等药，则以滋补为类。"清代本草中对药物记载中"功效"一词多次出现，具不完全统计在 19 本书中出现。如清·赵学敏《本草纲目拾遗》"天生磺，…… 故功效远过于石硫黄也。"

In the classics of Qing Dynasty, such as *Bencao Beiyao*, *Bencao Qiuzhen (Seeking Truth from the Grass)*, etc., efficacy was either recorded under the name of the medicinal, or noted in the paper header. This is the beginning of the efficacy as special division, and also laid foundation for the model establishment of efficacy as special division in modern Chinese materia medica. *Bencao Qiuzhen* written by Huanggongxiu of Qing Dynasty is a monograph among the existing works with perfect classification of efficacy in herbal classics. It begins with a clear meaning in every case: 'it is the preparation and listing of medicinals that are similar in Qi and as one kind smell. For example, the medicinals for tonifying fire are in the same category, and the medicinals for nourishing effect are in the same category. The word "efficacy" appeared many times in the herbal classics In the Qing Dynasty, as least appeared in 19 books with incomplete statistics. Such as in the book of *Bencao Gangmu Shiyi (Supplement to the Compendium of Materia Medica)* written by Zhao Xuemin, it was recorded that the efficacy of Tianshenghuang is far stronger than that of Shiliuhuang (Sulfur).

二、中药功效的近、现代发展
2 Development of Efficacy of Chinese Medicinals in Modern Times

近现代主要是《中华临床中药学》《临床中药学》等专著及教材中将药物功效独立进行论

述，对功效含义、分类、历史沿革等进行详细的阐述。2013 出版了《中药功效学》，是第一部中药功效学专书，对功效进行了较为全面的讨论，并强调了功效理论在中药学中的重要地位。

In modern times, it is mainly in the monographs and teaching materials such as *China Clinical Materia Medica, Clinical Chinese Materia Medica* that describes the medicinal efficacy independently, and elaborates the concept, classification and history of efficacy in detail. In 2013, the works *Efficacy of Materia Medica* was published, which is the first monograph on efficacy of Chinese Materia Medica. The book has a comprehensive discussion on efficacy and emphasizes the important role of efficacy theory in Chinese materia medica.

第三节　中药功效的现代研究
Section 3　Modern Research on Chinese Medicinal Efficacy

随着现代科学的发展，借助中药药理学、中药化学、药代动力学、细胞生物学、分子生物学、计算机科学等现代科学技术与方法，对中药功效进行全方位的研究，包括对中药功效宏观上、整体上研究，也包括在细胞、基因等微观水平对中药功效机理进行研究。

With the development of modern science and technology, the efficacy research of Chinese medicine, which includes macro and overall research, as well as research on the mechanism of it at the micro level of cells and genes can be comprehensively studied with the help of Chinese medicine pharmacology, Chinese medicine chemistry, pharmacokinetics, cell biology, molecular biology, computer science and other modern sciences and technologies.

一、中药功效研究现代概况
1 Study Overview on the Efficacy of Chinese Medicinals

中药的功效来源于对主治病证的归纳与提炼，功效的应用离不开临床，因此中药功效的研究需要在中医基础理论指导下从临床出发，依据对证、症、病功效的不同，建立中医证候模型、病证结合模型对中药功效进行研究。

The efficacy of Chinese medicine derives from the generalization and abstraction of the main symptoms, and the application of efficacy is inseparable from clinical practice, thus the study of the efficacy of Chinese medicine needs to start from the clinic work under the guidance of the basic theory of Chinese medicine, establishing the Chinese medicine syndrome model and disease syndrome combination model according to various effects of syndrome, symptom and disease.

1. **治疗功效的研究**　中药的治疗作用是中药功效的主流。治疗功效是中药针对疾病发挥的改善作用，包括对因治疗作用和对症治疗作用。

1.1 Study of the Therapeutic Efficacy

The therapeutic efficacy is the predominant function in efficacy. Therapeutic efficacy is the ameliorating effect of Chinese medicine on indications, including the etiological treatment effect and symptomatic treatment effect.

2. **保健功效的研究**　保健功效的研究主要包括预防作用和养生作用。中药预防作用是治疗作用的延伸，属于中药治未病的范畴。中药养生作用指中药用以增强人体适应能力，强身健体，调理情志，养护脏腑，延缓衰老等方面的作用。

1.2 Study of the Health Care Efficacy

The research on health care efficacy mainly contains preventive effect and health preserving effect. The preventive effect is extension of the therapeutic efficacy, and belongs to the category of preventive treatment of disease in Chinese medicine. And the health preserving effect refers to the functions of enhancing the adaptability of the human body, strengthening the body, regulating emotions, maintaining viscera, delaying aging, and so on.

二、中药功效的现代研究
2 Modern Research on the Efficacy of Chinese Medicinals

（一）中药新功效的发现
2.1 Discovery of New Efficacy of Chinese Medicinals

　　当中药的研究中不断引入新方法、新手段、新仪器及新剂型时，中药的新功效不断被发现被认识。如苦参升白细胞，青皮、枳实升压抗休克，泽泻、山楂降血脂，罗布麻降血压，砒霜抗癌等。这些功效逐渐被吸收到中药传统功效中，而且在临床中被应用。另一方面，发现新功效也是中药现代研究的重要目的之一，以期能扩大中药临床应用范围和提高临床疗效。

　　With the continuous introduction of new methods, new means, new instruments and new pharmaceutical forms in the research of Chinese medicine, the new efficacy has been constantly discovered and recognized. For instance, Kushen can increase the content of leukocyte, Qingpi and Zhishi can elevate blood pressure to exert the anti-shock effect, Zexie and Shanzha downregulate the blood lipid, Luobuma possesses hypotensive effect, Pishuang has anti-tumor activity. These functions are absorbed into the traditional functions of Chinese medicine gradually and applied in clinical practice. On the other hand, discovering new efficacy for Chinese medicine is one of the significant purposes in modern research, which is expected to expand the scope of clinical application of Chinese medicine and improve its clinical efficacy.

（二）中药功效术语的规范
2.2 Standardization of the Terms of Chinese Medicine Efficacy

　　中药功效名词术语存在不少弊端，诸如相似中药功效术语纷繁，如化瘀、消瘀、逐瘀、散瘀、行瘀及破瘀等，此类情况较多，不利于初学者学习掌握，也不利于临床医生准确理解和应用，阻碍了中药学的发展。为改变这一现状，促进中药学发展，中药功效术语规范化研究成为中药功效研究的重要内容。目前已经进行了部分中药功效术语规范化研究。成都中医药大学张廷模教授对中药功效术语规范化研究的必要性、提出功效术语规范性研究的方案并对部分中药功效术语进行了规范性研究。

　　There exist many flaus in Chinese medicine efficacy terms, such as plentiful similar terms of efficacy, like "resolving blood stasis" "dissipating blood stasis" "dispelling blood stasis" "diffusing blood stasis" "moving blood stasis" "breaking blood stasis" and so on. This kind of situation is numerous, which are not only difficult for beginners to learn, but also affect the accurate comprehension and application for clinicians, eventually blocking the development of traditional Chinese Materia Medica. The standardization of Chinese medicine efficacy terms has become a crucial part of Chinese medicine efficacy research for changing this situation and promoting the development of Chinese medicine, and some studies on it have been carried out presently. Professor ZhangTingmo of Chengdu university of TCM stated the necessity of standardizing the terms of efficacy of Chinese medicines, proposed the research program for standardized efficacy terms and conducted the normative research on some terms.

（三）中药功效与药性关系的相关研究
2.3 Study on the Relationship between Efficacy and Characteristics of Chinese Medicinals

　　如前所述，中药功效与药性具有个性与共性的关系，因此针对中药功效与药性之间的联系进行研究是认识中药功效的另一手段。当前主要开展了中药四气、五味药性与中药功效的关系研究。如研究认为寒热中药对寒热体质和寒热证候的干预作用是不同的，开展中药功效与寒热药性相关性研究应以采取证候模型的研究方法为主。有学者对中药功效与五味之间的关联进行研究，对《中华本草》所载 8980 味中药的五味数据及关联的药物功效进行分析，发现具有生津止渴、补气、补阴、润肺、补肺、润肺止咳、补血、润燥、除烦、补脾益气功能的中药其药味多为"甘"；具有发散风寒、解表、温中、散寒止痛功能的中药其药味多为"辛"；具有消肿止痛、清热解毒、清热泻火、清热燥湿、化瘀止血、杀虫功能的中药其药味多为"苦"。

As mentioned above, the relationship between efficacy and characteristics of Chinese medicine is like that between individuality and commonality, therefore, the study on the relationship between them is a means to recognize the efficacy of Chinese medicine. At present, the research on the relationship between four qi, five flavors and the efficacy of Chinese medicines are mainly carried out. For example, the research indicates that the intervention effects of cold and hot medicinal on cold and hot constitution are different from it on cold and hot syndrome, and the research on the correlation between efficacy of Chinese medicine and the cold and hot natures should be primarily conducted with Chinese medicine syndrome model. In addition, some scholars studied the relationship between the efficacy of Chinese medicine and the five flavors by analyzing the flavors and efficacy of 8980 medicinals recorded in *Chinese Materia Medica*, finding that the medicinals with efficacies of promoting the production of body fluid to relieve thirst, tonifying qi, invigorating yin, moistening lung, nourishing lung, nourishing lung to relieve cough, tonifying blood, moisturizing dryness, relieving dysphoria, tonifying spleen and invigorating qi are mostly sweet, inflavor while the medicinals with efficacies of dispersing pathogenic wind-cold, relieving exterior syndromes warming the middle energizer and dispersing cold to relieve pain are mostly pungent inflavor, and the medicinal with efficacies of subduing swelling to relieve pain, clearing heat to eliminate toxicity, clearing heat to purge fire, clearing heat and dampness, stopping bleeding by removing the blood stasis and destroying intestinal parasites are mostly bitter inflavor.

（四）中药功效网络的研究
2.4 Study on the Efficacy Network of Chinese Medicinals

有学者认为中药功效相关的多成分、多靶点、多环节之间组成了密切联系、相互协同与制约的复杂网络，发现这一复杂网络的内在联系，揭示各成分间相互协同的机理，明确这一复杂作用关系的整体效应，对于基本清楚中药的物质基础和作用机理具有关键作用，是中药学理论与现代研究成果相融合的基本途径。因此有研究人员提出并探讨了中药功效网络的基本概念，提出中药功效网络的三个层次，分别为中药功效的分子网络、模块网络和概念网络。提出中药功效网络构建的三种基本途径，分别为基于中药作用靶点辨识、基于药理指标相关作用环节和基于中医理论与中药基本信息的网络构建，并以活血化瘀功效网络为例探讨了中药功效网络可能的应用途径。

Some scholars believe that the multi-components, multi-targets and multi-links related to the efficacy of Chinese medicine constitute a complex network of close contact, mutual cooperation and restriction. The discovery of the internal connection of this complex network, the disclosure of the mechanism of mutual cooperation among the components, and the clarification of the overall effect of this complex interaction relationship play a key role in the basic understanding of the material basis and the active mechanism of Chinese medicine, which is an essential way to integrate the theory of Chinese medicine with modern research results. Therefore, some researchers proposed and discussed the basic notion of Chinese medicine efficacy network, and then three levels of Chinese medicine efficacy network have been put forward, namely molecular network, module network and concept network of Chinese medicine efficacy. They also came up with three basic approaches of Chinese medicine efficacy network construction, which are based on target identification, pharmacological indexes, Chinese medicine theory and basic information. In addition, they explored the possible application channels of the efficacy network of Chinese medicine by taking the network of promoting blood circulation and relieving blood stasis as an example.

（五）中药功效相关动物模型研究

2.5 Study on the Animal Models Concerning Efficacy of Chinese Medicinals

中药功效中多数功效是对证功效，因此对其研究的突破口是建立中医"证"的模型。中医证候动物模型最早建立阳虚模型，随后逐步建立起了阴虚、肾虚、脾气虚、血瘀等证候模型。通过建立中医证候动物模型，用相应的中药反证治疗，从而研究了中药的功效及其科学内涵。如用脾虚动物模型探讨人参、黄芪、党参、白术、山药、大枣的补脾气、健脾功效[7]。此外，也可根据需要选用现代医学的疾病动物模型和方法，间接研究其功效作用，这也是中药功效现代研究的常用的方法。

The therapeutic effect on syndrome is the majority in efficacy of Chinese medicines, so the breakthrough for this research is to establish models of Chinese medicine syndrome. The animal model of yang deficiency was first established, followed by syndrome model of yin deficiency, kidney deficiency, spleen deficiency, blood stasis, and so on. The efficacy and scientific connotation of Chinese medicine were certified through applying the corresponding medicinals to exert countervailing syndrome treatment. For example, the spleen deficiency animal model can be applied to study the effects of tonifying spleen qi and nourishing spleen of Renshen, Huangqi, Dangshen, Baizhu, Shanyao, and Dazao (Jujubae Fructus). Moreover, the animal models of modern diseases and modern methods can also be selected according to the needs to indirectly explore the efficacy of Chinese medicine, which is also a common method of modern research on the efficacy of Chinese medicine as well.

（六）中药保健功效研究

2.6 Study on the Health Care Efficacy of Chinese Medicinals

中药保健功效的现代研究，主要是根据国家

关于保健品开发的相关文件和指南，及养生、康复等现代研究理论、技术和方法开展研究。

The modern research on the health care efficacy of Chinese medicine is mainly carried out according to the relevant national documents and guidelines about the development of health care products, as well as the modern research theories, technologies and methods of health maintenance and rehabilitation

总之，在中药学的发展中，中药功效的内容是研究和临床应用的核心。目前对中药功效的研究还需要结合临床，结合药理深入对证模型研究，加强对功效术语的规范研究。随着对功效研究的深入，新的功效将不断被发现和使用；同时，随着医学发展和社会的发展，疾病谱发生改变，现有中药的部分功效会失去实用价值而被遗忘；而人们对中药常用功效的认识和应用，也会更加深入。因此，对中药功效的认识是不断发展的过程，中药功效是开放的，纳新的，并不断完善的。

In short, the content of efficacy of Chinese medicines is the core of research and clinical application in the progress of Chinese medicine. At present, the research on efficacy of Chinese medicine still needs deep studies on the syndrome model combined with clinical practice and pharmacology, as well as strengthening normative studies on the efficacy terms. With the further research of efficacy, new efficacy will be discovered and applied constantly. At the same time, with the advancement of medicine and society, the spectrum of diseases changes, and part of efficacy of Chinese medicine may lose its practical value and be forgotten, and people's cognition and application of the commonly used efficacy of Chinese medicine will be going deeper. Hence, the understanding of the efficacy of Chinese medicines is a continuously developing process. The efficacy of Chinese medicines is open, updated and constantly improved.

第七章　中药的应用
Chapter 7　Application of Chinese Medicinals

为了充分发挥中药的治疗效应，确保临床用药安全，需全面掌握中药的应用知识，根据病情、药性及治疗要求合理选择、准确应用。

To maximize the efficacy and ensure the clinical safety, the application knowledge of Chinese medicinals should be fully mastered, and the disease condition, nature of medicinals and needs of treatment should be considered comprehensively to achieve the purpose of accurate treatment.

第一节　中药应用的含义
Section 1　The Meaning of Chinese Medicinal Application

与临床疗效、用药安全密切相关的中药应用方法包括中药配伍、用药禁忌、用药剂量、给药途径、煎煮与服用方法等。

The methods of Chinese medicinal application include Chinese medicinal compatibility, medication contraindications, dosage, route of administration, method of decoction and administration, etc. of Chinese medicinal.

一、中药配伍
1 Compatibility of Chinese Medicinals

配伍是指根据病情需要及药物的特点，将两种或两种以上中药进行合理组合，调其偏性，制其毒性，增强或改变原有功效，消除或缓解对人体的不良影响的应用方法。《神农本草经·序言》将单味药的应用和药与药之间的配伍关系归纳为七个方面，即："有单行者，有相须者，有相使者，有相畏者，有相恶者，有相反者，有相杀者。凡此七情，合和视之。"这就是中药配伍应用的"七情"关系，包括单行、相须、相使、相畏、相恶、相反和相杀。

Compatibility refers to the application method of rationally combining two or more Chinese medicinal according to the needs of the disease and the properties of medicines, adjusting their bias, restricting their toxicities, increasing or changing the original efficacy, and eliminating or mitigating the adverse effects on the human body. The preface of *Shengnong Bencao Jing* summarizes the application of a single Chinese medicinal and the relationship of Chinese medicinal compatibility into seven aspects, namely: the application of a single medicinal, the mutual reinforcement, the mutual assistance, the mutual restraint, the mutual inhibition, the mutual antagosism, and the mutual suppression, which are called Qiqing relationship (seven emotional relationship) and required to take into full consideration while applying Chinese medicinals.

（一）七情的含义

1.1 Meaning of Qiqing (Seven Emotions)

1. **单行** 是指单用一味中药治疗疾病的应用方法。对于病情比较单纯，选用一味针对性较强的药物即能达到治疗目的。如清金散，即单用黄芩治肺热咳嗽；独参汤，重用单味人参治元气虚脱之危候。

1.1.1 Single Application

Single application means the method of only using one medicinal to treat disease. For the condition which is relatively simple, the use of only one targeted medicine can achieve the purpose of treatment. For example, Qingjin San (Powder), Huangqin is solely used to treat lung heat cough. Dushen Tang (Decoction) only containing Renshen (Ginseng Radix et Rhizoma in big dose), is used to treat the severe qi deficiency.

2. **相须、相使** 相须是指性能功效相似的药物配合应用，可以增强其原有功效。如麻黄配桂枝，能增强发汗解表，祛风散寒功效；石膏配知母，能增强清热泻火功效；大黄配芒硝，能增强攻下泻热功效等。相使是指在性能功效方面具有某些共性或治疗目的一致的药物配伍应用，以一种药物为主，另一种药物为辅，辅药可以提高主药的功效。如补气利水的黄芪与利水健脾之茯苓配伍用于脾虚水肿，茯苓可以提高黄芪补气利水功效；清热燥湿止痢的黄连与调中行气止痛之木香配伍用于湿热泻痢腹痛，木香可增加黄连清热燥湿止痢功效。相须、相使配伍可以起到协同增效作用，是中药配伍应用的主要形式。

1.1.2 Mutual Reinforcement, Mutual Assistance

Mutual reinforcement refers to the combination of medicinals with similar functions to strengthen their therapeutic actions. For example, Mahuang combined with Guizhi can enhance the effect of sweating and releasing the exterior, dispersing wind cold. Shigao combined with Zhimu can enhance the effect of clearing heat fire. Dahuang with Mangxiao can enhance the effect of attacking and purging heat downward. Mutual assistance refers to the compatibility of certain medicinals (one as the dominator and the other as an adjuvant) that have some commonalities or consistent therapeutic purposes in properties and efficacy. Take one medicine as the main medicine and the other medicine as the supplement, and the auxiliary medicine can improve the efficacy of the main medicine. For example, Huangqi with the effects of tonifying the qi and promoting urination combined with Fuling, with the effects of promoting urination and strengthening the spleen, can be used for spleen deficiency with edema, and Fuling can improve the effect of Huangqi on supplementing qi and promoting urination function. Huanglian for clearing heat and drying dampness and stopping dysentery Muxiang with qi-regulating and analgesic effects are combined for treating dysentery and diarrhea due to damp heat. With Muxiang, the effect of Huanglian on clearing heat, dampness and inhibiting diarrhea can be increased. Coordinative and synergistic effects by the actions of mutual reinforcement and mutual assistance are the main forms of the Chinese medicinal compatibility.

3. **相畏、相杀** 相畏指二药合用，一药的不良反应被另一药减轻或消除的配伍关系。相杀指二药合用，一药能减轻或消除另一药的不良反应的配伍关系。

1.1.3 Mutual Restraint, Mutual Detoxication

Mutual restraint means the combination of two medicines in which the adverse reactions of one medicinal are reduced or eliminated by another. Mutual suppression is a combination in which one medicinal can reduce or eliminate the side effects of another.

《神农本草经·序录》言"若有毒宜制，可用相畏、相杀者"，可知相畏、相杀配伍是二药合用使不良反应降低或消除。《本草纲目》云：

"相畏者，受彼之制也"、"相杀者，制彼之毒也"。可见相畏与相杀涉及的是同一药对，是同一配伍关系的两种提法，只是两者立场不同，相对而言的。如生半夏和生南星的不良反应能被生姜减轻或消除，其配伍关系表达为：生半夏和生南星畏生姜，生姜杀生半夏和生南星的"毒"。

The preface of *Shennong Bencao Jing* stated that the Chinese medicinals with toxic substance should be processed and use, mutual restraint or mutual suppression medicinals. That is to say, Mutual restraint and mutual suppression are the combined usage of two medicinals to reduce or eliminate adverse reactions. It is said in *Bencao Gangmu* that mutual restraint means the function of one medicinal are influenced by the other one, while mutual suppression means restricting toxin of each other. It can be seen that mutual restraint and mutual suppression are dual descriptions about the same medicine they are discribed in the same compatibility relationship. Only different stances comparatively. For example, the adverse reaction of Shengbanxia (raw) and Shengnanxing (raw) can be reduced or eliminated by Shengjiang. The compatibility relationship is expressed as follows: the toxicity of Shengbanxia and Shengnanxing is suppressed by Shengjiang, and Shengjiang counteracts the toxicity of Shengbanxia and Shengnanxing.

4. 相恶、相反　相恶是指合用后可致一药或二药某方面或某几方面治疗效应减弱甚至丧失的两味药之间的配伍关系。《神农本草经》也未对相恶做具体解释，但其序录中指出"勿用相恶、相反者"。之所以勿用，不外乎可能会使治疗效应降低、毒害效应增强或产生新的毒害效应。二药相恶，可能只是其中一药的治疗效应减弱或丧失，如人参恶莱菔子，人参的补气作用能被莱菔子减弱；也可能两败俱伤，二药的治疗效应都被削弱，如生姜恶黄芩，即黄芩的清肺、清胃功效与生姜的温肺、温胃功效相互拮抗而使各自的治疗效应降低。相反是指合用后不良反应增强，或产生新的不良反应的两

味药之间的配伍关系。《神农本草经》提出"勿用相恶、相反"的原则，虽未对相反做具体解释，但以相恶为减低治疗效应，相反为增加不良反应，已形成共识。历代本草所举七情药例涉及相反者多为"十八反""十九畏"，实际上相反也是一种广泛存在的配伍关系。二药合用后，只要其不良反应增强了，即属包含相反配伍关系。随着配伍对中药药理毒理效应及药代动力学影响研究的不断深入，将会发现更多的具有相反配伍关系的药对。

1.1.4 Mutual Inhibition, Mutual Antagonism

Mutual inhibition means after combined use, the compatibility relationship between the medicines are reduced or even lost. *Shennong Bencao Jing* did not explain the mutual inhibition in details, but its preface pointed out that mutual inhibition and mutual antagonism should not be used. The reason for not using these combinations is that it may reduce the therapeutic effect, increase the toxicity or produce new toxic effects. The mutual inhibition of medicinals may be the minimizing or lossing the therapeutic effect of one medicinal. For example, Renshen is inhibited with Laifuzi, because the qi-tonifying effects of Renshen can be reduced by Laifuzi. Inhibition can also influence both of medicines, and the therapeutic effects of the two medicines are minimized. For example, Shengjiang is inhibited with Huangqin, since the lung-clearing and stomach-clearing efficacy of Huangqin antagonizes the lung-warming. And stomach-warming efficacy of Shengjiang which decreasing therapeatic effects produced. Mutual antagonism means the combination of two substances can give rise to the adverse reactions or cause new adverse reactions. It is pointed out that the principle of mutual inhibition and mutual antagonism could not be used in Shennong Bencao Jing. Although no specific explanation is given to mutual antagonism, it is agreed that mutual inhibition is can reduce the efficacy and using mutual antagonism can increase the adverse reactions of medicines. The seven emotions examples about mutual antagonism in ancient Materia Medica mostly are "Shibafan" (eighteen antagonisms) and "Shijiuwei" (nineteen incompatibilities). In fact, the mutual antagonism is also a widely existing compatibility relationship. After the combination of two medicinals, once the adverse reactions are increased, it belongs to the mutual antagonism relationship. With the development of the research on the pharmacological and toxicological effects and pharmacokinetics of the compatibility of Chinese medicine, more medicinal pairs in a mutual antagonism relationship will be discovered.

（二）配伍七情的相对性与复杂性

1.2 The Relativity and Complexity of the "Qiqing" Compatibility

七情中各"情"均有的固定的含义，但具体药对中，药物之间的七情关系则是相对的。二药合用存在什么样的七情关系，应落实到具体病证来确定。若二药合用某些效应增强，对甲病而言，增强的是治疗效应，则配伍关系为相须（或相使）；但对乙病而言，可能增强的是不良反应，其配伍关系则属相反。若二药合用某些效应减弱，对甲病而言，减弱的是治疗效应，则配伍关系为相恶；但对乙病而言，可能减弱的是不良反应，则配伍关系属。

Each "emotion" in the Qiqing ("seven emotions") has a fixed meaning, but in a specific medicinal pair, the "seven emotions" relationship of medicines is relative. What kind of Qiqing relationship exists in the combination of two medicinals should be determined by a specific disease. If certain effects of the two combined medicinals are increased, for disease A, the therapeutic effect is increased, then the compatibility relationship is mutual reinforcement (or mutual assistant); but for disease B, the adverse reactions may be increased, and the compatibility relationship is mutual antagonism. If some effects of two combined medicines are minimized, for disease A, the therapeutic effect is minimized, then the combination is mutual inhibition; but for disease B, the adverse effects may be reduced, then the compatibility relationship is mutual restraint, or mutual suppression.

中药常常是多成分、多靶点、多途径作用于机体的，同一药对中复杂的中药成分相对于复杂的病理过程，可能兼有多种配伍关系，既可能产生增强（相须或相使）或减弱（相恶）治疗效应，亦可能产生增强（相反）或减弱（相畏或相杀）不良反应。

Chinese medicinals often acts on the body with multiple components, multiple targets, and multiple pathways. In relation with the complicated pathological process, the complex Chinese medicinal components in a medicinal pair may have multiple combination relationships, which may result in increased (mutual reinforcement or assitance) or decreased (mutual inhibition) effects, or induce increased (mutual antagonism) or decreased (mutual restraint, mutual suppression) adverse reactions.

综上，中药配伍可以进一步归纳为：相须、相使可提高治疗效应，相畏、相杀可降低或消除不良反应，是用药时应充分利用的配伍关系；相恶会使治疗效应下降，相反会使不良反应增强，是用药时应尽量避免的配伍关系。

In summary, the compatibility of Chinese medicinals can be further summarized as follows: mutual reinforcement and mutual assistance can improve the therapeutic effects, and mutual restraint and mutual suppression can reduce or eliminate adverse reactions. These compatibility relationships should be fully utilized in medication. Mutual inhibition will reduce the therapeutic effects, and mutual antagonism will increase the adverse reactions. These compatibility relationships should be avoided in medication.

二、用药禁忌
2 Contraindications of Medication

用药禁忌，为禁用、忌用、慎用的泛称，三者之间有程度上差异：禁用程度最重，意即"禁止"；忌用程度次之，可理解为"有所顾忌"；慎用程度最轻，可理解为"不宜太过"。用药禁忌包括病证用药禁忌、配伍禁忌、妊娠用药禁忌、服药食忌等内容。

Contraindication is a broad concept including medication with prohibition, contraindication, and caution, and these three terms are different in degree. The degree of prohibition is highest, meaning "forbidden". The degree of contraindication is the second, which can be understood as "can be used in some specific conditions". Caution is the lowest degree which can be understood as "can't be used widely". Medication contraindications include the contraindications of disease syndrome medication, compatibility contraindications, pregnancy medication contraindications, medication food contraindications, etc.

（一）病证用药禁忌
2.1 Contraindications for Disease and Syndrome Medication

病证用药禁忌的内容涉及范围较广，与药物性能功效密切相关。原则上，凡药不对证，可能导致病情加重、恶化者均属禁忌范围。如里寒证忌用寒凉伤阳的清热药；阴虚内热者还须慎用苦寒药，以免苦寒化燥伤阴；脾虚便溏者忌用泻下药，以免损伤脾胃；实热证及阴虚火旺者忌用助热伤阴的温里药和补阳药等。此外，还有一些与具体药物特性有关的病证用药禁忌。如青光眼患者忌用有扩散瞳孔作用的洋金花；胃炎及胃溃疡患者慎用对胃刺激较强的皂荚、远志；胃酸过多者不宜服用酸味很浓的五味子、山茱萸等。

The content of contraindications for disease and syndrome medication covers a wide range and is closely related to the medicinal property and efficacy. In principle, the condition that medicinals are not proper for syndromes and result in disease worsening belongs to contraindications. For example, cold and yang-impairing medicinals that clear heat can't be used to treat inner cold syndrome. Medicinals bitter and cold in nature should be cautiously used to treat yin deficiency syndrome, since the bitter and cold impair yin by the production of dryness. Spleen-deficiency patient with loose stool can't use downward-draining medicinals, in order to avoid harming spleen and stomach. Medicinals that warm the interior and medicinals that tonify the yang are forbidden for excess heat and hyperactivity of fire due to yin deficiency. In addition, there are some contraindications for disease related to specific medicinals characteristics. For example, patients with glaucoma can't use Yangjinhua (Daturae Flos) with mydriasis effects. Patients with gastritis and gastric ulcer should not use Zaojiao (Gleditsiae Fructus) and Yuanzhi which can stimulate the stomach. Those suffering from hyperacidity should not take Wuweizi, Shanzhuyu (Corni Fructus) etc..

（二）配伍禁忌
2.2 Contraindications for Compatibility

原则上凡是合用后会使疗效下降或使毒副效应增强者均属配伍禁忌。目前，约定俗成，共同认可的配伍禁忌主要是"十八反""十九畏"所涉及的药对。

In principle, any case which will decrease the curative effect or increase the side effects after combined use belong to contraindications for compatibity. At present, the conventional and commonly recognized compatibility contraindications are mainly the medicine pairs involved in "eighteen antagonism" and "nineteen mutual inhibitions".

1. **配伍禁忌溯源** 《神农本草经》序录即提出配伍禁忌的原则："勿用相恶、相反"，但未见相反药例。陶弘景在《本草经集注》中所列相反药例，包括"甘草反甘遂""人参反藜芦""乌头反贝母"等，共涉及药物19种（乌喙与乌头合计为一种），药对16对，与后世流传的"十八反"所涉及药物、药对完全相同。金元时期张从正《儒门事亲》的"十八反歌"的文字简练易记，流传至今。明·刘纯《医经小学》最早记载"十九畏"歌诀。

2.2.1 Origin of Compatibility Contraindications

The preface of *Shengnong Bencao Jing* puts forward the taboo principle of compatibility: "do not use the inhibition and antagonism", but there is no example of that.Tao Hongjing in *Bencaojing Jizhu (Collective Commentaries on Classics of Materia Medica)* listed the antognized medicinal examples, including "Gancao compatibe with Gansui" "Renshen antagonism Lilu (veratrum Nigrum)" and "Wutou anti Beimu". There are 19 species involved (Wuhui and Wutou counting as one species), which are the same as the later popularized " eighteen antagonisms " involved in medicinals. In the Jin Yuan Dynasties, The characters of " eighteen antagonisms-songs" written by Zhang Congzheng in *Rumen Shiqin (Confucian Family Affairs)* are concise and easy to remember, which have been handed down to this day.In Ming dynasty, Liu Chun's *Yijing Xiaoxue (Medical Classics Primary School)* is the earliest record of "nineteen antagonisms".

目前，一般认为"十八反"中各药对之间的配伍关系均为"相反"，而且"十八反"是相反配伍的主体，不仅是约定俗成、共同认可的配伍禁忌，而且为《中华人民共和国药典》认可，而成为法定配伍禁忌。此外，《中国药典》（2015年版，一部）还规定："十八反"中，不宜与乌头同用的药扩大为不宜与乌头类药材同用；附子不宜与半夏、瓜蒌、贝母、白及同用；人参叶、北沙参、党参均不宜与藜芦同用；平贝母、伊贝母、浙贝母均不宜与乌头类药材同用。至于"十九畏"中各药对之间究竟存在何种"七情"关系，至今尚未形成统一认识。但目前"十九畏"同"十八反"一样，成为约定俗成，共同认可的配伍禁忌。"十九畏"中部分内容亦为《中国药典》认可，而成为法定配伍禁忌。

At present, it is generally believed that the combination relationship of the medicinal pairs in the "eighteen antagonisms" is "mutual antagonism", and the "eighteen antagonisms" is not only conventional and commonly recognized combination contraindications, but also a legal contraindication confirmed by the *Pharmacopoeia of the People's Republic of China*. In addition, the *Pharmacopoeia of the People's Republic of China (Part One)* stipulates that: in the "eighteen antagonisms", the medicinals that are not suitable for use with Wutou are expanded to be unsuitable for use with Aconiti Radix homologues. Fuzi is not suitable for use with Banxia, Gualou (Trichosanthis Fructus), Chuanbeimu, and Baiji. Renshenye (Ginseng Polium), Beishashen (Glehniae Radix), Dangshen should not be used together with Lilu. Pingbeimu (Fritillariae Ussuriensis Bulbus), Yibeimu (Fritillariae Pallidiflorae Bulbus), Zhebeimu should not be used together with Aconiti Radix homologues. As to what kind of "qiqing (seven-emotion)" relationship exists in the medicinal pairs in "nineteen antagonisms", there is not a uniform understanding yet. However, the "nineteen antagonisms" like the "eighteen antagonisms" have become a commonly recognized combination contraindication. Part content of "nineteen antagonisms" is recorded in the Pharmacopoeia of the People's Republic of China, and has become a legally stipulated combination contraindication.

2. 配伍禁忌的相对性 从七情的角度而言，"相恶"会降低治疗效应，"相反"会增强不良反应，均应列入配伍禁忌。然配伍禁忌是有条件的，具有相对性。将"相恶""相反"列为配伍禁忌的本意是强调配伍用药时，应尽量避免或杜绝减低治疗效应、增强不良反应的情况发生，而不是在任何条件下都禁止配伍使用。如《本草新编》在人参项下强调"人参恶莱菔子"，又于莱菔子项下提出"莱菔子得人参其功更神"，是配伍禁忌具有相对性的典型例证。前者是将人参用于单纯气虚之证，莱菔子有耗气之弊，会影响人参补气之功，因此两者相恶；后者是针对气虚患者食积气滞之证，但用人参无益于食积气滞，但用莱菔子又有更虚其气之虞。两者合用，既消食行气，又补益其虚，相辅相成。此时，人参与莱菔子同用，并非相恶，而属于"相畏相杀"的关系。

2.2.2 Relativity of Compatibility Contraindications

From the point of view of "seven emotions", "mutual inhibition" will reduce the therapeutic effects, and "mutual antagonism" will enhance adverse reactions, which should be all included in the compatibility contraindications. However, compatibility taboos are conditional and relative. "Mutual inhibition" and "mutual antagonism" being listed as compatibility contraindications is to emphasize that compatibility contraindications should be avoided or eliminated, to enhance the occurrence of adverse reactions, rather than prohibiting using these combinations under any conditions. For example, in the *Bencao Xinbian (Renew Materia Medica)* it is emphasized that "Renshen and Laifuzi are incompatible" when described the Renshen, but it is proposed that "Laifuzi exerts greater efficacy combined with Renshen" when described the Renshen. This is a typical example to show the relativity of combination contraindications. The former used Renshen for the qi-deficiency syndrome. Laifuzi has the disadvantage of consuming qi, which will affect the tonifying qi function of Renshen, so they are the mutual inhibition. The latter is for the stagnation of food and qi syndromes in qi deficiency patients. Renshen is useless to food accumulation and qi stagnation. Although Laifuzi can alleviate them, it will aggravate the deficiency of qi. Combination of the two, not only eliminates food and promotes qi, but also replenishes its deficiency and complements each other. However, these problems can be solved by combination of the two medicinals. At this time, the combination is not mutual inhibition, but belongs to the relationship of "mutual restraint or suppression"

基于以上配伍禁忌相对性的理解，可以认为：配伍禁忌既不应局限于"十八反"、"十九畏"所涉药物，亦不宜盲目扩大范围；"十八反"、"十九畏"所涉药物，既非百无禁忌，亦不是绝对不能配伍使用的。但十八反、十九畏所涉药对已然成为约定俗成且为《中国药典》认可的配伍禁忌，使这些本不属于绝对配伍禁忌的药对应用受到限制。当前为弄清这些药对的七情关系，特别是是否具有相反配伍关系，药对相反的特定条件及可能产生的不良后果，已开展了大量研究，尚待得出科学的结论。多版全国高等医药院校中医中药专业《中药学》教材和《中国药典》都曾有扩大十八反内容的现象存在：将与半、蒌、贝、蔹、及相反的乌头扩大到"乌头类"；将"十八反歌"中的"诸参"由五参扩大到八参。特别是往反藜芦的"诸参"中加入北沙参、西洋参、党参实无依据：这三参是清代以后才正式入药的，金元时期编成的"十八反"歌诀中的"诸参"不可能包括它们。

Based on the understanding of the relativity of compatibility contraindications, it can be considered that the compatibility contraindications should neither be limited to the medicinals involved in "eighteen antagonisms" and "nineteen incompatibilities", nor be blindly expanded. These medicines in "eighteen antagonisms" and "nineteen mutual inhibitions" are not absolutely incompatible. Because the medicinals involved in "eighteen antagonisms" and "nineteen incompatibilities" have already accepted by the popular and the official, the application of these incompatible contraindications is restricted. A lot of research has been carried out to clarify the "seven emotions" of these medicinal pairs, especially whether they have mutual antagonism relationships, specific conditions that mutual antagonism appears, and possible adverse consequences. Scientific conclusions have not been drawn. Several versions of the textbook Traditional Chinese Medicine used in Chinese medicine specialty in medicinal colleges and universities and the *Pharmacopoeia of the People's Republic of China* expanded the contents of "eighteen antagonisms". The medicines that were not suitable for use with Wutou are expanded to be unsuitable for use with Aconiti Radix homologues. "Various Ginsengs" in the "eighteen antagonisms-song" is expanded from five to eight kinds. In particular, Beishashen, Xiyangshen, and Dangshen were added into the "Various Ginsengs" which are incompatible with Lilu. This is lack of evidence, because these three medicinals were used as medicinals until the Qing Dynasty. It's impossible to include them in "eighteen antagonisms-song" wrote during the Jin and Yuan Dynasties.

（三）妊娠用药禁忌

2.3 Contraindications for Pregnancy

妊娠用药禁忌，主要讨论妇女妊娠期，除中断妊娠以外，禁忌使用的药物。

Contraindications for pregnancy, mainly discusses the medicinals that are prohibited to use for pregnant woman, except medicinals for the interruption of pregnancy.

1. 妊娠用药禁忌溯源 古代医药家很早就对妊娠用药禁忌有所认识，《神农本草经》记载具堕胎作用的药6种。《本草经集注》中设"堕胎"项，载堕胎药41种。此后历代本草对堕胎药多有补充。至《证类本草》达55种，《本草纲目》增至72种。虽然《神农本草经》《本草经集注》中并无"妊娠禁忌药"的提法，但从历史的角度来说，在我国古代堕胎是违反传统道德观念的，所以前人记载堕胎药，除用以催生、下死胎外，可能主要还是从妊娠禁忌的角度来认识、对待堕胎药的。故《神农本草经》应是最早记录妊娠禁忌药者。现存文献最早汇集妊娠禁忌药者当属南宋·朱端章《卫生家宝产科备要》，列举产前所忌药物78种。明·缪希雍《炮炙大法》列举妊娠禁服药92种。20世纪初，陆晋笙据《沈尧封女科辑要》增补本收入妊娠用药禁忌124种；至《全国中草药汇编》《中药大辞典》分别记载妊娠禁用或慎用药196种和365种。随着对妊娠禁忌药的认识不断发展，妊娠禁忌药的数量可能还会增多。

2.3.1 Source of Contraindications for Pregnancy

Ancient Chinese medical practitioners understood early contraindications for pregnancy. *Shennong Bencao Jing (Shennong's Classic of Materia Medica)* described 6 medicines that have the abortion effect. The *Bencaojing Jizhu (Collective Commentaries on Classics of Materia Medica)* contained the "Abortion" item in the content, which contains 41 kinds of abortion medicines. Since then, many abortion medicines were supplemented into ancient materia medica. There are 55 kinds in *Zhenglei Bencao (Materia Medica Arranged According to Pattern)*, and 72 kinds of medicinals were added into *Bencao Gangmu (Compendium of Materia Medica)*. The *Shennong Bencao Jing (Shennong's Classic of Materia Medica)* and the *Bencaojing Jizhu (Collective Commentaries on Classics of Materia Medica)* do not contain a term of "the medicinals that are prohibited in pregnancy". Abortion in ancient China was against traditional moral concepts in a historical perspective. Therefore, the predecessors recorded abortion medicines was used to induce birth and stillbirth, it may be mainly used to understand and treat abortion medicine from the perspective of pregnancy contraindications. Therefore, *Shennong Bencao Jing (Shennong's Classic of Materia Medica)* might be the earliest record of contraindications for pregnancy. The earliest existing literature on contraindications for pregnancy is Zhu Duanzhang's *Weisheng Jiabao Chanke Beiyao (Treasured Household Prescriptions for Health)* in Southern Song Dynasty, which lists 78 types of prenatal contraindications. In the *Paozhidafa (Main Solution of Processing)* wrote by Miu Xiyong in Ming Dynasty, 92 kinds of medicines forbidden during pregnancy were recorded. In the beginning of the 20th century, Lu Jinsheng added 124 contraindications for pregnancy according to the *Shen Yaofeng Nvke Jiyao (Shen Yaofeng's Collection of Women's Studies)* Supplement. The *Quanguo Zhongcaoyao Huibian* and the *Traditional Chinese Medicine Dictionary* contained 196 and 365 contraindications for pregnancy, respectively.

With the development of understanding on contraindications for pregnancy, the number of contraindications may increase.

2. **妊娠用药禁忌内容**　妊娠禁忌药除禁用具体药物外，前人还从功效、药性的角度提出妊娠用药应忌破气、破血、升散、辛热、辛燥之药（《本草汇》）。还主张勿犯金石，勿近毒药，大热、大燥、大攻、大表、大寒、大凉、走窜、迅疾、泄利之品，咸宜禁止（《产孕集》）。近代则多根据临床应用实际，将妊娠禁忌药分为禁用与慎用两大类。妊娠禁用药多系剧毒药，或堕胎作用强的药，及药性作用峻猛之品，包括砒霜、水银、雄黄、轻粉、斑蝥、马钱子、蟾酥、川乌、草乌、藜芦、胆矾、瓜蒂、巴豆、甘遂、大戟、芫花、牵牛子、商陆、麝香、干漆、水蛭、虻虫、三棱、莪术等。妊娠慎用药则主要是部分活血化瘀药、行气药、攻下药、温里药，包括牛膝、川芎、红花、桃仁、姜黄、牡丹皮、枳实、枳壳、大黄、番泻叶、芦荟、芒硝、附子、肉桂等。

2.3.2 The Contents of Contraindications for Pregnancy

In addition to the specific contraindication medicinals for pregnancy, predecessors proposed that pregnancy contraindications from perspective of efficacy and medicinal properties. During pregnancy, the medicinals with characteristics like breaking qi, breaking blood, ascending, dispersing, pungent heat, and pungent dryness, should be prohibited to use, which is recorded in *Bencao Hui (Treasury of Words on Materia Medica)*. It was also advocated that we should neither use mineral medicinals with metal nature, nor use toxic medicinals with strong properties, such as extremely hot, dry, offensive, exterior, cold, extreme cold, migratory, quick, purgative products [*Chanyun Ji (Maternity and Pregnancy Collection)*]. In modern times, according to the actual clinical application, pregnancy contraindication medicinals are mainly divided into two categories, the forbidden one and the one used with caution. The forbidden-used medicinals during pregnancy are mostly highly toxic ones, or medicinals with strong abortion effects, or medicinals with drastic properties, including Pishuang, Shuiyin (Hydrargyrum), Xionghuang, Qingfen (Calomelas), Banmao, Maqianzi, Chansu (Bufonis Venenum), Chuanwu, Caowu, Lilu, Danfan (Blue Vitriol), Guadi (Melo Pedicellus), Badou, Gansui, Daji (Cirsii Japonici Herba), Yuanhua, Qianniuzi (Pharbitidis Semen), Shanglu (Phytolaccae Radix), Shexiang, Ganqi (Toxicodendri Resina), Shuizhi (Hirudo), Mengchong (Tabanus), Sanleng (Sparganii Rhizoma), Ezhu (Curcumae Rhizoma), etc.. Medicinals for pregnancy used with caution are mainly including medicinals that promote blood circulation to dispel blood stasis, medicinals that regulate the qi, downward-draining medicinals, and medicinals that warm the interior, such as Niuxi, Chuanxiong, Honghua, Taoren (Persicae Semen), Jianghuang (Curcumae Longae Rhizoma), Mudanpi (Moutan Cortex), Zhishi, Zhiqiao (Aurantii Fructus), Dahuang, Fanxieye (Sennae Folium), Luhui, Mangxiao, Fuzi, Rougui, etc..

3. **妊娠用药禁忌依据**　引起堕胎是早期妊娠用药禁忌的主要依据。此外，有的药还可能因不利于孕妇，或不利于胎儿，或不利于产程而列入。近年的相关研究揭示了妊娠妇女禁用或慎用某些中药的科学依据。如砒霜、水银、轻粉、斑蝥等属剧毒药，对孕妇及胎儿损伤极大；巴豆、牵牛子、甘遂、大戟、芫花、大黄等峻下泻利之品，能造成盆腔充血，甚至堕胎；麝香、红花、牛膝、姜黄等对妊娠子宫有兴奋收缩作用，可能引起流产；莪术、牡丹皮、雄黄等药具有抗早孕作用；甘遂、水蛭、姜黄等药具有终止妊娠作用；桃仁、杏仁、郁李仁、苦参等所含的某些活性成分有致畸胎作用。

2.3.3 The Basis of Contraindications for Pregnancy

Abortion-induced is the main basis of judging medication contraindications in early pregnancy. In addition, some medicinals are included because they are not good for pregnant women, the fetus, or stages of labor.

Relevant studies in recent years have revealed the scientific basis for forbidden or careful-used Chinese medicinals in pregnant women, such as Pishuang, Shuiyin, Qingfen, Banmao, etc.. Those are highly toxic medicinals, which can cause great damage to pregnant women and fetuses. Badou, Qianniuzi, Gansui, Daji, Yuanhua, Dahuang and other downward-draining medicinals can cause intrapelvic venous congestion, and even cause abortion. Shexiang, Honghua, Niuxi, Jianghuang, etc., can stimulate the contraction of the pregnant uterus, which may cause miscarriage. Ezhu, Mudanpi, Xionghuang, and other medicinals have anti-pregnant effects. Gansui (Kansui Radix), Shuizhi (Hirudo), Jianghuang and other medicinals can terminate pregnancy. Some active ingredients in Taoren, Xingren, Yuliren (Pruni Semen), Kushen, etc., have teratogenic effects.

综上，在历代文献提出的众多妊娠禁忌药中，是否应该全部列入禁忌，值得商榷。但其中确有一些药物被证明可能对妊娠产生危害，应给予足够重视，尽量避免使用。

In summary, it is worth to further study that whether all of the contraindicative medicinals for pregnancy proposed in the literature in the past should be listed as contraindications. However, sufficient attention should be given to those medicinals have been shown to be harmful to pregnancy, which should be avoided to use.

（三）服药食忌

2.4 Contraindications for Food taking

服药食忌，指服用药品时对某些食物的禁忌，俗称忌口。

Contraindications for food refer to diatary contraindications when taking some medicinals, commonly known as food taboo.

1. 服药食忌溯源 汉·张仲景《金匮要略·禽兽虫鱼禁忌并治第二十四》云："所食之味，有与病相宜，有与身为害，若得宜则益体，害则成疾，以此致危，例皆难疗。"《伤寒论》于

桂枝汤方后注明："禁生冷、粘滑、肉面、五辛、酒酪、臭恶等物。"现存本草中，最早记载服药食忌的是南朝梁代《本草经集注》。《本草经集注》云："服药不可多食肥猪、犬肉、肥羹及鱼臊脍"，指出了在服药期间一般应忌食生冷、油腻、腥膻、有刺激性食物。

2.4.1 Traceability on Contraindications for Food

It is described in *Jingui Yaolue, Qinshou Chongyu Jinji Bingzhi Twenty-fourth (Synopsis of Golden Chamber)* writtern by Zhang Zhongjing in Han Dynasty that the food taken could be good for the disease, or harm the body; the good food will benefit body, while the bad one will cause disease, even danger, or difficulty to cure. In latter part of Guizhi Tang (Decoction) in *Shanghan Zabing Lun*, it is noted that the crude, the cold, the sticky, meat, flour, five acrid flavouring, liquor, butter, the smelly and other foodstuffs are forbidden after taking Guizhi Tang (Decoction). Among the existing herbal books, the *Bencaojing Jizhu* in the Liang of Southern Dynasties is the earliest book that it documented food taboo of taking medicinals. The original description in *Bencaojing Jizhu* [*(Collective Commentaries on Classics of Materia Medica)* recorded that fat pork, dog meat, fat soup and fish maw were forbidden to have too much when taking medicinals. It also pointed out that crude, cold, greasy, fishy, and irritating foodstuffs should be avoided when taking medicines.

2. 服药食忌依据 古代文献中有关服药食忌的理由大致可归纳为：诱发药物的不良反应、影响疗效、加剧病情、导致新病。虽然这些解释大多缺乏科学依据，但服药期间需要避免进食某些食物还是有一定道理的。首先，某些食物本身亦为药用，食物与药物之间可能存在相恶或相反的配伍关系。如服皂矾应忌茶，因为皂矾为低价铁盐，遇茶中的鞣质易生成不溶于水的鞣酸铁，失去原有疗效。其次，生冷、多脂、黏腻、腥臭等食物会妨碍脾胃功能，而影响药物的吸收。其

三，某些食物对某些病证不利，亦会影响药物的疗效。如生冷食物对脾胃虚寒证不利；辛热食物对热证不利；食油过多，会加重发热症状；食盐过多，会加重水肿。

2.4.2 The Basis of Contraindications for Food taking

The reasons for food taboo of taking medicines in ancient literature can be roughly summarized as follows, inducing adverse reactions, affecting curative effects, exacerbating conditions, and causing new diseases. Although most of these explanations lacked scientific evidence, it is reasonable to avoid eating certain foodstuffs while taking medicinals. First of all, some foods are also medicinal in nature, and there may be an inhibitory or antagonizing relationship between the food and medicinals. Tea should be avoided if taking Zaofan (Alum Soap), because Zaofan, a low-cost iron salt, easily generates water-insoluble iron tannate when reacting with tannin in tea, thereby losing its original curative effect. Secondly, cold, fatty, sticky, and stinky foods can attenuate the functions of the spleen and stomach resulting in the absorption obstacle of medicines. Thirdly, some foods are not good for certain diseases and symptoms, and will affect the efficacy of the medicinals. For example, crude and cold foodstuffs are unfavorable for spleen and stomach deficiency syndrome; Spicy and hot food is not good for heat syndrome; too much oil can aggravate fever symptoms; too much salt can worsen edema.

三、中药的剂量
3 Dosage of Chinese Medicinals

（一）剂量的含义
3.1 The Meaning of Dosage

剂量即药剂的用量。中药大多是以复方制剂应用，因此，中药的剂量实际包括单味药的常用有效量、方剂中各药的相对用量、药物的实际利用量三方面含义。

A dosage is the amount of medicine. Therefore, the dosage of Chinese medicinals actually includes 3 meanings, the commonly useful effective amount of a single medicine, the relative amount of each medicine in a prescription, and the actual utilization of a medicine.

1. 单味药的常用有效量　为了使临床用药有效而安全，必须把单味药的用量规定在一定范围内。一般中药文献中各具体药物用量项下所标用量，除特别注明的以外，都是指干燥饮片在汤剂中，成人一天内服的常用有效量。这是临床确定单味药用量时的参考依据。

3.1.1 A Commonly Used Effective Dosage of Single Medicinal

To maximize the efficacy and ensure the clinical safety, the dosage of single medicinal must be specified within a certain range. Except for some limited special situations, the standard dosages marked for medicinals was recorded in the literatures of Chinese medicinals, refers to the commonly useful effective amount of dried medicinals decoction slices, orally taken by an adult per day. This is the reference basis for determination of single-dosage medicinal amount in clinics.

2. 方剂中各药的相对用量　在方剂中，单味药的剂量还涉及对其他药物作用的影响，以及与其他药物配合后产生共同效应的需要量。临床处方用药，应注意使方剂中药物与药物之间在用量方面符合一定的比例，以适应病情的需要。一般来说，复方中主要药物的用量可较大，辅助性药物的用量可较小。

3.1.2 The Relative Dosage of each Medicinal in Prescriptions

In prescriptions, the dosage of each medicinal also depends on its effect on other medicines, and the required amount for producing a common effect when combined with other medicines. For clinical prescriptions, we should notice that the dosage of medicinals must be in a certain proportion in order to meet the needs of disease. In general, the dosage of the main medicinals in compound can be used in large quantities, and the dosage of the auxiliary medicinals can be used in small quantities.

3. 药物的实际利用量　由于药材质量、炮制、剂型、制剂、服法等多种因素的影响，同一味药，药用剂量相同，其实际利用量却有可能不同（这里主要从生物活性物质的角度而言）。临床用药和评价药物疗效时，应充分考虑到各种因素对实际利用量的影响。

3.1.3 Actual Dosage of a Medicinal

Due to various factors such as the quality of medicinal materials, processing, pharmaceutical forms, preparations, and methods of administration, the actual utilization amount may be different in the same medicinal with the same dose (Here we elaborates it mainly from the perspective of biologically active substances). For the clinical application and the efficacy evaluation, the various factors that affect the actual utilization should be fully considered.

（二）计量单位

3.2 Unit of Measurement

中药的计量，古代曾用长度、容量、重量等多种计量方法量取不同药物。

Methods for the measurement of Chinese medicinals, such as length, capacity and weight were used in ancient China.

常用长度单位有寸、尺。其进制是 10 寸为 1 尺。中药以长度计量，主要是在汉方、晋方中应用。因以长度计量药物准确性差，随着历史发展，长度在中药剂量表示中渐趋消失。

Common length units are cun (寸, cùn) and chi (尺, chǐ), and 10 cun is equal to 1 chi. This length measurement method for Chinese medicinals was mainly used in Han and Jin Dynasty. Due to the poor accuracy, the method was gradually disappeared with the development of civilization.

古代容量单位有勺、合、升、斗、斛，其进制为：10 勺为 1 合，10 合为 1 升，10 升为 1 斗，10 斗为 1 斛（南宋曾改 5 斗为 1 斛）。唐以后的方书中，用容积表示剂量的渐少。

The ancient capacity units are shao (shao), ge (ge), sheng (sheng), dou (dou), and hu (hu). 10 shao is equal to 1 ge, 10 ge is equal to 1 sheng, 10 sheng is equal to 1 dou, 10 dou is equal to 1 hu (5 dou was equal to 1 hu in South Song Dynasty). In the recipes book after the Tang Dynasty, the method of volume measurement was rarely decreased.

古代药量衡制基本上分两类：宋以前用古制，即药称，亦即唐代的小称；宋以后则统一用国家规定的衡制，直到清代，很少变易。

Ancient system to measure the weight of medicinals was basically divided into 2 categories. Before the Song Dynasty, the weight was measured by medicine balance (yao cheng), also named minor balance in Tang Dynasty. After the Song Dynasty, state-stipulated standards weighing system (heng zhi) were used until the Qing Dynasty without obvious changes.

重量的计量单位，古代有黍、累、铢、分、两、斤。据文献记载，初唐铸开元钱时规定，每十钱重一两，以致晚唐时期，民间以一钱作为等于十分之一两的单位名称。五代时期，十钱为两，十分为钱之制，被官府确认为权衡定制，以代替以铢为单位的旧制。五代以后确定重量单位为毫、厘、分、钱、两、斤。其进制为 10 毫为 1 厘，10 厘为 1 分，10 分为 1 钱，10 钱为 1 两，16 两为 1 斤。

In aucient time, there were following units of measurement of weight like (shu), lei (lei), zhu (zhu), fen (fen), liang (liang), catty (jin). It is recorded that 10 qian (qian) was equal to 1 liang in Kaiyuan Reign Period in the early Tang Dynasty. The ancients regard 1 qian as one tenth of liang, and this unit was used in the Later Tang Dynasty. During the Five Dynasties period, 10 qian is equaled to 1 liang, and 10 fen is equaled to 1 qian. This was confirmed by the government as a trade-off standard to replace the zhu system used in previously. After the Five Dynasties, the weight units were determined as hao (hao), li (li), fen (fen), qian (qian), liang (liang), catty (jin). 10 hao is 1 li, 10 li is 1 fen, 10 fen is 1 qian, 10 qian is 1 liang, and

16 liang for 1 Jin.

宋以前的方书剂量，除特别标明大斤两者外，都可按每两14g计。宋以后至民国初年，法定衡制基本未变，都可按每两37g计。民国年间至中华人民共和国成立初期曾用市称：每市斤为500g，每斤16两，每两为31.25g。1956年6月25日国务院命令，市称改为十进制，每斤为10两，每两为50g。但中药调剂仍用每斤为16两的衡制。直至1984年2月27日国务院颁布《关于在我国统一实行法定计量单位的命令》，1986年7月1日起实施1984年6月9日国家计量局公布的《中华人民共和国法定计量单位使用方法》，全国才改为按十进制市称调配中药。

Before Song Dynasty, the dosage of medicinals in prescriptions was calculated by the rule that 1 liang was equal to 14g, except for the medicinals specifically marked for large dose. From the Song Dynasty to the beginning of the Republic of China, the statutory system of measurement remained basically unchanged, and 1 liang was equal to 37 g. From the Republic of China to the beginning of the founding of the People's Republic of China, the (wnit of Shi Cheng) was used: 500 g was equal to 1 Shi Cheng, 16 liang was equal to 1 Jin, and 31.25g was equal to 1 liang. Ordered by the State Council on June 25, 1956, the Shi Cheng cheng was changed to decimal, namely, 10 liang was equal to 1 Jin and 50g was equal to 1 liang. However, the dosage of Chinese medicinals still used the measurent that 16 liang was equal to 1 Jin. Until February 27, 1984, the State Council promulgated *the Order on the Unified Implementation of Legal Units of Measurement in the People's Republic of China.* Mean while, *the Using Methods of Legal Units of the People's Republic of China* promulgated by the National Metrology Bureau on June 9, 1984, was implemented from July 1, 1986. Since then, the decimal system was used wildly in Chinese medicinal measurement.

按国家计量局规定的"中药剂量（新旧市称与法定计量单位）的换算"：16两制1斤等于500g，1两为30g，1钱为3g，1分为0.3g。按此规定，累计16两只有480g，比规定的500g少20g，但由于处方剂量一般不用斤，影响不大。

According to the Conversion of Chinese medicine dosage (new and old Shi Cheng and legal unit of measurement) stipulated by the National Metrology Bureau, 1 Jin in 16 liang system is equal to 500g, 1 liang is 30g, 1 qian is 3g, and 1 fen is 0.3g. According to this standard, 16 liang is 480g, which is 20g less than the prescribed 500g. Nevertheless, medicinal weight above 1 Jin is rarely used in the prescription, so such a small weighting loss has little effect on the curative effect.

古代，除用度量、容量、重量等计量方法量取药物外，还用拟量、估量、数量等较粗略的计量方法量取药物，但因都很难保证剂量的准确性，逐渐为法定度量衡取代。

In ancient times, medicinals were also measured by rougher methods such as mimic quantity, estimation, and number, except for length, capacity, and weight. However, due to the lack of accuracy of dosage, these methods had gradually replaced by legal metrology.

（三）确定剂量的依据

3.3 The Basis for Determining Dosage

各种中药书籍中所标中药的剂量均为参考用量，临床应用时加减幅度较大。除峻烈药、毒性药和某些精制药外，一般中药的干燥品或炮制品入汤剂时成人一日内服的常用有效量为5~10g。部分常用量较大的药为15~20g。临床上主要依据所用药物的特性，临床应用的需要，以及患者的具体情况来确定用量。

The dosage listed in various Chinese materia medica books is a reference dose, and the modified clinical dosage of medicinals varies greatly. Except the medicinals of drastic medicinals, toxic medicinals, or purified medicinals, the common effective dosage of dried or processed products for adults in a day is 5~10g. Some in a larger dose of commonly medicinals are 15~20g. Clinically, the dosage depends on the properties of used medicinals, the demands of clinical application, and the specific conditions of patients.

1. 药物方面 药材质量有优劣之分，质次者药力不足，用量可酌情加大。花叶类质地较轻的药用量宜轻，无毒药一般用量为3~10g；金石、贝壳类质重的药用量宜重，无毒药一般用量为10~30g；鲜品无毒药一般用量为30~60g。药性较弱，作用温和，药味较淡者，用量可稍重；药性较强，作用强烈，药味较浓者，用量则宜轻。常用有效剂量内无毒者用量可稍重；有毒者应将用量严格控制在安全范围内。

3.3.1 Medicinals Aspects

The quality of medicinal materials can be classified into good or bad. Medicinals with poor quality exerts insufficient efficacy, and the dosage should be increased. Medicinal materials such flowers and leaves with light quality should be used in a small dose, and the general dosage of non-toxic medicinals among them is 3~10g. Medicinal materials such as stones and shells with heavy quality should be used in a large dose. The general dosage of the non-toxic medicinals is 10-30g, and the general dosage of fresh products with non-toxic is 30~60g. The medicinals with weak properties, mild action and lighter taste and can be used in a biger dose. Namely, those medicinals with strong properties, action and thicker taste, should be used in a lighter dose. The commonly effective dosage of non-toxic medicinals can be slightly heavier, or else should be strictly controlled in a safe range.

2. 应用方面 单味应用时用量可较大；入复方时用量可略小。同一药物在复方中做主药时一般较之做辅药用量为重。多数药物作汤剂用量一般较之作丸、散剂时的服用量为重。同一药物治疗目的不同，用量可能有异。如槟榔，用以消积、行气、利水时，常用剂量不过6~15g；而用以杀姜片虫、绦虫时，即需用到60~120g。

3.3.2 Application Aspects

The dosage can be larger when using single, and slightly smaller when combining with others.

The dosage for sovereign medicinal should be larger and the dosage for minister medicinal should be smaller in different prescriptions. The dosage of most medicinals used in decoctions is generally larger than that used as pills or powders. Different purposes of the same medicinal make the dosage vary. For example, Binglang is used to eliminate accumulation, activate the qi, promote urination, the commonly dosage is only 6~15g, and when it is used to kill fasciolopsiasis, tapeworms, 60~120g of Binglang should be used.

3. 患者方面 体质强壮者，用量可重；体质虚弱者，用量宜轻。小儿、老人对药物的耐受力较差，作用峻猛易伤正气的药物用量应低于青壮年的用药量。新病正气旺者，用量可重；久病正气虚者，用量宜轻。病急病重者，用量宜重；病缓病轻者用量宜轻。妇女在月经期、妊娠期，用活血化瘀、通经药用量不宜过大。

3.3.3 Patient Aspects

The large dosage should be used for those with strong constitution, the small dosage should be used for those with weak constitution. Children and the elderly are less tolerant to the medicine, and the medicine that acts violently and impairs qi easily can be used less than that of young adults. If the patient just falls ill with certain vitality, the medicinals can be used in a high dosage. If the patient is sick for a long time with the deficiency of vitality, the medicinals should be used in a low dosage. The medicinals in a high dosage should be used for patients who get sick fast and hard, and the medicinals in a low dosage should be used for those the syndromes are alleviated or light. The amount of medicinals with the efficacy of invigorating blood, dispelling blood stasis, and unblock the meridian should be used in an appropriate dose for women during menstruation or pregnancy.

此外，确定用药剂量还应考虑到季节、气候，以及患者居处的自然环境等方面的差异，充分权衡，力求安全效彰。

Additionally, determination of medicinal

dosage should also consider the differences in seasons, climate, and the environments where the patient lives. And full balance of these factors can make safety and effectiveness.

四、中药的用法
4 Administration of Chinese Medicinals

（一）中药的给药途径
4.1 Administration Route of Chinese Medicinals

给药途径的选择是影响中药疗效的重要因素之一。中药的传统给药途径，除口服和皮肤给药两种主要途径外，还有吸入、舌下给药、直肠给药、鼻腔给药、阴道给药等多种途径。现代又增添了皮下注射、肌内注射、穴位注射和静脉注射等。

The choice of the route of administration is one of the important factors affecting the efficacy of Chinese medicinal. In addition to the oral and dermal administration, there are various routes, including inhalation, sublingual administration, rectal administration, nasal administration, and vaginal administration. In modern medicine, subcutaneous, intramuscular, acupoint and intravenous injections are added.

1. 口服给药 口服是中药应用最广泛的给药途径，具有简便、安全等优点。但诸如昏迷患者不能主动吞服，部分药物消化道刺激较大，小儿依从性差等因素也使口服给药受到一定的限制。

4.1.1 Oral Administration

Oral administration is the most widely used route of administration of Chinese medicinal, which has the advantages of simplicity and safety. But factors such as unconscious patients cannot swallow initiatively, some medicines have great irritation for digestive tract, and poor compliance for children, etc, also make certain restrictions on oral administration.

2. 皮肤给药 皮肤给药不仅可以发挥局部作用，也可被吸收而产生全身作用。清代医家吴师机认为外治法与内治法有"殊途同归"之妙，

"内外可以同效"。在传统的皮肤给药方法中，除在病变部位施治外，还主张循经络穴位涂、贴、灸、熨。如涂足心引上病而下之以降火，用治口疮、鼻衄、头痛；贴肚脐以通壅闭，疗大小便不通等，颇具特色，也极有效验。

4.1.2 Transdermal Administration

Transdermal administration can not only exert a local effect, but also be absorbed to produce a systemic effect. Wu Shiji, a doctor in the Qing Dynasty, believed that both external and internal therapies achieve the same effects internally and externally had the same purpose, and they could achieve the same effects internally and externally. Traditional methods of dermal administration like smearing, pasting, moxibustion, and ironing on the meridian points were proposed to apply clinically, not only treating at the local diseased area, but also long the meridians. For instance, coating medicinals on the sole of the foot can guide the upper fire purging downward, which is applied to aphtha, epistaxis, and headache. Pasting medicinals on the navel can open the blockage to treat constipation and urinary obstruction. These treatment methods are quite unique and very effective.

皮肤给药具有以下优点：影响中药的吸收速度及吸收量的因素较口服给药少，能够维持较恒定持久的血药浓度；可避免肝脏的首过效应；避免口服药消化道刺激及注射给药的潜在危险；可减少给药次数，方便患者；皮肤给药一旦感觉不适，可方便除去而保证用药安全。还有研究表明，通过皮肤给药治疗内脏或全身疾病，宜在耳背部、脐部、穴位施药。因耳背部、脐部皮下脂肪少，角质层薄，血液供应丰富，药物容易透皮吸收。而在穴位体表用药，除可通过局部皮肤吸收药物外，还可通过药物对穴位的刺激，产生类似针灸的特殊治疗作用。

Skin administration has the following advantages. Fewer factors affect the absorption rate and amount of dermal administration than that of oral administration, which can maintain a relatively constant concentration of medicinals in blood. Skin administration can avoid the first-pass effect of the liver. It can avoid oral gastrointestinal irritation and potential dangers of the injection. Skin administration can reduce the frequency of administration, which is convenient for patients. Once the skin administration makes patient feeling uncomfortable, medicinals can be easily removed to ensure the medicinal administration safety. Other studies have shown that the medicinals administered subcutaneously through the back of ear, umbilical region, and acupoints for the treatment of visceral or systemic diseases can be easily absorbed, because of less fat, thin cuticle and abundant blood supply in these regions. Medicinals administered on the surface of the acupuncture points can not only be absorbed by the local skin, but also by the meridians, like acupuncture-similar effects through stimulus on the acupoints, producing special treatment similar to acupuncture.

3. **黏膜表面给药** 黏膜给药的范围较广，包括消化道、呼吸道和体腔给药。通常所说的黏膜给药主要是指为了产生局部作用的黏膜表面给药，如从眼结膜、口腔、咽喉、阴道和尿道给药等。但不可忽视的是，黏膜的吸收能力较强，常能产生吸收作用。如《备急千金要方》以巴豆霜吹喉，治疗喉闭痰涎壅盛；现代用滴鼻液治小儿高热等。

4.1.3 Mucosal Surface Administration

Mucosal administration ranges widely, including digestive, respiratory and body cavity administration. Generally speaking, the mucosal administration mainly refers to the administration of the mucosal surface that can produce local effects, such as administration from the conjunctiva, oral cavity, throat, vagina and urethra etc.. However, it cannot be ignored that the mucosa has a strong absorptive capacity and can absorb medicinals. For example, *Beiji Qianjin Yaofang* described that croton cream was blow to the throat to treat excessive phlegm and saliva induced by throat closure. In modern medicine, nasal drops are used to treat high fever in children.

黏膜的吸收能力强弱不一，鼻腔给药，更具特色。鼻腔黏膜表面积约为150cm²，黏膜下分

布着丰富的血管、毛细血管和毛细淋巴管网，黏膜上众多的细绒毛大大地增加了药物吸收的有效面积。且鼻腔与鼻旁窦、咽喉、口腔、耳、眼均有腔道相通，鼻腔给药，除可治疗鼻腔局部疾病外，还可以治疗鼻旁窦、咽喉、口腔、耳、眼乃至全身疾病。

The absorption capacity of the mucosa is different. Nasal administration is more distinctive. The nasal mucosa has surface area about 150 cm², and submucosa exerts abundant blood vessels, capillaries, and capillary lymphatic networks. Numerous villi on the mucosa greatly increase the effective area for medicine absorption. And the nasal cavity and the paranasal sinuses, throat, oral cavity, ears, eyes have channels communicated. Therefore, nasal administration, in addition to treating local nasal diseases, can also treat paranasal sinus, throat, mouth, ear, eye and even systemic diseases.

4. **直肠内给药** 直肠内给药在古代应用较局限，主要是蜂蜜、猪胆汁、土瓜根等用以通导大便。现在研究发现直肠内给药具有许多优点：避免药物对胃黏膜的刺激；避免消化液中酸碱度、酶类对药物的影响和破坏作用；通过直肠黏膜吸收的药物有50%~70%可避免肝脏的首过效应；直肠给药比口服给药吸收影响因素少，吸收更有规律；药物作用时间较口服给药更长。基于以上认识，近年直肠内给药应用范围有所扩大，如治疗急性肾衰竭采用直肠灌注给药，疗效比口服更佳。

4.1.4 Rectal Administration

In ancient times, application of rectal administration was limited anciontly. Usually, Honey, Zhudanzhi (Sus Scrofa Domestica Brisson), and Tugua Gen (Trichosanthes Radix) are used to remove the bowels. Modern studies have found that there are many advantages of rectal administration, such as, avoiding the irritation for gastric mucosa; avoiding the influence and destructive actions produced by pH values and enzymes in the digestive juice on medicinals; about 50% - 70% of medicinals can avoid the liver first pass effect; rectal administration has less influential factors for absorption and more regular absorption than oral administration, and the medicinals of rectal administration can act longer than that of oral administration. Based on the above knowledge, the scope of rectal administration has expanded in recent years. For example, rectal perfusion is used to treat acute renal failure, and the effect is better than that of oral administration.

5. 舌下给药 舌下给药是黏膜表面给药的一种特殊形式。早在东汉《金匮要略》就记载有将桂屑着舌下的用法。现代研究认为，舌下血管丰富，药物置于舌下可由口腔黏膜迅速吸收而发挥作用。舌下给药方法简便，且能避免药物被肝脏和胃肠消化液破坏。但舌下给药只适用于少数能被口腔黏膜吸收的药物。如近代将麝香做成丸剂舌下含服，治疗冠心病可收速效。

4.1.5 Sublingual Administration

Sublingual administration is a special form of mucosal surface administration. As early as in the Eastern Han Dynasty, the *Jingui Yaolue* recorded that put the cinnamon scraps under the tongue. Modern research suggests that sublingual capillaries are abundant, and medicines placed under the tongue can be quickly absorbed by the oral mucosa and then exert the therapeutic effect. The method of sublingual administration is simple and can prevent the medicinals from being destroyed by the liver and gastrointestinal digestive fluid. However, sublingual administration is only suitable for a few medicinals that can be absorbed by the oral mucosa. For example, Shexiang is made into pills and absorbed through sublingual administration to treat coronary heart disease in modern times.

6. 吸入给药 呼吸道吸收面积大，毛细血管丰富、致密，药物吸收快，吸收速率仅次于静脉注射。受制剂条件等限制，古代吸入给药比较简单。或以烧烟吸入，如《外科十三方考》以洋金花等药合烟丝，如寻常吸烟法吸之治哮喘；或以芳香药物煎煮，吸入药物芳香之气以治鼻渊头痛或感冒鼻塞；或佩带香囊、香袋，吸入药气以辟秽防疫或醒脑强身。吸入气雾剂的出现，可将

中药呈雾状喷出，吸入给药，扩大了临床应用。

4.1.6 Inhalation Administration

The respiratory tract has a large absorption area, rich and dense capillaries, resulting the fast absorption rate, which is second to the intravenous injection. Due to the limitation of preparation conditions, ancient inhalation was relatively simple. Inhale burning smokes, recorded in *Waike Shisanfang Kao (Thirteen Prescriptions of Surgery)*, that Yangjinhua and other medicinals combined with tobacoo, slices was smoked to treat asthma. Inhale the aromatic flavor when decocting the aromatic medicinals to treat nasosinusitis, headache, cold and nasal obstruction. Inhale the aromatic smell by wear sachets to prevent epidemics or refresh the body. The emergence of inhalation aerosols allow Chinese medicinals spray in a mist form, which expands the clinical applications of Chinese medicinals.

7. 注射给药 中药做成注射剂给药的历史不长，注射给药具有吸收快、奏效快、作用强等特点。中药注射给药分皮下注射、肌内注射、静脉注射、穴位注射等方式。皮下注射是将药物注射于真皮与肌肉之间的松软组织内，皮下注射痛感明显，吸收较缓，中药制剂应用较少。肌内注射是将药物注射于肌肉组织中。肌肉血管丰富，药物吸收迅速；肌肉内神经末梢分布较少，注射刺激性较小，是目前应用较广的注射给药方式。静脉注射是将药物直接注射入静脉血管内，因不需经过吸收阶段，奏效迅速。为了使药物缓缓进入血流，以便较长时间维持药物在血中的浓度，可采用静脉滴注法。穴位注射是特殊的肌内注射，既可产生药物的全身治疗作用，亦可通过药物对特定穴位的刺激而产生类似针灸的特殊疗效。

4.1.7 Injection Administration

The history of Chinese medicinals by injection administration is not long. Injection administration is characterized by fast absorption, quick and strong effects. Chinese medicinals injection is divided into subcutaneous injection, intramuscular injection, intravenous injection and acupoint injection and other methods.

Subcutaneous injection means that medicines are inject into the soft tissue between the dermis and muscle. It brings obvious pain, has slow absorption, and are quite few applicable medicinal preparations. Intramuscular injection means that medicinals are injected into muscle tissues. Muscle has abundant blood vessels and the medicinal is absorbed quickly. Meanwhile, muscles have less nerve endings and smaller injection irritation, thus intramuscular injection is widely used currently. Intravenous injection is a method that a medicinals is directly injected into a venous vessel, which works quickly because it does not need to go through the absorption stage. To make the medicinals slowly enter the bloodstream, and maintain the concentration of the medicinals in the blood for a long time, an intravenous drip method can be used. Acupoint injection is a special intramuscular injection, by which medicinals can produce systemic therapeutic effects, and also can produce special effects similar to acupuncture by stimulating specific points.

（二）中药的煎煮方法

4.2 Decoction Methods of Chinese Medicinals

中药的疗效还与制剂工艺有着密切关系。中药汤剂目前仍然是中药临床应用的主要方式，且多由病家自制，若制不得法，自然会影响疗效与用药安全。为保证临床疗效与用药安全，应将汤剂的正确煎煮方法向病家交代清楚。

The efficacy of Chinese medicinals is also closely related to the preparation technology. Decoctions are still the main application form of Chinese medicinals, and mostly made by patients themselves. Improperly decocting will decrease the efficacy and medication safety. In order to ensure the clinical efficacy and medication safety, the correct method of decoction should be explained in details to the patients.

1. **煎煮器具** 煎药宜用砂锅、砂罐等陶瓷器具，其化学性质稳定，不易与药物成分发生化学反应，且导热均匀，保暖性能好。金属器具易与药液中的成分发生化学反应，可能使疗效降低，甚至产生毒副作用。

4.2.1 Decoction Appliance

Decoction should be performed in ceramics such as casseroles and pots. Their chemical properties are stable, not easy to react with the medicinal ingredients. Furthermore, ceramics have uniform heat conduction and good thermal performance. Metal pots are susceptible to have chemical reactions with the components in the medicinal solution, which may reduce the efficacy and even have toxic and side effects.

2. **煎药用水** 煎药用水须无异味，洁净澄清，含矿物质、杂质少。一般来说，凡人们生活上可饮用的水都可用以煎药。

4.2.2 Decoction Water

The water for decoction must have no odor, be clean and clear, and contain few minerals and no impurities. In general, all drinkable water can be used for decoction.

3. **加水量** 煎药加水用量宜适量。加水太少，药物有效成分溶解不充分，且容易干锅、熬焦。加水太多，煎时过长，部分有效成分可能被破坏。应根据饮片质地疏密、吸水性能、煎煮时间长短来确定加水多少。一般用水量为将饮片适当加压后，液面淹没过饮片约2厘米。质地坚硬、黏稠或需久煎的药，加水量可较一般药略多；质地疏松或有效成分易挥散，煎时较短的药，则液面淹没药物即可。

4.2.3 The Amount of Decoction Water

The amount of decoction water should be appropriate. Adding too little water, the active ingredients of the medicine are not fully dissolved, and it is easy to dry and be burned. It needs more time when adding too much water which cause the damage of active ingredients. The amount of water added depends on the texture of the pieces, the performance of water absorption, and the decoction time. After pressing the decoction pieces slightly, add water to make the liquid surface submerge the decoction pieces beyond about 2 cm. Medicines that are hard, sticky or need to be cooked for a long time can be added with more water than ordinary medicines. For medicines with loose textures, active ingredients that are easy to disperse, or medicines that need a short decoction time, it is appropriate to add water to just submerge the decoction pieces.

4. 煎前浸泡 煎煮前适当浸泡，有利于药物有效成分煎出。如饮片不经浸泡，直接加热煎煮，会因药物表面的淀粉、蛋白质膨胀，阻塞毛细管道，使水分难于进入饮片内部，饮片中有效成分又难向外扩散。多数药宜冷水或温水浸泡20~30分钟。

4.2.4 Soaking before Decoction

Appropriately soaking before decoction is conducive to boiling out the active ingredients of the medicine. If the decoction pieces are directly heated and boiled without being soaked, the starch and protein on the surface of the medicinals will swell to block the capillary channels. This phenomenon makes it difficult for water to enter the decoction pieces and for the active ingredients in the decoction pieces to diffuse outward. Most medicines should be soaked in cold or warm water for 20-30 minutes.

5. 煎煮火候 火候是指火力大小与煎煮时间长短。煎药一般宜先用武火使药液尽快煮沸，以节约时间；后用文火继续煎煮，以免药汁溢出，或过快熬干。解表药及其他含挥发性有效成分的药，宜用武火煎沸，改用文火维持20分钟。有效成分不易煎出的矿物、骨角、贝壳、甲壳类药，煮沸后宜文火久煎（60分钟左右），使有效成分充分溶出。一般药物煮沸后，改用文火维持30分钟即可。

4.2.5 Duration and Degree of Boiling

The duration and degree of heating refers to the strength of fire and the boiling time. The decoction should generally be boiled as soon as possible with Wuhuo (strong fire) to save time, then continue to cook with Wenhuo (mild fire) to prevent the juice from overflowing or drying too quickly. Antipyretics and other medicinals containing volatile active ingredients should be

boiled first with strong fire and replaced with mild fire for 20 minutes. Minerals, bone horns, shells, and crustaceans that are not easy to boil out the active ingredients, should be cooked with mild fire for a long time (about 60 minutes) after boiling, so that the active ingredients are fully dissolved. In general, after boiling, we switch to mild fire to cook for other 30 minutes.

6. 及时滤汁 中药煎好应趁热及时滤汁。药物溶解是个动态平衡过程，在药液温度降低时，有效成分又会反向渗入药渣，影响实际利用量。古人还主张汤剂煎成后要绞榨取汁以减少有效成分损失。有实验表明，从绞榨药渣中得到的有效成分约相当于原方含量的1/3。

4.2.6 Filter the Juice Timely

Filter the juice timely after decoction. Medicinal dissolution is a dynamic equilibrium process. When the temperature of the medicinal solution is lowered, the effective ingredients will infiltrate into the medicinal residues and affect the actual utilization. The ancients also advocated squeezing the residues to get more the remaining decoction, which can reduce the loss of effective ingredients. Experiments have shown that the effective ingredients obtained from the squeezed residue are equivalent to about 1/3 of the original content.

7. 煎煮次数 一般来说，一剂药可煎三次，最少煎两次。因煎药时，有效成分会先溶解在进入药材组织内的水液中，然后再通过分子运动扩散到药材外部的水液中。当药材内外溶液的浓度达到平衡时，因渗透压平衡，有效成分就不再扩散了，这时，只有将药液滤出，重新加水煎煮，有效成分才会继续溶解。有人测量发现，第二、三次煎液中仍有不少有效成分，若将二、三煎液合并，其煎出物总量还超过第一煎液。为了充分利用药材，避免浪费，一剂药最好煎煮三次。

4.2.7 Decoction Times

In general, one dosage of medicinals can be cooked three times, or at least twice. When decocting medicines, the active ingredients will dissolve in the water that enters the tissue of the medicinal material, and then diffuse into the water outside the medicinal material through molecular movement. When the concentration of the solution inside and outside the medicinal material reaches equilibrium, the active ingredient will no longer diffuse due to the osmotic pressure balance. At this time, the active ingredient will continue to dissolve only by filtering out the medicinal solution and re-cooking it with water. Some people have found that there are still many active ingredients in the second and third decoctions. If the second and third decoctions are combined, the total amount of active ingredients does exceed that in the first decoction. In order to make full use of medicinal materials and avoid waste, it is better to cook three times for one dose of medicines.

8. 特殊煎煮及入药方法

一般情况下中药可同时入煎。但部分药因其性状、性能、临床用途不同，其所需煎煮时间及入药方法亦有差异。兹分述如下：

4.2.8 Special Decoction and Treating Methods

Generally, Chinese medicinals can be cooked together at the same time. However, due to their different properties, and clinical uses, some medicinals require different decoction times and methods. It is described below.

（1）先煎 有效成分不容易煎出的药物与其他药物共作汤剂时，应先煎一定时间（具体时间因药而异）后，再入其他药同煎。一般来说，动物角、甲、壳类药（如水牛角、鹿角、龟甲、鳖甲、石决明、牡蛎、珍珠母等），矿物类药（如石膏、花蕊石、青礞石、磁石、紫石英等）大多需要先煎半小时左右。部分有毒植物药久煎可使其毒性降低，亦应先煎（制川、草乌，制附子宜先煎半小时以上至不麻口为度）以减低毒性。

(1) Decoct first (先煎, xiān jiān) When medicines whose active ingredients are not easy to decoctbeed are used decoctions with other medicines, together they should be in first decocted for a certain period of time (the specific time varies depending on the medicine), and then the other medicines should be decocted together. In general, animal horns, nails, and shell medicines [such as Shuiniujiao (Bubali Cornu), Lujiao (Cervi Cornu), Guijia, Biejia (Trionycis Carapax), Shijueming (Haliotidis Concha), Zhenzhumu (Margaritifera Concha), etc], mineral medicines [such as Shigao, Huaruishi (Ophicalcitum), Qingmengshi (Chloriti Lapis), Cishi (Magnetitum), Zishiying (Fluoritum), etc] need to be decocted for about half an hour before other medicines are put in. Some poisonous medicinals should be decocted for a long time to reduce their toxicities. Such as prepared Zhichuanwu (prepared Aconiti Radix), Zhicaowu (prepared Aconiti Kusnezoffii Radix), and Zhifuzi (prepared Aconiti Lateralis Radix Praeparata), they should be decocted for more than half an hour until removal of numb state.

（2）后下 含挥发性有效成分，久煎容易挥发散失的药（如金银花、连翘、鱼腥草、徐长卿、肉桂、沉香、檀香、降香、月季花及解表药、化湿药中的大部分药物）和有效成分不耐煎煮或久煎发生变化影响疗效的药（如青蒿、大黄、番泻叶、麦芽、钩藤、决明子等）宜后下微煎。

(2) Decoct later (后下, hòu xià) Medicinals containing volatile active ingredients, which can be easily lost after long time decoction such as Jinyinhua, Lianqiao (Forsythiae Fructus), Yuxingcao, Xuchangqing (Cynanchi Paniculati Radix et Rhizoma), Rougui, Chenxiang (Aquilariae Lignum Resinatum), Tanxiang (Santali Albi Lignum), Jiangxiang (Dalbergiae Odoriferae Lignum), Yuejihua (Rosae Chinensis Flos) and most of medicines that relieve exterior syndrome and medicines that resdving dampness and medicinals that are not resistant to long-time boiling such as Qinghao, Dahuang, Fanxieye, Maiya (Hordei Fructus Germinatus), Gouteng (Uncariae Ramulus cum Uncis), Juemingzi (Cassiae Semen), etc. All of them should be decocted latterly.

（3）包煎 药材有毛，漂浮液面不便煎煮的药（如辛夷、旋覆花等），药材呈粉末状或煎后容易使煎液混浊的药（如海金沙、蒲黄、儿茶、五灵脂等），及煎后药液黏稠，不便滤取药汁的药（如车前子等），作汤剂时都宜用纱布包裹入煎。

(3) Decocted in gauze (包煎, bāo jiān) Medicinal materials are hairy and easily float on liquid surface such as Xinyi (Magnoliae Flos), Xuanfuhua (Inulae Flos), etc.; The medicinal materials are powdery or the medicines are easy to muddle up the decoction such as Haijinsha (Lygodii Spora), Puhuang (Typhae Pollen), Ercha (Catechu), Wulingzhi (Trogopterori Faeces) etc.; Medicinals are sticky after decoction, which are not convenient for filtering the juice such as Cheqianzi (Plantaginis Semen), etc.; they should be wrapped in gauze and then decocted.

（4）另煎 贵重药材（如人参、西洋参、羚羊角等）作汤剂时，宜另煎取汁，以免煎出的有效成分被同剂中其他药物的药渣吸附，造成贵重药材的浪费。

(4) Decoct separately (另煎, lìng jiān) When decocting precious medicinal materials such as Renshen, Xiyangshen, Lingyangjiao, etc with others, it is advisable to decoct them separately, so as to avoid the effective ingredients are absorb by other, resulting in the waste of precious medicinals.

（5）烊化（加热熔化）胶类药材（如阿胶、鹿角胶、龟甲胶等）如与其他药同煎，容易粘锅、熬焦，还会黏附于其他药材上，既造成胶类药的浪费，又影响其他药的有效成分溶出，因此宜单独烊化兑服。

(5) Melt by heat (烊化, yáng huà) If gum medicinal materials such as Ejiao, Lujiaojiao, Guijiajiao (Testudinis Carapacis et Plastri Colla), etc. are decocted with other medicines, they will easily stick to the pan, burn, and stick to other medicinals, which leads to the waste of gum medicinals, and affects the dissolution of the active ingredients of other medicinals. So, they should be decocted separately.

（6）冲服 入水即化的药（如芒硝等），液汁类药（如竹沥、蜂蜜、饴糖等），及羚羊角、沉香等加水磨取的药汁，不需入煎，宜直接用开水或药汁冲服。

(6) Take drenched (冲服, chōng fú) Medicinals that are ready to dissolve in water such as Mangxiao, etc., liquid juice medicines such as Zhuli (Bamboo Leaches), Honey, Yitang (Saccharum Granorum), etc., and Lingyangjiao, Chenxiang, and other medicinals that are ground with water, they can be taken directly with water or juice without decocting.

（三）中药的服用方法

4.3 Medication time

口服是临床使用中药的主要给药途径，口服给药的效果，除受到剂型、制剂方法等因素的影响外，还与服药时间、服药的多少及服药的冷热等服药方法有关。

Oral administration is the main route of Chinese medicine in clinical. The effect of oral administration is not only affected by factors such as pharmaceutical form and preparation methods, but also related to time, amount, and the temperature of taking medicines.

1. 服药时间 适时服药，也是合理用药的重要方面，具体服药时间应根据胃肠的状况、病情的需要及药物特性来确定。空腹服药可避免与食物混合，能迅速入肠充分发挥药效。驱虫药、峻下逐水药、攻下药及其他治疗肠道疾病、需要在肠内保持较高浓度的药，宜空腹时服药。饭后胃中存有较多食物，药物与食物混合可减轻其对胃肠的刺激，故对胃肠道有刺激性的药物宜饭后服。消食药宜饭后及时服用，使药物与食物充分混合，以利充分发挥药效。一般药物无论饭前或饭后服，服药与进食都应间隔1小时左右，以免影响药物与食物的消化吸收及药效的发挥。此外，为了使药物能充分发挥作用，有的药还应在特定的时间服用：安神药用于安神安眠，宜在睡前半小时至1小时服药；缓下剂亦宜睡前服用，以便翌日清晨排便；涩精止遗药应晚间服药；急性病、呕吐、惊厥等则不拘时服药。

4.3.1 Time of medication Taken medicinal at the right time is also an important aspect of reasonable medicating. The specific time should be determined depending on the gastrointestinal conditions, the disease conditions, and the property of the medicinals. Taking medicinals on an empty stomach can avoid mixing medicinals with food, and enable medicinals quickly enter the intestine and achieve better therapeutic effects. Medicinals for expelling Parasites, downward-draining, purging and other medicinals that treat intestinal diseases should be taken on an empty stomach to keep a high concentration of medicinals in the intestine. Mixing medicinals with food can reduce its irritation to the gastrointestinal tract, so medicinals that are irritating to the gastrointestinal tract should be taken after meals. Digestant medicinals should be taken in time after meals, for mixing well with food can exert better efficacy. Whether the medicinal is taken before or after meals, the interval time between taking the medicinal and meals should be about 1 hour to avoid influencing on absorption and digestion of the medicinal or food, and the activity of the medicinal. In addition, to achieve better therapeutic effects, some medicinals should also be taken at specific time: tranquilizers are used for calming the spirit and promote good sleep and it should be taken half to one hour before bedtime. Purgative medicinals are taken before bedtime so as to make it easier to defecate in the next day. Medicinal for arresting nocturnal emission or spermatorrhea should be taken at night. Medicinals for acute illness, vomiting, and convulsions can be taken any necessary time.

2. 服药多少 一般疾病服药多采用每日一剂，每剂分两次或三次服。病情急重者，可每隔4小时左右服药一次，使药力持续，利于顿挫病势。应用发汗药、泻下药时，如药力较强，服药应适可而止，不必拘泥于定时服药。一般以得汗、得下为度，不必尽剂，以免汗下太过，损伤正气。

4.3.2 Amount of medication For common diseases, medicinals should be taken a dose per day, and two or three times for each dose. Those in serious condition can take the medicine every four hours to maintain a longer-persisting action of medicinals, which instantly frustrating the disease. When using sweating medicinals and purgative medicinals, in case their efficacy is strong, the medicine should be used flexibly, instead of not sticking to the fixed time. That is to say, once sweating and bowel moving onset, people should stop taking them although the decoction is not completed yet since too much sweating and purging can injury healthy qi.

3. 服药冷热 一般汤药多宜温服。但临床用药时，服药的冷热应具体分析，区别对待。如治寒证用热药宜于热服，特别是辛温发汗解表药用于外感风寒表实证，不仅药宜热服，服药后还需温覆取汗。至于治热病用寒药，如热在胃肠，患者欲冷饮者，可凉服；如热在其他脏腑，患者不欲冷饮者，寒药仍以温服为宜。对于丸、散等固体药剂，除特别规定者外，一般都宜用温开水送服。

4.3.3 Temperature of medication Generally, decoctions should be taking while being warm. However, the temperature of decoction-taking should be specifically analyzed. For example, hot-nature medicinals used to treat cold syndrome should be taken as they are hot. Particularly, the pungent warm exterior-releasing medicinals are used for treating wind cold exterior excessive syndrome; they should be taken while hot. Moreover, people should keep warm to facilitate sweating. As for cold medicinals used for treating hot syndrome, when heat is in the stomach and intestines, and patient are favor of the cold one, then the medicinals can be cool; if the heat is in other organs, and patients do not want to drink cold, the medicines should be warm. Pills, powders and other solid medicinals are generally taken with warm water, except for special provisions.

Section 2　Development of Chinese Medicinal Application

随着时代的变迁，社会的进步，医药知识日趋丰富，人们对中药应用的认识在传承与创新中不断发展。

With the changes of the times, the development of the society, and the enrichment of medical knowledge, the understanding of the application of Chinese medicinals continually develops in the process of inheritance and innovation.

一、古代本草论中药应用
1 Application of Chinese Medicinals in Ancient Materia Medica

先秦时期，开始发现并应用中药。先民在采食植物时候发现了植物药，在狩猎活动中，发现了动物药。原始社会后期，随着采矿和冶炼的产生，矿物药逐渐被发现并应用。

During the pre-Qin period, Chinese medicines were discovered and used. The ancestors discovered botanical medicine when getting foodstuffs from plants and animal medicine during hunting. In hunting activities, animal medicine was discovered. In the later period of primitive society, with the emergence of mining and smelting, mineral medicine was gradually discovered and applied.

殷商时期，酿酒技术的产生，促进了药物的使用，酒能温经、活血、助溶，被称为"百药之长"，将酒与药有机结合形成酒剂，方便药物的应用，提高药物的疗效，推动医药的发展。夏商时期，人们将药物用水煎煮后作为汤剂应用。西周时已有专业的"医师"。《诗经》《山海经》等书籍中均有植物和动物药物的记载。长沙马王堆汉墓出土的《五十二病方》是我国现存最古的医方书，载药240余种，方280多个，所治疾病涉及内、外、妇、儿、五官各科疾病，并记载有丸、散、膏、丹等成药的传统剂型。春秋战国时期《黄帝内经》是我国现存最早的医学典籍，该书奠定了中医理论的基础，收载成方13首，其中汤剂4首，其余9种为成药，包括丸、散、膏、丹、酒等多种剂型。

During the Yin Shang Dynasties, the production of liquor-making technology promoted the use of medicines. Wine can be used to warm channels, invigorate blood, and promote dissolving of the medicines. It is called "the leader of medicines". Formula generated from the combination of liquor and medicine can facilate the application of medicines and improve the efficacy of medicines and promote the development of medicine. In the Xia and Shang Dynasties, people used a decoction after boiling medicines with water. In Western Zhou Dynasty, there was a professional "physician". Plants and animal medicines were recorded in *Shi Jing* and *Shanhai Jing*. *Wushier Bingfang*, unearthed from the Mawangdui Han Tomb in Changsha, is the oldest existing medical book in China. It contains more than 240 kinds of medicinals and more than 280 prescriptions. The diseases involved internal, external, women, children, and the five sense organs (ears, eyes, lips, nose and tongue), and the traditional pharmaceutical forms of pills, powders, syrups, special or vermillion pills and other medicines were recorded. *Huang Di Nei Jing* written in the Spring and Autumn Period and the Warring States Period, is the earliest existing medical classics in China. This book lays the foundation of the theory of Chinese medicine, collects 13 prescriptions including 4 decoctions and 9 prepared medicines, such as pills, powders, syrups, special or vermillion pills, liquor and other pharmaceutical forms.

秦汉时期，人们对中药的认识进一步发展，并形成了详细的文字记载。《神农本草经》系统总结了汉以前的药学成就，是最早的药学专著，其"序例"部分初步奠定了药学理论的基础，载药365种，并记载了丸、散、膏、酒等多种成药剂型。东汉末年，张仲景《伤寒论》确立了中医理法方药辨证论治体系。《伤寒论》收载成方113首，其中成药11种，《金匮要略》收载成方258首，其中成药50余种，剂型有丸剂、散剂、酒剂、软膏剂、滴耳剂、洗剂、熏洗剂、灌肠剂、肛门栓剂、阴道栓剂等10余种。

During the Qin and Han Dynasties, the understanding of Chinese Medicinal was further developed, and detailed written records were formed. *Shennong Bencao Jing* systematically summarizes the pharmaceutical achievements before Han Dynasty, which is the earliest pharmaceutical monograph. Its prologue part preliminarily lays the foundation of pharmaceutical theory, containing 365 kinds of medicinals, and a variety of pharmaceutical forms, such as pills, powders, syrups, liquor, etc. In the late Eastern Han Dynasty, Zhang Zhongjing's *Shanghan Zabing Lun* established a syndrome differentiation and treatment system for Chinese medicine. This book contains 113 prescriptions, including 11 kinds of Chinese patent medicines. *Jingui Yaolue* contains 258 prescriptions, including more than 50 kinds of Chinese patent medicinals, and more than 10 forms of Chinese medicinals doses, such as pills, powders, liquor, ointments, ear drops, lotions, fumigants, enemas, anal suppositories, vaginal suppositories etc.

魏晋南北朝时期，对《神农本草经》认识有进一步拓展与补充。梁·陶弘景所辑《本草经集注》对《神农本草经》加以注释、发挥，补充了采收、鉴别、炮制、制剂等方面的理论和操作原则，增列了"诸病通用药""解百毒及金石等毒例""服药食忌例"等。此时诞生的《雷公炮炙论》是我国现存第一部炮制学专论。晋代葛洪《肘后备急方》首次提出"成剂药"概念，最先把成药列为专卷，称"丸散膏

诸方"，成为我国最早成药方的配本。该书收载成药数十种，且对丸、散、膏剂的制备有较为详细的描述。

During the Wei, Jin, Southern and Northern Dynasties, there was further expansion and supplement of the understanding on *Shennong Bencao Jing*. In Liang Dynasty, Tao Hongjing in his book *Bencaojing Jizhu* made supplements and modification based on *Shennong Bencao Jing* from the following aspects including the theories and operating principles based on harvesting, identification, processing, preparation of Chinese medicinals etc. Besides, he added geneneral medicinals for various diseases, examples of detoxifying medicinals and mineral medicinals, examples of contraindicated food while taking medicinals. At the same time, the first monograph on processing science in China was born, which is *Leigong Paozhi Lun*. In the Jin Dynasty, Ge Hong in his *Zhouhou Beiji Fang* firstly proposed the concept of prepared medicinals, and for which he made a special volume, being called as prescriptions of pills, powders, syrups. This is the earliest collection book of prepared prescriptions in China. This book contains dozens of kinds of prescriptions, and has detailed descriptions on the preparation of pills, powders, and syrups.

隋唐时期，医药学有较大发展。唐显庆四年颁行了由李勣、苏敬等主持编纂的《新修本草》，是我国历史上第一部官修本草，奠定了我国编纂大型本草的格局。开元年间，陈藏器编成《本草拾遗》，将各种药物功用概括为十类，即宣、通、补、泻、轻、重、滑、涩、燥、湿十种，为中药按临床功效分类的发端。孙思邈著《千金要方》和《千金翼方》、王焘著《外台秘要》均收载了大量方剂。

During the Sui and Tang Dynasties, Great progress has been made in pharmacy. In the fourth year of the reign of Xian Qing of the Tang Dynasty, *Xinxiu Bencao* was compiled by Li Xun and Su Jing. It is the first official authorized herbal medicine book in the Chinese history and laid the foundation for the great compilation of medicinals. During the years of the reign of Kaiyuan, Chen Cangqi compiled the *Bencao Shiyi*, which summarized the functions of various medicines into ten categories, namely dissipating (xuan), unblocking (tong), tonifying (bu), purging (xie), light (qing), heavy (zhong), lubricating (hua), astringent (se), drying (zao), and dampness (shi), that was the beginning of classification of Chinese medicines efficacy. In the books of *Beiji Qianjin Yaofang* and *Qianjin Yifang*, written by Sunsimiao, and *Waitai Miyao* written by Wang Tao, a large number of prescriptions were recorded.

宋代社会经济的发展，尤其是雕板印刷技术的普遍应用，促进了本草、方书的编纂。《开宝本草》《嘉佑补注本草》《本草图经》等大型本草促进了中药学的发展。《本草图经》所附900多幅药图，是我国现存最早的版刻本草图谱，是本草考证的重要依据。唐慎微的《经史证类备急本草》，载药1500余种，附方3000多首，保存了宋以前许多本草资料，具有很高的学术价值、实用价值和文献价值。1076年，宋太医院设立了专门制售中成药的太平惠民和剂局，包括惠民局与和剂局。惠民局相当于药店，和剂局即制药工场，由和剂局制药供给惠民局出售。同时颁布了历史上第一部由官方编纂的成药典《太平惠民和剂局方》，收载成药配方788首，涉及临床各科，大大促进了中成药的使用和发展。其中逍遥散、平胃散、藿香正气散、凉膈散等至今仍在临床广泛使用。金元时期，出现了各具特色的医学流派如金元四大家，形成了火热论、攻邪论、补土论、养阴论等理论创见，创制了大量有效方剂及中成药，从不同角度丰富了中医药的内容，开创了中医学发展的新局面，促进了中药配伍理论、治则治法、方剂学、中药成药的发展。

The development of society and economy in Song Dynasty, especially the widespread application of the engraving printing technology, promoted the compilation of material medica and prescription books. Great materia medica books such as *Kaibao Bencao*, the *Jiayou Buzhu Shennong Bencao*, and the *Bencao Tujing (Identification of Drug Production) Illustrative Classic of Materia Medica*) accelerated the development of Chinese materia medica. More than 900 medicinal pictures were attached in the *Bencao Tujing* which is the earliest engraving material medica pictures in China, and is an important basis for the textual research on materia medica. In Tang Shenwei's *Jingshi Zhenglei Beiji Bencao* more than 1,500 kinds of Chinese medicinals and more than 3,000 prescriptions were recorded, preserving many materials about materia medica before Song Dynasty, and has high academic, practical and literatrue value. In 1076, Song Royal Hospital set up Taiping People's Welfare Bureau, which specialized in the manufacture and salement of prepared medicinals. The Bureau included Huimin Bureau and Heji Bureau. Huimin Bureau is a sort of pharmacy store, and Heji Bureau is a pharmaceutical factory. Medicinals were prepared by Heji Bureau and sold by Huimin Bureau. At the same time, the first official Chinese patent medicine pharmacopoeia in the history, *Taiping Huimin Hejiju Fang (The Prescriptions of the Bureau of Taiping People's Welfare Pharamacy)* was promulgated. The book contained 788 prescriptions of Chinese patent medicine medicinals, involving all clinical departments, promoting the use and development of Chinese patent medicines greatly. Among the formulas, Xiaoyao San (Powder), Pingwei San (Powder), Huoxiangzhengqi San (Powder) and Liangge San (Powder) are still widely used in clinics. During the Jin and Yuan Dynasties, various medical schools such as the Jin and Yuan medical schools appeared with different characteristics, forming theoretical ideas such as pathogenic fire theory, pathogen-attacking theory, earth-tonifying (spleen-invigorating) theory, and yin-nourishing theory, creating a large number of effective prescriptions and Chinese patent medicines. All these theories enriched the contents of Chinese medicine, creating a new situation in the development of Chinese medicine and promoting the improvement of the rules of Chinese medicine compatibility, the principles of treatment and therapy, science of Chinese medicinal formulae, and Chinese patent medicine.

明代社会经济发展迅速，医药知识不断丰富。李时珍著《本草纲目》，全面总结了明以前药物临床应用理论，收载药物 1892 种，方剂 13000 余首，集传统中药之大成。其后《炮炙大法》《普济方》《金匮要略方论衍义》《金镜内台方义》《医方考》《景岳全书》《外科正宗》《寿世保元》等记载了大量中药和方剂的内容，其中有大量的中成药品种至今在临床上使用。

With the rapid social and economic development in Ming Dynasty, medical knowledge was constantly enriched. Li Shizhen's Bencao Gangmu comprehensively summarized the clinical application theory of Chinese medicinals before Ming Dynasty, containing 1,892 medicinals and more than 13,000 prescriptions, which is a collection of Chinese medicinals. After that, *Paozhidafa, Puji Fang (Preions for Universal Relief), Jingui Yaolue Fanglun Yanyi (Synopsis of Prescriptions of the Golden Chamber), Jinjing Neitai Fangyi (Taiwan Justice in the Teritory of Jin), Yifangkao (Textual Research of Medical Prescriptions), Jingyue Quanshu (Jingyue's Complete Works), Waike Zhengzong (Orthodox Manual of External Medicine), Shoushi Baoyuan (Longevity and Life Preservation)* and other books recorded a large number of Chinese medicinals and prescriptions, which are widely used in clinical practice currently.

清代多次瘟疫流行，温病学派壮大。《温热论》《温病条辨》等对温病的发生、发展、传变进行归纳总结，创立了卫气营血辨证、三焦辨证，创造了诸多治疗温病的有效方剂，有的也制成中成药在临床广泛使用。

In the Qing Dynasty, plagues occurred in many times, promoting the generation of the academic school of warm disease. *Wenre Lun (Treatise on Warm-Heat Diseases)*, the *Wenbing Tiaobian*, etc, summarized the occurrence, development, transmisson and changes of warm disease, established the theory of "defensive-Qi-nutritive-blood syndrome" differentiation and syndrome differentiation, and created many effective prescriptions for treating warm diseases. Some are prepared into patent Chinese medicines and widely used in clinical practice.

二、中药应用的近现代发展
2 Modern Development of Chinese Medicinal Application

民国时期，由于西方医学的传入，我国医学发展的总体格局是中西医药并存。一些学者尝试在中医药理论指导下，运用现代方法开展中药功效研究。出现了前店后厂的中成药经营模式，引入西药的制剂工艺，丰富了中药的剂型，为近代中成药制药产业的发展与现代中成药的应用奠定了基础。

During the Republic of China, with the introduction of Western medicine, the overall pattern of China's medical development was the coexistence of Chinese and Western medicine. Some scholars have tried to use modern methods to carry out the efficacy of Chinese medicinals under the guidance of Chinese medicine theory. "Front Shop, Back Factory" business model for running Chinese patent medicines business appeared. The introduction of Western preparation technology enriched the pharmaceutical forms of Chinese medicinals, laying the foundation for the development Chinese patent medicine industry and application of the modern Chinese patent medicine.

新中国成立以后，国家高度重视中医药事业，制定一系列促进中医药发展的政策和措施，兴办中医药高等教育，开展中医药现代研究，使中医药事业走上了健康发展的轨道，对中药、中成药合理用药、剂型、不良反应方面都有了进一步的认识，促进了中药应用的科学发展。

After the founding of the People's Republic of China, we attached a great importance to Chinese medicine, and formulated a series of policies and measures to promote the development of Chinese medicine. Thus many Chinese medicine universities and colleges have been established, and modern researches on Chinese medicine have been carried out, putting Chinese medicine on the track of healthy development, getting further acknowledgement on rational administrations, pharmaceutical forms, and adverse reactions, etc., and acquiring a promotion for the scientific development of Chinese medicinal applications.

第三节　中药应用的现代研究
Section 3　Modern Research on Chinese Medicinal Application

在现阶段，中药主要是以饮片与中成药的形式应用于临床。人们关注在中医药理论指导下，运用现代科学方法，揭示中药防治疾病的机理，为更好的应用中药提供现代科学依据。

At present, Chinese medicinals are mainly used in clinic in the forms of decoction pieces and Chinese patent medicine. People focus on revealing the mechanisms of Chinese medicinals in the prevention and treatment of diseases by using modern scientific methods under the guidance of Chinese medicine theories, in order to provide rationales for a better application of Chinese medicinals.

一、中药饮片应用的研究
1 Research on the Application of Chinese Medicinal Decoction Pieces

（一）中药饮片现代研究概况
1.1 Overview of Modern Research on Chinese Medicinal Decoction Pieces

有关中药饮片现代研究，总体思路是在中医药理论指导下，将传统的本草研究与现代实验研究相结合，为中药应用的安全、有效提供现代科学依据。本章文献中蕴含着大量历代中医药学家对中药应用的宝贵经验，采用传统及现代文献研究手段加以整理、挖掘，将为临床应用提供线索。运用中药化学、药效学、药代动力学、生物信息学等现代科学技术，揭示中药的药理效应、作用机制及药效物质基础，为临床应用提供实验依据。

Combination of traditional medicinal research with modern experimental research under the guidance of Chinese medicine theory is the basic thoughts of modern research on Chinese medicine decoction pieces, which can provide the modern scientific basis for the safe and effective application of Chinese medicine. Literatures of materia medica contain a large number of valuable experience and thoughts from Chinese medicine scientists. Using traditional and modern literature research methods to sort out and explore ancient medicine books can provide clues for clinical application. The modern scientific research technologies as chemistry of Chinese medicinals, pharmacodynamics, pharmacokinetics, and bioinformatics are used in revealing the pharmacological effects, mechanisms of action and substance basis of medicinal efficacy, which can provide experimental basis for the clinical application.

（二）中药饮片应用的现代研究

1.2 Modern Research on the Application of Chinese Medicine Decoction Pieces

中药饮片的现代研究所涉内容较广，与临床应用密切相关的因素大体包括中药的品种、产地、采收季节、炮制、贮藏、剂型与制剂、剂量、配伍等方面，相关研究成果对于中药临床应用具指导作用。如目前国家标准及各级地方标准的正品中药，多品种入药现象仍然普遍。即使"正品"中药，品种不同，化学成分、药理效应、临床疗效亦有差异。有关道地药材道地性研究结果表明，同种药物，不同产地，品质及疗效差异较大。中药（特别是植物药）有一定的生长和成熟周期，其有效成分的含量高低与生长期关系密切。因而，原则上药物应在其有效成分含量最高时采集方能获得良好疗效。炮制影响中药化学成分，药理作用和临床疗效也会发生相应的变化，临床应用宜根据病情选择恰当的炮制品。不同的贮藏时间、贮藏温度、贮藏湿度对中药成分的含量有较大影响，中药的贮藏保管条件可直接影响饮片的质量与疗效。同一中药，如果制成不同的剂型，由于制剂工艺的不同，给药途径不同，往往影响药物的吸收、分布、代谢等，影响药理作用的强度及性质，继而影响疗效。在一定范围内，药物剂量大小与血药浓度的高低及其作用强度呈依赖关系，选择最合适剂量是临床安全、有效的保障。配伍是中医用药的特点，从经典配伍实例研究中获得中药配伍的规律性认识：相须、相使配伍，通过相加协同，能够增强药效；相畏、相杀配伍，通过制约，减轻或消除别的药物的毒副作用；相恶、相反配伍，通过拮抗，可能增毒减效。

The modern research content of Chinese medicinal decoction pieces is very wide and mainly focuses on such factors being closely related to the clinical application including the varieties of Chinese medicinals, production origin, harvest seasons, processing, storage, pharmaceutical forms and preparations, compatibility, etc. Research results have a guiding effect on the clinical application of Chinese medicinals. It is common that many different species of Chinese medicinals are included in national standard and local standard as authorized medicinals. Even for the authorized medicinals, the varieties, the chemical compositions, pharmacological effects, clinical efficacy might be different. The research on genuine regional medicinal shows that the quality and efficacy of the same medicinal from different origins are different. Chinese medicinal (especially herbs) has a certain growth and maturity cycle, which is closely related to the concentration of its active ingredients. Therefore, in principle, the medicinals should be collected when the concentration of its active ingredients is the highest in order to obtain a good effect. As we know, the processing affects the chemical composition of Chinese medicine. Accordingly, the pharmacological effects and the clinical effects will also change. It is appropriate to choose proper processed products depending on clinical needs. Different storage time, temperature, and humidity have a great effect on the ingredients of medicinals. The storage conditions of medicinals can directly affect the quality and efficacy of decoction pieces. The same medicinal is made into different pharmaceutical forms through different preparation processes, and applied in different administration routes, that will affect the absorption, distribution, and metabolism of the medicines. Further influencing its pharmacological actions and the efficacy are influenced. Within a certain range, the concentration in blood and the therapeutic effect depends on the dose of the medicine. So, choosing an appropriate dose is a guarantee for clinical efficacy and safety. Compatibility is one of the major features in Chinese medicinals. The rule of Chinese medicine compatibility is obtained from classic compatibility cases: mutual reinforcement, mutual assistance synergically enhance medicinal efficacy through adding coordination; mutual restraint and mutual suppression reduce or eliminate the toxic and side effects through restricting each other; mutual inhibition and mutual antagonism may increase the toxicity and reduce the treatment effect through antagonizing each other.

二、中成药应用的研究
2 Research on the Application of Chinese Patent Medicines

（一）中成药应用研究概况
2.1 Overview of Chinese Patent Medicines Application Research

中成药是中药应用的主要形式之一，目前中成药的研究与应用取得了显著的进步与重要成就。以科技创新为引领，以临床需求为导向，一大批不同类别的中成药成功上市，整体提高了中成药的研发与应用水平，推动了中药产业的快速发展，为临床提供了疗效更加确切、安全性更加可靠，质量更加可控的中成药。目前我国老龄化日趋严重，重大疾病发病率逐年上升，中药在老年性疾病、代谢性疾病、退行性疾病等方面具有一定优势，有着良好的应用前景。

Chinese patent medicines are the main forms of the Chinese medicinals application. At present, research and clinical usage of Chinese patent medicine make a remarkable progress and important achievement. Guided by scientific and technological innovation and clinical needs, a large number of different types of Chinese patent medicines are successfully marketed, which improve the levels of research, development and application of Chinese patent medicines, promote the rapid development of the Chinese medicinal industry. All these technologies make Chinese medicine with effects more accurate safty wore reliable, quality more controllable than before. At present, China's aging is getting more and more serious, and the incidence of major diseases is increasing year by year. Hence, Chinese medicinals have some advantages for future in treatment of senile diseases, metabolic diseases, and degenerative diseases, have a bright application future.

（二）中成药应用的现代研究
2.2 Modern Research on the Application of Chinese Patent Medicines

目前我国中成药的研究和生产发展迅速，品种丰富。据统计中成药在心血管、泌尿、呼吸、骨骼肌肉系统等疾病的治疗中占比达30%。临床内、外、妇、儿、伤、五官等各科均有各种中成药在临床应用。中成药在心脑血管疾病、病毒感染性、肿瘤等重大疾病防治方面具有优势与特色。

At present, the research and production of Chinese medicinals in China are developing rapidly and the abundant varieties. According to statistics, Chinese patent medicines account for 30% medicines in the treatment of cardiovascular, urinary, respiratory, and skeletomuscular diseases. Various Chinese patent medicines are applied in different clinical departments, such as internal and external medicine, gynecology, pediatrics, surgery, ophthalmology and otorhinolaryngology. Chinese medicinals have advantages and features in the prevention and treatment of serious diseases such as cardio-cerebro vascular and cerebrovascular diseases, viral infection, and cancers.

心脑血管病多为慢性久病，心脑血管疾病中成药多具有保护心功能、保护脑细胞、抗缺血缺氧、抗心衰、抗休克等作用，如速效救心丸、复方丹参滴丸、参附注射液、生脉注射液等大量中成药产品在冠心病、心肌缺血、心绞痛等疾病中广泛应用。安宫牛黄丸、脑心通丸、益脑宁片、血塞通注射液、红花注射液、清开灵注射液等在脑血管疾病中亦有广泛应用。

Cardio-cerebro vascular diseases are chronic diseases. Mostly Chinese patent medicines for these diseases have the functions of cerebroprotection, cardioprotection, and have antiischemia and antihypoxia, anti-heart failure, anti-shock effects. A large number of Chinese patent medicines, such as Suxiao

Jiuxin Wan, Fufang Danshen Diwan, Shenfu Zhusheye and Shengmai Zhusheye are widely used to treat coronary heart disease, myocardial ischemia and angina pectoris, etc. Angong Niuhuang Wan, Naoxintong Pian, Yinaoning Pian, Xuesaitong Zhusheye, Honghua Zhusheye, Qingkailing Zhusheye, etc, are also widely used in cerebrovascular diseases.

用于感染性疾病中成药多具有抗病毒、抑菌、抗炎等多方面作用，应用于包括呼吸系统、消化系统、循环系统、泌尿系统等的多种疾病。如感冒灵颗粒、板蓝根冲剂、连花清瘟胶囊、喜炎平注射液等在流行性感冒、呼吸道感染等疾病中应用广泛。

Chinese patent medicines used for infectious diseases have antiviral, antibacterial, anti-inflammatory and other functions and are used for diseases in respiratory system, digestive system, circulatory system, urinary system, et al. Ganmaoling Keli, Banlangen Chongji, Lianhua Qingwen Jiaonang, Xiyanping Zhusheye, etc, are widely used in influenza, respiratory infections and other diseases.

中医防治肿瘤的常用治法包括祛邪和扶正，通过扶助正气，提高生活质量。目前开发大量的中成药产品如：以薏苡仁油为主要成分的康莱特注射液，以蟾衣为主要成分制成华蟾素注射液，以莪术油为主要成分的莪术油注射液，以鸦胆子油为主要成分的鸦胆子油注射液，以苦参、当归等为主要成分的复方苦参注射液等中成药品种以抑制肿瘤为主。还有大量的辅助正气的品种，广泛用于肿瘤的治疗或辅助手术、放化疗，如参麦注射液、槐耳颗粒、参芪片、贞芪扶正胶囊、灵芝片等。

The common therapelltic methods of Chinese medicine in prevention and treatments of cancer are strengthening vital qi to eliminate pathogenic factor, by which improve the patients' life quality. At present, a large number of Chinese patent medicines mainly used to suppress the growth of tumors have been developed, such as: Kanglaite Zhusheye mainly containing Yiyiren You (Oil), Huachansu Zhusheye using Chanyi (Bufonis Periostracum, toad skin) as the main component, E'zhu You Zhusheye mainly containing E'zhu (Curcumae Rhizoma) oil, Yadanzi You Zhusheye with Bruceae Fructus oil as the main component, and Fufang Kushen Zhusheye with Kushen and Danggui (Angelicae Sinensis Radix) as the main medicinals. There are also a large number of Chinese patent medicines which can strengthen vitality are widely used in cancer treatment or as adjuvants for surgery, radiotherapy and chemotherapy, such as Shenmai Zhusheye, Huaier Keli, Shenqi Pian (Tablets), Zhenqi Fuzheng Jiaonang, Lingzhi (Ganoderma) Pian and so on.

中成药临床应用广泛，疗效肯定，不仅中医使用，越来越多的西医亦在使用。应更多地利用和借鉴新理论、新技术，研发中成药新品种，提升中成药科学内涵，更好地服务临床，造福全人类。

Because of the wide ranged application and credible curative effects, Chinese patent medicines are wildly used not only by Chinese medicine doctors, but also by more and more western medicine doctors. More new theories and technologies should be learned and applied in developing new varieties of Chinese patent medicines, and exalting the scientific connotation of Chinese patent medicines, to make it work better for clinical work and serve human beings.

各 论
Monograph

第八章 解 表 药
Chapter 8　Exterior-releasing Medicinals

凡以发散表邪为主要功效，主治表证的药物，称为解表药，又叫发表药。此类药物多轻扬辛散，作用趋向以升浮为主，善行肌表，疏达腠理，促进肌体发汗，使表邪由汗出而解或从外而散，即《黄帝内经》所谓："其在皮者，汗而发之"。主要用于治疗恶寒发热、头身疼痛、无汗或有汗不畅、苔薄脉浮之外感表证，或用于水肿、咳喘、麻疹、风疹、风湿痹痛、疮疡初起等兼有表证者。解表药一般分为发散风寒药（辛温解表药）和发散风热药（辛凉解表药）两类，多含挥发性成分，入汤剂不宜久煎。解表药一般具有发汗、解热、镇痛、抗炎、抗病原微生物、调节免疫功能等作用。常见的解表药有麻黄、桂枝、防风、薄荷、柴胡、菊花等。

Exterior-releasing medicinals, are also called exterior-effusing medicinals, refer to the medicines that can disperse exterior pathogens and treat exterior syndromes. The properties of these medicines are mostly light, pungent and divergent. The main trend is up-bearing and floating, flowing on the skin, dispersing the interstices, promoting the sweating of the body, dispelling the exterior pathogens along with sweating or spreading from the outside, as it is said that "if the disease is located on the skin, sweating it out." in *Huang Di Nei Jing*. They are mainly used to treat exterior syndromes induced by exterior pathogens, such as aversion to cold with fever, pain in the head and body, no sweating or unsmooth sweating, thin fur and floating pulse, or to treat edema, cough and dyspnea, measles, rubella, wind-dampness impediment, emerging sores and so on at the early stage acconpnied by exterior syndromes. Generally, the exterior-releasing medicinals have two categories, namely wind-cold-dispersing medicinals (pungent-warm exterior-releasing medicine) and wind-heat dispersing medicinals (pungent-cool exterior-releasing medicine). Most of these medicinals contain volatile components so that they should not be decocted for a long time. The exterior-releasing medicinals generally have the effects of promoting sweating, being antipyretic analgesic anti-inflammation, anti-pathogenic microorganisms, regulating immune and so on. The exterior-releasing medicinals such as Mahuang, Guizhi, Fangfeng (Saposhnikoviae Radix), Bohe, Chaihu (Bupleuri Radix), and Juhua are commonly used.

麻　黄

Mahuang

(Ephedrae Herba)

麻黄是山西道地药材。临床常用炮制品有麻黄与蜜麻黄两种。麻黄味辛、微苦，性温，归肺、膀胱经，具发汗散寒，宣肺平喘，利水消肿的功效，主治风寒感冒，胸闷喘咳，风水浮肿。蜜麻黄润肺止咳，多用于表证已解，气喘咳嗽。麻黄主要含生物碱、挥发油等成分，有发汗、平喘、利尿、抗病原微生物、解热、抗炎、镇痛、止咳等药理作用，可用于治疗感冒、肺炎、支气管炎、哮喘、急性肾炎、风湿性关节炎等属风寒表实证者。

Mahuang is a genuine regional medicinal in Shanxi Province. Common processed products are Mahuang and Mimahuang (processed with honey). Mahuang is warm in nature and pungent and mild bitter in flavor, and it enters the lung and bladder meridians. It has the effect of sweating for dispelling cold, ventilating the lungs and relieving dyspnea and inducing diuresis for removing edema, and to treat wind-cold common cold, oppression in the chest, dyspnea, cough, and edema caused by wind and water retention. Mimahuang (processed with honey) has the effect of moistening the lung to suppress cough, and it is mostly used to treat dyspnea and cough with exterior syndrome released. Mahuang mainly contains alkaloids, volatile oils and other ingredients with the pharmacological effects of promoting sweating, calming panting, diuresis, anti-pathogenic microorganisms, being antipyretic, anti- inflammation, relieving pain, and suppressing cough etc. It can be used for the treatment of wind-cold exterior excess syndromes including common cold, pneumonia, bronchitis, asthma, acute nephritis, rheumatoid arthritis and so on.

【品种品质】
[Variety and Quality]

一、基原品种与品质
I Origin Varieties and Quality

1. **品种概况**　来源于麻黄科植物草麻黄 *Ephedra sinica* Stapf、中麻黄 *Ephedra intermedia* Schrenk et C. A. Mey. 或木贼麻黄 *Ephedra equisetina* Bge. 的干燥草质茎。

1 Variety

Mahuang is the dried herbaceous stem of *Ephedra sinica* Stapf, *Ephedra intermedia* Schrenk et C.A. Mey. or *Ephedra equisetina* Bge.

麻黄首载于《神农本草经》,《酉阳杂俎》描述麻黄"茎端开花，花小而黄，丛生。子（果实）如覆盆子，可食。至冬枯死如草，及春却青"，与今草麻黄植物形态一致。

Mahuang is first recorded in the book of *Shennong Bencao Jing*. It was described as "Fasciculate, the flower blooms in stem apex, small and yellow in cluster. The fruit is like Fupenzi (Rubi Fructus), and is edible. It withers like dried grass in winter, but turns green in spring." in the book of *Youyang Zazu (YawYang Essays)*. The morphology of the Mahuang plant described in the book is consistent with that of the plant of *E. sinica* in nowadays.

2. **种植采收**　麻黄既有野生也有人工种植，人工种植的麻黄主要为草麻黄，主产于山西、内蒙古、陕西、宁夏、吉林、辽宁、河北、甘肃、新疆等省区。麻黄种植多采用育苗移栽的方式，采收期对麻黄质量影响较大，一般于移栽 3 年后采收，于秋季割取地上绿色草质茎，晒干。

2 Planting and Harvesting

Mahuang is both wild and artificial cultivated. The planted Mahuang is mainly *E. sinica*, and mainly produced in provinces of Shanxi, Inner Mongolia, Shaanxi, Ningxia, Jilin, Liaoning, Hebei, Gansu, Xinjiang, etc. The cultivation of Mahuang adopts the way of seedling transplanting. The time of harvest plays an important role in the quality. Generally, to ensure good quality, people harvest Mahuang after three years of transplanting seedlings, and the ground green herbaceous stems are collected in autumn and dried in the sun.

3. 道地性及品质评价　据本草考证，麻黄"生晋地（山西境内）及河东（河北境内），荥阳、中牟（河南境内）者为胜"，其道地产区经历了由河南到山西的变迁，自民国初至今，麻黄产于"西北各省，大同产佳"，以山西大同为道地产区。麻黄性状评价以干燥、茎粗、淡绿色、内心充实、味苦涩者为佳。

3 Genuineness and Quality Evaluation

According to herbal textual records, Mahuang "grows in Jindi (in Shanxi province), Hedong (in Hebei province), Yingyang and Zhongmu (in Henan province) is better". Its genuine producing areas changed from Henan province to Shanxi province. Since the beginning of the Republic of China, Mahuang is produced "in the northwest provinces, and the best is in thus Datong", Datong in Shanxi province is the best producing area". Currently, the high-qualified Mahuang are dry, with thick stem, pale green, dense in center and bitter taste.

麻黄主要含有生物碱类成分，以麻黄碱和伪麻黄碱为主，主要存在于草质茎髓部，此外还含有挥发油与鞣质等。生物碱与挥发油是麻黄的主要药效物质基础，其中麻黄碱、伪麻黄碱和挥发油是麻黄平喘的主要物质基础，挥发油是其发汗的主要成分，D-伪麻黄碱是利尿的主要成分。麻黄中多种成分均有抗炎作用。《中国药典》规定麻黄药材中含盐酸麻黄碱和盐酸伪麻黄碱的总量不得少于0.80%。

Mahuang mainly contains alkaloids, which are mainly ephedrine and pseudoephedrine, and the most of these existing in the pith of the stems. In addition, It also contains volatile oils and tannin etc. The alkaloids and volatile oils are the main therapeutic material basis of Mahuang. Ephedrine, pseudoephedrine and volatile oils are the main material basis of Mahuang to relieve the dyspnea. Volatile oils are the main components for sweating, and D-pseudoephedrine is the main material for diuresis. Many components in Mahuang have anti-inflammatory effect. *Pharmacopoeia of the People's Republic of China* regulates that the total amount of ephedrine hydrochloride and pseudoephedrine hydrochloride in Mahuang shall not be less than 0.80%.

二、炮制品种与品质
II Processed Varieties and Quality

麻黄的炮制品种有20多个，临床常用品种近10种，包括麻黄、蜜麻黄等。麻黄以干燥、茎粗、表面淡绿或黄绿，内心充实、色红棕，有细纵脊线，气微香，味苦涩者为佳。蜜麻黄以表面深黄色，微有光泽，略具黏性，有蜜香气，味甜者为佳。《中国药典》规定麻黄和蜜麻黄的含量测定同药材。

There are more than 20 processed products of Mahuang. Nearly 10 clinical varieties are commonly used in clinical practice, which involves Mahuang and Mimahuang (processed with honey), etc. The good Mahuang is characterized by dry, thick stems, pale or yellow green on surface, full reddish brown in center, slender longitudinal line in ridge, slightly fragrant in flavor, and bitter in taste. Mimahuang is good with deep yellow surface, slightly glossy, a little viscosity, honey aroma, sweet in taste. According to *Pharmacopoeia of the People's Republic of China*, the content determination of Mahuang and Mimahuang (processed with honey) is the same as that of the raw medicinals.

三、中成药品种与品质
III Varieties and Quality of Chinese Patent Medicines

含有麻黄或其炮制品的中成药有 280 余个，其中《中国药典》收载含有麻黄的中成药 70 余个。以麻黄为君药或主药的品种有三拗片、止喘灵注射液、小青龙合剂等。在质量控制中多采用薄层色谱法确定麻黄的存在，采用含量测定法进行指标成分限量。如三拗片以 HPLC 含量测定法限定盐酸麻黄碱和盐酸伪麻黄碱总量；止喘灵注射液以薄层色谱法检测盐酸麻黄碱的存在，以滴定法测定麻黄总生物碱含量，以保证药品质量稳定。非以麻黄为君药的制剂，葛根汤片、鼻渊通窍颗粒、芩芷鼻炎糖浆等通过薄层鉴别盐酸麻黄碱、麻黄对照药材提取液以确定含有麻黄。

There are more than 280 Chinese patent medicines containing Mahuang or its processed products, and among them, over 70 Mahuang patent medicines are recorded in *Pharmacopoeia of the People's Republic of China*. Mahuang is served as the sovereign or main medicine in many formulas, such as in San' ao Pian, Zhichuanling Zhusheye and Xiaoqinglong Heji (Mixture), etc. TLC is used to identify the existence of Mahuang, and content determination is used to make the limit of index components. For example, the total content of ephedrine hydrochloride and pseudoephedrine hydrochloride are detected by HPLC for San'ao Pian (Tablets). In Zhichuanling Zhusheye, the existence of ephedrine hydrochloride is detected by TLC, and the content of total alkaloids is measured with titration to ensure its stable quality. In the preparations in which Mahuang is not applied as sovereign medicinal, such as Gegentang Pian (Tablets), Biyuan Tongqiao Keli, Qinzhi Biyan Tangiang (Syrup), Mahuang is identified by TCL to determine the existence of Mahuang by differentiating ephedrine hydrochloride contained and contrasting with the extracted solution of raw medicinal.

【制药】
[Pharmacy]

一、产地加工
I Processing in Production Area

麻黄于秋季割取绿色草质茎，除去杂草、残茎、须根及泥沙，扎成小把，在通风处晾至 7~8 成干时再晒干。其曝晒或烘烤过久色发黄，受霜冻色变红，均影响质量，应注意避免。

The green herbaceous stems of Mahuang are collected in autumn; the weeds, residual stems, fibrous roots, and silt removed, tied into small bundles, dried in a ventilated place until 70% to 80% dry, afterwards dried in the sun. Mahuang turning yellow after solarization or baking for a long time, or turning red after frost frozen that will affect its quality and should be avoided.

二、饮片炮制
II Processing of Decoction Pieces

麻黄的炮制方法，经历了许多转变。古籍记载有"去节汤泡""酒熬成膏""姜汁浸""去根节，蜜酒煮黑"等。现行有麻黄、蜜麻黄、麻黄绒、密麻黄绒等炮制方法，《中国药典》载有麻黄与蜜麻黄两种炮制饮片。麻黄经炮制后挥发油和生物碱含量下降，其中 L- 麻黄碱及 d- 伪麻黄碱含量以炒麻黄降低最多，蜜炙品次之。现代研究证明麻黄绒较麻黄作用缓和是麻黄总生物碱含量较低的原因。

The processing methods of Mahuang have experienced many changes. Ancient books record "removing stems and soaking in the water", "boiling with liquor into paste", "soaking with ginger solution", "removing joint and root, boiling with honey liquor into black" and so on. The present processing methods have Mahuang, Mimahuang (proccssed with honey), Mahuangrong (fine fiber), Mimahuangrong (fine fiber and processed with honey), etc. *Pharmacopoeia of the People's Republic of China* records two decoction pieces of Mahuang and Mimahuang (processed with honey). After Mahuang being processed, its content of volatile oil and alkaloids decreases, and Chaomahuang (stir-frying) reduces the content of L-ephedrine and d-pseudoephedrine in Chaomahuang (stir-frying) is decreased more than that decreased in Mimahuang (processed with honey). Modern research proves that the effect of Mahuangrong (fine fiber) is gentler than Mahuang due to the lower content of total alkaloid.

三、中成药制药
III Pharmacy of Chinese Patent Medicines

麻黄传统中药制剂多选用麻黄、麻黄绒入汤剂。现代制剂中，多选用生品煎煮或打粉入药，如三拗片、清肺消炎丸等。此外，还有使用麻黄提取物入药的，如复方川贝精片，以麻黄浸膏投料。

In traditional preparations of Chinese materia medica, Mahuang and Mahuangrong (fine fiber) are more chosen to be used in decoctions. In modern preparations, the raw Mahuang is decocted or powdered to be used in medicine, such as, San'ao Pian (Tablets) and Qingfei Xiaoyan Wan, etc. In addition, the extracts of Mahuang are also used into medicine, such as in Fufang Chuanbeijing Pian (Tablets), which are applied for decoction.

如以麻黄为君药的清肺消炎丸，其制备过程采用麻黄细粉入药，制成的蜜丸在体内溶解缓慢，而使麻黄能够缓慢而持久的发挥辛温解表、宣肺平喘作用。再如在止喘灵注射液制剂工艺中，因麻黄中的生物碱类成分可溶于水与醇类溶剂中，故麻黄采用水煎法提取，随后采用乙醇沉淀处理和冷藏的方法除去醇不溶性成分，同时保留醇溶性成分，达到注射剂制剂要求。

For example, in Qingfei Xiaoyan Wan, as the sovereign medicine, Mahuang is crushed into honey pills, and dissolves slowly in the body, thus enable Mahuang exerting its effects of relieving the exterior with pungent-warm nature and ventilating lung qi slowly and durably for stopping

asthma. In the preparation of Zhichuanling Zhusheye, because the alkaloids of Mahuang are soluble in water and alcohol solvents, Mahuang is extracted with water decoction, and then alcohol-insoluble components are removed with ethanol precipitation and refrigeration. At the same time, alcohol-soluble components are retained to meet the requirements of injection preparations.

【性能功效】
[Property and Efficacy]

一、性能
I Property

麻黄辛、微苦，温；归肺、膀胱经。
Mahuang is pungent and slightly bitter in flavor, warm in nature, and enters the lungs and bladder meridians.

二、功效
II Efficacy

1. 发汗散寒　麻黄辛温发散、轻清上浮，能祛散侵袭肌表的风寒邪气，开泄腠理、透发毛窍。其功效的发挥与发汗、解热、抗炎、抗病原微生物等药理作用密切相关。麻黄发汗散寒的有效物质基础主要是挥发油与生物碱类成分，通过调节中枢和外周神经系统功能，阻碍汗腺导管对钠离子的重吸收、扩张汗腺导管发挥发汗作用。

1 Sweating for Dispelling Cold
The properties of Mahuang are pungent, warm, divergent, light and up-flowing. It can dispel the wind-cold pathogenic qi that invade the surface, open and disperse interstices, and ventilate hair orifices. Its effectiveness is closely related to pharmacological effects such as sweating, relieving heat and anti-inflammatory, anti-pathogenic microorganisms, etc. The volatile oils and alkaloids are the main effective material basis for the sweating for dispelling cold. They regulate the central and peripheral nervous system function,

obstruct sweat gland catheter to reabsorb sodium ions, and dilate sweat gland duct, for performing the sweating function.

2. **宣肺平喘** 麻黄辛散而微苦，则兼苦降之性，主入肺经，宣发肺气，止咳平喘。其功效的发挥与平喘等药理作用密切相关。麻黄平喘的有药效物质基础主要是麻黄碱、伪麻黄碱和挥发油，通过拟肾上腺素样作用，松弛支气管平滑肌，抑制抗体产生发挥平喘作用。

2 Ventilating the Lung Qi for Relieving Dyspnea

Mahuang is pungent, divergent and slightly bitter and is bitter and downward in nature, and the main meridian entry is the lung. It can diffuse lung qi, relieve cough and calm asthma. Its efficacy is closely related to its anti-asthmatic effect and other pharmacological effects. Ephedrine, pseudoephedrine and volatile oils are the main pharmacodynamics substances of calming panting in Mahuang. Through adrenergic effect, relaxing bronchial smooth muscle and inhibition of antibodies, they extert anti-asthmatic effects.

3. **利水消肿** 麻黄上宣肺气，下利膀胱，可通调水道，利尿消肿。其功效的发挥与利尿、保护肾功能等药理作用密切相关。麻黄利尿的有效物质基础主要是 D- 伪麻黄碱，通过扩张肾血管使肾血流增加，并阻碍肾小管对钠离子重吸收发挥利尿作用。

3 Inducing Diuresis for Removing Edema

Mahuang diffuses the lung qi upward, relieves the bladder pathogen downward, and can regulate the waterways, induce diuresis to reduce edema. These functions of Mahuang are closely related to pharmacological functions as diuresis and the protection of kidney functions. The effective material basis for the diuretic effect of Mahuang is D-pseudoephedrine through dilating the renal blood vessels to increase the renal blood flow, and blocking the reabsorption of sodium ions in renal tubules, to exert it diuretic effect.

【应用】
[Application]

一、主治病证
I Indications

1. **风寒表证** 本品辛能发散，温可去寒，为发汗解表第一要药，长于开泄腠理，发汗散邪，尤宜于风寒表证表实无汗者。治疗外感风寒，恶寒、发热、无汗，头身疼痛、脉浮紧等，并常与桂枝相须为用，增强发汗解表之力，如《伤寒论》麻黄汤。

1 Wind Cold Exterior Syndrome

Mahuang, being pungent to disperse, warm, to dispel being the cold pathogen, it is the first key medicine for sweating and releasing exterior. Mahuang is good at opening muscular interstices, sweating to remove the exterior evil, and is especially suitable for those who have no sweating with wind-cold exterior excess syndrome. It can be used to treat exogenous wind-cold, aversion to cold, fever, anhidrosis, head and body pain, with floating and tightening pulse, etc. It is often used in combination with Guizhi (Cinnamomi Ramulus) to enhance the ability of sweating and resolving the exterior syndrome, such as in Mahuang Tang (Decoction) in *Shanghan Zabing Lun*.

现代临床，麻黄配伍常用于治疗外感风寒所致普通感冒、流行性感冒及小儿因感冒、扁桃体炎等导致的高热等风寒表实证者。如麻黄汤、小儿清热止咳合剂等。

In modern clinical practice, Mahuang compatibility is often used to treat common cold, influenza and children high fever caused by cold and tonsillitis and other illnesses from wind-cold exterior excess syndrome, such as in Mahuang Tang (Decoction), Xiaoer Qingre Zhike Heji, etc.

2. **胸闷喘咳** 本品辛散 苦泄，开宣肺气，凡邪气壅肺，胸闷喘咳，常以本品为主药。治疗风寒外束，肺气壅遏的喘咳实证，常与苦杏仁、甘草合用，如《太平惠民和剂局方》三拗汤。治疗寒痰停饮，咳嗽气喘，痰多清稀者，常与细辛、干姜、半夏等同用，如《伤寒论》小青龙汤。若肺热壅盛，高热喘急者，常与石膏为伍，如《伤寒论》麻杏甘石汤。

2 Chest Oppression and Wheezing Cough Syndrome

This product is pungent for dispersing and bitter for discharging, and diffuses the lung qi. Mahuang is often used as the main medicinal to treat the diseases of evil obstructing the lung, chest stuffiness and panting cough. Mahuang with Kuxingren and Gancao is often used to wheezing cough excess syndrome lung qi congestion with due to exogenous wind-cold and, such as San'ao decoction in *Taiping Huimin Heji Ju Fang*. With Xixin, Ganjiang, Banxia, etc., Mahuang is used to treat the diseases of water-retention due to cold phlegm, cough, wheeze, asthma, profuse thin phlegm, as in Xiaoqinglong Tang (Decoction) (small green dragon decoction) in *Shanghan Zabing Lun*. If the diseases are characterized by lung-heat excessive congestion and high fever with asthma, it is often used with Shigao, such as Maxing Ganshi Tang (Decoction) in *Shanghan Zabing Lun*.

现代临床，麻黄配伍常用于治疗肺炎、急慢性支气管炎、支气管哮喘、喉源性咳嗽、过敏性鼻炎属于风寒表证、咳喘病症者，如三拗片、克咳片、急支糖浆等。

In modern clinical practice, Mahuang compatibility is commonly used for pneumonia, acute and chronic bronchitis, bronchial asthma, laryngeal cough and allergic rhinitis, with with cough or asthma belonging to the wind-cold exterior syndrome, as in San'ao Pian (Tablets), Keke Pian (Tablets), Jizhi Tangjiang (Syrup), etc.

3. 风水浮肿　本品开腠发汗，使肌肤之水湿从毛窍外散，又能宣散肺气，通调水道，下输膀胱，而有消肿利水之效。常用于风邪袭表，肺失宣降的水肿、小便不利兼有表证者，每与甘草同

用，如《金匮要略》甘草麻黄汤。如再配伍生姜、白术等发汗解表、利水退肿药，则疗效更佳，如《金匮要略》越婢加术汤。

3 Wind-water Edema

Mahuang can open interstices to sweating, make the muscle and skin moisture dispersing from the hair orifice, and can also ventilate the lung qi, regulate the water passages, and transport water into the bladder to induce diuresis and edema. It is often used together with Gancao for the treatment of wind evil assailing the exterior, the edema due to lung dysfunction dispersing and descending, and difficulty in urination with exterior syndrome, such as in Gancao Mahuang Tang (Decoction) in *Jingui Yaolue*. If it is combined with Shengjiang, Baizhu and other medicinals with the function of sweating, dispelling exogenous evils, and inducing diuresis to alleviate edema, the curative effect will be better, as in Yuebi Jiazhu Tang (Decoction) in *Jingui Yaolue*.

现代临床，麻黄配伍常用于治疗急性肾炎初期、慢性肾炎、前列腺增生、小儿遗尿症等属于水肿兼表证者，如金利油软胶囊、麻黄连翘赤小豆汤等。

In modern clinical practice, Mahuang compatibility is commonly used in the treatment for edema with exterior syndrome of initial-stage acute nephritis, chronic nephritis, prostatic hyperplasia, infantile enuresis, etc., as in Jinliyou Ruanjiaonang (Soft Capsules), Mahuanglianqiao Chixiaodou Tang (Decoction), etc.

此外，取麻黄散寒通滞之功，麻黄配伍还可用于治疗风湿痹证、阴疽、痰核。相当于现代临床治疗风湿性关节炎与类风湿性关节炎等，如骨苓通痹丸、寒热痹颗粒等。

In addition, with the effects of Mahuang can be dispeling coldness and smoothing stagnation, it combination with other medicinals to treat wind-dampness impediment syndrome, yin gangrene and phlegm nodule. Those are equivalent to the modern clinical treatment of rheumatic and rheumatoid arthritis, etc., as in Guling Tongbi

Wan, Hanrebi Keli, etc.

二、用法用量
II Administration and Dosage

煎服，2~10g。
2~10g, water decoction.

三、注意事项
III Precautions

1. 本品发汗力强，性温燥，故表虚自汗、阴虚盗汗、虚喘及头痛者不宜使用。

1 This herb has strong sweating efficacy, and is warm and dry dryness in nature, so it is not suitable for the patients with spontaneous perspiration due to exterior deficiency, night sweat due to yin deficiency, asthenia asthma and headache due to deficiency.

2. 麻黄所含麻黄碱可引起中枢神经和交感神经兴奋，并可使血压上升，故失眠及高血压患者慎用。

2 The ephedrines contained in Mahuang can cause central and sympathetic nerve excitation, and make blood pressure rise, so that it should be paid great caution when applying for patients with insomnia and hypertension.

【知识拓展】
[Knowledge Extension]

麻黄药用历史悠久，国内因中医使用麻黄

而产生毒副作用的情况鲜见。但国外近年来将麻黄制剂用于减肥和提高运动成绩，使麻黄毒副作用增多。大剂量使用麻黄能够引起失眠、神经过敏、焦虑不安、震颤、心律失常、血压升高、眩晕、头痛等。麻黄药效物质麻黄碱是制造冰毒（甲基苯丙胺）的前体，具有药物依赖性，过多服用会使人上瘾，因而国家对麻黄的种植、采收、销售、运输等各个环节有明确的监管规定，确保麻黄及其制剂既能满足防治疾病的需要，又不致流入非法渠道。

Mahuang has a long history of medicinal use and only few reports show its toxic and side effect in China. However, in recent years, the preparations containing Mahuang are used to reduce weight and improve sports performance in foreign countries, so that its toxic and side effects increase. Mahuang can stimulate the central nervous system, and large doses of use can cause insomnia, nervousness, willies, tremor, arrhythmia, blood pressure rise, dizziness, headache, etc. Ephedrine, as the pharmacodynamics substance in Mahuang, is the precursor for making meth (methamphetamine), with medicinal dependence, excess dosage makes people addictive. Therefore, China and other countries have made clear regulations on the cultivation, harvesting, marketing, transportation, etc., so as to ensure Mahuang and its preparations can not only meet the needs of diseases prevention and treatment, but also not flow into illegal channels.

桂 枝

Guizhi
(Cinnamomi Ramulus)

桂枝是广西、广东道地药材。桂枝性温，味辛、甘、归心、肺、膀胱经，具发汗解肌，温通经脉，助阳化气，平冲降气的功效，主治风寒感冒，脘腹冷痛，血寒经闭，关节痹痛，痰饮，水肿，心悸，奔豚。桂枝中主要含有挥发油、有机酸、多糖、香豆素及鞣质等成分，有解热、扩张血管、促进发汗、抗病原微生物、改善心血管功能、镇痛、抗炎、抗过敏等药理作用，可用于治疗感冒、上呼吸道感染、支气管炎、支气管哮喘等风寒表证者，水肿、小便不利等阳虚水肿，痰饮证，骨关节炎、风湿或类风湿关节炎、骨质增生等风湿痹证者，痛经、产后腹痛等寒凝血滞证者，冠心病、心绞痛、心肌梗死等心阳不振、心脉瘀阻者。

Guizhi is a genuine regional medicinal in Guangxi and Guangdong Provinces. Guizhi is warm in nature, pungent and sweet in flavor, and it enters the heart, lung and bladder meridians. It has the effect of sweating to expel pathogenic factors from the muscles, warming the meridian vessels, assisting yang transforming into qi and directing qi downward. It mainly treats the diseases of wind-cold common cold, cold pain in the stomach and abdomen, amenorrhea due to coldness in blood, joint impediment diseases, phlegm and fluid retention, edema, palpitations, and kidney amassment running-pig sensation (bentun). Guizhi mainly contains volatile oil, organic acids, polysaccharides, coumarin and tannins, which possess various pharmacological effects, including relieving fever, expanding blood vessels, promoting sweating, anti-pathogenic microorganisms, improving cardiovascular function, analgesia, anti-inflammation and antianaphylaxis etc. Guizhi can treat common cold, upper respiratory tract infection, bronchitis, bronchial asthma, etc. with such exterior wind-cold syndrome, edema or dysuria, or phlegm-fluid retention such yang deficiency syndrome, osteoarthritis, rheumatic or rheumatoid arthritis, osteoproliferation such wind-dampnessbi syndrome, dysmenorrhea, postpartum abdominal pain such blood stasis syndrome due to cold coagulation, and coronary artery heart disease, angina pectoris, myocardial infarction, etc such syndrome of devitalization of heart yang or blockage of heart vessel.

【品种品质】
[Variety and Quality]

一、基原品种与品质
I Origin Varieties and Quality

1. **品种概况** 来源于樟科植物肉桂 *Cinnamomum cassia* Presl. 的干燥嫩枝。

桂枝首载于《神农本草经》。北宋《重广补注神农本草并图经》记载"仲景《伤寒论》发汗用桂枝。桂枝者，枝条，非身干也。取其轻薄而能发散。今又有一种柳桂，乃桂之嫩小枝条也"，其描述与樟科植物肉桂的嫩枝相同。

1 Variety

Guizhi is the dried young twigs of *Cinnamomum cassia* Presl.

It is first recorded in the book of *Shennong Bencao Jing*. According to *Chongguang Buzhu Shennong Bencao Bingtu Jing (intensive and Extensive Supplementary Note of Shennong Herbal and Map Classics)* written in Northern Song Dynasty, "Guizhi is used to sweat as recorded in *Shanghan Zabing Lun* by Zhang Zhongjing. Guizhi is the young twig, not the trunk, but with the feature of being light and can diperse. Now, a young small *Liu*,the tender and fine twing of Guizhi, and its description is the same as young twig of *Cinnamomum Cassia* Presl.

2. 种植采收 桂枝主要来自于人工种植，主产于广西、广东、云南、福建等省区，多为栽培，属半阴树种，种子寿命短，多随采即播。桂枝采收宜于3~7月剪取嫩枝。

2 Planting and Harvesting

It is mainly produced in provinces including Guangxi, Guangdong, Yunnan, Fujian, etc. and mostly cultivated and is the semi-shade specie. Its seeds have a short lifespan, so they are sown immediately after harvest. The young Guizhi twigs are suitable to be harvested from March to July.

3. 道地性评价及品质评价 《新修本草》云"桂今出广州湛慧为好，湘州、始兴、桂阳县即是小桂，亦有，而不如广州者，交州、桂州者亦好"，说明自唐代起，便明确了两广产桂枝品质为佳。现代仍以广西产者质量最佳，特别是平南、藤县所产者，被誉为"六陈玉桂"和"西江桂"。形态上桂枝以枝条嫩细均匀，色红棕，香气浓者为佳。

3. Genuineness and Quality Evaluation

According to the *Xinxiu Bencao*, "Gui from Zhanhui in Guangzhou has good quality now, the ones in Xiangzhou, Shixing and Guiyang countics are called Xiaogui, whoes quality is not as good as those from Guangzhou, and those in Jiaozhou and Guizhou is also good". This shows the quality of Guizhi is good from Guangdong and Guangxi provinces since the Tang Dynasty. In modern times, Guizhi produced in Guangxi still has the best quality, especially in Pingnan and Teng counties, which are known as "Liuchen Yugui" and "Xijiang Gui", respectively. Guizhi, with tender, evenfine twigs, red-brown color and strong aroma, are considered to have good quality.

桂枝中主要含有挥发油类成分，其中桂皮醛与桂皮酸（肉桂酸）为主要有效成分。桂皮醛是桂枝抗血小板聚集、防止心肌损害、抗病毒、抗肿瘤的有效物质，桂皮酸与桂枝解热作用正相关。此外，桂枝中含有的缩合类鞣质是其强抗过敏组分。《中国药典》规定桂枝中桂皮醛含量不得少于1.0%。

The main components in Guizhi are volatile oils, among them cinnamaldehyde and cinnamic acid are the main active ingredients. Cinnamaldehyde is an effective substance for anti-platelet aggregation, preventing myocardial damage, anti-virus and anti-tumor. Cinnamic acid is positively related to the antipyretic effect of Guizhi. In addition, the condensed tannins contained in Guizhi are its strong anti-allergic components. *Pharmacopoeia of the People's Republic of China* records the content of cinnamaldehyde in Guizhi shall be not less than 1.0%.

二、炮制品种与品质
II Processed Varieties and Quality

桂枝炮制方法清代之前有净制和切制的记载，自清代开始有焙制、甘草汁制、蜜炙等炮制方法。目前临床常用品种主要为桂枝与蜜桂枝两种。桂枝以枝嫩、色红、去净叶及杂质者为佳。蜜桂枝以形如桂枝片，表面老黄色，微有光泽，略带黏性，香气减弱，味甜微辛为佳。《中国药典》规定桂枝饮片含量测定同药材。

Before the Qing Dynasty, Guizhi's processing methods were cleaning and cutting. Since the Qing Dynasty, its processing methods include baking, processing with Gancao juice, stir-frying with honey and so on. At present, the varieties in the clinical practices are mainly Guizhi and Miguizhi (stir-frying with honey). High-qualitied Guizhi is considered to be young twigs, red color, without leaves and impurities. High-qualitied Miguizhi (stir-frying with honey) is characterized by a similar shape of Guizhi decoction pieces, deep yellow on surface, mild luster, slight stickiness, weakened aroma, and sweet and thinly pungent flavor. According to *Pharmacopoeia of the People's Republic of*

China, the content determination of processed Guizhi pieces is the same as required for the raw material medica.

三、中成药品种与品质
III Varieties and Quality of Chinese Patent Medicines

《中国药典》收载含有桂枝的中成药共计67种。以桂枝为君药或主药的品种有小建中片（合剂、颗粒）、桂龙咳喘宁胶囊（颗粒）、桂枝茯苓丸（片、胶囊）等。在中成药的品质控制中多采用薄层色谱法确定桂枝的存在，采用含量测定法进行指标成分限量。如小建中片以 HPLC 法测定桂皮醛含量以限定每片含桂枝的量，桂龙咳喘宁胶囊以薄层色谱法检测桂皮醛的存在，以 HPLC 法测定肉桂酸含量以限定每粒含桂枝的量，以保证药品质量稳定。

There are more than 67 kinds of Chinese patent medicines containing Guizhi recorded in the *Pharmacopoeia of the People's Republic of China*. As the sovereign medicine or the main medicine, Guizhi can be found in prescriptions like Xiaojianzhong Pian (Tablets) (Heji, Keli), Guilong Kechuanning Jiaonang, and Keli, Guizhi Fuling Wan and Pian(Tablets), Jiaonang, etc. In the quality control of Chinese patent medicines, TLC is often used to determine the existence of Guizhi and the content determination is used to measure the limit the components. For example, the content of cinnamaldehyde is determined by HPLC to restrict the amount of Guizhi in each tablet of Xiaojianzhong Pian (Tablets). The existence of cinnamaldehyde is identified by TLC, and the content of cinnamic acid is determined by HPLC to limit the amount of each capsule to ensure the stable quality of Guilong Kechuanning Jiaonang.

【制药】
[Pharmacy]

一、产地加工
I Processing in Production Area

除去叶，鲜时切段，晒干。

While being fresh, remove leaves, cut into thick slices and dry them.

二、饮片炮制
II Processing of Decoction Pieces

桂枝的炮制方法，古籍记载有净制、蜜炙等。现行主要有桂枝、蜜桂枝两种，以生用为主。生品辛散温通作用较强，长于发汗解表，温经通阳。蜜桂枝辛通作用减弱，长于温中补虚，散寒止痛。《中国药典》载有桂枝一种炮制饮片。

According to historical records, the processing method of Guizhi mainly includes jingzhi (cleaning), mizhi (stir-frying with honey), etc. Nowadays, the processing products of Guizhi mainly include Guizhi, Miguizhi (stir-frying with honey), and raw Guizhi is mainly used. Raw Guizhi has a better function of pungent dispersing and warming the body, and it is good at promoting sweating to release the exterior, warming the meridian and activating yang. The effects of Miguizhi (stir-frying with honey) decrease in pungency dispersion and warming channels, but increase in warming spleen and stomach for tonifying deficiency and dissipating cold to relieve pain. *Pharmacopoeia of the People's Republic of China* records prepared Guizhi decoction slices.

三、中成药制药
III Pharmacy of Chinese Patent Medicines

桂枝在现代制剂中，提取工艺多为先提取挥

发油后再煎煮药渣，如小儿柴桂退热口服液、外感风寒颗粒等；也有直接打粉入药或煎煮入药，如乌梅丸、心荣口服液等；还有通过浸渍渗漉入药的，如消肿止痛酊。

In modern Chinese pharmaceutical preparations, the extraction process is mostly to extract the volatile oil first and then decoct the residue of Guizhi, such as in Xiaoer Chaigui Tuire Koufuye, Waigan Fenghan Keli, etc.; Guizhi is also directly powdered or decocted into medicine, such as in Wumei Wan, Xinrong Koufuye, etc. After Guizhi is steeped and percolated, the extractive is also used as medicine, such as in Xiaozhong Zhitong Ting (Tincture), etc.

如以桂枝为君药的桂龙咳喘宁胶囊，其制备过程采用桂枝细粉入药，制成的胶囊在体内溶解缓慢，使桂枝能够缓慢而持久地发挥助阳化气、降气平喘的作用。在小建中片制剂工艺中，桂枝所含挥发油是该中成药重要的有效物质，直接水煎易造成挥发油的损失，故先对其蒸馏提取挥发油，再与其他药合煎。

For example, in Guilong Kechuanning Jiaonang, Guizhi is used as the sovereign medicinal, and its fine powder are made into capsules, that makes the active components of Guizhi play a slow and lasting release role and keeps its function of reinforcing yang to transform qi and depressing qi to relieve asthma. In processing technology of Xiaojianzhong Pian (Tablets), the volatile oil of Guizhi is the important active material component, direct decocting in water will easily cause the loss of volatile oil. Therefore, it is extracted with distillation first, and then the residue is decocted with other medicinals.

【性能功效】
[Property and Efficacy]

一、性能
I Property

桂枝辛、甘，温；归心、肺、膀胱经。

Guizhi is pungent and sweet in flavor, warm in nature, and enters the heart, lung and bladder meridians.

二、功效
II Efficacy

1. **发汗解肌** 本品辛甘温煦，甘温通阳扶卫，开腠理发汗之力较麻黄缓和，长于宣阳气于卫分，畅营阴于肌表，使汗液蒸化有源。其功效的发挥与解热、抗病原微生物、抗炎、抗过敏等药理作用密切相关，这些作用的物质基础主要是挥发油和多酚类成分。桂枝可通过扩张皮肤血管发挥解热作用；通过抑制花生四烯酸代谢，影响炎症因子生成和抗氧化发挥抗炎、抗过敏作用；通过影响 Toll 样受体 7 的信号转导发挥抗病原微生物作用。

1 Sweating for Expelling Pathogenic Factors from Muscles

Guizhi is pungent, sweet and warm, activates yang and strengthens defensive qi, and its functions of sweating and opening muscular interstices are milder than those of Mahuang. Guizhi is good at dispersing yang qi to defense aspect, enriching yin in fleshy exterior to enable source of evaporation of sweating. Its effect is closely related to the pharmacological actions of releasing heat, anti-pathogenic microorganism, anti-inflammation and anti-allergy, etc. The material bases of these pharmacological effects are mainly the volatile oil and polyphenols. Guzhi can exert antipyretic effect by expanding skin blood vessels, inhibit the metabolism of arachidonic acid to influence inflammatory factors and anti-oxidation to exert anti-inflammatory and anti-allergic effects, and affect signal transduction of Toll-like receptor 7 to carry out anti-pathogenic microorganism effects.

2 **温通经脉** 桂枝辛甘性温，善入血分，能助心阳，通血脉。其功效的发挥与抗血小板聚集、抗凝血、改善心血管系统等药理作用密切相关。桂枝抗血小板聚集、抗凝血的有效物质基础主要是桂皮醛。

2 Warming and Dredging Collaterals

Guizhi is pungent and sweet in flavor, warm in nature, easy take effect in blood aspect, can help heart yang to dredge blood vessel. Its efficacy is closely related to the functions of anti-platelet aggregation, anti-coagulation, and improvement of cardiovascular system, etc. The cinnamaldehyde is the main ingredient for antiplatelet aggregation and anticoagulant effects in Guizhi.

3. 助阳化气 桂枝甘温，上助心阳以通脉，中助脾阳以运水，下助膀胱以行水。其功效的发挥与利尿等药理作用密切相关。

3 Assisting Yang Transforming into Qi

Guizhi is sweet and warm, can help heart yang to dredge the channel (blood vessels) in the upper body, promote the spleen yang to transport water in the middle body, and aid bladder to carry water in the low body. Its effect is closely related to diuresis of Guizhi.

4. 平冲降气 桂枝辛甘性温，能助心阳，通血脉，止悸动，故能平冲降逆。其功效的发挥与镇静、抗焦虑等药理作用密切相关，这些作用的物质基础主要是挥发油与桂皮醛。

4 Assuaging Flutter and Depressing Qi

Guizhi is pungent and sweet in flavor, warm in nature, helps the heart yang to circulate blood vessel and restrains palpitation, so it can assuage flutter and reduce the adverse qi. Its effect is closely related to the pharmacological activity of sedation, antianxiety, etc. The volatile oil and cinnamaldehyde are the main material bases of effects of Guizhi.

【应用】

[Application]

一、主治病证

I Indications

1. 风寒感冒 治疗外感风寒，表实无汗者，常与麻黄配伍，如《伤寒论》麻黄汤，与葛根配伍，如《伤寒论》葛根汤；治疗表虚有汗者，常

与敛阴止汗之白芍配伍，如《伤寒论》桂枝汤。

1 Common Cold of Wind-cold Syndrome

The compatibility of Guizhi or often treats the patients who have exogenous wind cold and no sweat with exterior excess, for example with Mahuang in Mahuang Tang (Decoction); with Gegen in Gegen Tang (Decoction) in *Shanghan Zabing Lun*. If the patients have sweat with exterior deficiency syndrome, Guizhi is often used together with Baishao which can astringe yin and stop sweating, such as Guizhi Tang (Decoction) in *Shanghan Zabing Lun*.

现代临床，桂枝配伍常用于治疗普通感冒、流行性感冒等风寒表实或营卫不和证，如外感风寒颗粒、表虚感冒颗粒等。

In modern clinical practice, Guizhi compatibility is often used in the treatment of common cold, influenza, etc., which are characterized by wind cold with exterior excess or disharmony between nutrient qi and defensive qi, such as Waigan Fenghan Keli and Biaoxu Ganmao Keli and so on.

2. 脘腹冷痛、血寒经闭，关节痹痛 治中焦虚寒之脘腹拘急疼痛，常与白芍、甘草配伍，如《金匮要略》小建中汤；治妇女寒凝胞宫证，可与吴茱萸、当归配伍，如《金匮要略》温经汤；治风寒湿痹，肩臂疼痛，与芍药、附子配伍，如《金匮要略》桂枝芍药知母汤；治营血不足的痹痛，常与黄芪、白芍配伍，如《金匮要略》黄芪桂枝五物汤。

2 Abdominal Cold Pain, Blood Cold Amenorrhea, and Joint Impediment Diseases

Guizhi together with Baishao and Gancao can treat acute abdominal cramping pain with deficient cold in middle energizer, such as Xiaojianzhong Tang (Decoction) in *Jingui Yaolue*. The compatibility of Guizhi, Wuzhuyu and Danggui treats the syndrome of coagulated cold in uterus, such as Wenjing Tang (Decoction) in *Jingui Yaolue*; Guizhi combined with Shaoyao and Fuzi treats wind-cold-dampnessbi, shoulder and arm pain, such as Guizhi Shaoyao

Zhimu Tang (Decoction) in *Jingui Yaolue*; The compatibility of Guizhi, Huangqi and Baishao treats arthralgia caused by nutrient-blood deficiency, such as Huangqi Guizhi Wuwu Tang (Decoction) in *Jingui Yaolue*.

现代临床，桂枝配伍常用于治疗胃炎、胃及十二指肠溃疡、月经不调、痛经、产后腹痛、骨关节炎、风湿或类风湿性关节炎及手足麻木、腰腿酸痛等属寒凝血滞诸痛证，可用安中片、桂枝茯苓丸、尪痹颗粒、冯了性风湿跌打药酒等。

In modern clinical practices, Guizhi compatibility is commonly used to various pains syndrome due to cold coagulation and blood stagnation, and treat gastritis, gastric and duodenal ulcer, irregular menstruation, dysmenorrhea, postpartum abdominal pain, osteoarthritis, rheumatic or rheumatoid arthritis, numbness of hands and feet, waist-leg sour pain, etc., For these cases Anzhong Pian, Guizhi Fuling Wan, Wangbi Keli, Fengliaoxing Fengshi Dieda Yaojiu (Medicinal Liquor), etc. can be applied.

3. 痰饮、水肿 治脾阳不运，水湿内停的痰饮眩晕、心悸、咳嗽，常与茯苓、白术配伍，以补益心脾，化湿利水，如《金匮要略》苓桂术甘汤；治肾阳不足，膀胱气化失司，见水肿、小便不利者，多与茯苓、泽泻等同用，如《伤寒论》五苓散。

3 Phlegm and Fluid Retention, Edema

Guizhi is often combined with Fuling and Baizhu to tonify the heart and spleen, to dissolve dampness and to improve diuresis, they compatibility treats phlegm and fluid retention, dizziness, palpitation and cough caused by the stagnation of spleen yang and water dampness, such as Linggui Zhugan Tang (Decoction) in *Jingui Yaolue*. Guizhi together with Fuling and Zexie treats kidney yang deficiency, dysfunction of bladder in qi transformation, edema and difficult urination, such as Wuling San (Powder) in *Shanghan Zabing Lun*.

现代临床，桂枝配伍常用于治疗上呼吸道感染、支气管哮喘、支气管炎、肾炎、水肿等，如桂枝加厚朴杏子汤、肾炎消肿片。

In modern clinical practices, Guizhi compatibility is often used to treat upper respiratory tract infection, bronchial asthma, bronchitis, nephritis, edema, etc., such as Guizhi Jiahoupo Xingzi Tang (Decoction), Shenyan Xiaozhong Pian (Tablets).

4. 心悸、奔豚 治疗心阳不振，不能宣通血脉，症见心悸动、脉结代者，多与炙甘草、人参同用，如《伤寒论》炙甘草汤；治疗阴寒内盛，引动下焦冲气，上凌心胸之奔豚者，常与芍药、生姜同用，如《伤寒论》桂枝加桂汤；治疗心阳不振或心失温养所致的心下悸动，常与甘草为伍，如《伤寒论》桂枝甘草汤。

4 Palpitations, Kidney Amassment (Running-pig Rushing up)

Guizhi combined with Zhigancao (processed) and Renshen is often used to the patients with palpitation and intermittent pulse, treat devitalization of heart yang and blood circulation obstacle, such as Zhigancao Tang (Decoction) in *Shanghan Zabing Lun*. Guizhi together with Shaoyao and Shengjiang is used to the patients with Bentun, (pig-running like rushing up), treats yin-cold internal exuberance, lower energizer qi up-rushing syndrome with bullying heart and chest, such as Guizhi Jiagui Tang (Decoction) in *Shanghan Zabing Lun*. Guizhi is often accompanied by Gancao to treat palpitation due to heart yang deficiency or heart malnutrition, such as Guizhi Gancao Decoction in *Shanghan Zabing Lun*.

现代临床，桂枝配伍常用于治疗冠心病、心绞痛、心肌梗死等心阳不振、心脉瘀阻者，如枳实薤白桂枝汤，参桂胶囊等。

In modern clinical practice, Guizhi compatibility is often used to treat devitalization of heart yang and blockage of heart vessel, such as coronary heart disease, angina pectoris, myocardial infarction, etc., like Zhishi Xiebai Guizhi Tang (Decoction) and Shengui Jiaonang, etc.

二、用法用量
II Administration and Dosage

3~10g，煎服。
3-10g each time, water decoction.

三、注意事项
III Precautions

本品性温助热，易伤阴动血，故外感热病、阴虚火旺、血热妄行者忌用。孕妇及月经过多者慎用。

This product is warm in nature but it is easy to injure yin and over-motivate blood. Therefore, it is forbidden to the patients who suffer from exogenous febrile disease, hyperactivity of fire due to yin deficiency and blood-heat bleeding. It should be carefully used for the pregnant women or women with menorrhagia.

柴　胡

Chaihu
(Bupleuri Radix)

柴胡是陕西、甘肃等地区著名的道地药材。临床常用炮制品有醋柴胡与酒柴胡。柴胡味辛、苦，微寒，归肝、胆、肺经，具疏散退热，疏肝解郁，升举阳气之功效，主治外感表证、寒热往来、中气下陷、肝郁气滞、骨蒸盗汗等。柴胡主要含柴胡皂苷、甾醇、挥发油、多糖等成分，有解热、镇静、抗炎、抗病毒、保肝利胆、增强免疫、抗肿瘤等药理作用，可用于治疗外感发热、寒热往来属少阳表证者，胸胁胀痛、月经失调属肝郁气滞证者，子宫脱垂，脱肛属中气下陷证者。

Chaihu is a noted genuine regional medicinal in Shaanxi and Gansu Provinces. The clinical used processed products are mainly Cuchaihu (vinegar processed) and Jiuchaihu (liquor processed). Chaihu is pungent and bitter in flavor, and slightly cold in nature and enters to the liver, gallbladder and lung meridians. Chaihu has the effect of dispersing and relieving fever, soothing the liver to relieve the depression, and raising yang qi. It is often used for treating the exterior syndromes, alternating chills and fever, collapse of middle qi, stagnation of liver qi, hectic fever with night sweating, etc. Chaihu mainly contains saikosaponins, sterols, volatile oil, polysaccharides and other chemical components, giving full play to the pharmacological effects of relieving fever, sedation, anti-inflammation, anti-virus, liver and gallbladder protection, immunity enhancement, anti-tumor and other pharmacological effects, which can be used for the treatment of exogenous fever, alternating chill and fever of shaoyang exterior syndrome, or chest distended pain, rib pain, menstrual disorders due to liver qi stagnation, or uterine prolapse, anal prolapse and other diseases due to middle qi collapse.

【品种品质】
[Variety and Quality]

一、基原品种与品质
I Origin varieties and quality

1. 品种概况　来源于伞形科植物柴胡 *Bupleurum chinense* DC. 或狭叶柴胡 *Bupleurum Scorzonerifolium* Willd. 的干燥根。

1 Variety

Chaihu is the dried root of *Bupleurum*

Chinense DC or *Bupleurum Scorzonerifolium* Willd of Umbelliferae.

柴胡始载于《神农本草经》，名为"茈胡"，《新修本草》提出茈胡之名因其根紫色而得，"茈"即古柴字，北宋《本草图经》始易其名为柴胡。自古以来柴胡入药品种繁多，主要源于伞形科柴胡属植物，如《证类本草》中记载有柴胡、狭叶柴胡、春柴胡、银柴胡等品种。现按其性状不同，分别习称"北柴胡"与"南柴胡"。

It is first recorded in the book of *Shennong Bencao Jing*, and classified its name as Zihu, which named after its purple root. It has been renamed as Chaihu in *Bencao Tujing* since Northern Song Dynasty, for Zi in Chinese Character is similiar as Chai in Chinese Character. From the records of materia medica in previous dynasties, it can be seen that there are many kinds of Chaihu used in medicine with more complex sources since ancient times, which are mostly generated from the genus *Bupleurum* of Umbelliferae, including Chaihu, Xiaye Chaihu, Chun Chaihu and Yin Chaihu etc., as recorded in *Zhenglei Bencao*. According to their different characters, they are commonly called "Beichaihu" (Northern Chinese Thorowax Root) and "Nanchaihu" (Southern Chinese Thorowax Root).

2. 种植采收 柴胡主要以种植为主，主产于甘肃、陕西、山西等地，柴胡种植继承了育苗移栽、种子直播的栽种技术。柴胡喜冷凉而温润的气候，较耐寒耐旱，忌高温和涝洼积水。一般春季播种，至秋季植株下部叶片开始枯萎时采收，采挖根部，抖去泥土，残茎除净。

2 Planting and Harvesting

Chaihu is mainly planted in Gansu, Shaanxi, Shanxi Provinces and other places. The cultivation of Chaihu inherits the planting technique of seedling transplanting and direct seeding. Chaihu prefers a cool and moist climate, and is more resistant to cold and drought but intolerant to high temperature and waterlogging. It is generally sowed in spring and harvested when the lower leaves of the plant begin to wither in autumn. As

soon as the roots are dug out, shake off the soil and remove the the residual stems.

3. 道地性及品质评价 北柴胡主产我国北部地区，陕西北部、甘肃等地是传统的道地产区，南柴胡主要产区集中在四川、湖北、云南等地。柴胡在形态上以主根粗长、分枝少、残留茎较少、质地柔软者为佳。

3 Genuineness and Quality Evaluation

"BeiChaihu" is a genuine regional medicinal in Northeast China including North Shaanxi and Gansu Provinces, while "NanChaihu" is a genuine regional medicinal in Sichuan, Hubei and Yunnan Provinces. Morphologically, the quality of Chaihu with thick and long main root, less branches and residual stem, and soft texture is better.

柴胡中主要含柴胡皂苷、甾醇、挥发油、多糖、黄酮等，其中柴胡皂苷是其抗炎、抗病毒、抗肿瘤、抗肝损伤的主要物质基础，所含挥发油是其解热的主要物质基础，柴胡多糖是抗辐射、增强免疫的主要物质基础。《中华人民共和国药典》2015 年版规定柴胡药材中含柴胡皂苷 a 和柴胡皂苷 d 的总量不得少于 0.30%。

Chaihu mainly contains saikosaponin, sterol, volatile oil, polysaccharide and flavonoid etc., in which saikosaponin is the main material basis for anti-inflammation, anti-virus, anti-tumor and anti-liver injury, and the volatile oil is the main material basis of antipyretic effects. Polysaccharide in Chaihu is the main material basis of anti-radiation and enhancing immunity. According to the *Pharmacopoeia of the People's Republic of China*, the total amount of saikosaponin a and saikosaponin d in Chaihu should not be less than 0.30%.

二、炮制品种与品质
II Processed Varieties and Quality

柴胡从古至今形成了系列炮制方法，仅在古代，其炮制方法多达 20 余种，沿用至今的有生柴胡、醋柴胡、蜜柴胡、酒柴胡等。《中国药典》收载了北柴胡、醋北柴胡、南柴胡、醋南柴胡等四个品种。柴胡饮片以呈不规则厚片，外表皮黑褐色或浅棕色，质硬，气微香，味微苦为佳；醋柴胡以形如柴胡片，色泽加深，微具醋香气者为佳，饮片的含量测定要求同药材。

It has formed a series of processing methods for Chaihu from ancient times to the present. In ancient times, there are more than 20 processing methods, including raw Chaihu, Cuchaihu (processed with vinegar), Michaihu (processe with honey),Jiuchaihu(processed with liquor) are still used today. *The Pharmacopoeia of the People's Republic of China* records four varieties, namely BeiChaihu, CuBeichaihu (vinegar processed), NanChaihu and CuNanChaihu (vinegar processed). Chaihu with irregular thick slices, dark brown or pale brown skin, hard in texture, slightly aroma and slightly bitter in flavor is with good quality. Cuchaihu with similar shape of the raw medicinal but the one in deeper color and with slightly vinegar aroma is better. The content determination requirements for processed products are the same as required for its raw material Medica of Chaihu.

三、中成药品种与品质
III Varieties and Quality of Chinese Patent Medicines

含有柴胡或其炮制品的中成药有 400 余个，《中国药典》收载 100 余个。以柴胡为君药的品种有小柴胡颗粒、柴胡注射液、逍遥丸等。在中成药质量控制中多采用显微鉴别或薄层色谱法确定柴胡的存在，中成药中少见测定其化学成分作为含量指标。如小柴胡颗粒以柴胡对照药材为对照，采用薄层色谱法确定柴胡的存在，补中益气丸以显微鉴别"油管含淡黄色或黄棕色条状物，直径 8~25μm"确定含有柴胡。

At present, there are more than 400 Chinese patent medicines containing Chaihu or its processed products and more than 100 Chinese patent medicines are recorded in the *Pharmacopoeia of the People's Republic of China*. Prescriptions with Chaihu as the sovereign medicinal are Xiaochaihu Keli, Chaihu Zhusheye, Xiaoyao Wan, etc. In the quality control of Chinese patent medicines, microscopic identification or TLC is often used to determine the existence of Chaihu. It is rare to determine its chemical components as content index in Chinese patent medicine. For example, In Xiaochaihu Keli, it takes Chaihu control medicinal to determine the existence of Chaihu by TLC, while whether Buzhong Yiqi Wan, the containing of Chaihu is determined by microscopic identification on "the tubing contains light yellow or yellowish brown strips with a diameter of 8~25μm".

【制药】
[Pharmacy]

一、产地加工
I Processing in Production Area

将采挖的鲜柴胡根以水冲洗干净后进行晾晒，当晒到 7~8 成干时，将须根去净，根条顺直，捆成小把再继续晒干，即可。

The fresh Chaihu root is usually washed by water and dried in the sun. When the root reaches 70%-80% dry, remove the fibrous root, straighten the root strip, tie it into a small handful bandle and continue to dry it.

二、饮片炮制
II Processing of Decoction Pieces

柴胡的主要炮制工序包括润透、切片，或再加辅料制。目前生柴胡、醋柴胡成为商品规格中的主流。另外尚有清炒、酒制、蜜制、鳖血制等炮制方法。

The main processing processes of Chaihu include moistening, slicing and adding auxiliary materials, from which the most commonly used varieties in clinical are Shengchaihu and CuChaihu. In addition, there are plain stir-fried Chaihu, liquor-processed Chaihu, honey-processed Chaihu, Chaihu processed with soft-shelled turtle blood and other varieties in use.

柴胡在醋制过程中，加热导致柴胡挥发油中正己醛、正庚醛等有效成分含量下降，而柴胡皂苷 a、d 在酸性环境中会转化为柴胡皂苷 b₁、b₂，部分皂苷水解为药理作用更强的苷元，而皂苷比例的变化和苷元含量的增加使醋柴胡的抗抑郁作用显著增强，而挥发油含量下降使其解表作用减弱。

In the process of vinegar preparation, heating will lead to the decrease of the effective contents of n-hexanal and n-heptanal in volatile oil of Chaihu, while saikosaponins a and saikosaponins d will be transformed into saikosaponins b_1 and saikosaponins b_2 in acidic environment. Some of the saponins are hydrolyzed into aglycone with stronger pharmacological effects, while the antidepressant effect of vinegar processed Chaihu is significantly enhanced by the change of the proportion of saponins and the increase of aglycone content, while the decrease of the content of volatile oil weakens the effect of releasing the exterior.

三、中成药制药
III Pharmacy of Chinese Patent Medicines

含柴胡的中成药剂型丰富，可单味药制成制剂，如柴胡注射液、柴胡口服液，但更多时候与其他药物以复方配伍形式应用，如逍遥丸、小柴胡颗粒、柴连口服液等。中成药中柴胡多以生品投料，传统丸剂常粉碎为用，如逍遥丸至今仍沿用传统制剂方法。而用于解热作用之柴胡注射液，采用水蒸气蒸馏法单独提取柴胡挥发油，通过加入增溶剂增加挥发油在水中的溶解度和稳定性，制成的柴胡注射液能够快速发挥药效。

Chinese patent medicines containing Chaihu have many dosage forms, which can be made into single-used preparations, such as Chaihu Zhusheye and Chaihu Koufuye, but it is more often used in the form of compound compatibility with other medicinals, such as Xiaoyao Wan, Xiaochaihu Keli, Chailian Koufuye and so on. Most of the

Chinese Patent medicines apply raw Chaihu materials, and the traditional pills often use the crushed Chaihu. For example, Xiaoyao Wan still use the traditional preparation method. For the antipyretic effect of Chaihu Zhusheye, the volatile oil of Chaihu was extracted by steam distillation, and the solubility and stability of volatile oil in water were increased by adding solubilizer, so that the Chaihu Zhusheye could exert its efficacy quickly.

【性能功效】
[Property and Efficacy]

一、性能
I Property

柴胡辛、苦，微寒；归肝、胆、肺经。
Chaihu is pungent and bitter in flavor, slightly cold in nature and enters the liver, gallbladder and lung meridians.

二、功效
II Efficacy

1. **疏散退热** 柴胡辛散苦泄，可升可散，且入肺经，故长于疏解半表半里之邪。其功效的发挥与其解热、抗炎、抗内毒素、抗病原微生物等药理作用密切相关。柴胡解热、抗炎、抗内毒素的有效物质基础主要是柴胡皂苷、皂苷元 A、柴胡挥发油，通过作用于下丘脑体温调节中枢，抑制体温调定点的上移而发挥解热作用；通过抑制炎性渗出、毛细血管通透性升高、炎症介质释放、白细胞游走等炎症途径发挥抗炎作用。

1 Dispersing and Relieving Fever
Chaihu is dispersing with the pungent nature and draining with the bitter nature which can float both up-bearing and disperse and enters into the lung meridian, so it is good at relieving the pathogen of half-exterior and half-interior. Its efficacy is closely related to its antipyretic, anti-inflammatory effects and pharmacological effects

of anti-endotoxin, anti-pathogenic microorganisms and others. The effective substance bases of antipyretic, anti-inflammatory and anti-endotoxin effect of Chaihu are mainly saikosaponin, sapogenin A and Bupleurum volatile oil. The main mechanism of action is to exert antipyretic effect by acting on the hypothalamic temperature regulation center and inhibiting the upward movement of the temperature setting point. It can play an anti-inflammatory role by inhibiting inflammatory exudation, increasing capillary permeability, releasing inflammatory mediators and migrating leukocytes.

2. **疏肝解郁**　柴胡入肝、胆经，辛行苦泄，主散，疏肝解郁。其功效的发挥与抗抑郁、保肝利胆等药理作用密切相关。柴胡抗抑郁、保肝利胆的有效物质基础主要是柴胡皂苷，通过刺激垂体-肾上腺皮质系统，增加内源性糖皮质激素分泌，促进抗体和干扰素的产生，抗过氧化损伤，抑制肝细胞凋亡等发挥保肝作用；并通过提高中枢 NE、DA、5-HT 浓度及抗氧化作用发挥抗抑郁作用。

2 Soothing the Liver and RelievingDepression

Chaihu enters the liver and gallbladder meridians, moving with the pungent and draining with the bitter but mainly dissipating, taking on the effects of soothing the liver and relieving depression. Its efficacy is closely related to the pharmacological effects such as anti-depression, liver protection and gallbladder protection. The effective material basis of Chaihu for antidepressant, liver protection and choleretic effects is saikosaponin, through stimulating pituitary-adrenal cortex system, increasing endogenous glucocorticoid secretion, to promote antibody and interferon production, resist peroxide damage and inhibit hepatocyte apoptosis. It can play an antidepressant action by increasing the concentration of NE, DA, 5-HT in the pivot and its antioxidant effect.

3. **升举阳气**　柴胡性辛主升发，故可升中焦脾胃之阳气。其升举阳气之功与增强免疫功

能、兴奋内脏平滑肌等药理作用密切相关。柴胡增强免疫功能、兴奋内脏平滑肌的物质基础主要是柴胡皂苷、柴胡多糖，通过增强库普佛（Kupffer）细胞吞噬功能，提高巨噬细胞、自然杀伤细胞（NK）的功能，提高淋巴细胞的转换率发挥增强免疫功能作用；并通过增强乙酰胆碱对肠肌的收缩发挥兴奋内脏平滑肌作用。

3 Raising Yang Qi

Chaihu, mainly ascending and dispering, pungent innature, can raise the *yang qi* of spleen and stomach in middle energizer. The function of raising *yang qi* is closely related to pharmocological effects as enhanceming immune function and exciting visceral smooth muscle. Saikosaponin and Bupleurum polysaccharide are the material basis for Chaihu exciting above effects, which strengthens immune function by enhancing phagocytosis of Kupffer cells, improving the functions of macrophages and natural killer cells (NK) and increasing the conversion rate of lymphocytes. It can stimulate visceral smooth muscle by enhancing the contraction of intestinal muscle by acetylcholine.

此外，柴胡还有抗惊厥、抗肿瘤、降血脂等作用。

In addition, Chaihu also has the effects of anti-convulsion, anti-tumor, reducing blood lipid and so on.

【应用】
[Application]

一、主治病证
I Indications

1. **外感发热、寒热往来**　对于感冒发热，无论风热、风寒表证，皆可使用。治疗风寒感冒，常与防风、生姜等药配伍，如《景岳全书》正柴胡饮。治外感风寒，寒邪入里化热，恶寒渐轻，身热增盛者，多与葛根、黄芩等配伍以解表清里，《伤寒六书》如柴葛解肌汤。治疗风热感冒，

可与菊花、薄荷等辛凉解表药同用。若伤寒邪在少阳，寒热往来、胸胁苦满，常与黄芩等配伍，如《伤寒论》小柴胡汤。

1　Fever due to Exterior Pathogen and Alternating Chills and Fever

Chaihu can be used for chills and fever for both wind-heat syndrome and wind-cold syndrome. Chaihu is often combined with Fangfeng, Shengjiang etc. for treating wind-cold fever, such as in Zhengchaihu Yin (Decoction) in *Jingyue Quanshu*. Chaihu is mostly combined with Gegen, Huangqin etc. for treating exterior wind-cold pathogen entering the interior to transform into heat with aversion to cold but gradually lighter and body heat increasing, to release the exterior and clear interior, such as used in Chaigejieji Tang (Decoction) in *Shanghan Liushu (Six Texts on Cold Damage)*. For the treatment of wind-heat common cold, it can be used with Juhua, Bohe and other pungent-cool exterior releasing medicinals. If cold pathogen is in shaoyang meridians, for patients suffering from alternating chills and fever, bitterness and fullness in chest and hypochondrium, it is often combined with Huangqin, such as shown in Xiaochaihu Tang (Decoction) in *Shanghan Zabing Lun*.

现代临床，柴胡常配伍用于感冒、肺炎、支气管炎、扁桃体炎、疟疾等引起的体温升高，临床采用柴胡注射液、柴胡口服液等均有较好效果。

In modern clinic, Chaihu compatibility is often used for high fever caused by common cold, pneumonia, bronchitis, tonsillitis, malaria and so on. Chaihu Zhusheye and Chaihu Koufuye have good effects in clinic.

2. **肝郁气滞证**　治肝失疏泄，气机郁滞所致的胸胁胀痛、情志抑郁及妇女月经不调、痛经等，可与香附、川芎等配伍，如《景岳全书》柴胡疏肝散；治肝郁血虚，脾失健运，症见胁肋作痛、神疲食少或月经不调，乳房胀痛者，常与当归、白芍等配伍，如《太平惠民和剂局方》逍遥散。治肝郁气滞，胸痞胀满，胃脘疼痛者，配伍延胡索、枳壳等，如气滞胃痛片《中华人民共和

国药典》。

2　Liver Depression and Qi Stagnation Syndrome

For the treatment of chest pain, emotional depression, irregular menstruation and dysmenorrhea in women caused by the failure of liver dispersing and draining and stagnation, Chaihu can be compatible with Xiangfu and Chuanxiong, such as in Chaihushugan San (Powder) in *Jingyue Quanshu*; for the treatment of syndromes such as rib pain, fatigue and poor oppetite or irregular menstruation, breast distension and pain caused by liver depression and blood deficiency, spleen failing in transportation, Chaihu is often compatible with Danggui and Baishao etc., such as Xiaoyao San (Powder) in *Taiping Huimin Heji Ju Fang*. For the treatment of chest stuffiness and fullness, epigastric fullness and pain caused by liver depression and qi stagnation, it can be compatible with Yanhusuo and Zhiqiao etc., such as in Qizhi Weitong Pian (Tablets) in *Pharmacopoeia of the People's Republic of China*.

现代临床，本药可配伍用于治疗急慢性肝炎、胃炎、肠易激综合征等属肝郁气滞证者，如小柴胡汤、柴胡疏肝散。

In modern clinical, Chaihu compatibility can be used to treat acute and chronic hepatitis, gastritis and irritable bowel syndrome belonging to liver depression and qi stagnation syndrome, such as Xiao Chaihu Tang (Decoction) and Chaihu Shugan San (Powder).

3. **脾虚气陷证**　治疗久泻脱肛，子宫下垂，胃下垂等内脏下垂，常与人参、黄芪、升麻等补气升阳药同用，如《脾胃论》补中益气汤。

3　Spleen Deficiency and Qi Collapse Syndrome

For the treatment of prolapse of the anus due to long-time diarrhea, uterine prolapse, gastroptosis and other visceral prolapse, Chaihu can be compatible with Renshen, Huangqi, Shengma and other *qi*-tonifying and upraising medicinals, such as in Buzhong Yiqi Tang (Decoction) in *Piwei Lun*

(Treatise on Spleen and Stomach).

现代临床，柴胡可配伍用于治疗痛经、脱肛等属中气下陷证的治疗。

In modern clinical practice, Chaihu can be combined for the treatment of dysmenorrheal and anal prolapse with the syndrome of middle qi collapse.

二、用法用量
II Administration and Dosage

3~10g，煎服，疏散退热宜生用，疏肝解郁宜醋炙。

3~10g each time, decocted for drink, use the raw medicinal for dispelling heat, while use the vinegar processed one for soothing the liver and relieving depression.

三、注意事项
III Precautions

1. 肝阳上亢，阴虚火旺及气机上逆者忌用。

1 It should not be used for those who has with the syndromes of liver yang hyperactivity, or yin deficiency with fire exuberance and upward reversal of qi activity.

2. 本品毒性较小，但口服较大剂量可出现嗜睡、工作效率下降，甚至出现深睡等现象，或出现腹胀、食欲减退等。

2 The toxin of Chaihu is mild, but a large oral dose can lead to drowsiness, decreased work efficiency, or even deep sleep, or abdominal distension, loss of appetite and so on.

葛 根

Gegen
(Puerariae Lobatae Radix)

葛根主产于陕西、湖北、湖南、四川等地。葛根味甘、辛，性凉，归脾、胃、肺经，具有解肌退热、生津止渴、透疹、升阳止泻、通经活络、解酒毒之功效，主治外感发热头痛，项背强痛，口渴，消渴，麻疹不透，热痢，泄泻，眩晕头痛，中风偏瘫，胸痹心痛，酒毒伤中。葛根主要含有黄酮类和香豆素类成分，另含三萜皂苷和生物碱类成分；有解热、降血糖、降血脂、抗心肌缺血、抗心律失常、扩张外周血管、降压等药理作用，临床可用于治疗普通感冒、流行性感冒等属风寒或风热表证者、神经性头痛、血管性头痛、偏头痛等表邪侵犯阳明经者。葛根素静脉给药对冠心病、心肌梗死、心律失常、脑梗死等疾病具有较好疗效。

Gegen is mainly produced in Shaanxi, Hubei, Hunan, Sichuan, etc. Gegen is sweet and pungent in flavor, and cool in nature which enters the spleen, stomach, and the lung meridians, functioning as releasing the muscle and dispersing the heat, promoting fluid production to quench thirst, promoting eruption, upraising *yang* and relieving diarrhea, unblocking the meridian, activating collaterals, and relieving alcoholism. It mainly treats exterior fever with headache, pain and stiffness in nape and neck, thirst, consumptive-thirst, measles without adequate eruption, heat dysentery, diarrhea, dizziness and headache, wind stroke with hemiplegia, chest impediment and heart pain, alcoholic poisoning injuring the middle. Gegen mainly contains flavonoids and coumarins, as well as triterpenoid saponins and alkaloids. It has the pharmacological effects of being antipyretic, hypoglycemic, hypolipidemic, anti-myocardial ischemia, anti-arrhythmia, dilating peripheral blood vessels, reducing blood pressure and so on. Gegen can be used to treat the common cold and influenza syndrome as wind-cold or wind-heat, as well as the neuropathic headache, vascular headache and migraine caused by exterior pathogen invading *yangming* meridian. Intravenous administration with puerarin has a good effect on coronary heart disease, myocardial infarction, cerebral arrhythmia, thrombosis, and other diseases.

【品种品质】
[Variety and Quality]

一、基原品种与品质
I Origin Varieties and Quality

1. **品种概况**　来源于豆科植物野葛 *Pueraria lobata (Willd.)* Ohwi 的干燥根。

1 Variety

Gegen is the dried root of *Puerarialobata (Willd.)* Ohwi of *Leguminosae*.

葛根首载于《神农本草经》。梁代陶弘景《本草经集注》记载葛根入药品种不止一种，并有可食用品种。李时珍《本草纲目》载其有野生和家种之分。综合历代本草记载，葛根来源主要有甘葛与野葛两种来源，在唐以前认为野葛入药最好，甘葛主要用于食疗。自《中华人民共和国药典》2005 年版始，将甘葛以粉葛单列，野葛即为葛根。

The medicinal use of Gegen was first listed in *Shennong Bencao Jing*. *Bencaojing Jizhu* written by Tao Hongjing in Liang Dynasty recorded that there was more than one variety of Gegen as medicine, besides edible varieties. *Bencao Gangmu* written by Li Shizhen records that there are wild and domestic species. From the records of *Materia Medica* in previous dynasties, it can be seen that Gegen mainly comes from *Pueraria thomsonii Benth.* and *Pueraria lobata (Willd.)* Ohwi (Kudzu). Before Tang Dynasty, Kudzu was the best specie for medicine while *Pueraria thomsonii Benth.* is mainly used for dietotherapy. Since *Pharmacopoeia of the People's Republic of China (2005 Edition)*, *Pueraria thomsonii Benth.* has been listed individually as Fenge (Puerariae Thomsonii Radix), and Kudzu is regarded as Gegen (Puerariae Lobatae Radix).

2. **种植采收**　葛根以野生为主，也有人工种植，主产于陕西、湖北、湖南、四川等地。人工种植一般于 3 月上旬移栽葛苗，2~3 年后秋、冬二季采挖，趁鲜切成厚片或小块，干燥。

2 Planting and Harvesting

Gegen is mainly wild, but also artificially planted. It is mainly planted in Shaanxi, Hubei, Hunan, Sichuan and other places. Gegen is generally planted by transplanting the Gegen seedlings in early March, harvested in autumn and winter 2-3 years later. Then cut it into thick slices or small pieces while fresh, and dry it.

3. **道地性及品质评价**　葛根道地产区不明确，在全国多数地区均产，一般认为以陕西、湖北、湖南等地所产质优。葛根以质地疏松、切面纤维性强者为佳。

3 Genuineness and Quality Evaluation

Gegen produced most parts of China, so the genuine regional producing area is not clear. Generally, the species grown in Shaanxi, Hubei, Hunan and other places are regarded with good quality. The one with loose texture and strong fiber in section is preferred.

葛根主要含有黄酮类和香豆素类成分，黄酮类成分主要包括葛根素、黄豆苷元、黄豆苷等。葛根发挥解热、降血糖、降血脂的有效成分为主要为葛根素，葛根总黄酮和葛根素是扩张冠状血管、扩张脑血管、改善微循环、抗心肌缺血的物质基础。此外，葛根还含有三萜皂苷和生物碱类等成分。《中国药典》规定葛根药材含葛根素不得少于 2.4%。

Gegen mainly contains flavonoids and coumarins, and flavonoids mainly include puerarin, daidzein, daidzin, etc. The active component of Gegen producing antipyretic, hypoglycemic and hypolipidemic effects is mainly puerarin. Total flavonoids and puerarin are the material bases of dilating coronary vessels, dilating cerebral vessels, improving microcirculation and anti-myocardial ischemia. In addition, Gegen also contains triterpenoid saponins and alkaloids. According to the *Pharmacopoeia of the People's Republic of China*, the content of puerarin in Gegen material medica should not be less than 2.4%.

二、炮制品种与品质
II Processed Varieties and Quality

葛根在临床上以生品最为常用,另有煨制品现临床少有应用。生品饮片呈不规则厚片、粗丝或小方块,切面浅黄棕色至棕黄色,以质韧,纤维性强为佳;煨葛根形如葛根,表面焦黄色,气微香。生品饮片的含量测定要求同药材。

Gegen is mainly used with the raw material, while the roasting products are rarely used clinically. The raw Gegen slices are irregular thick slices, thick silk or small squares in shape, and light yellowish brown to brown in section. The one in good quality is hard in texture, and with strong fiber. The roasting processed Gegen is shaped like raw one, but the surface is scorched yellow and is slightly fragrant in flavor. The content determination requirements of rew Chaihu deloction slices are the same as the raw meterial medica.

三、中成药品种与品质
III Varieties and Quality of Chinese Patent Medicines

含有葛根的中成药有300余个,其中《中国药典》收载80多个。以葛根为君药的品种有葛根芩连丸、小儿泻痢片、葛根汤颗粒等。在质量控制多采用显微鉴别和薄层色谱法确定葛根的存在,采用高效液相色谱法等对制剂中葛根素的含量进行测定,也有采用特征图谱对制剂中葛根特征性成分进行控制。如葛根芩连片采用高效液相色谱法和指维图谱双重控制制剂中葛根的质量;再造丸、脑得生丸等通过显微鉴别"纤维成束,

周围细胞中含草酸钙方晶,形成晶纤维,含晶细胞的壁木化增厚"确定含有葛根;葛根汤颗粒以葛根对照药材和葛根素为对照品,采用薄层色谱法确定含有葛根。

There are more than 300 kinds of Chinese patent medicine containing Gegen, of which over 80 kinds are included in *Pharmacopoeia of the People's Republic of China*. The representative varieties of Gegen serving as sovereign medicine are Gegen Qinlian Wan, Xiaoer Xieli Pian (Tablets), Gegentang Keli and so on. In the quality control, microscopic identification and TLC are used to determine the existence of Gegen, HPLC is used to determine the content of puerarin in the preparations containing Gegen, and characteristic atlas is also used to control the characteristic components of Gegen in the preparations. For example, in Gegen Qinlian Pian, the quality of Gegen was dually controlled by both HPLC and the fingerprints. In preparations such as Zaizao Wan and Naodesheng Wan, Gegen was identified by microscopic identification on the characteristics like "fiber bundles, calcium oxalate square crystals in the surrounding cells, forming of crystal fibers, and thickening of the walls of crystal cells" to ensure containing of Gegen. Gegen in Gegentang Keli was determined by TLC by taking Gegen medica material and puerarin as reference substance.

【制药】
[Pharmacy]

一、产地加工
I Processing in Production Area

将采挖的葛根以水洗净表面泥沙及杂物,剪去两端根茎、尾根及周围的细根,刮去粗皮,趁鲜纵切为长方形或小方块,烘干。

The Gegen is washed with water after digging out to remove the sand and imparities, cut off the rhizome and root of the both ends and the surrounding fine roots, and scrape off the rough skin. Then it was cut into rectangles or small squares by longitudinal while fresh, then roasted to dry.

二、饮片炮制
II Processing of Decoction Pieces

葛根炮制历史悠久，在唐代有蒸制，宋代出现了醋制、炙、焙制等炮制方法，明代还有炒制为用，清代新增煨法。目前，除生品饮片外，主要炮制方法以煨法为主，包括湿纸煨和麦麸煨两种。湿纸煨是将葛根以湿纸包好，埋入无烟热火灰中，煨至纸呈焦黑色，葛根呈微黄色时即可。麦麸煨是将麦麸撒于热炒药锅中，加热，锅中冒烟时加入葛根，翻炒至药面呈焦黄色即可。

The processing of Gegen has a long history, including steaming in the Tang Dynasty, vinegar processing, stir-baking with adjuvant and baking in the Song Dynasty, stir-frying in the Ming Dynasty and a new method roasting in the Qing Dynasty. Nowadays except for raw decoction slices, Gegen is mainly processed by roasting, including wet paper roasting and wheat bran roasting. To roast it with wet paper, Gegen is wrapped in the wet paper, buried in smokeless hot ash, and roasted until the paper is scorched black, then is taken out while it turns yellowish. To roast it with the wheat bran, firstly put the wheat bran in the hot pot, continue to heat, and add Gegen pieces when the pot has smoke, and then stir-fry it until the medicine is scorched yellow.

麸煨可使葛根中葛根素、大豆苷元等黄酮类有效成分含量增加。同时，麸煨的加热操作，使凉性的葛根转为温性，清热作用减弱而温脾实肠作用增强，实现"煨熟可以厚肠止泻"的效果。

After Gegen is roasted with wheat bran, the contents of flavonoids such as puerarin and daidzein are significantly higher than those in raw products. At the same time, the heating operation makes the cool property of Gegen turn into warm, and its effect of clearing heat is weakened, while the effect of warming spleen and invigorating intestines is enhanced, realizing the effect of "roasted product can check diarrhea by invigorating intestines".

三、中成药制药
III Pharmacy of Chinese Patent Medicines

含葛根的中成药剂型丰富，涵盖了固体、液体与半固体剂型。传统剂型中多采用葛根原粉投料，现代制剂中，葛根多以提取后制剂或以葛根提取物投料，也有以部分粉碎、部分提取后投料，从而体现中药制剂"药辅合一"特色，也可以有效成分葛根素直接制备制剂，如葛根素注射液。

There are many kinds of pharmaceutical forms of patent Chinese medicines containing Gegen, including solid, liquid and semi-solid forms. The raw powder of Gegen is often used in traditional pharmaceutical forms, but in modern preparations, Gegen is mostly used after extraction as the extract or extract preparations, also in the form of partially crushed and partially extracted, which reflects the characteristics of Chinese pharmaceutical preparation—"the combination of medicine and auxiliary". Puerarin can also be prepared directly, such as Puerarin Zhusheye.

如葛根芩连片，将部分葛根粉碎成细粉，剩余葛根与其他饮片进行提取，将提取物和葛根细粉混合后进行制剂，葛根粉碎部分不但作为制剂的药物组成，同时作为制剂辅料（可发挥稀释剂、崩解剂作用），减少外加辅料的用量，同时，制剂中原粉和提取物中有效成分的溶出速度不同，使药物的作用时间延长。多数含葛根的制剂如小儿泻痢片、心可舒片等主要通过水提或醇提等工艺，提取葛根中以葛根素为代表的黄酮类有效成分。

For example, in the preparation process of Gegen Qinlian Pian (Tablets), part of Gegen is crushed into fine powder and the rest is extracted with other medicinals, both of which are mixed for preparation. In this way, the fine powder of Gegen is not only part of the medicinal composition, but also the auxiliary material of the preparation (serving as diluent and dis-integrant), which saves the amount of additional excipients. The dissolution rates of the active components in the original powder and the extract are different, which prolongs the action time of the preparation. Most of the preparations containing Gegen, such as Xiaoer Xieli Pian (Tablets) and Xinkeshu Pian (Tablets), Gegen is mainly extracted by water or alcohol to obtain the effective components of flavonoids represented by puerarin.

【性能功效】
[Property and Efficacy]

一、性能
I Property

葛根味甘、辛，性凉，归脾、胃、肺经。

Gegen is sweet and pungent in flavor, cool in nature, and enters the spleen, stomach and lung meridians.

二、功效
II Efficacy

1. **解肌退热，透疹**　葛根甘辛性凉，轻扬升散，有发表散邪，解肌退热，透发麻疹之功，凡外感表证无论寒热，均可用本品。其功效的发挥与解热、改善血液流变学、调节平滑肌活动等药理作用密切相关。葛根解热、改善血液流变学的有效物质基础主要是葛根素、葛根总黄酮，可通过阻断中枢部位的 β 受体而使 cAMP 生成减少，扩张皮肤血管发挥解热作用，并通过促进血液循环而加快散热。

1 Releasing the Flesh and Dispersing the Heat, and Promoting Eruption

Gegen is sweet and pungent in taste, and cool in nature, with raising and dispersing in property. It acts as releasing the flesh and dispersing the heat, and promoting eruption. Gegen can be used for all exterior syndromes, regardless of cold and heat, and its efficacy is closely related to its pharmacological effects of being antipyretic, improving hemorheology and regulating smooth muscle activity. The effective material bases for dispersing heat and improving hemorheology are puerarin and its total flavonoids, they can block the β-receptor in the central region to reduce the production of cAMP, expand skin blood vessels to relieve fever, and promote blood circulation to accelerate heat dissipation.

2. **生津止渴**　本品甘凉，于清热之中，又能鼓舞脾胃清阳之气上升，而有生津止渴之功。其功效的发挥与降血糖等药理作用密切相关。葛根降血糖的有效物质基础主要是葛根素，通过增加脑垂体、胰腺组织 β 内啡肽（β-EP）合成，增加胰岛素分泌，上调骨骼肌组织葡萄糖转运体 4（GLUT4）的表达，促进葡萄糖摄取，并降低炎性因子 TNF-α 水平和单核细胞趋化蛋白（MCP）水平，改善微循环发挥降血糖作用。

2 Promoting Fluid Production to Quench Thirst

Gegen is sweet in taste and cool in nature, which can inspire the the clear *yang qi* of spleen and stomach while dispersing the heat, and has the function of promoting fluid production to quench thirst. Its efficacy is closely related to the hypoglycemic pharmacological effect of Gegen. Puerarin is the effective material basis of Gegen in lowering blood sugar, the main mechanism of which is increasing the synthesis of β-endorphin (β-EP) in pituitary and pancreas, increasing insulin secretion, up-regulating the expression of glucose transporter 4 (GLUT4) in skeletal muscle tissues, promoting glucose uptake, as well as reducing the levels of inflammatory factor TNF-α and monocyte chemo-attractant protein (MCP) and improving microcirculation.

3. **升阳止泻**　葛根味辛升发，能升发清阳，鼓舞脾胃清阳之气上升而奏止泻痢之效。其功效的发挥与内脏平滑肌的调节等药理作用密切相关。葛根调节内脏平滑肌的有效物质基础主要是葛根素、大豆苷元，通过抑制胃排空和小肠推进率发挥调节内脏平滑肌作用。

3 Raising Yang and Checking Diarrhea

Gegen is pungent in taste, with rising and dispersing effect, therefore it can inspire the clear *yang qi* of spleen and stomach to control diarrhea. Its efficacy is mainly related to its effect on regulating visceral smooth muscle. Both puerarin and daidzein are the effective substance bases of Gegen in regulating visceral smooth muscle, which works by inhibiting gastric emptying and intestinal propulsion rate.

4. **通经活络** 葛根味辛能行，能调经活络。其功效的发挥与抗心肌缺血、抗心律失常、降血压、降血脂、改善血液流变性抗血栓形成、抗氧化等药理作用密切相关。葛根抗心肌缺血、抗心律失常、降血压、改善血液流变性、抗血栓的有效物质基础主要是葛根素，通过降低心肌消耗量，减少心肌乳酸产生发挥抗心肌缺血作用；通过延长心肌细胞动作电位时程抑制延迟整流钾电流发挥抗心律失常作用；通过抑制肾素 - 血管紧张素系统活性、降低儿茶酚胺的含量发挥降压作用；并通过抑制血小板聚集发挥抗血栓作用。

4 Unblocking the Meridian and Activating Collaterals

With pungent taste, Gegen is featured with moving effect, therefore it can unblock the meridian and activate collaterals. Its efficacy is closely related to its pharmacological effects, such as anti-myocardial ischemia, anti-arrhythmia, lowering blood pressure, lowering blood lipids, improving hemorheology, anti-thrombosis, antioxidation and so on. The main effective substance of Gegen to play the role of resisting myocardial ischemia, arrhythmia and thrombosis formation, lowering blood pressure, and improving hemorheology is puerarin; among which, the anti-myocardial ischemia effect is achieved by reducing myocardial consumption and lactic acid production. The anti-arrhythmia effect is achieved by inhibiting delayed rectifier potassium current and prolonging action potential duration of myocardial cells. The blood pressure lowering effect is achieved by inhibiting the activity of renin-angiotensin system and reducing the content of catecholamine. And the antithrombotic function is achieved by inhibiting platelet aggregation.

5. **解酒毒** 葛根味甘能解酒毒，其功效的发挥与调节免疫功能、抗氧化、保肝及对中枢神经系统的保护等药理作用密切相关。葛根保护神经系统的有效物质基础主要是葛根总黄酮、葛根素。

5 Relieving Alcoholism

Gegen is sweet in flavor which can be used for relieving alcoholism. The effect may be closely related to its actions on regulating immune function, antioxidation, liver protection and central nervous system protection. The main effective substances of Gegen to play the role of protecting the nervous system are puerarin and total flavonoids.

此外，葛根还有抗骨质疏松、雌激素样作用、抗肿瘤、保护胃黏膜等作用。

In addition, Gegen has anti-osteoporosis and estrogen-like effects, and anti-tumor effects, and it can also protect gastric mucosa.

【应用】
[Application]

一、主治病证
I Indications

1. **外感发热头痛、项背强痛** 葛根可与薄荷、菊花等配伍治疗风热感冒，发热、头痛等症；也可与柴胡、黄芩等配伍治疗风寒感冒，如《伤寒六书》柴葛解肌汤。

1 Fever, Headache, and Pain and Stiffness of Neck and Back due to Exogenous Attack

Gegen can be compatible with Bohe and Juhua to treat wind-heat common cold, fever, headache and other diseases. Combining with Chaihu and Huangqin, it can treat wind-cold common cold, such as Chaige Jieji Tang (Decoction) in *Shanghan Liushu*.

现代临床，葛根配伍常用于普通感冒、流行

性感冒、颈椎病等属于风寒表证或风热表证者，如葛根汤、柴葛解肌汤；配伍用于神经性头痛、血管性头痛、偏头痛等属于表邪侵犯阳明经者，如升麻芷葛汤。

In modern clinical practice, Gegen compatibility is often used for treating common cold, influenza, cervical spondylosis and other diseases belonging to wind-cold or wind-heat exterior syndromes, such as Gegen Tang (Decoction), Chaige Jieji Tang (Decoction); For neurogenic headache, vascular headache, migraine and other cases due to exterior pathogen invading *Yangming* meridian, Gegen is used in combination, such as Shengma Zhige Tang (Decoction).

2. **热病口渴、消渴** 治疗热病津伤口渴，常与芦根、天花粉等同用。治疗消渴证属阴津不足者，可与天花粉、麦门冬等配伍。若内热消渴、口渴多饮，体瘦乏力，气阴不足者，可用《沈氏尊生书》玉泉丸。

2 Thirst in Febrile Diseases, and Consumptive-thirst

Gegen can be combined with Lugen (Phragmitis Rhizoma) and Tianhuafen to treat febrile diseases with thirst due to fluid injury. For the treatment of consumptive-thirst due to the deficiency of *yin* fluid, Gegen can be combined with Tianhuafen, Maimendong (Ophiopogonis Radix) and so on. For those with consumptive-thirst, and thirst with polydipsia due to interior heat, thin and lack of strength, deficiency of *qi* and *yin*, Yuquan Wan in *Shenshi Zunsheng Shu (Shen's Book that Honors Life)* can be used.

现代临床，葛根配伍常用于糖尿病等属气阴两虚症者，如玉液汤。

In modern clinical practice, Gegen compatibility is often used for diabetes patients with deficiency of both qi and yin, such as Yuye Tang (Decoction).

3. **麻疹不透** 与他药配伍可治麻疹初起，表邪外束，疹出不畅，如《阎氏小儿方论》升麻葛根汤。如麻疹初起，已现麻疹，但疹出不畅，见发热咳嗽，或乍冷乍热者，可配伍牛蒡子、荆芥等。

3 Measles without Adequate Eruption

Gegen is combined with other medicinals for treating measles at the initial stage, showing as fetter of exterior pathogen limiting measles from eruption, such as Shengma Gegen Tang (Decoction) in *Yanshi Xiaoer Fanglun (Yanshi Children's Prescription)*. For those at the initial stage have measles without adequate eruption, accompanied with fever and cough, or alternative chills and fever, Gegen can be combined with Niubangzi (Arctii Fructus), Jingjie and so on.

现代临床，葛根配伍常用于出疹性疾病的初期，如升麻葛根汤。

In modern clinical practice, Gegen compatibility is often used in the early stage of rashes, such as Shengma Gegen Tang (Decoction).

4. **热泻热痢、脾虚泄泻** 用治表证未解，邪热入里，身热，下利臭秽，肛门有灼热感，苔黄脉数，或湿热泻痢，热重于湿者，可用《伤寒论》葛根芩连汤。若脾虚泄泻，可用《小儿药证直诀》七味白术散。

4 Heat Diarrhea and Dysentery, and Diarrhea due to Spleen Deficiency

For the treatment of symptoms caused by exterior heat pathogen unsolved entering into the interior, manifested as fever, diarrhea with smelly excrement, burning sensation of the anus, and yellowish tongue coating and rapid pulse, or for the treatment of dampness-heat diarrhea and dysentery with heavier heat than dampness, Gegen Qinlian Tang (Decoction) in *Shanghan Zabing Lun* can be used. For diarrhea caused by spleen deficiency, Qiwei Baizhusan in *Xiaoer Yaozheng Zhijue (Key to Diagnosis and Treatment of Children's Diseases)* can be used.

现代临床，葛根配伍常用于痢疾、小儿夏季腹泻等属于表证未解，邪热入里者，如葛根芩连汤。

In modern clinical practice, Gegen compatibility is often used for dysentery, children's summer diarrhea and other diseases which are caused by the unsolved exterior syndrome invading into the interior, such as Gegen Qinlian Tang (Decoction).

5. **中风偏瘫、胸痹心痛、眩晕头痛**　用治中风偏瘫、胸痹心痛、眩晕头痛，可与三七、丹参、川芎等配伍。

5　Stroke with Hemiplegia, Chest Impediment with Cardiodynia, Dizziness and Headache

For the treatment of stroke with hemiplegia, chest impediment with cardiodynia, dizziness and headache, Gegen can be combined with Sanqi, Danshen, Chuanxiong, etc.

现代临床，葛根单味药制剂或配伍复方可用于治疗高血压病、冠心病、脑梗死、突发性耳聋等症见胸痹心痛、眩晕、头痛、偏瘫者，可用中成药葛根素片、葛根素注射液等。

In modern clinical practice, preparations with only Gegen or its combinations can be used to treat hypertension, coronary heart disease, cerebral infarction, sudden deafness and other diseases manifested as chest impediment with cardiodynia, vertigo, headache and hemiplegia, such as Chinese patent medicines Gegensu Pian (Tablets) and Gegensu Zhusheye.

6. **酒毒伤中**　对酒毒伤中症见恶心呕吐、脘腹痞满者，常与陈皮、白豆蔻、枳椇子等理气化湿、解酒毒药同用。

6　Alcoholic Poisoning Injuring the Middle Energizer

For treatment of alcoholic poisoning injuring the middle which manifests as nausea, vomiting and epigastric fullness, Gegen can be combined with Chenpi (Citri Reticulatae Pericarpium), Baidoukou (Amomi Rotundus Fructus), Zhijuzi (Hoveniae Semen) and other qi-regulating, dampness-resolving and alcoholic poisoning-removing medicine.

现代临床，葛根也常用作解酒药、解酒保健品和功能茶饮料的原料；对于酒精中毒才是可用葛根

素注射液、葛根枳椇子栀子胶囊等中成药。

In modern clinical practice, Gegen is often used as the raw material of antialcoholic medicinals, antialcoholic health-care products and functional tea drinks; for alcoholism, Gegensu Zhusheye, Gegen Zhijuzi Zhizi Jiaonang and other Chinese patent medicines can be used.

二、用法用量
II　Administration and Dosage

10~15g，煎服。
10~15g, water decoction.

三、注意事项
III　Precautions

葛根的药物开发较好，现已形成系列中成药广泛用于临床，但也存在一些不良反应，用药时宜警惕。如临床少数患者口服葛根片后有头胀感，减量后可消失。葛根素注射液可引起发热、过敏反应（药疹、药物性皮炎、严重者致过敏性休克）、丙氨酸转氨酶升高、肾绞痛等不良反应。

Gegen is well developed and applied, and now a series of its Chinese patent medicines have been widely used in clinic, but there are also some adverse reactions that should be vigilant when taking them. For example, a small number of patients have a feeling of distension in the head after oral administration of Gegen Pian (Tablets), which can disappear along with dose reduction. Gegensu Zhusheye can cause adverse reactions including fever, allergic reactions (medicinal eruption, medicinal-induced dermatitis, and anaphylactic shock in severe cases), elevated alanine aminotransferase, and renal colic.

第九章　清　热　药
Chapter 9　Heat-clearing Medicinals

凡以清里热为主要作用的药物，称为清热药，根据其功效特点又可分为清热泻火、清热燥湿、清热解毒、清热凉血和清虚热五大类清热药。本类药物药性寒凉，主要用于表证已解、里热炽盛而无积滞的里热病证，包括外感热病、湿热证、热毒内盛证、血分实热证和虚热证。使用清热药时，需辨别热证虚实，同时还应注意有无兼证。另，本类药物药性寒凉，易伤脾胃，凡脾胃气虚，食少便溏者慎用，阴虚者亦需慎用，而阴盛格阳、真寒假热者禁用。现代研究表明，清热药具有抗病原微生物、解热、抗炎、抗毒素、调节免疫功能、抗肿瘤等作用。

Medicinals that have key function of clearing interior heat are called Qingreyao (heat-clearing medicinals), which are divided into 5 categories as heat-clearing and fire-purging, heat-clearing and dampness-drying, heat-clearing and detoxicating, heat-clearing and blood-cooling, and deficiency heat-clearing medicinals according to the efficacy. These medicinals are cold or cool in nature and are mainly used to treat interior heat syndromes with excessive interior heat but no stagnancy, yet the exterior syndrome and stagnancy, including heat disease caused by exterior evil, dampness-heat syndrome, dominance of toxic heat in interior, blood-heat syndrome and deficiency heat syndrome. When application with Meat-clearing medicinals sighificant to differentiate excess heat from deficiency heat, and with or without accompanying syndromes. Moreover, these medicinals with cold or cool in nature are easy to injure the spleen and the stomach, so patients with qi deficiency of spleen and stomach, or with syndromes of anorexia and loose stool, should use carefully. Patients with yin deficiency also need careful use. Patients with syndromes of yin exuberance with yang debilitation, or true cold with false heat are forbidden to use them. Modern studies indicate that Qingreyao have such effects as anti-pathogen microorganism, antipyretic, anti-inflammatory, anti-toxin, regulating immune function, anti-tumor, etc.

常用的清热药有石膏、知母、天花粉、金银花、连翘、板兰根、黄芩、黄连、黄柏、地黄、玄参、青蒿、白薇、地骨皮等。

Commonly used heat-clearing medicinals include Shigao, Zhimu, Tianhuafen, Jinyinhua, Lianqiao, Banlangen, Huangqin, Huanglian, Huangbo, Dihuang, Xuanshen, Qinghao, Baiwei (Cynanchi Atrati Radix Et Rhizoma), Digupi (Lycii Cortex),and so on.

知　母

Zhimu
(Anemarrhena Rhizoma)

知母为河北的道地药材，知母炮制品有知母和盐知母。知母味苦甘，性寒，归肺、胃、肾经，具有清热泻火、滋阴润燥的功效，主治外感热病，高热烦渴，肺热燥咳，骨蒸潮热，内热消渴，肠燥便秘等。知母主要含有甾体皂苷、双苯吡酮类、木脂素类等成分，有抗病原微生物、解热、抗炎、降血糖等作用。知母性寒润肠，脾胃虚寒，大便溏泻者禁服。

Zhimu is a genuine regional medicinal in Hebei Province. The main processed products used in clinical are Zhimu and Yanzhimu (salty Zhimu). Zhimu is bitter and sweet in flavor as well as cold in nature, and enters the lung, stomach and kidney meridians. It has the effects of clearing heat and purging fire, nourishing yin to moisten dryness, which is used for treating the syndromes of exogenous fever, high fever and polydipsia, lung heat and dry cough, bone steaming and hot flashes, internal heat and thirst, dry intestines and constipation caused by intestinal dryness etc.. Zhimu mainly contains steroidal saponins, diphenpyrone, lignans components, which possess the pharmacological effects of anti-pathogenic microorganisms, antipyretic, anti-inflammatory, hypoglycemic etc. Zhimu is cold and moisturizing the intestines, those with the spleen and stomach insufficiency cold, and with loose stools are forbidden to take it.

【品种品质】
[Variety and Quality]

一、基原品种与品质
I Origins

1. **品种概况**　来源于百合科植物知母 *Anemarrhena asphodeloides* Bge. 的干燥根茎。

1 Variety

Zhimu is the dried rhizome of Anemarrhena asphodeloides Bge.

知母首载于《神农本草经》列为中品，《本草图经》载："知母，根黄色，似菖蒲而柔润，叶至难死，掘出随生，须燥乃止。四月开青花如韭花，八月结实"。其对知母原植物的描述与今用知母基本相符。

Zhimu was first recorded in the book of *Shennong Bencao Jing*. According to the book of *Bencao Tujing*, "The root of Zhimu is yellow, soft and moistening like Changpu (Acori Tatarinowii Rhizoma), and its leaves are hard to wither that they keep alive even being dug out only until its root dry. In April, it blossoms the blue and white flowers like leek flowers, and bears fruits in August. The description of the original plant of Zhimu is basically consistent with that of today.

2. **种植采收**　河北安国、博野，安徽亳州有种植。知母一般采用种子繁殖和分株繁殖。种子繁殖是在 4 月中旬进行播种；分株繁殖宜在秋冬季植株休眠期至翌年早春萌发前进行。一般在栽植后 2~3 年采收为宜，春秋两季采挖。

2 Planting and Harvesting

Zhimu was planted in Anguo, Boye in Hebei Province, and Bozhou in Anhui Province. Zhimu generally adopts seed propagation and branch propagation. Seed reproduction is carried out in mid-April. Branching reproduction should be carried out during the dormancy period of autumn and winter of the plants and before the germination of early spring the following year. Generally, it is advisable to harvest in spring and autumn 2 to 3 years after planting.

3. 道地性及品质评价 历代本草记载，河北易县为其道地产区，品质最佳，称"西陵知母"。古人从形、色、气、味等方面提出了知母性状评价指标，以"条肥大""质硬""断面黄白"为佳。

3 Genuineness and Quality Evaluation

According to the historical records, Yixian of Hebei Province is the genuine regional producing area of Zhimu, it is at the best quality and was called "Xiling Zhimu". The ancients proposed evaluation indexes of characters of Zhimu from the aspects of shape, color, flavour and taste. The one with hypertrophic shape, hard texture, yellow and white section is the best.

知母中主要含有皂苷（知母皂苷 BⅡ 和知母皂苷 AⅢ）、木脂素类（扁柏树脂酚类）、双苯吡酮类（芒果苷）等，其中，芒果苷、知母皂苷 BⅡ 和知母皂苷 AⅢ 等是抗炎的主要物质基础，知母的水提物、甾体皂苷、皂苷元及芒果苷为其降血糖、抗肿瘤的主要物质基础。此外知母还含有生物碱、蒽醌、有机酸、低聚糖、微量元素等成分。《中国药典》规定含芒果苷不得少于 0.70%，含知母皂苷 BⅡ 不得少于 3.0%。

Zhimu mainly contains saponin (timosaponin BⅡ and timosaponin AⅢ), lignans (hinoki resin phenols), bisbenzene pyridones (mangiferin) etc. Among which, mangiferin, timosaponin BⅡ and timosaponin AⅢ are the material bases of anti-inflammation. Water extract of Zhimu, steroidal saponin, saponin and mangiferin are the major material bases for lowering blood sugar and anti-tumor effect. In addition, Zhimu also contains alkaloids, anthraquinones, organic acids, oligosaccharides and trace elements etc. The *Pharmacopoeia of the People's Republic of China* regulated that the content of mangiferin should not be less than 0.7% (ml/g) of, and timosaponin BⅡ should not be less than 3.0% in Zhimu.

二、炮制品种与品质
II Processed Varieties and Quality

知母的炮制品种主要有知母、酒炒知母、麸炒知母、盐知母等。其中药典收载主要为知母和盐知母。

Processed products of Zhimu are mainly Zhimu, Jiuchaozhimu (stir-frying with liquor), Fuchaozhimu (stir-frying with bran) and Yanzhimu (stir-frying with salt) etc. among which, Zhimu and Yanzhimu are recorded in the *Pharmacopoeia of the People's Republic of China*.

知母以不规则类圆形的厚片，外表皮黄棕色或棕色，气微，味微甜、略苦，嚼之带黏性为佳。盐知母以色黄或微带焦斑，味微咸为佳。《中国药典》规定知母含芒果苷（$C_{19}H_{18}O_{11}$）不得少于 0.50%，含知母皂苷 BⅡ（$C_{45}H_{76}O_{19}$）不得少于 3.0%；盐知母含芒果苷不得少于 0.40%，含知母皂苷 BⅡ 不得少于 2.0%。

Good quality of Zhimu is that with irregular round slabs, surface in yellow-brown or brown, slightly odour, slightly taste sweet and bitterish and while chewing viscosity. Yan Zhimu (stir-frying with salt) with yellow or scorched spots and slightly salty are considered to have better quality. According to *Pharmacopoeia of the People's Republic of China*, the total contents of Mangiferin ($C_{19}H_{18}O_{11}$) shall not be lower than 0.50%, the contents of timosaponin BII ($C_{45}H_{76}O_{19}$) shall not be lower than 3.0%, the total contents of Mangiferin ($C_{19}H_{18}O_{11}$) of Yanzhimu (stir-frying with salt) shall not be lower than 0.40%, and the contents of timosaponin BII ($C_{19}H_{18}O_{11}$) shall not be lower than 2.0% to ensure the stability and controllability of quality.

三、中成药品种与品质
III Varieties and Quality of Chinese Patent Medicines

含有知母或其炮制品的中成药有 240 余个，其中药典收载含有知母的中成药 40 余个。以知母为君药或主药的品种有知柏地黄丸、大补阴丸、养阴清胃颗粒等。质量控制多采用显微鉴别确定知母的存在，采用薄层色谱法以对照药材和芒果苷对照品进行定性鉴别，如大补阴丸。非以知母为君药的制剂，如清胃黄连丸、益血生胶囊、润肺止嗽丸、清肺抑火丸等通过显微鉴别特征"草酸钙针晶成束或散在"确定含有知母。

At present, there are more than 240 Chinese patent medicines containing Zhimu or its processed products and 40 are recorded in *Pharmacopoeia of the People's Republic of China*. Among of which, prescriptions with Zhimu as sovereign are Zhibai Dihuang Wan, Dabuyin Wan, Yangyin Qingwei Keli etc. In quality control, the existence of Zhimu is mainly determined by microscopic identification, and the control medicinals and mangioferin reference substance are qualitively identified by TLC in Dabuyin Wan. In the preparations not taking Zhimu as sovereign medicine, such as Qingwei Huanglian Wan, Yixuesheng Jiaonang, Runfei Zhike Wan, Qingfei Yihuo Wan are identified by microscopic identifying the characteristics of "calcium oxalate needles bunched or scattered" to determine the existence of Zhimu.

【制药】
[Pharmacy]

一、产地加工
I Processing in Production Area

除去茎苗及须根，保留黄绒毛和浅黄色的叶痕及茎痕晒干者，为"毛知母"；趁鲜时剥去栓皮晒干者为"光知母"。

Removing stems and fibrous root, remaining yellow fluff, yellow light leaf and stem marks, it is known as "Maozhimu"; or peeling off the cork and then drying it when it is fresh, it is called "Guangzhimu".

二、饮片炮制
II Processing of Decoction Pieces

知母以润透、切片、盐炙为主要加工工序，

由此生产的知母、盐知母是商品中的主流品种。

The main processing procedure of Zhimu is moistening, sectioning and salt processing, through which processed Zhimu and Yanzhimu (stir-frying with salt solution adjuvant) are the major varieties of comercial products.

知母盐炙后引药下行，增强滋阴润燥作用。其炮制原理是盐炙过程中，清热成分新芒果苷转化为芒果苷，含量降低；降糖成分知母皂苷 AⅢ、知母皂苷 BⅢ、芒果苷、菝葜皂苷元、总多糖含量增加，使降糖作用增强。

The Zhimu processed with salt has the effects of conducting medicinals downward, and its effect of nourishing yin and moisturizing was enhanced. The processing principle is that during the processing, the heat-clearing composition of neo-mangiferin is converted to mangiferin, making its content decreased. Hypoglycemic constituents such as timosaponin-A Ⅲ, timosaponin B Ⅲ, mangiferin, saponin, and total polysaccharide content are increased, which enhances the hypoglycemic effect.

三、中成药制药
III Pharmacy of Chinese Patent Medicines

含知母的中成药剂型丰富，涵盖了固体、液体剂型。在含知母的中成药制剂中多制成丸剂。如知柏地黄丸，全方饮片细粉直接泛丸制成水蜜丸或蜜丸，而水蜜丸或蜜丸在制剂过程中相对其他剂型来说在温度较低的情况下操作，能有效避免药材中有效成分流失，使药效更佳。

Chinese patent medicines containing Zhimu are rich in preparation, covering solid and liquid dosage forms. Chinese patent medicines containing Zhimu are mostly made into pills. For example, Zhibai Dihuang Wan, the whole fine powder of prescription decoction pieces is directly made into water honey pill or honey pill, which is operated under the condition of low temperature, compared with other dosage forms, can effectively avoid the loss of effective ingredients and ensure better efficacy.

【性能功效】
[Property and Efficacy]

一、性能
I Property

知母苦、甘、寒，质润；归肺、胃、肾经。

Zhimu is bitter, sweet and cold in flavor, moist in texure, and enters the lung, stomach and kidney meridians.

二、功效
II Efficacy

1. 清热泻火　知母苦寒之性善入肺、胃二经，以清肺胃实热。其功效的发挥与解热、抗炎、抗病原微生物等药理作用密切相关。知母的解热、抗炎、抗病原微生物作用的有效物质基础主要是皂苷类和双苯吡酮类，通过抑制细胞膜上 Na⁺-K⁺-ATP 酶活性，减少 5- 羟色胺的代谢；抑制环氧化酶，减少前列腺素的合成，进而影响体温调节中枢发挥解热作用；并通过促进肾上腺分泌糖皮质激素及抑制炎症组织 PGE 的合成或释放发挥抗炎作用。

1 Clearing Heat and Purging Fire

Zhimu is cold in nature and bitter in flavor and enters the lungs and stomach meridians to clear the lungs and stomach heat. Its efficacy is closely related to pharmacological effects such as antipyretic, anti-inflammatory effects and anti-pathogenic microorganisms. The effective material basis for the antipyretic and anti-pathogenic microorganisms is mainly saponins and diphenpyrone. Its mechanism of action is by inhibiting the Na⁺-K⁺-ATP enzemy activity on the cell membrane and reducing the metabolism of serotonin, inhibiting the cyclooxygenase and reducing the synthesis of prostaglandins, then affecting the body's temperature regulation center

to play the antipyretic role. At the same time，it plays an anti-inflammatory role by promoting the secretion of glucocorticoids by adrenal glands and inhibiting the synthesis or release of PGE in inflammatory tissues.

2. 滋阴润燥　知母苦寒清热，泻火存阴，可滋肾水而益肺胃。其功效的发挥与降血糖、下调 β - 肾上腺素受体 -cAMP 系统功能等药理作用密切相关，知母降血糖的有效物质基础主要是知母皂苷和知母多糖，通过抑制 α - 葡萄糖苷酶活性发挥降血糖作用。

2 Nourishing Yin for Moistening Dryness

Zhimu is cold and bitter, clearing heat, purging fire and keeping yin, which can nourish kidney water and benefit lungs and stomach. Its effect is closely related to the pharmacological effects such as lowering blood sugar and inhibiting sympathetic nerve-β receptor function. The effective material bases of its hypoglycemic are mainly timosaponin and timosa polysaccharide, which play a role by inhibiting α-glucosidase activity.

此外，知母还有抗肿瘤、改善老年性痴呆症状、改善骨质疏松症状、抗抑郁等作用。

In addition, Zhimu also has the effects of anti-tumor, improving the symptoms of senile dementia and the symptoms of osteoporosis, as well as antidepress, etc..

【应用】
[Applications]

一、主治病证
I Indications

1. 气分实热　治疗外感热病，高热烦渴者，知母常与石膏配伍以滋胃阴而生津止渴，如《伤寒论》白虎汤；治温疟但热不寒，口渴喜冷饮，呕不能食者，可与鳖甲、常山、青蒿配伍以清热养阴，如《延年方》知母鳖甲汤。

1 Qi Aspect Excess Heat

Zhimu is used to treat exogenous febrile disease, high fever and polydipsia and thirst, and it is often combined with Shigao to nourish the stomach yin and quench thirst, such as Baihu Tang (Decoction) in *Shanghan Zabing Lun*; curing malaria with heat but not cold, thirsty like cold drinks, vomiting and unable to take food, it also can be compatible with Biejia, Changshan, Qinghao to clear the heat and nourish the yin such as Zhimu BiejiaTang (Decoction) in *Yannian Fang (Macrobiotic Prescription)*.

现代临床，知母配伍常用于治疗口腔溃疡及咽喉肿痛、中暑、感冒等属于气分实热，如白虎汤和川升麻散。

In modern clinical practice, Zhimu compatibility is often used for the treatment of oral ulcers and sore throats, sammer heat stroke, colds, etc., such as Baihu Tang (Decoction) and Chuanshengma San (Powder).

2. **肺热燥咳证** 治肺热燥咳，肺燥久嗽气急者，治食积火郁，咳嗽痰多者，知母多配伍贝母、桃仁、茯苓等以化痰润燥，如《妇人大全良方》二母散。

2 Lung Heat and Dry Cough Syndrome

Syndrome Treatment of dry cough due to lung heat, longtime cough with shortness of breath due to dryness of the lungs accumulation of fire due to food stagnation, and cough and sputum, Zhimu is compatible with Beimu, Taoren, Fuling etc. Such as Ermu San (Powder) in *Furen Liangfang Daquan*.

现代临床，知母配伍常用于治疗急性肺部感染等肺热燥咳证，如知石清解注射液。

In modern clinical practice, Zhimu compatibility is used for dry cough caused by lung heat, like acute lung infections, such as Zhishi Qingjie Zhusheye.

3. **阴虚证** 治阴虚火旺所致骨蒸潮热、盗汗、心烦等，知母可与黄柏、地黄、山药配伍以滋阴降火，如《医宗金鉴》知柏地黄丸；治温病后期，邪伏阴分，夜热早凉者，可以青蒿、鳖甲等配伍以养阴透热，如《温病条辨》青蒿鳖甲汤。

3 Yin Deficiency Syndrome

Zhimu is often combined with other medicinals to treat bone-steaming and tidal fever, night sweats, and irritability caused by yin deficiency with effulgent fire. For instance, Zhimu can be compatible with Huangbo, Dihuang and Shanyao to nourish yin and lower fire, such as Zhibai Dihuang Wan in *Yizong Jinjian (Golden Mirror of Medicine)*. Zhimu also can be compatible with Qinghao, Biejia, to nourish the yin and clearing the heat such as Qinghao Biejia Tang (Decoction) in *Wenbing Tiaobian*.

现代临床，知母常配伍用于肺结核等阴虚证、治疗糖皮质激素副作用，如知柏地黄丸。更年期综合征，如百合地黄汤和百合知母汤；风湿性关节炎、类风湿性关节炎如桂枝芍药知母汤。

In modern clinical practice, it is often combined for treating yin deficiency syndrome such as tuberculosis and the side effects of glucocorticoids, such as in Zhibai Dihuang Wan; treating menopause syndromes, such as in Baihe Dihuang Tang (Decoction) and Baihe Zhimu Tang (Decoction); treating rheumatic arthritis, and rheumatoid arthritis such as in Guizhi Shaoyao Zhimu Tang (Decoction).

4. **内热消渴证** 治疗阴虚内热之消渴证，知母可与山药、黄芪、鸡内金等配伍升元气以治消渴，如《医学衷中参西录》玉液汤。

4 Internal Heat Consumptive Thirst Syndrome

Zhimu can be used to treat yin deficiency and internal heat consumptive thirst syndrome, by combining with Shanyao, Huangqi, Jineijin (Galli Gigerii Endothelium Corneum) to boost Original Qi (vitality) to quench thirst such as Yuye Tang (Decoction) from *Yixue Zhongzhong Canxi Lu (Records of Traditional Chinese and Western Medicine in Combination)*.

现代临床，知母配伍常用于治疗糖尿病等消

渴证，如石膏知母汤。

In modern clinical practice, Zhimu compatibility is often used to treat consumptive thirst syndromes like diabetes, such as Zhimu Shigao Tang (Decoction).

5. **肠燥便秘** 知母可与其它药物配伍治疗治阴虚肠燥便秘证，常配生地黄、玄参等药用。

5 Intestinal Dryness Constipation

Zhimu can be combined with other medicinals to treat constipation and intestinal dryness syndrome caused by yin deficiency, such as Shengdihuang, Xuanshen etc.

二、用法用量
II Administration and Dosage

6~12g。

三、注意事项
III Precautions

脾胃虚寒，大便溏泻者禁服。

For those with the spleen and stomach deficiency and cold, with loose stool or diarrhea, it is forbidden to take it.

黄 芩

Huangqin
(Scutellariae Radix)

黄芩为河北承德道地药材。临床常用炮制品主要为生黄芩、酒黄芩、炒黄芩、黄芩炭等。黄芩味苦，性寒，归肺、胆、脾、大肠、小肠经，有清热燥湿、泻火解毒、止血、安胎的功效，主治湿温，暑湿，胸闷呕恶，湿热痞满，泻痢、黄疸，肺热咳嗽、高热烦渴，血热吐衄，痈肿疮毒，胎动不安。黄芩中主要含有黄酮、挥发油、多糖等成分，有抗病原微生物、抗毒素、抗肿瘤、抗炎、解热、抗变态反应等作用，可用于治疗上呼吸道感染、急性支气管炎等属外感风热、温病初起者及急性肠炎、病毒性肝炎等属湿热内胜者。

Huangqin is a genuine regional medicinal from Chengde in Hebei Province. The mainly processed products used in clinical are raw Huangqin, Jiuhuangqin (liquor processed), Chaohuangqin (stir-frying), and Huangqintan (carbonized), etc.. The medicinal properties of Huangqin are bitter and cold and the meridians entered of Huangqin are the lungs, gallbladder, spleen, large intestine and small intestine. It has the function of clearing heat, drying dampness, detoxication and purging fire, hemostasis and tranquilizing fetus to prevent miscarriage. It is used to treat the syndromes of dampness-warm, summer heat-dampness, chest distress, vomiting, dampness-heat, nausea, epigastric distension, diarrhea, jaundice, lung-heat cough, high fever, thirst, blood-heat, hematemesis, carbuncle, abscess, soreness and fetal irritability. Huangqin mainly contains flavonoids, volatile oil and polysaccharide, and exerts broad pharmacological effects, such as anti-pathogenic microorganisms, anti-toxin, anti-tumor, anti-inflammation, antipyresis and anti-anaphylaxis. Hence, it can be applied to treat the exogenous wind-heat syndrome and warmdisease of the early stage, such as respiratory infection and acute bronchitis, and the excessive dampness-heat syndrome, such as acute enteritis and viral hepatitis, etc..

【品种品质】
[Variety and Quality]

一、基原品种与品质
I Origin Variety and Quality

1. 品种概况 来源于唇形科植物黄芩 *Scutellaria baicalensis* Georgi 的干燥根。

1 Variety

Huangqin belongs to the labiform plants, which is the dried root of *Scutellaria baicalensis* Georgi.

黄芩始载于《神农本草经》。《新修本草》云："叶细长，两叶相对，作丛生，亦有独茎者。"《证类本草》绘有"耀州黄芩""潞州黄芩"药图，大致可认为今用唇形科黄芩一直是主流品种。但古用黄芩饮片似非一种，《本草纲目》即有"西芩""北芩"之分，应是根据产地划分者，其北芩当为今用正品。

Huangqin was first recorded in the *Shennong Bencao Jing*. The *Xinxiu Bencao* described that Huangqin has long and thin leaves with leaves opposite, and growing in cluster or alone. It is concluded that the labiform plants Huangqin used today has been the mainstream variety according to the pictures of "Yaozhou Huangqin" and "Luzhou Huangqin" recorded in the *Zhenglei Bencao (Classified Materia Medica)*. However, prepared Huangqin used in ancient time are quite different. Huangqin in the *Bencao Gangmu* were divided into "Xiqin" and "Beiqin", which might be classified by the original area. Actually, "Beiqin" is the current genuine product.

2. 种植采收 黄芩主产于河北、内蒙古、山西、山东、东北等地区。商品药以栽培为主，在栽培上采用种子、扦插或分株繁殖。栽培2~3年可采收，以生长3年的黄芩药材质量为佳。

2 Planting and Harvesting

Huangqin is mainly planted in Hebei Province, Inner Mongolia, Shanxi Province, Shandong Province, northeast and other regions. The commercial medicinal materials are cultivated by seed, cuttings or division propagation. Huangqin can be harvested after 2~3 years cultivation and those growing for 3 years have good quality.

3. 道地性及品质评价 历代本草记载表明，黄芩在湖北秭归、山东菏泽、江苏彭城等均有种植。现今山西产量大，以河北承德质量优。形态上以条长、质坚实、色黄者为佳。

3 Genuineness and Quality Evaluation

According to historical herbal records, Huangqin was from Zigui City in Hubei Province, Heze City in Shandong Province and Pengcheng City in Jiangsu Province. At present, output of Huangqin in Shanxi Province is the largest, but the one with good quality is from Chengde City, Hebei Province, it has long shape, hard texure, and yellow rcolor.

黄芩主要含有黄酮类成分，包括黄芩苷、黄芩素、汉黄芩素、汉黄芩苷、千层纸素A等。该类成分为黄芩的主要药效物质。此外，黄芩还含有挥发油、多糖及萜类化合物等。《中国药典》规定黄芩药材中黄芩苷含量不得少于9.0%。

Huangqin mainly contains flavonoids, such as baicalin, baicalein, wogonin, wogonoside, oroxylin A, etc. They are major active components of Huangqin. Besides, Huangqin also contain volatile oils, polysaccharides and terpenes, etc. According to the *Pharmacopoeia of the People's Republic of China*, baicalin content in Huangqin should not be less than 9.0%.

二、炮制品种与品质
II Processed Varieties and Quality

黄芩的炮制品种有炒制、蜜制、姜制、酒制黄芩等。目前，临床常用为黄芩饮片、酒黄芩、炒黄芩、黄芩炭。黄芩饮片以类圆形或不规则形薄片，外表皮黄棕色或棕褐色，具放射状纹理为佳；酒黄芩以形如黄芩片，略带焦斑，微有酒香气为佳。黄芩片、酒黄芩的品质评价方法同药材且黄芩苷含量不得少于8.0%。

Processing methods of Huangqin include simple stir-frying and stir-frying with honey, ginger, and liquor. At present, Huangqin decoction pieces and Jiuhuangqin (liquor processed), Chaohuangqin (stir-frying) and Huangqintan (carbonized) are most frequently used in clinic. Huangqin decoction pieces with good quality are round or irregular thin slices with yellowish-brown or reddish-brown epidermis and radial textures. The Jiuhuangqin (liquor processed) at good guality is similar to Huangqin decoction pieces in shape, and has little burnt spots and liquor aroma. The quality evaluation of Huangqin decoction pieces and Jiuhuangqin (liquor processed) is the same as that of the Huangqin materia medica, and baicalin content should not be less than 8.0%.

三、中成药品种与品质
III Varieties and Quality of Chinese Patent Medicines

含有黄芩或其炮制品的中成药近 1000 个，其中药典收载 230 余个。常见含黄芩的中成药有双黄连口服液（片）、一清颗粒等。在质量控制多采用薄层色谱法和液相色谱含量测定法进行指标成分（黄芩苷）测定。

There are nearly 1000 Chinese patent medicines containing Huangqin or its processed products, of which almost 230 are recorded in the *Pharmacopoeia of the People's Republic of China*. Shuanghuanglian Koufuye/Pian (Mixture/Tablets), Yiqing Jiaonang (Granules) are common Chinese patent medicines containing Huangqin. In quality control, the TLC and liquid chromatography (LC) were frequently used to determine index composition (baicalin).

【制药】
[Pharmacy]

一、产地加工
I Processing in Production Area

采挖后去掉杂质及泥土，堆闷 1~2 天，至外层粗皮稍干，即可撞皮，后晒干即可。

After dug out, the impurity and soil cleaned, Huangqin is piled up for 1–2 days until its outer layer is slightly dry, then bumped to remove the scarfskin, finally dried in the sun.

二、饮片炮制
II Processing of Decoction Pieces

唐代以前，黄芩主要生用；自宋代起，陆续出现酒制、炒制、制炭等多种方法；至清代其炮制方法已达 20 余种。目前临床主要为黄芩片和酒黄芩。

Before the Tang Dynasty, raw Huangqin was widely used. Since the Song Dynasty, there have been many processing methods such as stir-frying with liquor, simple stir-frying and carbonizing by stir-frying, etc. In the Qing Dynasty, there were more than 20 processing methods. At present, Huangqin decoction pieces and Jiuhuangqin (liquor processed) are the mainstream of commercial specifications.

黄芩根中含有黄芩酶，在一定条件下能促使黄芩苷和汉黄芩苷水解，生成黄芩素和汉黄芩素。黄芩素性质不稳定，易被氧化成不溶于水的醌类衍生物，沉积在黄芩表面而显绿色，导致药材药效降低。因此，采用蒸切、煮切法，一方面可软化药材，便于切制；另一方面也可减少酶活性，避免有效成分的损失。此外，酒炒有利于有效成分的溶出。

Baicalin and wogonoside can be hydrolyzed to baicalein and wogonin in certain condition by enzymes contained in the root of Huangqin. For baicalein is unstable and easily oxidized to water-insoluble quinone derivatives, which gathering superficially and displaying green, it lowers efficacy of Huangqin. Therefore, steaming and boiling are applied to not only soften medicinal materials, and easy for cutting, but also reduce enzyme activity to avoid the loss of effective ingredients. Besides, stir-frying with liquor is also used to facilitate the solution of active components of Huangqin.

三、中成药制药
III Phamacy of Chinese Patent Medicines

黄芩单味药物制成的制剂，如黄芩片。含黄芩的中成药剂型十分丰富，涵盖了固体、液体与半固体剂型。不同中成药中炮制品的选用原则基本遵循清热泻火解毒选生黄芩，如一清颗粒、三黄片、双黄连口服液、银黄颗粒；清上焦之热多用酒黄芩，如清肺化痰丸、二母清肺丸；凉血止血多选黄芩炭，如荷叶丸。

Huangqin Pian (Tablets) is made of Huangqin alone. Additionally, Chinese patent medicines containing Huangqin are rich in pharmaceutical forms as the following: solid, liquid and semi-solid dosage forms. The selection principles of different processed Huangqin in Chinese medicines are as the following: raw material is selected for clearing heat, purging fire and resolving toxicity, such as Yiqing Keli, Sanhuang Pian (Tablets), Shuanghuanglian Koufuye and Yinhuang Keli. Jiuhuangqin (liquor processed) is often used to clear the heat in the upper energizer such as Qingfei Huatan Wan and Ermu Qingfei Wan. For cooling the blood and stopping bleeding, charcoalized Huangqin can be used, such as Heye Wan.

黄芩的主要有效成分黄芩苷，在热水中有较好的溶解度，且较为稳定，可采用水煎煮法制备。当水煎液加酸调节 pH 至 1~2 时，可使黄芩苷从水溶液中析出，这也是目前制备黄芩浸膏和黄芩苷的主要方法。如，一清颗粒、一清胶囊，为避免方中黄芩与黄连混合煎煮时黄芩苷类黄酮与小檗碱类生物碱发生络合反应，生成难溶性沉淀，降低药效，常将两者分开提取后混合，完成后面的制剂工艺。

Baicalin, the main effective component of Huangqin, has a good solubility and stable state in hot water, so it can be prepared by water decoction. When the value of pH is adjusted to 1~2 by adding acid, baicalin can be precipitated from the aqueous solution, that is also the main method to prepare Huangqin extract and baicalin. In order to avoid the complexation reaction of flavonoids from Huangqin and berberine alkaloid from Huanglian when being decocted together and avoid the generation of insoluble precipitates and the reduction of the efficacy, these two medicinals are extracted, respectively, then mixed in the later technology.

【性能功效】
[Property and Efficacy]

一、性能
I Property

黄芩苦，寒；归肺、胆、胃、大肠、小肠经。
Huangqin is bitter and cold, and enters the lung, gallbladder, stomach, large intestine, and small intestine meridians.

二、功效
II Efficacy

1. **清热燥湿** 黄芩能清肺胃、肝胆、大肠等湿热，尤善清中上焦湿热。其功效的发挥与解热、抗病原微生物、抗炎、抗过敏、保肝等药理作用密切相关。黄芩发挥上述药理作用的主要物质基础为黄酮类成分，如黄芩苷。黄芩通过降低 IL-1β、IL-6、NO 的含量，抑制 PGE_2 和 cAMP 的合成发挥解热作用；通过减少组胺、慢反应物质（SRS-A）等过敏介质的释放发挥抗过敏作用；黄芩抗炎的作用机制与抑制花生四烯酸的代谢和调节白细胞的功能有关。

1 Clearing Heat and Eliminating Dampness
Huangqin clears the dampness-heat in the lung, stomach, liver, gallbladder and large intestine, especially good at clearing heat in the middle and upper energizer. The efficacy is closely correlated to the pharmacological effects such as antipyresis, antipathogenic microorganisms, anti-inflammation, anti-allergy and liver protection. It is flavonoids-like components to exert the

above effects, such as baicalin. The antipyretic mechanisms are associated with the decrease of IL-1β, IL-6 and NO, and the inhibition of PGE$_2$ and cAMP synthesis. Through reducing the release of histamine, slow reaction substances (SRA-A) and other allergenic mediators, Huangqin plays an antiallergic role. The anti-inflammatory mechanisms are associated with inhibiting the metabolism of arachidonic acid and regulating the function of leukocytes.

2. 泻火解毒　黄芩苦寒泄泻，清肃沉降，善解热毒而疗疮痈。其功效的发挥与抗病毒、抗内毒素等药理作用密切相关，主要药效物质基础为黄酮类成分，如黄芩苷。黄芩抗内毒素的机制与减少 TNF-α、NO、E- 选择素和 NO 的表达有关。

2 Clearing Heat and Detoxication

Huangqin is bitter and cold in nature. It can clear heat, descend lung qi, which is good at relieving heat-toxicity and treating sores and carbuncles. Its efficacy is closely related to pharmacological effects such as anti-viral and anti-endotoxin. The major active components are flavonoids, such as baicalin. The anti-endotoxin mechanisms are associated with the decrease of TNF-α, NO, E-selectin and the expressing of NO.

3. 止血安胎　黄芩苦寒，善止血安胎。其功效的发挥与抗血小板聚集、抑制子宫收缩等药理作用密切相关。黄芩抗血小板聚集的有效物质基础主要是黄酮类成分。

3 Stopping Bleeding and Tranquilizing Fetus to Prevent Miscarriage

Huangqin excels in stopping bleeding and soothing fetus due to its cold and bitter nature. Its function is in connection with the inhibition of the aggregation of blood platelet and uterine contraction. Flavonoids-like substances are the effective material bases of Huangqin in anti-aggregation of blood platelet.

此外，现代研究显示黄芩具有降血压、降血脂、抗血小板聚集等作用。

In addition, modern research reveals that Huangqin also has hypotensive, hypolipidemic effects and the effect of anti-aggregation of blood platelet.

【应用】
[Applications]

一、主治病证
I Indications

1. 湿温暑湿，胸闷呕恶，湿热痞满，泻痢，黄疸　黄芩可与他药配伍治疗湿温或暑湿初起，身热不扬，胸脘痞闷，舌苔黄腻等症，方如《温病条辨》黄芩滑石汤；治湿热中阻，痞满呕吐，方如《伤寒论》半夏泻心汤；治湿热泻痢，方如《医学六书》芍药汤；治湿热黄疸，须配伍茵陈、栀子等药。

1 Dampness Warm and Summer Heatdampness, Chest Distress, Vomit, Nausea, Distention and Fullness Caused by Dampness Warm, Diarrhea, Jaundice

The combination of Huangqin and other medicines can treat the syndromes of dampness warm, summer heat-dampness, chest distress, with yellow greasy tongue coating, such as Huangqin Huashi Tang (Decoction) in the *Wenbing Tiaobian* (*Datailed Analysis of Warm Diseases*); For the syndromes of dampness-heat encumbering with chest tightness and vomit, such as Banxia Xiexin Tang (Decoction) in the *Shanghan Zabing Lun*; For dampness-heat diarrhea, such as Shaoyao Tang (Decoction) in the *Yixue Liushu (Six Books of Medicine)*. It is combined with Yinchen and Zhizi can treat dampness-heat jaundice.

在现代临床黄芩配伍常用于治疗急性肠炎、流行性腹泻、急性菌痢、病毒性肝炎等湿热内胜者，如葛根芩连汤、黄芩汤。

In modern clinical practice, Huangqin compatibility is often applied for acute enteritis, epidemic diarrhea, acute bacillary dysentery, and viral hepatitis caused by interiorly excessive dampness-heat, such as Gegen Qinlian Tang.

2. **肺热咳嗽，高热烦渴**　本品单用即可治肺热咳嗽，即《丹溪心法》清金丸；与他药配伍治疗痰热咳嗽，方如《医方考》清气化痰丸；治外感热病，邪郁于内之高热烦渴，尿赤便秘者，方如《太平惠民和剂局方》凉膈散；若邪在少阳，往来寒热，可配伍柴胡，方如《伤寒论》小柴胡汤。

2 Lung-heat Cough, High Fever and Polydipsia

Huangqin alone can be used to relieve lung-heat cough, such as Qingjin Wan in *Danxi Xinfa* (*Danxi's Experiential Therapy*). When combined with other medicinals, it can be used for cough due to phlegm-heat, such as Qingqi Huatan Wan in *Yifang Kao*; for relieving the syndromes of exogenous high fever, thirst, deep-colored urine and constipation, such as Liangge San (Powder) in *Taiping Huimin Heji Ju Fang*; The combination of Huangqin and Chaihu is used for alternating chill and fever, and the evil lying in Shaoyang, such as Xiaochaihu Tang (Decoction) in *Shanghan Zabing Lun*.

3. **痈肿疮毒**　黄芩可与他药配伍治疗痈肿疮毒，方如《外台秘要》黄连解毒汤。

3 Sores and Abscesses

Huangqin could be combined with other medicinals to treat carbuncles, swellings and sores, such as Huanglian Jiedu Tang (Decoction) in *Waitai Miyao*.

在现代临床黄芩配伍常用于治疗急慢性咽炎、腮腺炎、上呼吸道感染等，如双黄连口服液、双黄连注射液、银黄注射液等。

In modern clinical prctice, Huangqin compatibility is often used for acute and chronic pharyngitis, mumps, upper respiratory tract infections, such as Shuang Huanglian Koufuye, Shuang Huanglian Zhusheye, Yin Huang Zhusheye and so on.

4. **血热出血证**　治血热盛迫血妄行之吐血，衄血，单用，如《太平圣惠方》黄芩散，或与大黄同用，如《圣济总录》大黄汤；治血热便血常配伍地榆、槐花。

4 Bleeding Due to Blood Heat

Huangqin can be used alone such as Huangqin San (Powder) in *Taiping Shenghui Fang* or combined with Dahuang such as Dahuang Tang (Decoction) in the *Sheng Ji Zonglu* (*General Records of Holy Universal Relief*) for blood vomiting or hematemesis due to blood heat. It is often combined with Diyu and Huaihua (Sophorae Flos) for hemafecia due to blood heat.

5. **胎动不安**　黄芩可与他药配伍治疗胎热之胎动不安，方如《金匮要略》当归散；治血虚有热之胎动不安，方如《寿世保元》安胎丸。

5 Excessive Fetal Movements

Huangqin compatibility is used for fetal restlessness caused by fetal heat, such as Danggui San (Powder) in *Jingui Yaolue*; or fetal restlessness caused by the blood deficiency, such as Antai Wan in *Shoushi Baoyuan*.

二、用法用量
II Administration and Dosage

3~10 g。

三、注意事项
III Precautions

脾胃虚寒者不宜使用。

It should not be used in the cases of deficiency cold in the spleen and stomach.

【知识拓展】
[Knowledge Development]

以黄芩为君药的黄芩汤（PHY906）与化疗药物联合使用，可明显减轻单用化疗药所致的腹泻、疲乏、腹痛等症状，并延长肝癌患者生存期，优于一线抗肝癌药物索拉菲尼。2018年8月，PHY906通过美国食品药品监督管理局（FDA）核准得到IND批件。

Huangqin Tang (PHY906 Decoction),

taking Huangqin as the sovereign medicinal, can being combined with chemotherapy agents, to significantly attenuate chemotherapy-induced diarrhea, fatigue, abdominal pain and other syndromes,and prolong the survival time. Its effect is better than that of first-line anti-hepatic cancer drug sorafenib . In August 2018, PHY906 received Investigational New Drug (IND) certificate approved by the U.S. Food and Drug Administration (FDA).

黄 连

Huanglian
(Coptidis Rhizoma)

黄连是著名的川产道地药材。常用的炮制品为酒黄连、姜黄连以及萸黄连等，黄连味苦性寒，归心、脾、胃、肝、胆、大肠经，具清热燥湿、泻火解毒功效，主治湿热痞满，呕吐吞酸，泻痢，黄疸，高热神昏，心火亢盛，心烦不寐，心悸不宁，血热吐衄，目赤，牙痛，消渴，痈肿疔疮；外治湿疹，湿疮，耳道流脓。黄连中主要含生物碱等成分，有抗菌、抗炎、抗病毒、利胆、降血糖、免疫调节等药理作用，可用于治疗湿热泻痢、湿疹、高热神昏、目赤肿痛、痈肿疔疮、消渴等。黄连苦寒之性强，脾胃虚寒者忌用，阴虚津伤者慎用。

Huanglian is a famous genuine regional medicinal produced in Sichuan. The commonly used processed products of Huanglian are Jiuhuanglian (liquor-processed), Jianghuanglian (ginger-processed), and Yuhuanglian (Wuzhuyu-processed). Huanglian is bitter in flavor and cold in nature, and enters the heart, spleen, stomach, liver, gallbladder and large intestine meridians. It has the effects of clearing heat, drying dampness, purging fire and detoxicating, and is mainly used for treating dampness-heat fullness, vomiting, acid regurgitation, diarrhea, jaundice, high fever, coma, hyperactivity of heart fire, restlessness, palpitation, dysphoria, hematemesis, conjunctival congestion, toothache, diabetes, carbuncle, swelling and furuncle. It is also used for the external treatment of eczema, wet sores, and ear canal abscess. Huanglian mainly contains alkaloids and other components, and has antibacterial, anti-inflammatory, antiviral, cholagogic, hypoglycemic, and immune-regulation pharmacological effects. It can be used for treating dampness-heat dysentery, eczema, hyperpyretic coma, conjunctival congestion, swelling and pain, carbuncle, furuncle, and diabetes. Because Huanglian has strong bitter flavor and cold nature, it should not be used for the patients with spleen and stomach deficiency and cold, and with caution for those with yin deficiency and fluid injury.

【品种品质】
[Variety and Quality]

一、基原品种与品质
I Origin Varieties and Quality

1. 品种概况 来源于毛茛科植物黄连 *Coptis chinensis* Franch.、三角叶黄连 *Coptis. deltoidea* C. Y. Cheng et Hsiao 或 云 连 *Coptis Coptis. teeta* Wall. 的干燥根茎。

1 Variety

It is derived from the dried rhizome of *Coptis chinensis* Franch., *Copti sdeltoidei* C. Y. Cheng et Hsiao or *Coptis teena*. Wall.

黄连始载于《神农本草经》。《名医别录》及《本草纲目》记载四川产者为良。《本草纲目》记载"味连""雅连"，前者原植物为黄连；后者原植物为三角叶黄连。《滇南本草》："滇连，一名云连，人多不识，生禹山（今云南省昆明市境内），形似车前，小细子，黄色根，连成条状"，其描述的形状特征与现今《中华人民共和国药典》一部规定的云连性状一致。

Huanglian was first recorded in *Shennong Bencao Jing*. *Mingyi Bielu* (*Miscellaneous Records of Famous Physicians*) and *Bencao Gangmu* record that Huanglian produced in Sichuan is the best. "Wei Lian" and "Ya Lian" were recorded in *Bencao Gangmu*. The original plant of the former is *Coptischinensis* and the original plant of the lalter is *Coptisdeltoides*. *Diannan Bencao* (*Materia Medica of South Yunnan*) recorded as: "Dianlian (Dian means Yunnan province) is also named Yunlian, which is not known by many people. It grows in Yushan (Kunming City, Yunnan Province), is shape like a Cheqian, with small and thin seed, yellow roots and is connecting as strips". this descriptions of the shape and characteristics are consistent with the Yunlian character stipulated in the current *Pharmacopoeia of the People's Republic of China*.

2. 种植采收　黄连以栽培品为主。味连主要产于重庆石柱、湖北利川等地，雅连主产于四川洪雅、峨眉等地，云连主产于云南德钦、碧江及西藏东南部。黄连常采用种子育苗移栽，于栽培5~6年后，在10~11月间采收。

2　Planting and Harvesting

Huanglian is mainly cultivated. Weilian is mainly produced in Shizhu in Chongqing, and Lichuan in Hubei. Yalian is mainly produced in Hongya, Sichuan and Emei in Sichuan province. Yunlian is mainly produced in Deqin, Yunnan and Bijiang in Yunnan province and southeast Tibet. Huanglian is usually transplanted by seed seedling and harvested in October to November after 5 to 6 years of cultivation.

3. 道地性及品质评价　历代本草记载四川是黄连的主产地。古人从形、色、气、味等方面提出了黄连的性状评价指标，味连以身干肥壮，

连珠形，质坚实，"过桥"短，无残茎、毛须，断面红黄色、有菊花心、味极苦者为佳；雅连以身干肥壮，质坚实，断面色黄色者为佳；云连以身干坚实，曲节多，须根少，色黄者为佳。川产黄连品种最优。

3　Genuineness and Quality Evaluation

Ancient materia medica literature records that Sichuan is the main producing area of Huanglian. The ancients put forward the evaluation index of Huanglian from the aspects of shape, color, and taste. The best quality of Weilian is characterized by dry, plump, beaded body, solid texture, short junction, free of residual stems and hairy whiskers, red and yellow in cross section, chrysanthemum-like heart and bitter in taste. The best quality of Yalian is characterized by a strong thick body, solid quality and yellow cross section. The best quality of Yunlian is characterized by dry firm, with many knots, few fibrous roots and yellow color. Huanglian from Sichuan is the best variety.

黄连的主要成分为多种生物碱，包括小檗碱、黄连碱、巴马汀、表小檗碱、药根碱和甲基黄连碱。一般认为总生物碱是黄连的药效物质基础，其中小檗碱、黄连碱、巴马汀、表小檗碱是抗炎、抗菌及止泻的主要成分。此外，还含有木兰花碱、阿魏酸落叶松脂素和反式阿魏酸对羟基苯乙酯等。《中国药典》规定味连含小檗碱以盐酸小檗碱计，不得少于5.5%，表小檗碱不得少于0.80%，黄连碱不得少于1.6%，巴马汀不得少于1.5%。雅连含小檗碱以盐酸小檗碱计，不得少于4.5%；云连不得少于7.0%。

The main components of Huanglian are various alkaloids, including berberine, coptisine, palmatine, epiberberine, jatrorrhizine and methyl coptisine. It generally believes that the total alkaloids are the pharmacodynamic material basis of Huanglian. Berberine, coptisine, palmatine and epiberberine are the main components for anti-inflammatory, antibacterial and anti-diarrheal effects. In addition, it also contains magnoflorine, ferulic acid deciduous rosins, trans ferulic acid p-hydroxybenzene ethyl ester, etc. *The Pharmacopoeia of the People's Republic of China* stipulates that the content of berberine in Weilian shall not be less than 5.5% counted by and based on berberine hydrochloride, epiberberine not less than 0.80%, coptisine not less than 1.6%, and palmatine not less than 1.5%. Content of berberine in Yalian shall not be less than 4.5% counted by berberine hydrochloride, that in Yunlian shall not be less than 7.0%.

二、炮制品种与品质
II Processed Varieties and Quality

黄连的炮制品种有 10 多个，临床常用品种有 8 种，如酒黄连、姜黄连等。黄连片呈不规则的薄片；外表皮灰黄色或黄褐色，具放射状纹理，气微，味极苦。酒黄连形如黄连片，色泽加深；略有酒香气。姜黄连表面棕黄色；有姜的辛辣味。萸黄连以粗壮、坚实、断面皮部橙红色，木部鲜黄色或橙黄色者为佳。饮片的品质评价同药材。

There are more than 10 processed varie- ties of Huanglian, 8 varieties of which are commonly used clinically, such as Jiuhuanglian (liquor-processed) Jianghuanglian (ginger-processed). The Huanlian Pian (decoction pieces) are irregular thin slices. Its outer skin is grayish yellow or yellowish brown, with a radial texture, slight smell and extremely bitter taste. The Jiuhuanglian (liquor-processed) is in similar shape with Huanlian Pian but deeper in color with a slight aroma of liquor. Jianghuanglian (ginger-processed) has a brownish yellow surface with pungent taste of ginger. The best quality of Yuhuanglian (Wuzhuyu-processed) is characterized by thick, firm, with orange-red section skin and bright yellow or orange-yellow xylem. The quality evaluation of decoction pieces is the same as that of medicinal materials.

三、中成药品种与品质
III Varieties and Quality of Chinese Patent Medicines

含有黄连或其炮制品的中成药有 513 种，其中《中国药典》记载 103 个，以黄连为君药或主药的品种有五黄养阴颗粒、心速宁胶囊、清胃黄连丸（大蜜丸）等。在相关中成药质量控制中常以黄连中小檗碱为指标成分进行了限量，如清胃黄连丸中即规定了每丸中黄连、黄柏以盐酸小檗碱的含量最低限。

There are 513 kinds of Chinese patent medicines containing Huanglian or its processed products, of which 103 are recorded in the *Pharmacopoeia of the People's Republic of China*. The varieties with Huanglian as the monarch (soveign) medicinal or main medicinal include Wuhuang Yangyin Keli, Xinsuning Jiaonang, Qingwei Huanglian Wan (Dami Pills), etc. In the quality control of related Chinese patent medicines, berberine in Huanglian is often as the index component with certain limit, such as the minimal limit of the berberine hydrochloride in Huanglian and Huangbo of each pill is stipulated in Qingwei Huanglian Wan.

【制药】
[Pharmacy]
一、产地加工
I Processing in Production Area

秋季采挖，除去须根及泥沙，干燥，撞去残留须根。

Dug out in autumn with fibrous roots and silt, removed Huanglian will be dried and knocked off.

二、饮片炮制
II Processing of Decoction Pieces

从古至今黄连形成了十多种炮制方法，以

"切制 - 酒炙 - 姜汁炙 - 吴茱萸制"为工艺，生黄连、酒黄连、姜黄连、萸黄连是商品规格的主流。

Since ancient time, Huanglian has formed more than ten processing methods. With the processing techniques of "cutting, stir-frying with liquor, stir-frying with ginger juice, processing with Wuzhuyu", raw Huanglian, Jiuhuanglian (liquor-processed), Jianghuanglian (ginger-processed) and Yuhuanglian (Wuzhuyu-processed) are the mainstreams of commercial specifications.

中药炮制中常用辅料姜、酒、吴茱萸是黄连炮中常用之品，可抑制黄连的苦寒之性，使其"去性存用"；而胆汁、醋、盐则可增加或增强黄连的寒凉、收敛、下行等药性。

Ginger, liquor and Wuzhuyu, commonly as auxiliary materials in the processing of Chinese medicinals, are commonly used in the processing of Huanglian, which can inhibit the bitter and cold nature of Huanglian and enable it to be "useful with nature removal"; meanwhile, the applying of bile, vinegar and salt in the processing of huanglian can increase or enhance the nature of cold, astringent and descending properties of Huanglian.

三、中成药制药
III Pharmacy of Chinese Patent Medicines

含黄连的中成药，剂型十分丰富，涵盖了固体、液体与半固体剂型，具体包括丸剂、散剂、颗粒剂、胶囊剂、片剂、合剂（口服液）等。在中成药中，黄连一般与其他药物以复方配伍形式应用，也有以黄连单味入药制成的胶囊（黄连胶囊）。若用于肝胆火旺、头晕目眩，宜选用酒黄连，如当归龙荟丸；若用于肝胃不和、胃失和降导致的腹痛、嗳气吞酸，宜选用姜黄连，如加味左金丸；若用于大肠湿热导致的痢疾、泄泻，宜选用萸黄连，如香连丸、香连片。这些中成药的制剂中要特别注意黄连中生物碱成分的提取和保留，常采用水提醇沉法，如香连丸。

Chinese patent medicines containing Huanglian are rich in pharmaceutical forms, including solid, liquid and semi-solid pharmaceutical forms. Specifically, these dosage forms have pills, powder, granules, capsules, tablets, mixture, etc. In Chinese patent medicines, Huanglian is commonly used in combination with other medicinals, and there are also capsules like Huanglian Jiaonang alone that uses Huanglian. For treating excessive fire of liver and gallbladder and dizziness, Jiuhuanglian (liquor-processed) should be selected, such as in Danggui Longhui Wan. For abdominal pain, belching and acid regurgitation caused by liver-stomach disharmony and failure of descending stomach disharmony, Jianghuanglian (ginger-processed) should be selected such as in Jiawei Zuojin Wan. For dysentery and diarrhea caused by dampness-heat in large intestine, Yuhuanglian (Wuzhuyu-processed) should be used, such as in Xianglian Wan and Xianglian Pian (Tablets), In the preparation of these Chinese patent medicines, special attention should be paid to the extraction and retention of alkaloids in Huanglian. Thus water extraction and alcohol precipitation are often used, such as Xianglian Wan.

【性能功效】
[Property and Efficacy]

一、性能
I Property

黄连苦，寒；归心、胃、肝、大肠经。
Huanglian is bitter in flavor and cold in nature, and enters the heart, spleen, stomach, liver, gallbladder and large intestine meridians.

二、功效
II Efficacy

1. **清热燥湿**　黄连大苦大寒，既可清热又能燥湿，又归心、脾、胃、肝、胆、大肠经，长于清泄中焦湿热，为治痢要药。其功效的发挥与抗病原微生物、抗炎、解热、止泻等药理作用密切相关。黄连抗病原微生物、抗炎、解热、止泻的有效物质基础主要是小檗碱，通过刺激皮质激素的释放发挥抑制炎症作用。

1 Heat-clearing and Dampness-drying

Huanglian, bitter in flavor, cold in nature, can clear heat and dry dampness, and enters to the heart, spleen, stomach, liver, gallbladder and large intestine meridians. It is good at clearing and purging heat and dampness in the middle energizer and is an essential medicinal for dysentery. The exertion of its efficacy is closely related to the pharmacological effects of anti-pathogenic micro-organisms, anti-inflammatory, antipyretic, anti-diarrheal effects, etc. The effective substance basis of Huanglian for anti-pathogenic micro-organism, anti-inflammatory, antipyretic and anti-diarrheal effects are berberine, which can inhibit inflammation by stimulating the release of cortical hormone.

2. **泻火解毒** 黄连清热泻火力强，尤善清心火。其功效的发挥与抗心律失常、抗心肌缺血、降血脂、降血糖、抗肿瘤等药理作用密切相关。黄连抗心律失常、抗心肌缺血、降血压、降血脂、降血糖、抗肿瘤的有效物质基础主要是小檗碱，通过延长心肌细胞的动作电位，拮抗肾上腺素的作用，抑制心肌 Na^+ 内流发挥抗心律失常作用；通过抑制糖原异生和促进糖酵解发挥降血糖作用。

2 Clearing Heat and Detoxication

Huanglian has a strong effect in clearing heat and purging fire, especially clearing the heart fire. The exertion of its efficacy is closely related to the pharmacological effects of anti-arrhythmia, anti-myocardial ischemia, lowering blood lipid, lowering blood sugar, anti-tumor, etc. The effective substance basis of those above-mentioned pharmacological effects is berberine, which plays anti-arrhythmic role by prolonging the action potential of myocardial cells, antagonizing the effect of epinephrine and inhibiting myocardial NA^+ influx, and reduces blood sugar by inhibiting

glycogenesis and promoting glycolysis.

【应用】
[Applications]

一、主治病证
I Indications

1. **湿热痞满、泻痢，呕吐吞酸** 治湿热阻滞中焦，气机不畅所致脘腹痞满、恶心呕吐，常配苏叶用，如方出《温热经纬》名见《中医妇科学》苏叶黄连汤，或配黄芩、干姜、半夏用，如《伤寒论》半夏泻心汤；若配人参、白术、干姜等药用，可治脾胃虚寒，呕吐酸水，如《症因脉治》连理汤。黄连为治泻痢要药，单用有效。若配木香，可治湿热泻痢，腹痛里急后重，如《兵部手集方》香连丸；若配乌梅，可治湿热下痢脓血日久，如《外台秘要》黄连丸。

1 Dampness-heat and Fullness, Diarrhea and Dysentery, Vomiting and Acid Regurgitation

For epigastric fullness, nausea and vomiting caused by dampness-heat blocking the middle energizer and qi stagnation, it is often combined with Suye, named as Suye Huanglian Tang in *Chinese Medicine Gynecology*, the prescription recorded in *Wenre Jingwei (Compendium on Epidemic Febrile Disease)*; or combined with Huangqin, Ganjiang and Banxia, such as Banxia Xiexin Tang (Decoction) in *Shanghan Zabing Lun*. If it is combined with Renshen, Baizhu, Ganjiang and other medicinals, it can be used to treat spleen and stomach deficiency cold, vomiting and acid water, such as Lian Li Tang (Decoction) from *Zhengyin Maizhi (Syndrome Identification, Pathogeny, Pulse Diagnosis and Treatment)*. Huanglian as an essential medicinal for treating diarrhea can be used in single. Being combined with Muxiang, it can treat dysentery due to dampness-heat diarrhea, abdominal pain with tenesmus, such as Xianglian Wan from the *Bingbu Shoujifang (Hand Set Square of the Ministry of War)*. Combined with Wumei, it can also be used to treat prolonged dysentery with bloody pus due to dampness-heat, such as Huanglian Wan from *Waitai Miyao*.

现代临床，黄连配伍可用于治疗消化系统疾病。如以黄连为主的复方（葛根芩连汤加味）常用于治疗湿热阻滞之腹痛腹泻，相对于现代医学的直肠炎属大肠湿热者。

In modern clinical practice, Huanglian compatibility can be used to treat digestive system diseases. For example, the compound prescription modified Gegen Qinlian Tang taking Huanglian as main medicinal is used to treat abdominal pain and diarrhea due to dampness-heat blockage, which is a large intestine dampness-heat type proctitis in modern medicine comparatively.

2. **高热神昏，心烦不寐，血热吐衄** 治心火亢盛所致神昏、烦躁之证。若配黄芩、黄柏、栀子，可治三焦热盛，高热烦燥；若配石膏、知母、玄参、丹皮等药用，可治高热神昏，如《疫疹一得》清瘟败毒饮；若配大黄、黄芩，可治邪火内炽，迫血妄行之吐衄，如《金匮要略》泻心汤。

2 High Fever and Coma, Vexation and Insomnia, Hematemesis and Epistaxis

Huanglian is used to treat coma and dysphoria caused by hyperactivity of heart fire. In the compatibility of Huangqin, Huangbo and Zhizi, Huanglian can be used to treat excessive heat in the triple energizer and dysphoria due to high fever. In the compatibility of Shigao, Zhimu, Xuanshen and Danpi, it can be used to treat hyperpyretic coma, such as Qingwen Baidu Yin recorded in *Yizhen Yide (Achievements Regarding Epidemic Rashes)*. In the compatibility of Dahuang and Huangqin, it can be used to treat vomiting and hematemesis caused by internal excessive pathogenic fire, such as Xiexin Tang (Decoction) from *Jingui Yaolue*.

现代临床，黄连配伍可用于治疗心血管系统疾病。如以黄连为主配朱砂、生地黄，治心火亢盛之心烦失眠。

In modern clinical practice, Huanglian compatibility can be used to treat cardiovascular

system diseases. For example, Huanglian is mainly combined with Zhusha and Shengdihuang to treat vexation and insomnia due to hyperactivity of heart fire.

3. **痈肿疔疮，目赤牙痛** 治痈肿疔毒，多与黄芩、黄柏、栀子同用，如《外台秘要》黄连解毒汤；若配淡竹叶，可治目赤肿痛，赤脉胬肉，如《普济方》黄连汤；若配生地黄、升麻、丹皮等药用，可治胃火上攻，牙痛难忍，如《兰室秘藏》清胃散。

3 Carbuncle, Swelling, Furuncle, Sore, Red Eyes and Toothache

For carbuncle, swelling and furuncle, Huanglian is usually combined with Huangqin, Huangbo and Zhizi, such as Huanglian Jiedu Tang (Decoction) from *Waitai Miyao*. Huanglian can be used to treat conjunctival congestion, swelling and pain, and red vein and pterygium in the combination with Danzhuye (Lophatheri Herba), such as Huanglian Tang (Decoction) in *Puji Fang*. In the compatibility of Sheng Dinghuang, Shengma and Dangpi, it can be used to treat stomach fire attack and unbearable toothache, such as Qing Wei San from *Lanshi Micang (Secret Book of the Orchid Chamber)*.

现代临床，黄连配伍可用于治疗五官科疾病。如以黄连为主配黄芩、大黄，治心火内炽，迫血妄行，吐血者。研细，外搽治疗牙缝出血。

In modern clinical practice, Huanglian compatibility can be used to treat diseases of five-senses departments (ENT departments). For example, Huanglian is mainly combined with Huangqin and Dahuang to treat hematemesis or vomitting blood due to heart fire force blood flowing drastically Huanglian can be ground and applied externally to treat gum bleeding.

4. **湿疹、湿疮、耳道流脓** 治皮肤湿疹、湿疮，取黄连浸汁涂患处，煎汁滴眼、耳，治疗眼目红肿、耳道流脓。

4 Eczema, Wet Sores, Ear Canal Abscess

For skin eczema and wet sores, Huanglian decoctionis to apply on the affected drea, and drip the decoction on eyes and ears to treat red swelling of eyes and pus in ear canal.

现代临床，黄连配伍可用于治疗化脓性痈肿、恶疮等外科疾病。如黄连为主配黄柏、乳香、龟甲为末研匀，香油调敷，治疗严重湿疹。

In modern clinical practice, Huanglian compatibility can be used to treat surgical diseases such as suppurative carbuncle, swelling and malignant sore. For example, Huanlian is mainly combined with Huangbo, Ruxiang and Guijia, evenly ground, and mixed with sesame oil and be applied them externally to treat severe eczema.

5. **消渴** 治消渴，如《普济方》消渴丸；或配黄柏用，以增强泻火之力，如《圣济总录》黄柏丸；若配生地黄，可用治肾阴不足，心胃火旺之消渴，如《外台秘要》黄连丸。

5 Consumptive Thirst or Diabetes

Huanglian can be used for Treating Consumptive Thirst or diabetes, such as Xiaoke Wan in *Puji Fang*, it can be combined with Huangbo to enhance the ability of purging fire, such as HuangboWan in *Sheng Ji Zonglu (General Records of Holy Universal Releif)*. For consumptive thirst or diabetes caused by deficiency of kidney *yin* and hyperactivity of heart and stomach fire, it can be combined with

Shengdihuang, such as Huanglian Wan from *Waitai Miyao*.

现代临床，黄连常用于治疗糖尿病属肺脾肾阴虚湿热内盛者。

In modern clinical practice, Huanglian is commonly used to treat diabetes mellitus due to *yin* deficiency of lung, spleen and kidney and internal excess of dampness heat.

二、用法用量
II Administration and Dosage

饮片：煎汤，2~5g。外用适量。

Decoction pieces: decoction, 2~5g. Appropriate amount for external use.

三、注意事项
III Precautions

1. 本品大苦大寒，脾胃虚寒者忌用。

1 This product is greatly bitter cold in nature, and should not be used for the patients with spleen-stomach deficiency cold.

2. 阴虚津伤者慎用。

2 Patients with yin deficiency and fluid depletion should use it with caution.

金 银 花

Jinyinhua
(Lonicerae Japonicae Flos)

金银花是河南、山东的著名道地药材。金银花味甘，性寒，归肺、心、胃经，有清热解毒、疏散风热的功效，主治热毒壅盛、痈疖、风热表证、温热卫分证等。金银花主要含有黄酮类、有机酸类、三萜皂苷、多糖等成分，有抗病原微生物、抗内毒素、抗炎、解热、抑制血小板聚集、抗氧化等作用，现代临床主要用于呼吸系统、消化系统、神经系统等感染性疾病属热毒壅盛或风

热表证、温病初起者。

Jinyinhua is a famous genuine regional medicinal both in Henan and Shangdong province. It is cold in nature and sweet in flavor, and enters the lung, heart and stomach meridians. It has the effects of clearing heat and detoxication, and dispersing wind-heat, so that it is traditionally used to treat syndromes of dominance of heat in interior,

Yongju (carbuncle and furuncle), exterior wind-heat syndrome, warm disease in Weifen defensive level, etc. Jinyinhua contains mainly, flavonoids, organic acids, triterpenoid saponins, polysaccharides. It has pharmacological effects of anti-pathogenic microorganism, anti-endotoxin, anti-inflammation, antipyretic, inhibition of platelet aggregation, anti-oxidation etc. In modern clinical practice, Jinyinhua is mainly applied to treat infectious diseases of respiratory system, digestive system and nervous system, etc. that are differentiated as dominance of heat heat toxin, or exterior wind-heat syndrome, or early stage of warm disease.

【品种品质】
[Variety and Quality]

一、基原品种与品质
I Origin Varieties and Quality

1. 品种概况 来源于忍冬科植物忍冬 *Lonicera japonica* Thunb. 的干燥花蕾或带初开花。

1 Variety

Jinyinhua is the dried bud or that with early blossoming flower of *Lonicera japonica* Thunb. of Caprifoliaceae.

金银花因其花蕾有黄、白两色而得名，始载于《名医别录》，称"忍冬"，《证类本草》载陶弘景谓其"今处处皆有，似藤生，凌冬不凋，故名忍冬"，沿用至清代。金银花的入药部位也有变迁，《本草纲目》载其全草入药，《救荒本草》首次明确花和花蕾入药，并称之为"金银花"。

Jinyinhua is named for it blooming yellow and white flowers. It was first recorded in the book of *Mingyi Bielu* with the name of "Rendong". As recorded in the book of *Zhenglei Bencao*, Tao Hongjing said that Jinyinhua distributed everywhere and liked a vine plant, not withering in winter, so it was called Rendong. The name used from then to the Qing Dynasty. The medicinal part of Jinyinhua also changed in history. According to the book of *Bencao Gangmu*, the whole grass was medicinal parts. The book of *Jiuhuang Bencao*

(Materia Medica of Famine Relief) first recorded that its definite medicinal parts are bud and flower, and its name is "Jinyinhua".

2. 种植采收 金银花的适应性强，在全国大部分地区均有分布，药用以种植为主，以山东和河南最为适宜。可通过种子繁殖和扦插繁殖进行育种，移栽。金银花应在花蕾尚未开放前采摘，一年可采摘多次，一日之中以清晨最佳。

2 Planting and Harvesting

The plant of Jinyinhua is well-adapted and distributes in most regions of China. However, the medicinal is produced mainly by cultivation and Shangdong province and Henan province are the optimum area. It can be bred or transplanted by seed propagation or cutting propagation. Jinyinhua should be collected before blossoming. It and can be collected for several times a year, and early morning is the best time in a day.

3. 道地性与品质评价 据明代《救荒本草》记载，河南是金银花的传统道地产区，称"怀银花"，又以密县者最佳，称"密银花"。此外，山东也是金银花的道地产区，称"济银花"。传统评价上金银花以花蕾多、色绿白、质柔软、气清香者为佳。

3 Genuineness and Quality Evaluation

According to the recording in book of *Jiuhuang Bencao* in the Ming Dynasty, Henan is the traditional genuine producing area of Jinyinhua, so it is called "Huaiyinhua". Jinyinhua produced in Mi County is of best quality and is called "Miyinhua". Besides, Shandong province is also the genuine producing area of Jinyinhua, which is called "Jiyinhua". Traditionally, Jinyinhua with the characters of many buds, green-white color, soft texture and fragrant smell is in high quality.

金银花主要含有有机酸类（主要含绿原酸、异绿原酸等）和黄酮类（如木犀草素、木犀草苷、木犀草素 -7-O- 葡萄糖苷、忍冬苷等），及挥发油、多糖、皂苷等。按《中国药典》规定，金银花中绿原酸、木犀草苷的含量分别不得少于1.5% 和 0.050%，且对其所含重金属和有害元素铅、镉、砷、汞、铜等有严格的限量。

Jinyinhua mainly contains organic acids (mainly containing chlorogenic acid, isochlorogenic acid, etc.), flavonoids (such as luteolin, luteoloside, luteolin -7-O-glucoside, lonicerin, etc.), volatile oil, polysaccharide and saponin. According to the regulation of *Pharmacopoeia of the People's Republic of China*, the content of chlorogenic acid and luteoloside in Jinyinhua should not less than 1.5% and 0.050% respectively, and contents of heavy metals and harmful elements, such as lead, cadmium, arsenic, mercury and copper, are strictly limited.

二、炮制品种与品质
II Processed Varieties and Quality

金银花经干燥即得金银花饮片。

Fresh Jinyinhua is collected and dried to get the decoction pecies of Jinyinhua.

三、中成药品种与品质
III Varieties and Quality of Chinese Patent Medicines

含金银花的中成药逾400个,《中国药典》收载70余个。金银花单制剂有金银花露、金银花糖浆、金银花颗粒等;以金银花为君药的复方制剂有双黄连口服液(颗粒、糖浆、注射液等)、抗感颗粒(口服液)、小儿咽扁颗粒等。中成药制药中多以花入药,也有以提取物为原料的,如茵栀黄系列。另外还有中西药复方制剂,如复方银翘氨敏胶囊。

There are more than 400 Chinese patent medicines containing Jinyinhua and 70 of them are recorded in *Pharmacopoeia of the People's Republic of China*. Among these medicinals, the products that made only from Jinyinhua include Jinyinhua Lu (Dew), Jinyinhua Tangjiang, Jinyinhua Keli, etc. Prescriptions with Jinyinhua as sovereign herb are as follows: Shuanghuanglian Koufuye (Keli, Tangjiang, Zhusheye, etc.),

Kanggan Keli, Xiaoer Yanbian Keli, etc.. In most Chinese patent preparations , it mostly applies the the flower part of Jinyinhua , while in the series products of Yinzhihuang,its extracts are also used as raw material. Besides, there are Chinese-western medicine compound preparations, such as Fufang Yinqiao Anmin Jiaonang (antiallergic Capsules).

金银花的中成药常用所金银花所含绿原酸为质量控制成分,因处方中金银花剂量、剂型、规格等的不同而限量不同,如双黄连不同制剂的最小规格中绿原酸含量限制不同,金噪散结丸的水蜜丸和大蜜丸每丸的含量要求也不同。另外,也可通过显微鉴别中金银花特征结构来控制质量。如金噪开音丸。

In Jinyinhua-contained prescriptions, chlorogenic acid is usually used as quality control component, and its content limit varies according to different dosages, forms, and specifications among different Chinese patent medicinals. For example, the limited contents of chlorogenic acid in minimum specifictions of Shuanghuanglian series in ravious dosage forms are different; the limited contents of chlorogenic acid ench pill in big honey pill and small honey pill of Jinzao Sanjie Wan vary. Besides, microscopic identification on characteristics of Jinyinhua is also applied for quality control, for example of Jinsan Kaiyin Wan.

【制药】
[Pharmacy]

一、产地加工
I Processing in Production Area

金银花采收后需除去梗、叶及杂质,及时干燥。干燥方法有晒干、阴干、烘干、杀青等不同初加工方法,但不同方法对黄酮、有机酸等成分含量影响较大,目前认为杀青烘干法较优且适于推广。

The raw medicinal is collected and dried in time after removal of steam, leaves and impurities.

Drying methods include sun drying, drying in the shade, roasting for removing green . The varieties of drying methods have great influence on the content of flavonoids and organic acids in Jinyinhua. At present, it is considered that green-removal drying method is better and suitable for spreading

二、饮片炮制
II Processing of Decoction Pieces

金银花自古以生用居多，明清时期开始出现酒制、炒制、酿制、制炭、制露等炮制方法。现以生用为主。

Jinyinhua was mainly used in raw since ancient times. During the Ming and Qing Dynasties, processing methods of Jinyinhua appeared, such as liquor processing, stir-frying, carbonizing and dew making. At present, the raw Jinyinhua is widely used.

三、中成药制药
III Pharmacy of Chinese Patent Medicines

在中成药制剂中，金银花可以单味药制药，如金银花露；但更多时候与其他药物配伍入药开发为多种剂型。金银花中有机酸等有效物质有一定的水溶解性，在热水中的溶解性增加。因而含金银花中成药制药中多采用水煎，如银黄片和茵栀黄泡腾片。而在注射剂中，为保留这些有机酸成分，常采用成盐再酸化收集的制药工艺。如银黄注射液制备过程中，使用 20% 石灰乳与金银花提取物反应使其中有机酸类成分成钙盐沉淀，再向沉淀中分别依次加入乙醇、50% 硫酸溶液使有机酸充分溶出、再浓缩，用于制剂工艺。

In the Chinese patent medicinals, Jinyinhua can be singly used, such as Jinyinhua Lu (Dew). Mostly, Jinyinhua is used in compatible with other medicinals to produce different pharmaceutical forms. The active ingredients in Jinyinhua such as organic acids have certain water solubility and become more soluble in hot water. Therefore, in most Chinese patent medicinals containing Jinyinhua, decoction method is often used, such as Yinhua Pian (Tablets) and Yinzhihuang Paotengpian (Effervescent tablets). While for injection, to keep these organic acids, the pharmaceutical process of salt forming and reacidification is often adopted. For example, in the pharmaceutical process of Yinhuang Zhusheye, 20% lime milk reacts with Jinyinhua extract to translate the seorganic acids into calcium salt precipitation and settled. Then ethanol and 50% sulfuric acid solution is added orderly into the precipitation to fully dissolute organic acids followed by concentration and further preparation.

【性能功效】
[Property and Efficacy]

一、性能
I Property

金银花苦、辛、甘，寒；归肺、心、胃、大肠经。

Jinyinhua is cold in nature and sweet in favor, enters the lung, heart, stomach and large intestine meridians.

二、功效
II Efficacy

1. **清热解毒** 金银花性寒可清热，又入卫、气、血分，故能清卫气血分之热，清热解毒，散痈消肿，为疮痈要药；又入肺经，芳香疏散，故善散肺经热邪。其功效的发挥与抗病原微生物、抗炎、解热、抗内毒素、调节免疫功能、抗血栓、抗氧化等药理作用密切相关。金银花抗病原微生物、调节免疫功能的有效物质基础主要是绿原酸。

1 Clearing away Heat and Detoxicating
As cold in nature, and entering to defense, qi, and blood aspects, Jinyinhua is good at reliving

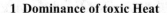

heat of defense, qi, and blood aspects, clearing away heat-toxin and dissipating carbuncle and relieving swelling, thus is a key medicinal for sore and carbuncle. It entering to lung meridian and being aromatic with dispersing laction, Jinyinhua is good at relieving heat in lung meridian. These functions are related to pharmacological actions of anti-microorganism, anti-inflammation, antipyretic, anti-endotoxin, regulating immune function, anti-thrombosis, antioxidanting, etc. Chlorogenic acid is the effective substance basis for anti-microorganism and regulating immune function.

2. **疏散风热** 金银花宣透发散，入卫、气分，可疏散风热。其功效的发挥与抗病原微生物、抗炎、解热、调节免疫功能、抗过敏等药理作用密切相关。

2 Dispersing Wind-heat

Jinyinhua, with characteristics of ventilating and divergence, entering the defense and qi aspects, has effects of dispersing wind heat, acting of which are related to pharmacological actions of anti-microorganism, anti-inflammation, antipyretic, regulating immune function, anti-allergy, etc.

【应用】
[Applications]

一、主治病证
I Indications

1. **热毒壅盛证** 金银花是治一切痈肿疔疮阳证的要药。初起红热肿痛者，可单用金银花浓煎内服或外敷，或与蒲公英、紫花地丁等配伍，如《医宗金鉴》五味消毒饮；若疮疡肿毒脓成未溃者，可与穿山甲、皂角刺等配伍，如《校注妇人良方》仙方活命饮；若温病热入营血症见高热神昏、烦躁不安，或斑疹隐隐，常与丹皮、生地、玄参等合用，如《温病条辨》清营汤。另金银花炭可单用浓煎内服或与他药配伍治疗热毒血痢。

1 Dominance of toxic Heat

Jinyinhua is a significant medicinal for treating all yang syndromes of carbuncle, boil、swelling and furuncle. At the early stage manifesting as red swelling and hot pain, Jinyinhua can be decocted alone to get concentrated decoction for internal or external application, or used in compatibility with other medicinals as Pugongying、Zihuadiding, for example Wuwei Xiaodu Yin (Decoction) recorded in *Yizong Jinjian*. For sore and ulcer without pus eruption, Jinyinhua is usually used with Chuanshanjia and Zaojiaoci (Gleditsiae Spina), such as Xianfang Huoming Yin (Decoction) from *Jiaozhu Furen Liangfang (Revised Good Remedies for Women)*. For warm disease with heat entering nutrientive-blood aspects, manifesting as high fever and unconsciousness, dysphoria and thirsty or unclear appearing of macule, it is combined with Danpi, Shengdi, Xuanshen, such as Qingying Tang (Decoction) from *Wenbing Tiaobian*. Besides, Jinyinhua is applied to treat bleeding dysentery due to toxic heat by thickly decocted alone for oral take or combined with other medicinals.

现代临床，金银花常配伍用于治疗各种感染性疾病属于热毒壅盛者，如化脓性扁桃体炎、蜂窝组织炎、急性乳腺炎、等，方如仙方活命饮、托里消毒散等。也可用于治疗流行性脑脊髓膜炎、乙型脑炎等属热入营血分者，如清营汤。

In modern clinical practice, Jinyinhua compatibility is often used to treat various infectious diseases belonging to excessive toxic heat, such as suppurative tonsillitis, cellulitis, acute mastitis, etc. formula such as Xianfang Huoming Yin and Tuoli Xiaodu San (Powder). It also can be used to treat epidemic cerebrospinal meningitis and Japanese encephalitis of heat entering nutrient-blood aspect syndrome, such as Qingying Tang (Decoction).

2. **外感风热表证或温病初起** 对外感风热表证或温病初起症见发热微恶寒，头身疼痛，常配伍连翘、菊花等，如《温病条辨》银翘散；对温病气分热盛者见高热烦渴，大汗出，脉洪大，可与石膏、知母、连翘配伍，如《中国中医秘方大全》银翘白虎汤；此外本品蒸馏制成银花露，还用于暑热烦渴。

2 Exterior Wind-heat Syndrome, Early Stage of Warm Diseases

Jinyinhua is combined with Lianqiao, Juhua and other medicinals to treat exterior wind-heat syndrome and early stage of warm disease, manifesting as fever with slight cold, pain in head and body, such as Yinqiao San recorded in *Wenbing Tiaobian*. For high fever with polydipsia, profuse sweating, and flood pulse caused by excessive heat in nutrient-blood aspect, Jinyinhua is used in compatibility with Shigao, Zhimu and Lianqiao, such as Yinqiao Baihu Tang (Decoction) recorded in *Secret Prescription Collection of Traditional Chinese Medicine in China*. Besides, it can be distilled into Jinyinhua Lu (Dew) to treat dysphoria and thirsty due to summer-heat.

现代临床，金银花配伍常用于治疗呼吸系统和头颈部感染性疾病属外感风热证或温病初起，如急性支气管炎、急慢性咽炎、感冒、腮腺炎等，方可用银翘散或中药成双黄连口服液、双黄连注射液等。

Nowadays, Jinyinhua is usually combined with other medicinals to treat infectious diseases in the respiratory system or in head and neck, belonging to exterior wind-heat syndrome or early stage of warm disease, such as acute bronchitis, acute and chronic pharyngitis, cold, mumps, etc. Yinqiao San (Powder) or the Chinese patent medicines such as Shuang Huanglian Koufuye/Zhusheye are suitable for them.

二、用法用量
II Administration and Dosage

煎汤，6~15g；或入丸、散。外用：适量，捣敷。

6~15g, for decoction, or Wan, or San (Powder). External use: appropriate amount for externally applying.

三、注意事项
III Precautions

1. 脾胃虚寒及气虚疮疡脓清者忌用。

1 It is taboo for the patients with deficiency cold of spleen and stomach, as well as sore and furuncle with thin pus due to qi deficiency.

2. 含有金银花的某些中成药可能引起过敏反应，如双黄连注射液、银黄注射液等，应仔细阅读说明书，谨慎使用。

2 Some Chinese patent medicines containing Jinyinhua, such as Shuang Huanglian Zhusheye, Yin Huang Zhusheye, may cause allergic reactions. It should be used in caution according to the reading of instructions.

【知识拓展】
[Knowledge Extension]

金银花的基原在既往有忍冬科植物忍冬 *Lonicera japonica* Thunb.、红腺忍冬 *Lonicera hypoglauca* Miq.、华南忍冬 *Lonicera confusa* DC. 和灰毡毛忍冬 *Lonicera* macranthoides Hand.-Mazz. 等，随着药典的修订，《中国药典》将后三种分列出来称"山银花"。忍冬科植物忍冬 *Lonicera japonica* Thunb. 的干燥茎枝是另外一个中药"忍冬藤"，功效与金银花相似，但通络作用增强。

In the past, the origin of Jinyinhua inclu-ded *Lonicera japonica* Thunb., *Lonicera hypoglauca* Miq., *Lonicera confusa* DC., *Lonicera* macranthoides Hand.-Mazz. of Caprifoliaceae. With constant revision of Chinese Pharmacopoeia, the last three spieces had been separated from Jinyinhua and named "Shanyinhua". The dried stem branches of *Lonicera japonica* Thunb. is another medicinal called "Rendongteng", which has similar efficacy to Jinyinhua, except enhanced action of dredging collaterals.

地 黄

Dihuang

(Rehmanniae Radix)

地黄是著名的"四大怀药"之一,自北魏以来形成了成熟的人工种植技术,临床常用炮制品有地黄和熟地黄。地黄味甘、苦,性寒,归心、肝、肺经,有清热凉血,止血,养阴生津的功效,主治热入营血分、血热妄行证和热病伤阴、津伤口渴证等。地黄主要含有多糖、苷类、环烯醚萜等,有抗缺血再灌注损伤、降血糖、增强免疫功能、镇静、促进造血功能、促凝血、调节内分泌等药理作用,可用于治疗血小板减少性紫癜、慢性肾炎、糖尿病等疾病属热入营血分、血热妄行证或热病伤阴证、津伤口渴证者。地黄性寒而滞,脾虚湿滞腹满便溏者,不宜使用。

Dihuang is one of the "Four Huai (Henan province) Chinese Medicinals". Mature artificial planting technology for it has been formed since the Northern Wei Dynasty. The unprocessed Dihuang and Shudihuang (prepared) are commonly used in clinical practice. Dihuang is sweet and bitter in flavor, cold in nature, enters the heart, liver and lung meridians, and has the effects of clearing heat and cooling blood, stopping bleeding, nourishing yin and generating fluid. It is mainly used for syndromes of heat entering nutrient-blood aspect, the syndrome of bleeding due to blood heat and syndrome of yin injured by heat and syndrome of fluidinjured thirst. Dihuang contains mainly polysaccharides, glycosides, iridoid terpenes, etc., with functions of anti-ischemic reperfusion injury, regulating blood sugar, enhancing immune function, sedation, promoting hematopoiesis, promoting blood coagulation, regulating endocrine system and other pharmacological effects. It can be used to treat thrombocytopenic purpura, chronic nephritis, diabetes belonging to the syndromes of heat entering nutrient-blood, bleeding due to blood heat, yin injured by heat and fluid-injured thirst.

As Dihuang is cold in nature and easy to induce stagnation, so it shouldn't be used for syndromes of abdominal distension and loose stool due to spleen insufficiency and dampness stagnation.

【品种品质】

[Variety and Quality]

一、基原品种与品质
I Origin Varieties and Quality

1. 品种概况 来源于玄参科植物地黄 *Rehmannia glutinosa* Libosch. 的新鲜或干燥块根。

1 Variety

Dihuang is the fresh or dried root tuber of *Rehmannia glutinosa* Libosch. of Family Scrophulariaceae.

地黄载于《神农本草经》,唐代《名医别录》谓"生者尤良",表明唐代兼用生品及干品。宋代《本草图经》载地黄"二月生叶,布地便出似车前,叶上有皱纹而不光,高者及尺余,低者三四寸,其花似油麻花而红紫色,亦有黄花者……"明代《本草纲目》记载与之一致,表明古今基原未发生变迁。

As a medicinal, Dihuang is recorded in *Shennong Bencao Jing*. It is recorded in *Mingyi Bielu* that the raw material is better, which indicated that both the unprocessed and dried Dihuang were used in Tang Dynasty. In *Bencao Tujing* of Song Dynasty, the plant of Dihuang is recorded as "leaves grow out in February, close to the ground like Cheqian (Plantaginis Herba). There are wrinkles on the leaf surface which is not smooth. The height of the plant can be more than one chi or nearly three to four cun. The flowers are similar with the shape of sesame flower but in reddish purple, and there are also yellow flowers..." The same records could be seen in *Bencao Gangmu* which indicates that the origin of Dihuang has changed since the ancient times.

2. 种植采收　自北魏以来地黄即已有成熟的人工种植技术，现代形成大规模化规范化种植。地黄一般采用根茎繁殖，秋季 10 月至 11 月当地上茎叶枯黄且带斑点时采挖。

2　Planting and Harvesting

The artificial planting technology of Dihuang has been developed mature since Northern Wei Dynasty. Today, the large-scale normalized cultivation of Dihuang is formed. It is usually propagated by rhizome. Generally, Dihuang is dug out and collected from October to November in autumn when the Dihuang is rhizome and leaves above ground are withered and yellow with spots.

3. 道地性及品质评价　《名医别录》载地黄"生咸阳川泽"，即指河南。随后《本草经集注》《新修本草》载地黄生"长安、彭城、历阳、江宁、周州"等地，即今之陕西、江苏、安徽等地。至明代《本草纲目》云"今人惟以怀庆地黄为上"，至今仍为公认，并称河南产地黄为"怀地黄"。鲜地黄以粗壮、色红黄者为佳，生地黄以块大、体重、断面乌黑者为佳。

3　Genuineness and Quality Evaluation

It is recorded in *Mingyi Bielu* "Dihuang grows in Xianyang Chuanze", which refers to Henan province today. In the subsequent works *Bencaojing Jizhu*, and *Xinxiu Bencao*, Dihuang is recorded growing in Chang'an, Pengcheng, Liyang, Jiangning, Zhouzhou, etc., referring to Shaanxi, Jiangsu and An'hui provinces, etc. In Ming Dynasty, the book of *Bencao Gangmu* describes "people today think Dihuang from Huaiqing is the best". This is widely accepted since then with the special name 'Huaidihuang' for Dihuang produced in Henan province. Xiandihuang (fresh) with thick, firm body and red-yellow-color are better in quality, and Shengdihuang (raw) with big size, heavy weight, and black cross-section are better.

地黄主要成分为环烯醚萜类（如梓醇、毛蕊花糖苷、地黄苷 D、地黄苷 A 等）和多糖，是地黄增强免疫功能、降血糖等作用的主要药效物质基础。此外还含有黄酮类、酚酸、氨基酸、微量元素等。《中华人民共和国药典》规定，生地黄按干燥品计算，含梓醇（$C_{15}H_{22}O_{10}$）和毛蕊花糖苷（$C_{29}H_{36}O_{15}$）分别不得少于 0.20%、0.020%。

The main components of Dihuang are iridoids, including catalpol, acteoside, martynoside A, D, and polysaccharide. Which are the main effective substance basis of enhancing immune function and reducing blood sugar, and so on. In addition, it also contains flavonoids, phenolic acids, amino acids, trace elements and so on. According to *Pharmacopoeia of the People's Republic of China*, the contents of catalpol ($C_{15}H_{22}O_{10}$) and acteoside ($C_{29}H_{36}O_{15}$) should be separately not less than 0.20% and 0.020% in the dried products.

二、炮制品种与品质
II　Processed Varieties and Quality

《中国药典》载有鲜地黄、生地黄和熟地黄三种饮片，以生地黄和熟地黄为临床常用。生地黄以外表皮棕黑色或棕灰色，极皱缩，切面棕黑色或乌黑色，有光泽，具黏性，气微，味微甜为佳。

Xiandihuang (fresh), Shengdihuang (raw), Shudihuang (processed), are collected in the current *Pharmacopoeia of the People's Republic of China*, in which the Shengdihuang (raw) and Shudihuang (processed) are most widely used in clinical practice. Shengdihuang (raw) whose outer surface is brown black or brown gray and extremely wrinkled, section surface is brown black or gray black, glossy, sticky, slight odor, and slight sweet taste is considered to have better quality.

三、中成药品种与品质
III　Varieties and Quality of Chinese Patent Medicines

含地黄的中成药约 650 余个，其中《中华人民共和国药典》现行版收载含地黄的中成药品种270余个，以地黄为君药或主药的品种有养阴清肺膏（糖浆、口服液、丸）、增液口服液、慢肝养阴胶囊等。在这些中成药的质量检测中基本无地黄相关的检测。

There are more than 650 Chinese patent medicines containing Dihuang of which about 270 are collected in the current *Pharmacopoeia of the People's Republic of China*. Medicines that contain Dihuang as the sovereign or main medicinal in prescriptions include Yangyin Qingfei Gao (Paste) Tangjiang, Koufuye or Wan, Zengye Koufuye, Mangan Yangyin Jiaonang etc. In the quality detection of these Chinese patent medicines, Dihuang is basically not set as a test indicator.

【制药】
[Pharmacy]

一、产地加工
I Processing in Production Area

地黄采收后，除去芦头、须根，洗净泥土，分开大小，即为鲜地黄；将鲜地黄切片或不切片置于火炕上发汗，至块根发软，内无硬核，颜色变黑，外皮变硬，即为生地黄。

After being collected, remove the residual parts and the fibrous root, clease soil ,sort out in big and small size, thenthe Xiandihuang (fresh) has been made . Then put the sliced Xiandihuang (fresh) or unsliced one on the heated brick bed for sweating until the root becomes soft without hard core inside, the color turns black, and the outer skin becomes hard, then it has been processed into Shengdihuang (raw).

二、饮片炮制
II Processing of Decoction Pieces

地黄的炮制方法在古代有20余种，南北朝时期形成了蒸焙、酒拌蒸等工艺。但生地黄以闷润、切片、干燥即可，主要便于保存。《中华人

民共和国药典》2020年版以酒炖法或蒸法由生地黄炮制熟地黄。经炮制后的熟地黄寒凉之性减弱，而滋补之功增强。

There are more than 20 kinds of processing methods of Dihuang in ancient times. In the Southern and Northern Dynasties period, there were processing methods of steaming, baking, and steaming with liquor mixture. Shengdihuang (raw) is processed by stewing for moistening, cutting into slices and drying so as to preserve it easily. It is recorded that Shudihuang (processed) is prepared from Shengdihuang (raw) by stewing with liquor, or steaming. After being processed, the cold property of Shudihuang (processed) becomes weak and nourishing effect is enhanced.

三、中成药制药
III Pharmacy of Chinese Patent Medicines

含地黄的中成药剂型十分丰富。用于清热凉血，养阴生津时，常用地黄，如养阴清肺膏、消渴丸、湿毒清胶囊等；用于凉血止血时，多以地黄炭入药，如止红肠澼丸。地黄有效成分多为水溶性或醇溶性，稳定性较好，在中成药制药中多与处方中其他中药一起水煎，如养阴清肺口服液、金果饮等，或醇提，如消银片；也可打粉入药，如在养阴清肺丸中为打粉入药制蜜丸。

Chinese patent medicines containing Dihuang are rich in pharmaceutical forms. Dihuang is often used to clear heat and cool blood, nourish *yin* and generate fluid, for example, in Yangyin Qingfei Gao (Paste), Xiaoke Wan, Shiduqing Jiaonang, etc. To cool blood and stop bleeding, Dihuangtan (carbonized) is usually applied, such as in Zhihong Changpi Wan. Most effective components of Dihuang are water-soluble or alcohol soluble with good stability. Therefore, it is decocted with other medicinals in water, such as Yangyin Qiingfei Koufuye and Jinguo Yin (Decoction), or extracted by alcohol, such as Xiaoyin Pian (Tablets), or powdered for honey processed pills, such as

Yangyin Qingfei Wan.

【性能功效】
[Property and Efficacy]

一、性能
I Property

地黄甘、苦，寒；归心、肝、胃、肾经。

Dihuang is sweet and bitter in flavor and cold in nature, and enters the heart, liver and kidney meridians.

二、功效
II Efficacy

1. **清热凉血、止血**　地黄苦寒能清热，尤善清血分热而凉血、止血，为清热凉血要药。其功效的发挥与镇静、促凝血等药理作用密切相关，地黄促凝血的有效物质基础主要是地黄苷A。

1 Clearing Heat to Cool the Blood and Stop Bleeding

Dihuang can clear heat for its bitter flavor and cold nature. It is especially good for clearing heat in blood aspect, cooling blood and stopping bleeding. The efficacy is closely related to pharmacological effects of sedation, promoting blood coagulation, etc. The effective material basis of Dihuang in promoting blood coagulation is mainly Rehmannia Glucoside A.

2. **养阴生津**　地黄甘寒质润，有养阴生津之功效。其功效的发挥与下调β-肾上腺素受体-cAMP系统功能、促进造血功能、增强免疫功能等药理作用密切相关，有效物质基础主要是地黄多糖、梓醇。地黄可促进骨髓造血干细胞增殖和多种造血生长因子的分泌；可激活淋巴系统增加B淋巴细胞分泌抗体和使T淋巴细胞致敏。

2 Nourishing Yin and Generating Fluid

With sweet, cold and moist quality, Dihuang has effect of nourishing *yin* to generate fluid, which is tightly related to its pharmacological actions of down regulating the function of β-adrenergic receptor-cAMP system, promoting hematopoiesis, reinforcing immune function, etc. Polysaccharides as well as catalpol in Dihuang are the active substance basis. Dihuang can promote the proliferation of bone marrow hematopoietic stem cells and help secreting multiple hematopoietic growth factors, and can activate the lymphatic system, increase the secretion of antibodies by B-type lymphocytes and stimulate T-type lymphocytes sensitization.

【应用】
[Applications]

一、主治病证
I Indications

1. **热入营血证、血热妄行证**　对入营血之壮热烦渴，神昏舌绛，常与水牛角、玄参等配伍，如《温病条辨》清营汤；也可用于热入营血致血热妄行之各种出血证，如《备急千金要方》犀角地黄汤用于吐血衄血、斑疹紫黑，《妇人良方》四生丸用于便血、崩漏下血，《医学心悟》生地黄汤用于吐血脉数。

1 Syndrome of Heat Entering Nutrient-blood, Syndrome of Bleeding Due to Blood Heat

Dihuang, combined with Shuiniujiao (Bubali Cornu) and Xuanshen can treat syndrome of heat entering nutrient-blood manifesting as hight fever, polydipsia unconsciousness with crimson tongue, such as Qingying Tang (Decoction) recorded in *Wenbing Tiaobian*. It can be also used to treat hemorrhage due to blood heat with heat entering nutrient-blood, such as Xijiao Dihuang Tang (Decoction) recorded in *Beiji Qianjin Yaofang,* which is used to treat such symptoms as hematemesis, bleeding or subcutaneous purple and black macula; Sisheng Wan in the book of *Furen Liangfang (Compendium of Effective Prescriptions for Women)* is used to treat hematochezia and metrorrhagia. The book *Yixue Xinwu (Comprehension of Medicine)* records that

Shengdihuang Tang (Decoction) is used to treat such symptoms as hematemesis and rapid pulse.

现代临床，地黄配伍常用于治疗原发性血小板减少性紫癜、慢性肾炎、慢性肝炎、白血病等属热入营血致出血证者，常用方剂如犀角地黄汤、清营汤等。

In modern clinical practice, Dihuang compatibility is often used to treat primary thrombocytopenic purpura, chronic nephritis, chronic hepatitis, leukaemia and other bleeding syndromes pertaining to syndrome of heat entering nutrient-blood, such as Xijiao Dihuang Tang (Decoction), Qingying Tang (Decoction), etc.

2. **热病伤阴证、津伤口渴证** 地黄可与他药配伍治疗温病后期热病伤阴、津伤口渴。对邪伏阴分，夜热早凉，舌红脉数者，常与鳖甲、青蒿等配伍，如《温病条辨》青蒿鳖甲汤；对阴虚火旺、盗汗不止者，常用黄柏、黄芪、浮小麦等配伍，如《景岳全书》生地黄煎；对骨蒸潮热者，可与丹皮、知母等配伍，如可《古今医统》地黄膏；对肺阴亏损，虚劳干咳咯血者，可与人参、茯苓等配伍，如《洪氏集验方》琼玉膏。对热病伤胃阴之口干咽燥、烦渴多饮者，常与玉竹、麦冬、沙参等配伍，如益胃汤；对肺热津伤之烦渴多饮者，常与天花粉、黄连等配伍，如《丹溪心法》消渴方；对暑热伤阴、口渴引饮者，可与黄连、乌梅、阿胶等配伍，如《温病条辨》连梅汤。对阳明温病症见热结伤津致大便燥结，咽干口渴，可与玄参、麦门冬配伍，如《温病条辨》增液汤。

2 Syndrome of Yin damage Due to Heat Disease, Thirst Due to Fluid Consumption

The compatibility of Dihuang with other medicinals can be applied for *yin* deficiency and fluid consumption with thirst in the late stage of warm diseases. In the case of pathogen retained in *yin* phase, night fever abating at dawn, reddish tongue and rapid pulse, it is often combined with Biejia, Qinghao etc. such as Qinghao Biejia Tang (Decoction) recorded in *Wenbing Tiaobian* is used; for those with hyperactivity of fire due to yin deficiency, constant night sweating, Dihuang

compatibility with Huangbo, Huangqi, Fuxiaomai, such as *Shengdihuang Jian* from *Jingyue Quanshu* can be used; for bone steaming and tidal fever, Dihuang combined with Danpi, Zhimu, such as Dihuang Gao in *Gujin Yitong (Medical Complete Book, Ancient and Modern)* can be used; for the lung yin deficiency manifesting as fatigue, dry cough and hemoptysis, Qiongyu Gao recorded in *Hongshi Jiyanfang (hong's Prescription)* can be used, in which Dihuang combined with Renshen and Fuling, etc. For stomach yin damaged by heat disease manifesting as dry mouth, polydipsia and thirsty polydrink, *Yiwei Tang* can be used. While Xiaoke Fang from *Danxi Xinfa* is effective for polydipsia and thirsty for polydrink caused by lung heat and fluid consumption, in which Dihuang is combined with Tianhuafen, Huanglian, etc.; thirsty for polydrink due to summer-heat damaging yin, *Lianmei Tang* from *Wenbing Tiaobian* is used of which Dihuang combined with Huanglian, Wumei, Ejiao etc. For yangming warm disease manifesting as heat accumulation injurying fluid, causing constipation, dry throat and thirst, *Zengye Tang* from *Wenbing Tiaobian* can be used, in which Xuanshen, Maimendong combined.

现代临床，地黄配伍常用于治疗糖尿病、更年期综合征、干眼症、肿瘤等属阴虚内热或气阴两虚证者，方可用增液汤、消渴方等，中成药可用养阴生血合剂等。

In modern clinical practice, Dihuang compatibility is usually used to treat diabetes, menopausal syndrome, ophthalmoxerosis, tumor, etc. pertaining to syndromes of *yin* deficiency with internal heat or deficiency of both qi and yin, such as Zengye Tang (Decoction), Xiaoke Fang (Formula), and so on.

二、用法用量
II Administration and Dosage

鲜地黄 12~30g。生地黄 10~15g。
12~30g for Xiandihuang (fresh); 10~15g for

Shengdihuang (raw)

使用。

三、注意事项
III Precautions

地黄性寒而滞，脾虚湿滞腹满便溏者，不宜

As Dihuang is cold in property and easy to induce stagnation, patients with abdominal distension and loose stool due to spleen insufficiency and dampness stagnation should not use it.

青 蒿

Qinghao
(Artemisiae Annuae Herba)

青蒿是重庆酉阳的道地药材，青蒿味苦、辛，性寒，归肝、胆经，有清虚热，除骨蒸，解暑热，截疟，退黄的功效，主治虚热证、暑邪发热、疟疾寒热、湿热黄疸证。青蒿中主要含青蒿素萜类、黄酮、挥发油等成分，有抗疟原虫、抗菌、抗病毒、抗炎解热镇痛等药理作用，可用于治疗疟疾、高热、黄疸、系统性红斑狼疮、银屑病、荨麻疹等属热证者。青蒿苦寒，脾胃虚弱者忌用。

Qinghao is a famous genuine regional medicinal in Youyang, Chongqing. It is bitter and pungent in flavor and cold in property, and enters liver and gallbladder meridians. It has the effects of clearing deficient heat, relieving bone steaming, releasing summer-heat, interrupting malaria and abating jaundice. It is mainly the syndrome of deficiency heat, fever induced by summer pathogen, malaria with cold and heat, dampness-heat jaundice. Qinghao mainly contains terpenes, flavonoids, volatile oils, etc. It has anti-plasmodium, antibacterial, antiviral, anti-inflammatory, antipyretic, analgesic and other pharmacological effects. It can be used for the treatment of malaria, high fever, jaundice, systemic lupus erythematosus, psoriasis, urticaria and other heat syndromes. Qinghao is bitter and cold, and should not be used for those with deficiency of spleen and stomach.

【品种品质】
[Variety and Quality]

一、基原品种与品质
I Origin Varieties and Quality

1. 品种概况　来源于菊科植物黄花蒿 *Artemisia annua* L. 的干燥地上部分。

1 Variety

Qinghao is the dried aerial part of *Artemisia annua* L (Fam. Compositae).

青蒿载于《神农本草经》，名草蒿，青蒿为别名。明代《本草纲目》载："青蒿，二月生苗，茎粗如指而肥软，茎叶色并深青。其叶微似茵陈，而面背俱青。其根白硬。七八月开细黄花颇香。结实大如麻子，中有细子。"结合历代本草所绘青蒿药图，所述即为今天的黄花蒿。

Qinghao was recorded in the book of *Shennong Bencao Jing*. It was named as Caohao, Qinghao is its another name.

The *Bencao Gangmu* in the Ming Dynasty described that seedling of Qinghao appears in February, its stem is thick like fingers, fat and soft, the color of stem and leaf are deep green. Its leaves slightly like Yinchen (Artemisiae Scopariae Herba), its face and back are both green. Its root is white and hard. Fine yellow flowers blossoning in July and August. Fruit are large like hemp fruit and with tiny seeds inside it. According to the Qinghao pictures of previous dynasties, the Qinghao described above is today's artemisia annua.

2. 种植采收　重庆酉阳、广西、广东等地有种植，采用种子和分株繁殖。主要在秋季花盛开时采收。

2 Planting and Harvesting

Qinghao is now mainly planted in Youyang of Chongqing, Guangdong and Guangxi provinces. Seed and division propagation are adopted in the planting of Qinghao. Qinghao is harvested mainly in autumn when the flowers are in full bloom.

3. 道地性评价及品质评价　历代本草记载荆州（今湖北）为青蒿的道地产区，现今青蒿最主要生产基地在重庆酉阳。以色绿、叶多、香气浓者为佳。

3 Genuineness and Quality Evaluation

According to historical records, Jingzhou of Hubei province is the genuine producing area of Qinghao. Nowadays, the main production base of Qinghao is located in Youyang, Chongqing. The good quality of Qinghao is characterized with many leaves, green in color, and strong aroma.

青蒿化学成分主要包括倍半萜类（青蒿素、氢化青蒿素、脱氧青蒿素）、黄酮类（猫眼草酚、紫花牡荆素、蒿黄素）、香豆素类（东莨菪内酯、滨蒿内酯），其中青蒿素是青蒿清虚热、截疟的药效成分。此外还含有挥发油、苯丙酸类、二萜类、三萜类等。现代主要以青蒿素含量为评价指标。

The chemical constituents of Qinghao mainly include sesquiterpenoids (artemisinin, hydrogenated artemisinin, deoxyartemisinin), flavonoids (chrysosplenol, casticin, artemetin), and coumarins (scopolamine, scoparone), among which artemisinin is the effective component of Qinghao for clearing deficiency heat and preventing malaria. In addition, it also contains volatile oil, phenylpropionic acid, diterpene, triterpene, etc. Modern clinical practice mainly uses artemisinin content as the evaluation index.

二、炮制品种与品质
II Processed Varieties and Quality

青蒿临床使用主要是青蒿生品，青蒿以不规则小段，茎、叶、花蕾混合，气香特异，味微苦为佳。

The clinical use of Qinghao is mainly raw products. The irregular small segments, stem, leaf, bud are all applicable. Those has unique fragrance, a little bitter taste in better quality.

三、中成药品种与品质
III Varieties and Quality of Chinese Patent Medicines

含青蒿的中成药有70余个，其中《中国药典》收载含有青蒿的中成药10余个。以青蒿为君药或主药的品种有青蒿鳖甲片、柴银口服液、小儿肺咳颗粒等。质量控制多采用薄层色谱法以对照药材为对照进行定性质量控制。

There are more than 70 Chinese patent medicines containing Qinghao, of which over 10 are included in the *Pharmacopoeia of the People's Republic of China*. Prescriptions with Qinghao as the sovereign medicinal are as follows: Qinghao Biejia Pian (Tablets), Chaiyin Koufuye, Xiaoer Feike Keli, etc. And its quality control is mainly to apply TLC to make qualitative discrimination through comparing with the reference Materia medica.

【制药】
[Pharmacy]

一、产地加工
I Processing in Production Area

除去老茎，阴干。

Qinghao is generally removed from older stem, and dried in shade.

二、饮片炮制
II Processing of Decoction Pieces

青蒿的炮制方法比较简单，在除去杂质后，喷淋清水，待稍微润湿，切成段，低温干燥或晾干为主要加工工序，由此生产的青蒿已成为主流商品。

The processing method of Qinghao is relatively simple. Spray water to slightly moisten it after removing impurities, and cut into sections, dry in low temperature or in shade, that is the main processing method. By this way, the processed production of Qinghao has become a mainstream commodity.

三、中成药制药
III Pharmacy of Chinese Patent Medicines

含青蒿的中成药，剂型十分丰富，涵盖了固体、液体制剂。在传统用药中，青蒿多入汤剂，或入丸、散，在外用时捣敷或研末调敷。现今为满足现代制剂处方成形性及减少服用剂量，一般制剂如片剂和胶囊剂等多以青蒿挥发油入制剂中。

There are various kinds of Chinese patent medicines containing Qinghao, covering solid and liquid preparations. In traditional medicines, Qinghao is often added into decoction, or added into pills and powder. For external application, it is mashed or ground . Nowadays, in order to satisfy the formability of modern preparation prescription and reduce the dosage, the volatile oil of Qinghao is often used in general preparations such as tablets and capsules.

如以青蒿为君药的青蒿鳖甲片，在制备过程中将青蒿提取挥发油，加入其他药物制备的颗粒中直接制片，最大程度保留了青蒿的有效成分，防止成分受热挥散。

For example, when processing Qinghao Biejia Pian (Teblets), Qinghao as the sovereign medicinal, volatile oil extracted from Qinghao is added into the granule preparation of other medicinals to directly prepare pills, which can remain the active ingredients of Qinghao to the greatest extent and prevent them from being volatilized by heating.

【性能功效】
[Property and Efficacy]

一、性能
I Property

青蒿苦、辛，寒；归肝、胆、肾经。

Qinghao are bitter and pungent in flavor, cold in nature, and enters the liver, kidney and gallbladder meridians.

二、功效
II Efficacy

1. **清虚热，除骨蒸** 青蒿苦寒之性，能清能透，可使阴分伏热透外而解，从而清虚热，除骨蒸。其功效的发挥与抗内毒素、解热、抗炎、抑制免疫功能等药理作用密切相关。青蒿抗内毒素、抗炎、抑制免疫功能的有效物质基础主要是青蒿素，通过抑制巨噬细胞释放 IL-6、TNF-α 等促炎细胞因子的产生发挥抗炎作用。

1 Clearing Deficient Heat and Relieving Bone Steaming

Qinghao, with a bitter flavor and cold property, can clear the exterior heat and also dispel the interior heat from inside our body. Particularly, it can drive the hidden heat pathogens out from innermost,so as to clear deficiency-heat and relieve bone steaming. Its effect is closely related to the pharmacological effects of anti-endotoxin, antipyretic effect, anti-inflammation and immune function suppression. Qinghao's effective material basis for anti-endotoxin, anti-inflammation and immune function suppression is mainly based on artemisinin, which exerts anti-inflammatory effects by inhibiting the production of pro-inflammatory cytokines such as IL-6 and TNF-α released by macrophages.

2. 解暑热　青蒿苦寒清热，又辛香而散暑湿，可外解暑热，内除湿热。其功效的发挥与解热、抗病原微生物、抗炎等药理作用密切相关。

2 Releasing Summer-heat

Qinghao is bitter and cold and can clean heat. Being pungent and fragrant for dispersing summer-heat dampness, it can relieve summer-heat outside and damp-heat inside. Its effect is related to antipyretic, anti-pathogenic microorganism, anti-inflammatory effects.

3. 截疟，退黄　青蒿性苦寒，入肝胆经，又气味芳香，可截疟和清肝胆湿热，故可截疟退黄，为治疟疾寒热的要药。其功效的发挥与抗疟原虫、抗炎、解热等药理作用密切相关。青蒿抗虐原虫的有效物质基础主要是青蒿素，通过抑制血红蛋白酶和产生大量自由基和活性氧，从而抑制疟原虫的生长或破坏疟原虫的膜系结构，导致疟原虫死亡发挥作用。

3 Preventing Malaria and Abating Jaundice

Qinghao is bitter and cold, and enter meridians of liver and gallbladder. Being good at clearing the dampness-heat of liver and gallbladder, it can prevent malaria and abating jaundice. Its effect is closely related to the anti-malaria, anti-inflammation, antipyretic and other pharmacological effects. Artemisinin is the effective material base of anti-malaria in Qinghao. Artemisinin can inhibit the growth or damage the membrane structure of plasmodium parasites by inhibiting hemoglobin protease and producing large amounts of free radicals and reactive oxygen species, leading to the death of plasmodium parasites.

【应用】
[Applications]

一、主治病证
I Indications

1. 虚热证　对骨蒸劳、体瘦、发渴、寒热

者，青蒿可与桃仁、甘草等配伍，如《太平圣惠方》青蒿圆。若虚劳，盗汗、烦热、口干，可与人参、麦冬等配伍，如《圣济总录》青蒿丸。

1 Deficiency-heat Syndrome

Qinghao combined with Taoren and Gancao can treat patients with bone steaming and consumptive fever, skinny body, thirst, in both cold and hot type, such as Qinghao Yuan (Decoction) recorded in *Taiping Shenghui Fang*. Patients with consumptive disease, night sweating, dysphoria with feverish sensation, dry mouth, Qinghao can be combined with Renshen, Maidong (Ophiopogonis Radix), such as Qinghao Wan (Pills) recorded in *Sheng Ji Zonglu*.

现代临床，青蒿配伍常用于治疗系统性红斑狼疮、银屑病、日光性皮炎及荨麻疹、老年性便秘等虚热证的治疗，如《温病条辨》青蒿鳖甲汤，清骨散等。

In modern clinical practice, Qinghao is often used in the treatment of systemic lupus erythematosus, psoriasis, solar dermatitis, urticaria, senile constipation and other diseases, such as Qinghao Biejia Tang (Decoction), Qinggu San (Powder), etc recorded in *Wenbing Tiaobian*.

2. 暑邪发热　对于外感暑热、头昏头痛、发热口渴者，可与连翘、茯苓配伍以清暑泄热，如清凉涤暑汤。

2 Fever Induced by Summer heat Pathogen

For summer-heat, dizziness, headache, fever and thirst, Qinghao can be combined with Lianqiao, Fuling to clear summer-heat and discharge heat, such as Qingliang Dishu Tang (Decoction).

现代临床，青蒿配伍常用于治疗中暑、外感高热等热证的治疗，如柴葛青蒿汤、青银注射液。

In modern clinical practice, Qinghao compatibility is often used to treat summer heat stroke, high fever by exopathogen, such as Chaige Qinghao Tang (Decoction), Qing Yin Zhusheye.

3. 疟疾寒热　治疟疾寒热，单用居多；针对虚劳久疟，可用酒剂；治疗少阳疟疾，可配伍

鳖甲、知母以养阴透热，如《温病条辨》青蒿鳖甲汤。

3 Malaria with Cold-heat Complex

Qinghao can be used alone to treat malaria and cold-heat alternations. For consumptive disease and chronic malaria, alcohol agent can be applied; Qinghao can also be used with Biejia (Trionycis Carapax) and Zhimu (Anemarrhenae Rhizoma) for yin nourishing and heat penetrating to treat Shaoyang malaria, such as Qinghao Biejia Tang (Decoction) recoded in *Wenbing Tiaobian*.

现代临床，青蒿配伍常用于治疗疟疾、痢疾等，如蒿豉丹。

In modern clinical practice, Qinghao is often used in the treatment of malaria and dysentery, such as Haochi Dan.

此外，现代研究还显示青蒿具有降血压等作用。

In addition, modern research also shows that Qinghao has the effect of lowering blood pressure and other effects.

二、用法用量
II Administration and Dosage

6~12g，后下。

6~12g, decocted later.

三、注意事项
III Precautions

产后脾胃薄弱，忌与当归、地黄同用；脾胃虚弱者，忌用。

It should not be used with Danggui, Dihuang when spleen and stomach are weak after delivery. It is a taboo for the patients with deficiency of spleen and stomach.

【知识拓展】
[Knowledge Extension]

青蒿素是从青蒿中提取的有效成分，有良好的抗疟疾作用，开发为产品后拯救了全球许多患者，该研究的主要负责人屠呦呦教授因该药对人类健康做出的巨大贡献，2015 年被授予诺贝尔生理学或医学奖，为我国第一个诺贝尔奖得主。

Artemisinin is an active ingredient extracted from Qinhao, has good anti-malaria effects. It has saved many patients around the world after it was developed as a product. Professor Tu You-you, the person in charge of this research, was awarded the Nobel Prize of Medicine and Physiology in 2015 for her great contribution to human health, who is the first Nobel Prize winner in China.

第十章 泻 下 药
Chapter 10　Purgative Medicinals

凡能攻积、逐水，引起腹泻，或润肠通便的药物，称为泻下药。此类药物多味苦性寒，具泻下通便作用，用于里实证。其主要功用有三：一通利大便，排除肠道内宿食积滞或燥屎及有害物质；二清热泻火，使实热壅滞通过泻下而解除；三逐水退肿，使水邪从大小便排除，以消退水肿，有些药兼具逐瘀、消癥瘕、杀虫等功效。根据泻下程度的不同，可分为峻下逐水药、攻下药及润下药三类。攻下药、峻下逐水药因作用峻猛，或具有毒性，应用时当奏效即止，以免伤正气及脾胃。对作用峻猛有毒性的泻下药，要严格炮制法度，控制用量，确保用药安全。现代研究表明，泻下药多通过刺激肠道黏膜分泌消化液或促进平滑肌蠕动而致泻，此外有利胆、抗菌、抗炎、抗肿瘤及增强免疫功能作用。常见的泻下药有大黄、芒硝、甘遂、巴豆、番泻叶、芦荟、火麻仁、郁李仁等。

Purgative Medicinals refer to the medicinals that can expel water and eliminate accumulations by purgation, or treat constipation by inducing diarrhea or lubricating the large intestine. These medicinals are commonly bitter in favor and cold in property, and are used for internal excess syndrome. Its main functions are as follows: ① promoting defecation by eliminating food retention, dry excrement and harmful substances in intestinal tract; ② clearing heat and purging fire, so that excess heat stagnation can be relieved by purging down; ③ relieving edema by eliminating water pathogen through defecation and urination. Some medicinals also have the effects of removing blood stasis, eliminating abdominal mass, killing parasites, etc. According to the degree of purgative effect, these medicinals can be divided into three types: drastic expelling water retention, offensive purgative and moistening purgative. Due to their strong action or toxicity, drastic expelling water retention and offensive purgative should be stopped immediately once they take effect, so as to avoid the overuse damaging vital qi, spleen and stomach. For those purgative medicinals with drastic effect and toxicity, their processing must be strictly carried out and the dosages should be controlled to ensure the medicinal safety. Modern research shows that purgatives mostly induce diarrhea by stimulating intestinal mucosa to secret digestive fluids, or by promoting smooth muscle peristalsis. In addition to purgative effect, they can also promote gallbladder function, and resist bacteria, inflammation and tumor, and enhance immune function as well. Common purgative medicinals include Dahuang, Mangxiao, Gansui, Badou, Fanxieye, Luhui, Huomaren (Cannabis Fructus), and Yuliren (Pruni Semen), etc.

大 黄

Dahuang
(Rhei Radix et Rhizoma)

大黄是著名的川产道地药材。生大黄泻下作用峻烈，易伤胃气，临床常用为酒大黄、熟大黄（酒蒸或酒炖）等。大黄味苦性寒，归脾、胃、大肠、肝、心包经，具泻下攻积，清热泻火，凉血解毒，逐瘀通经，利湿退黄等功效，主治胃肠积滞、大便燥结等症。大黄主要含蒽醌类衍生物、鞣质类、二苯乙烯苷类、苯酚苷类和苯丁酮类等成分，有增加肠蠕动、促进排便、抗感染、抗病原微生物、扩张血管、利尿、保肝利胆、止血、降血脂等药理作用。可用于润肠通便、抑菌、促进胆汁分泌、降脂、降压等。大黄具有一定的肝、肾毒性，可通过依法炮制、辨证用药、合理配伍、控制剂量和用药周期等达到控毒增效。

Dahuang is a famous genuine regional medicinal produced in Sichuan Province. The Shengdahuang (raw) has strong purgative effect and is easy to damage stomach *qi*. Therefore, when using in clinical practice, it is often, Jiudahuang (liquor-processed) or Shudahuang (liquor-steamed or stewed, prepared). Dahuang is bitter in favor and cold in property, and enters the meridians of the spleen, stomach, large intestines, liver and pericardium. It has the effects of eliminating accumulation by purgation, clearing heat and purging fire, cooling blood and detoxicating, expelling blood stasis and dredging meridians, and eliminating dampness to remove jaundice. It is mainly used for gastrointestinal stagnation, dry excrement and constipation. Dahuang mainly contains anthraquinone derivatives, tannins, stilbene glycosides, phenol glycosides, butyl ketone benzene and other components, and has pharmacological effects of increasing intestinal peristalsis, promoting defecation, resisting infection, resisting pathogenic microorganisms, dilating blood vessels, inducing diuresis, protecting liver, promoting gallbladder functions, stopping bleeding, and reducing blood lipid. It can be used for relaxing bowels, inhibiting bacteria, promoting bile secretion, reducing blood lipid, lowering blood pressure, etc. Dahuang has certain liver and kidney toxicity, which can be controlled by regulated processing according methods, medication according to syndrome differentiation, reasonable compatibility, the dosage control and medication cycle.

【品种品质】
[Variety and Quality]

一、基原品种与品质
I Origin Varieties and Quality

1. **品种概况** 来源于蓼科植物掌叶大黄 *Rheum palmatum* L.、唐古特大黄 *Rheum tanguticum* Maxim. ex Balf. 或药用大黄 *Rheum officinale* Baill. 的干燥根及根茎。

1 Variety

Dahuang is derived from the dried roots and rhizomes of *Rheum palmatum* L., *Rheum tanguticum* Maxim.ex Balf or *Rheum officinale* Baill of Polygonaceae.

大黄首载于《神农本草经》。《证类本草》曰："大黄，其色也。将军之号，但其骏快也"；《吴普本草》对大黄的植物形态描述可见所指大黄为大黄属 *Rheum* 掌叶组 *Sect. Palmata* 植物，《本草纲目》及《植物名实图考》中大黄的附图，其叶片均有接近中裂的掌状分裂，可以推断历代本草所指的大黄主要指的是掌叶大黄 *Rheum palmatum*。但根据产地分析，唐古特大黄 *Rheum. tanguticum*、药用大黄 *Rheum officinale*

两个品种应该包括在内。

Dahuang is first recorded in *Shennong Bencao Jing*. As recorded in *Zhenglei Bencao (Materia Medica Arranged According to Pattern)*: "Dahuang, yellow in color, possesses the characteristics like a general, whose function is strong and fast". The plant morphology of Dahuang described in *Wupu Bencao (Wu Pu's Materia Medica)* is the plant of *Rheum palmatum* (Sect. Palmata). In the attached drawings of Dahuang in *Bencao Gangmu* and *Zhiwu Mingshi Tukao (Illustrated Reference of Botanical Nomenclature)*, the leaves are all drawn with palmation close to median split, from which it can be inferred that the Dahuang mentioned in previous generations of materia medica is mainly *Rheum palmatum*. However, according to the analysis of its producing area, *Rheum tanguticum* and *Rheum officinale* should have also been included.

2. 种植采收　大黄既有野生也有人工种植。主产于四川、青海、甘肃等地。多采用种子繁殖、育苗移栽或直播。定植后一般于第三年或第四年秋末冬初时采收，先割去地上部分，将根及根茎全部掘起。

2 Planting and Harvesting

Dahuang can be both wild and planted. It is mainly produced in Sichuan, Qinghai, and Gansu. Seed propagation, seedling transplanting or direct seedings are often used. After planting, it is generally harvested at the end of autumn and the beginning of winter in the third or fourth year. First, the overground part is cut off and then the root and its rhizome are all dug up.

3. 道地性及品质评价　自古以来四川、甘肃、青海是大黄的道地产区。其中掌叶大黄、唐古特大黄以甘肃、青海为道地产区，药用大黄以四川为道地产区以身干，外表黄棕色，质坚实分重，断面呈现锦纹及星点明显，红棕色，有油性，气清香味苦而不涩，嚼之发粘者为佳。大黄主要含有蒽醌类，包括游离型及结合型蒽醌类衍生物等，其中番泻苷及结合型蒽醌，苷类是其泻

下的主要物质基础，没食子酸等鞣质是其止血、收敛的主要物质基础，鞣质及游离蒽醌衍生物是其抑菌的主要物质基础。此外，还有二苯乙烯苷类、鞣质及多酚类化合物等。《中国药典》列有生大黄、酒大黄、熟大黄、大黄炭4种炮制品。规定饮片生大黄，游离蒽醌以芦荟大黄素、大黄酸、大黄素、大黄酚和大黄素甲醚的总量计，不得少于0.35%，酒大黄、熟大黄，游离蒽醌不得少于0.5%，大黄炭，游离蒽醌不得少于0.5%，总蒽醌，不得少于0.9%。

3 Genuineness and Quality Evaluation

Sichuan, Gansu and Qinghai have been the genuine producing areas of Dahuang since ancient times. Gansu and Qinghai are the genuine producing areas of *Rheum palmatum* L. and *Rheum tanguticum* L., and Sichuan is the genuine producing area of *Rheum officinale* L., and that with yellow-brown appearance, solid and heavy quality, obvious brocade and star spots on the cross section, reddish brown, oily, delicate fragrance, bitter but not astringent, and sticky when chewing is preferred. Dahuang mainly contains anthraquinones, including free and binding anthraquinones derivatives, among which sennoside and binding anthraquinones, and glycosides are the main material bases for its purgative effect, tannins such as gallic acid are the main material bases for its hemostasis and convergence effects, while tannins and free anthraquinones derivatives are the main material bases for its bacteriostasis effect. In addition, there are stilbene glycosides, tannins and polyphenol compounds. In *Pharmacopoeia of the People's Republic of China*, it lists 4 processed products, namely Shengdahuang (raw), Jiudahuang (liquor-processed), Shudahuang (prepared), and Dahuangtan (carbonized). It is stipulated that the free anthraquinone in Shengdahuang (raw) slices shall not be less than 0.35% based on the total amount of aloe-emodin, rhein, emodin, chrysophanol and physcion, the free anthraquinone in Jiudahuang (liquor-processed) and Shudahuang (prepared) shall not be less than 0.5%, while in Dahuangtan (carbonized), free anthraquinone shall not be less than 0.5% and total anthraquinone not less than 0.9%.

二、炮制品种与品质
II Processed Varieties and Quality

大黄的炮制品种有 20 多个，临床常用品种有 10 种，如生大黄、酒大黄、熟大黄、大黄炭等。生大黄以断面黄棕色或黄褐色，具有锦纹，气清香，味苦而微涩，嚼之粘牙，有沙粒感为佳；酒大黄以表面深棕色或棕褐色，偶有焦斑，内部呈浅棕色，略具酒香气为佳；熟大黄以内外呈均匀黑褐色，有特异芳香气为佳。饮片的品质评价同药材。

There are more than 20 processed varieties of Dahuang and 10 of them are commonly used in clinical practice, such as Shengdahuang (raw), Jiudahuang (liquor-processed), Shudahuang (prepared), and Dahuangtan (carbonized). For Shengdahuang (raw), that with yellow-brown cross section, brocade pattern, fragrant smell, bitter and slightly astringent taste, sticky when chewing, and a sense of sand grains is preferred. For Jiudahuang (liquor-processed), those with dark brown or chocolat-brown surface and occasional scorch spots, light brown inside, and slightly liquor-like aroma is preferred. For Shudahuang (prepared), those with black and brown inside and outside, and special aroma are preferred. The quality evaluation of decoction pieces is the same as that of materia medica.

三、中成药品种与品质
III Varieties and Quality of Chinese Patent Medicines

含有大黄或其炮制品的中成药有 776 个，其中药典收载 110 余个。以大黄为君药或主药的品种有一捻金、一清胶囊等。在质量控制多采用薄层色谱法和含量测定法。如薄层鉴别，分光光度

法对一捻金中大黄总蒽醌的检测，薄层扫描法测定一捻金中大黄素含量，高效液相色谱法测定一清胶囊大黄素、大黄酚、大黄酸、大黄素甲醚、芦荟大黄素等成分。非以大黄为君药的制剂，有十一味能消丸、十香止痛丸、十滴水、十滴水软胶囊、八正合剂、九味肝泰胶囊等。

There are 776 Chinese patent medicines containing Dahuang or its processed products, of which more than 110 have been recorded in the Pharmacopoeia. The varieties with Dahuang as sovereign medicinal or main medicinal include Yinianjin, Yiqing Jiaonang, etc. In quality control, TLC and content determination are mostly used. For example, thin-layer identification and spectrophotometry for detection of total anthraquinone of Dahuang in Yinianjin, thin-layer scanning method for determination of emodin content in Yinianjin, and HPLC for determination of emodin, chrysophanol, rhein, physcion, aloe-emodin and other components in Yiqing Jiaonang. There are also preparations not using Dahuang as the sovereign medicinal, such as Shiyiwei Nengxiao Wan, Shixiang Zhitong Wan, Shidi Shui, Shidishui Ruanjiaonang (Soft capsules), Bazheng Heji and Jiuwei Gantai Jiaonang.

【制药】
[Pharmacy]

一、产地加工
I Processing in Production Area

刚挖出的大黄除去泥土，切去茎叶及细根，用瓷片刮去粗皮及顶芽（忌用铁器，以免变黑）切成片、瓣或圆柱形，晒干、炕干、暗火烟熏干燥或阴干，以防腐烂。出口外销商品有的还放在滚筒或竹笼中撞光。

Dig up Dahuang and remove soil, cut off stems, leaves and fine fibrous roots, then use Porcelin Chip to scrape off its rough skin and terminal buds, then cut into pieces, petals or cylinders (Irons are not allowed to use to avoid

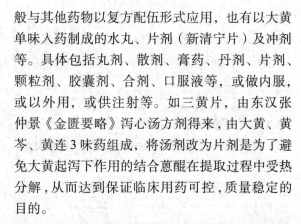

blackening). After that, dry it in the sun, or oven, or smoke and dry it with the dark fire; or dry it in the shade so as to prevent decay. Some export commodities are filled into rollers or bamboo cages to smash off the scarfskin.

二、饮片炮制
II Processing of Decoction Pieces

从古至今形成了 20 多种大黄炮制方法，主要包括酒制和炭制。目前生大黄、酒大黄、熟大黄、大黄炭成为商品规格中的主流。

More than 20 processing methods of Dahuang have been formed since ancient times, mainly including liquor processing and carbonized processing. At present, Shengdahuang (raw), Jiudahuang (liquor-processed), Shudahuang (prepared) and Dahuangtan (carbonized) have become the mainstream of commercial specifications.

大黄泻下作用峻烈，易伤胃气，经炮制后可以缓和泻下作用和增加抑菌，其原理是：加工炮制后，总蒽醌、结合型蒽醌含量较生品明显下降，游离型蒽醌含量有所增加。因此蒸、炒等均可缓和泻下作用及增加抑菌作用。

Dahuang has strong purgative effect and is easy to damage stomach *qi*. The processing one can alleviate purgative effect and increase bacteriostasis. The mechanism is that the content of total anthraquinone and binding anthraquinone is significantly lower than that of raw products after processing, while the content of free anthraquinone is increased. Therefore, steaming and stir-frying can abate purgative effect and increase bacteriostasis effect.

三、中成药制药
III Pharmacy of Chinese Patent Medicines

含大黄的中成药，剂型十分丰富，涵盖了固体、液体、半固体、气体等多种剂型。大黄一

般与其他药物以复方配伍形式应用，也有以大黄单味入药制成的水丸、片剂（新清宁片）及冲剂等。具体包括丸剂、散剂、膏药、丹剂、片剂、颗粒剂、胶囊剂、合剂、口服液等，或做内服，或以外用，或供注射等。如三黄片，由东汉张仲景《金匮要略》泻心汤方剂得来，由大黄、黄芩、黄连 3 味药组成，将汤剂改为片剂是为了避免大黄起泻下作用的结合蒽醌在提取过程中受热分解，从而达到保证临床用药可控，质量稳定的目的。

Chinese patent medicines containing Dahuang are rich in pharmaceutical forms, covering solid, liquid, semisolid, gas and other pharmaceutical forms. Dahuang is commonly used in combination with other medicinals, and there are also water pills, tablets (Xinqingning Tablets) and granules made from Dahuang alone. Specifically, the pharmaceutical form includes pill, powder, plaster, pellet, tablet, granule, capsule, and mixture as well as oral liquid, etc. for oral administration, external use, or for injection. For example, Sanhuang Pian (Tablets) is derived from Xiexin Tang (Decoction) in *Jinkui Yaolue (Synopsis of the Golden Chamber)* by Zhang Zhongjing of the Eastern Han Dynasty. It consists of Dahuang, Huangqin and Huanglian. The purpose of changing the decoction into tablets is to avoid the decomposition of combined anthraquinones, of its purgative effect working, by heating in the process of extraction, so as to achieve the purpose of ensuring clinical medication controllability and stable quality.

【性能功效】
[Property and Efficacy]

一、性能
I Property

大黄苦，寒；归脾、胃、大肠、肝、心包经。

Dahuang is bitter in favor and cold in nature. It enters the spleen, stomach, large intestine, liver and pericardium meridians.

二、功效
II Efficacy

1. **泻下攻积** 大黄苦寒沉降，入脾、胃、大肠经，能荡涤肠胃，推陈致新，为泻下攻积之要药，尤善治实热积滞便秘。其功效的发挥与泻下等药理作用密切相关。大黄致泻的有效物质基础主要是结合型蒽醌苷、二蒽酮苷，通过刺激肠黏膜及肠壁肌层内神经丛，并兴奋肠平滑肌上 M 胆碱受体，从而使结肠蠕动发挥作用。

1 Eliminating Accumulation by Purgation

Dahuang is bitter and cold, and sinking and descending in property. It enters meridians of spleen, stomach and large intestine, which can cleanse intestines and stomach, bring forth the new through the old. It is an essential medicinal for eliminating accumulation by purgation, especially good at treating constipation due to accumulation of excessive heat. The exertion of its efficacy is closely related to the pharmacological effects such as diarrhea. The binding anthraquinone glycoside and anthrone glycoside are the main effective substance bases of Dahuang inducing diarrhea, which works by promoting colon peristalsis through stimulating intestinal mucosa and nerve plexus in intestinal wall muscle layer, and exciting M choline receptor on intestinal smooth muscle.

2. **清热泻火** 大黄苦寒沉降，既能折上炎之火，也能导热下行，行清热泻火之功效。其功效的发挥与抗病原微生物、抗炎等药理作用密切相关。大黄素抗病原微生物、抗炎的有效物质基础主要是游离苷元、蒽醌类成分，通过抑制细菌核酸和蛋白质合成，及抑制糖代谢发挥抗病原微生物作用；并通过抑制花生四烯酸的代谢，从而减少前列腺素和白三烯生成发挥抗炎作用。

2 Clearing Heat and Purging Fire

Dahuang is bitter and cold, and sinking and descending in property, which can not only break up the fire flaming upward, but also conduct heat downward, so as to play the role of clearing heat and purging fire. The exertion of its efficacy is closely related to the pharmacological effects of anti-pathogenic microorganisms and anti-inflammation. The effective substance bases of emodin in resisting pathogenic microorganism and inflammation are mainly free aglycone and anthraquinone components. Its anti-pathogenic microorganism effect is achieved by inhibiting bacterial nucleic acid and protein synthesis and inhibiting sugar metabolism. While the anti-inflammatory effect is playing through inhibiting the metabolism of arachidonic acid, thereby reducing the production of prostaglandins and leukotrienes.

3. **凉血解毒** 大黄苦寒之性可入血分，清血分热，具有凉血止血功效；同时又善解疮疡热毒，共奏凉血解毒之功。其功效的发挥与抗炎、抗病原微生物、止血等药理作用密切相关。大黄止血的有效物质基础主要是 d- 儿茶素、没食子酸、大黄酚、大黄素甲醚，通过收缩损伤局部血管，降低毛细血管的通透性，增加血小板数量，促进血小板粘附和聚集，降低抗凝血酶Ⅲ（AT-Ⅲ）的活性和纤溶酶活性发挥止血作用。

3 Cooling Blood and Detoxifying

Dahuang is bitter and cold, which can enter the blood aspect to clear away its heat by cooling blood and stopping bleeding. At the same time, it is also good at relieving sore and ulcer due to heat toxin, showing as cooling blood and removing toxin. The acting of its efficacy is closely related to its pharmacological effects of anti-inflammation, anti-pathogenic microorganisms, hemostasis, etc. The effective substance bases of Dahuang functioning as hemostasis are mainly d-catechin, gallic acid, chrysophanol and physcion, and it takes effect by contracting damaged local blood vessels to reduce capillary permeability, increasing platelet quantity, promoting platelet adhesion and aggregation, and reducing antithrombin Ⅲ (AT-Ⅲ) activity and fibrinolytic enzyme activity.

4. **逐瘀通经** 大黄味苦入血分，具有活血化瘀通经之功，正如《医学衷中参西录》载大黄能

"破一切瘀血"。其功效的发挥与改善微循环、抗肿瘤等药理作用密切相关。大黄抗肿瘤的有效物质基础主要是大黄酸、大黄素、芦荟大黄素，通过抑制细胞膜 Na$^+$-K$^+$-ATP 酶活性提高血浆渗透压，补充血容量，降低血液黏度发挥改善微循环作用；并通过阻止细胞周期进程，抑制肿瘤细胞增殖、转移，诱导肿瘤细胞凋亡发挥抗肿瘤作用。

4 Expelling Blood Stasis to Dredge Channels

Dahuang tastes bitter and enters the blood aspect, possessing the functions of promoting blood circulation, removing blood stasis and dredging channels. Just as the book *Yixue Zhongzhong Canxi Lu* recorded, Dahuang can "eliminate all kinds of blood stasis". Its efficacy is closely related to its improvement of microcirculation, anti-tumor and other pharmacological effects. Rhein, emodin and aloe-emodin are the effective substance bases of Dahuang for its anti-tumor effect, which can improve plasma osmotic pressure by inhibiting Na$^+$-K$^+$-ATP enzyme activity of cell membrane to supplement blood volume, and reduce blood viscosity so as to improve microcirculation. It can also inhibit the proliferation and metastasis of tumor cells by preventing the cell cycle progression and induce apoptosis of tumor cells so as to play an anti-tumor role.

5. 利湿退黄　大黄苦寒入肝经，能清泻肝胆湿热，利湿退黄。其功效的发挥与保肝、利胆、利尿、抗病毒、抗炎等药理作用密切相关。大黄保肝利胆、利尿的有效物质基础主要是大黄蒽醌衍生物，通过疏通肝内毛细胆管，促进胆汁分泌和排泄发挥保肝利胆作用；并通过抑制肾髓质 Na$^+$-K$^+$-ATP 酶发挥利尿作用。

5 Eliminating Dampness to Remove Jaundice

Dahuang is bitter and cold and enters the liver meridian, which can clear away dampness-heat of liver and gallbladder, and eliminat dampness to remove jaundice. The exertion of its efficacy is closely related to the pharmacological effects of protecting liver, promoting gallbladder functions, diuresis, resisting virus, resisting inflammation, etc. The effective substance basis for Dahuang to protect liver, and promote gallbladder functions and djuresis is mainly rhubarb anthraquinone derivatives, which play the role of protecting liver and promoting gallbladder functions by promoting bile secretion and excretion through dredging intrahepatic bile capillary. It plays a diuretic role by inhibiting Na$^+$-K$^+$-ATP enzyme in renal medulla.

【应用】
[Applications]

一、主治病证
I Indications

1. **实热积滞便秘**　治疗实热积滞之便秘尤为适宜，常与芒硝、厚朴、枳实等配伍，以增强泻下攻积之力，用治阳明腑实证，如大承气汤《伤寒论》。若大黄用量太轻，则泻下力缓和，与麻仁、苦杏仁、蜂蜜等润肠药同用，如麻子仁丸《伤寒论》。若里实热结而正气虚者，当与补虚药配伍，以攻补兼施，标本并顾。如配人参、当归等药，可治里实热结而气血不足者，如黄龙汤《伤寒六书》；如配麦冬、生地、玄参等，可治热结津伤者，如增液承气汤《温病条辨》；若与附子、干姜等配伍，可治脾阳不足，冷积便秘，如温脾汤《千金要方》。

1 Constipation Due to Accumulation of Excessive Heat

It is especially suitable for the constipation due to accumulation of excessive heat. It is often combined with Mangxiao, Houpo, and Zhishi to strengthen the ability of purgation and accumulation elimination to treat syndrome of excess of Yangming fu-viscera, such as Da Chengqi Tang (Decoction) in *Shanghan Zabing Lun*. With small dosage, the strong purgative effect of Dahuang will be relieved, and then it can be combined with intestine-moistening medicinals such as Maren (Cannabis Fructus), Xingren and Fengmi (Mel), such as Maziren Wan in *Shanghan Zabing Lun*. If excess heat in the interior is accumulated and vital *qi* is deficient, deficiency-tonifying medicinals should be combined to treat both manifestation and root causes through reinforcement and elimination in combination. For instance, if combined with Renshen, Danggui and other medicinals, it can treat excessive heat accumulation in the interior and deficiency of *qi* and blood, such as in Huanglong Tang (Decoction) in *Shanghan Liushu*. If combined with Maidong, Shengdi and Xuanshen, it can treat the injured fluid due to heat accumulation, such as Zengye Chengqi Tang (Decoction) in *Wenbing Tiaobian (Detailed Analysis of Warm Diseases)*; If combined with Fuzi and Ganjiang, it can be used to treat deficiency of spleen *yang* and constipation due to cold accumulation, such as in Wenpi Tang (Decoction) in *Qianjin Yaofang*.

现代临床，大黄配伍还可用于治疗消化系统疾病（肠梗阻、便秘、急性胆囊炎、急性胰腺炎等）属于阳明腑实证者。如以大黄为主的复方（大承气汤）。

In modern clinical practice, Dahuang compatibility can also be used to treat the digestive system diseases (intestinal obstruction, constipation, acute cholecystitis, acute pancreatitis, etc.) with the syndrome belonging to excess of Yangming fu-viscera, such as the compound prescription Dachengqi Tang (Decoction) mainly composed of Dahuang.

2. **血热吐衄，目赤咽肿，牙龈肿痛**　治疗血热妄行之吐血、衄血、咳血，常与黄连、黄芩等同用，如泻心汤《金匮要略》。

2 Hematemesis and Epistaxis Due to Blood Heat, Red Eyes, Swollen Pharynx, and Swelling and Pain in Gums

For hematemesis, epistaxis and hemoptysis caused by blood heat, Dahuang is often combined with Huanglian and Huangqin, such as Xiexin Tang (Decoction) in *Jinkui Yaolue*.

现代临床，单用大黄粉治疗上消化道出血，有较好治疗。若治火邪上炎所致的目赤、咽喉肿痛、牙龈肿痛等证，还可与黄芩、栀子等药同用，如《太平惠民和剂局方》凉膈散。

In modern clinical practice, Dahuang powder used alone is good for upper gastrointestinal hemorrhage. For red eyes, sore throat and gingival swelling and pain caused by pathogenic fire ascending, it can be treated by Dahuang combining with Huangqin, Zhizi and other medicinals, such as Liangge San (Powder) in *Taiping Huimin Heji Ju Fang*.

3. **痈肿疔疮，肠痈腹痛**　治热毒痈肿疔疮，常与金银花、蒲公英、连翘等同用；治疗肠痈腹痛，可与牡丹皮、桃仁、芒硝等同用，如大黄牡丹汤《金匮要略》。本品外用也能泻火解毒，凉血消肿，治热毒痈肿疔疮，《妇人良方》以之与生甘草共研末，酒熬成膏外敷；《太平圣惠方》用治口疮糜烂，以之与枯矾等分为末擦患处。

3 Swelling Carbuncle and Furuncle, Intestinal Carbuncle with Abdominal Pain

For swelling carbuncle and furuncle due to heat-toxicity, Dahuang is often used with Jinyinhua, Pugongying (Taraxaci Herba) and Lianqiao. For intestinal carbuncle with abdominal pain, it can be combined with Mudanpi (Moutan Cortex), Taoren and Mangxiao, such as Dahuang Mudan Tang (Decoction) in *Jinkui Yaolue*. For external use, Dahuang can also purge fire and remove toxin, cool blood and reduce swelling to treat swelling carbuncle and furuncle due to heat toxin. In *Furen Liangfang (Fine Formulas for Women)*, Dahuang was recorded for external application by being ground together with Shenggancao (Glycyrrhizae Radix, raw) and decocted with liquor into paste. In *Taiping Shenghui Fang*, Dahuang was recorded for treating oral aphthae with erosion by applying the powder of Dahuang and Kufan (Alumen) in the same dose to the affected part.

现代临床，大黄配伍治疗胃脘胀痛，如大柴胡汤。

In modern clinical practice, Dahuang compatibility is used to treat gastric distending pain, such as Dachaihu Tang (Decoction).

4. 瘀血经闭，产后瘀阻，跌打损伤　治妇女产后瘀阻腹痛、恶露不尽者，常与桃仁、土鳖虫等同用，如下瘀血汤《金匮要略》；治妇女瘀血经闭，可与桃仁、桂枝等配伍，如桃核承气汤《伤寒论》；治跌打损伤，瘀血肿痛，常与当归、红花、穿山甲等同用，如复元活血汤《医学发明》。

4 Amenorrhea Due to Blood Stasis, Postpartum Blood Stasis, and Traumatic Injury

For postpartum abdominal pain due to blood stasis and persistent lochia, Dahuang is often combined with Taoren and Tubiechong (Eupolyphaga Steleophaga), as shown in Xiayuxue Tang (Decoction) from *Jinkui Yaolue*. For women with amenorrhea due to stagnant blood, Dahuang can be used with Taoren and Guizhi, such as in Taohe Chengqi Tang (Decoction) in *Shanghan Zabing Lun*. For traumatic injury and swelling and pain due to blood stasis, it is often combined with Danggui, Honghua and Chuanshanjia, such as in Fuyuan Huoxue Tang (Decoction) in *Yixue Faming (Medical Invention)*.

现代临床，大黄配伍治疗治疗寒积里实证（胆绞痛、慢性痢疾、尿毒症等属于寒积里实者），如以大黄为主的复方（大黄附子汤）。

In modern clinical practice, Dahuang compatibility is used to treat interior excess due to cold accumulation (biliary colic, chronic dysentery, and uremia with the syndrome of interior excess due to cold accumulation), such as in the compound prescription Dahuang Fuzi Tang (Decoction) mainly composed of Dahuang.

5. 湿热痢疾，黄疸尿赤，淋证，水肿　治肠道湿热积滞之痢疾，可与黄连、黄芩、芍药等同用；用治肝胆湿热蕴结之黄疸、尿赤者，常配茵陈、栀子，如茵陈蒿汤《伤寒论》；若治湿热淋证，水肿，小便不利，常配伍木通、车前子、栀子等，如八正散《太平惠民和剂局方》。

5 Dampness-heat Dysentery, Jaundice, Reddish (bloody) Urination, Stranguria and Edema

For dysentery due to retention of dampness-heat in intestinal tract, Dahuang can be used with Huanglian, Huangqin and Shaoyao. For jaundice and bloody urination due to dampness-heat accumulation in liver and gallbladder, it is often combined with Yinchen and Zhizi, such as in Yinchenhao Tang (Decoction) in *Shanghan Zabing Lun*. For dampness-heat stranguria, edema and dysuria, it is often combined with Mutong (Akebiae Caulis), Cheqianzi, Zhizi, etc., such as in Bazheng San (Powder) in *Taiping Huimin Heji Ju Fang*.

现代临床，治疗泌尿系统疾病（慢性肾功能衰竭、慢性肾功能不全、糖尿病肾病、尿毒症、泌尿系统）结石属于阳虚水泛证者，如以大黄为主的复方（大黄附子汤等）。治疗热淋证（急慢性前列腺炎、前列腺增生肥大、急慢性肾盂肾炎、膀胱炎、尿道炎等）属于热淋证者，以大黄为主的复方（如八正合剂、分清五淋丸等）。

In modern clinical practice, it is used for treatment of urinary system diseases (chronic renal failure, chronic renal insufficiency, diabetic nephropathy, uremia, and stone in urinary system) belonging to the syndrome of edema due to yang deficiency, such as the compound prescription Dahuang Fuzi Tang (Decoction) mainly composed of Dahuang. For the treatment of acute and chronic prostatitis, prostatic hyperplasia, acute and chronic pyelonephritis, cystitis, urethritis, etc. with the syndrome of heat stranguria, Dahuang-based compounds, such as Bazheng Heji, Fenqing Wulin Wan, can be used.

6. 烧烫伤　现代临床，治疗皮肤疾病。如外用治烧烫伤，可单用粉，或配地榆粉，麻油调敷患处。

6 Burn and Scald

In modern clinical practice, Dahuang can be used for skin diseases, especially externally using for burn and scald; it can be applied to the affected part with its powder alone or mixing with Diyu

(Sanguisorbae Radix) powder and sesame oil.

二、用法用量
II Administration and Dosage

饮片：煎汤，3~15g；用于泻下不宜久煎。外用适量，研末敷于患处。

Decoction pieces: water decoction, 3-15g; when it is used for purgation, it should not be decocted for too long. Appropriate amount for external use, ground it into power and applied it to the affected part.

三、注意事项
III Precautions

1. 孕妇及月经期、哺乳期妇女应慎用。因其成分易从乳汁排泄，导致婴幼儿不明原因的腹泻，故哺乳期妇女不宜使用大黄。

1 Pregnant women and women during menstruation and lactation should use Dahuang with great caution. Because its components are easy to excrete from milk, leading to unexplained diarrhea in infants, Dahuang is not suitable for women during lactation.

2. 本品苦寒，易伤胃气，脾胃虚弱者应慎用。

2 Dahuang is bitter in flavor and cold in nature, which is easy to hurt stomach *qi*, so it should be used with caution for patients with deficiency of spleen and stomach.

第十一章 祛风湿药
Chapter 11　Wind-Dampness-Dispelling Medicinals

凡以祛除风湿、解除痹痛为主要作用的药物，称为祛风湿药。此类药物多辛香苦燥走散，功善祛除留着肌表、经络的风湿，部分药物可止痹痛、通经络、强筋骨，故可用于治疗风湿痹痛、筋脉拘挛、麻木不仁、半身不遂、腰膝酸痛、下肢痿弱等证。部分祛风湿药辛香苦燥，易耗伤阴血，故阴虚血亏者应慎用。根据功效及药性不同，可分为祛风湿散寒药、祛风湿清热药和祛风湿强筋骨药。现代研究表明，祛风湿药多具有抗炎、镇痛、免疫调节等药理作用。常见的祛风湿药有独活、川乌、威灵仙、防己、雷公藤、秦艽、五加皮、桑寄生、狗脊等。

Wind-dampness-dispelling medicinals take removing wind-dampness and relieving arthralgia and pain as main functions. Most of these medicinals being pungent and bitter in taste , aromatic and drying in property, therefore could dispel the wind and dampness from the skin and meridians. Some could relieve arthralgia and pain, remove obstruction in meridians and strengthen tendon and bone. Thus, Wind-dampness-dispelling medicinals could be used to treat arthralgia aggravated by wind and dampness, muscle and tendon crispation, sequela of apoplexy, hemiplegia, soreness and weakness of waist and knees and other syndromes. It should be used with cautions in patients with syndrome/pattern of yin deficiency and blood inadequacy because the dry bitter and pungent property of some of the medicinal readily injuring the *yin* and blood. According to the differences of efficacy and properties, it can be divided into the wind-dampness-dispelling and cold-dispelling medicinal, the wind-dampness-dispelling and heat-clearing medicinal, and the wind-dampness-dispelling and tendon-bone-strengthening medicinal. Modern research suggests that most of wind-dampness-dispelling medicinals have pharmacological effects of anti-inflammation, analgesia, immune regulation and so on. Representative medicinals include Duhuo (Angelicae Pubescentis Radix), Chuanwu, Weilingxian (Clematidis Radix Et Rhizoma), Fangji (Stephaniae Tetrandrae Radix), Leigongteng (Tripterygium wilfordii), Qinjiao, Wujiapi (Acanthopanacis Cortex), Sangjisheng, Gouji, and so on.

独　活

Duhuo
(Angelicae Pubescentis Radix)

独活为川产道地药材。独活味辛、苦，性微温，归肾、膀胱经，有祛风除湿，通痹止痛的功效，主治风寒湿痹、腰膝疼痛、少阴伏风头痛、风寒夹湿头痛等证。独活主要含有挥发油、香豆素等，有抗炎、镇痛、抑制血小板聚集、抗血栓形成等活性，可用于治疗风湿性、类分湿性关节炎，腰椎间盘突出症，坐骨神经痛等属风湿痹证、头风头痛、风寒表证及表证夹湿者。服用独活可能会导致日光性皮炎。

Duhuo is a genuine regional medicinal in Sichuan Province. Duhuo is pungent and bitter in favor, and slightly warm in property, and it enters into the kidney meridian and the bladder meridian, functioning in dispelling wind-dampness, relieving arthralgia and pain. It could be used to treat syndrome of wind-cold-dampness arthralgia, to relieve the pain of waist and knees, to relieve the headache due to wind pathogens of Shaoyin disease , and to relieve the headache due to wind-cold mixed with dampness, and other syndromes. Volatile oils and coumarins are major components of Duhuo which possess various pharmacological effects, such as anti-inflammation, relieving pain, inhibiting platelet aggregation and anti-thrombosis. It could be used to treat rheumatic arthritis, rheumatoid arthritis, prolapse of lumbar intervertebral disc, and sciatica pertaining to the syndrome of wind-dampness arthralgia, head-wind headache, exterior syndrome of wind-cold and the exterior syndrome mixed with wind-dampness. Taking Duhuo may cause solar dermatitis.

【品种品质】
[Variety and Quality]

一、基原品种与品质
I Origin Varieties and Quality

1. 品种概况

为伞形科植物重齿毛当 *Angeliea pubescens* Maxim. f. *biserrata* Shan et Yuan 的干燥根。

独活始载于《神农本草经》。《本草经集注》云："出益州北部、西川者为独活，色微白，形虚大……其一茎独上，不为风摇，故名独活。"《证类本草》绘有风翔府独活、茂州独活、文州独活等5幅药图。茂州独活颇接近今用正品独活重齿毛当归。从品种来源上分析，宋代独活药材的原植物已基本与今用品种相一致。

1 Variety

Duhuo is the dry root of *Angeliea pubescens* Maxim. f. *biserrata* Shan et Yuan.

Duhuo is first recorded in the book *Shennong Bencao Jing*. According to the description of the *Bencaojing Jizhu*, Duhuo growsin the northern part of Yizhou and Xichuan, with a slight white color and a large puffy shape. One sole stem,wind-blowing unshakable, so it was called Duhuo. The *Zhenglei Bencao* (*Classified Materia Medica*) recorded five medicinal pictures, including Fengxiangfu Duhuo, Maozhou Duhuo, and Wenzhou Duhuo. Among them, the Maozhou Duhuo is quite similar to the genuine Duhuo (*Angeliea pubescens* Maxim. f. *biserrata* Shan et

Yuan). The original plant of Duhuo in the Song Dynasty has basically been consistent with that used today by the analysis of the source of the variety.

2. 种植采收　独活主产于四川。在栽培上采用种子繁殖、根芽繁殖及育苗移栽，播种分春播和秋播。育苗移栽的独活在当年 10~11 月即可收获，直播的独活在生长 2 年后可收获。独活收获时先割去地上茎叶，再挖出根部。

2 Planting and Harvesting

Duhuo is mainly planted in Sichuan Province and cultivated by seed, shoot root but pagation and seedling transplanting, which can be in spring and autumn. Seedling transplanting Duhuo can be harvested from October to November in the same year, while the direct sowing one can be harvested after two years. Before digging out Duhuo at harvest time, firstly remove its aerial stems and leaves.

3. 道地性及品质评价　自古以来四川是独活的道地产区。以"圆柱形，根头大，圆锥状，多横皱纹，表面灰褐色或棕褐色，断面皮部灰白色，有多数散在的棕色油室，木部灰黄色至黄棕色，形成层环棕色为佳，有特异香气，味苦、辛，微麻舌。

独活主要含有香豆素类，包括东莨菪素、蛇床子素、二氢欧山芹醇、二氢欧山芹醇乙酸酯、二氢欧山芹素等。该类成分为独活的主要活性成分。此外，独活还含有挥发油、当归酸等。《中国药典》规定独活药材中蛇床子素含量不得少于 0.50%，二氢欧山芹醇当归酸酯不得少于 0.080%。

3 Genuineness and Quality Evaluation

Sichuan Province is the genuine producing area of Duhuo. It is better to have "cylinder, large roots, conical" in shape and "transverse wrinkles", and "taupe- or sepia-colored surface, gray-white cortex with many dispersed brown oil chambers, and gray-yellow to brown corpus lignosum, and brown cambium ring" in color. Duhuo has a strongly aromatic fragrance, is bitter and pungent in flavor and causes slight numbness of tongue.

Duhuo contains coumarins, including scopoletin, osthole, columbianetin, columbianetin acetate, columbianadin, *et al*. They are the main active component of Duhuo. It also contains volatile oils, angelic acids and so on. The *Pharmacopoeia of the People's Republic of China* regulates that the content of osthole in Duhuo should not be less than 0.50%, and the content of columbianetin should not be less than 0.080%.

二、炮制品种与品质
II Processed Varieties and Quality

独活的炮制品种有淫羊藿制、炒制、盐制、酒制等。目前，临床常用为饮片。独活饮片以呈类圆形薄片，形成层环棕色，有特异香气，味苦、辛，微麻舌为佳。饮片的品质评价同药材。

Duhuo can be processed by the following methods including processing by Yinyanghuo (Epimedii Herba), by stir-frying, by salt and by liquor. At present, the main type of processed products is the decoction pieces. Duhuo decoction pieces in good quality are the quasi-circular slices with a brown cambium ring, and has umgue fragrance, are bitter and pungent in flavor and cause feeling of slight numbness of tongue. The quality evaluation of Duhuo decoction pieces is the same as that of the Duhuo material medica.

三、中成药品种与品质
III Varieties and Quality of Chinese Patent Medicines

含有独活的中成药有 230 余个，其中药典收载 20 余个。以独活为君药或主药的品种有独活寄生丸、独活寄生合剂等。在质量控制多采用薄层色谱法对照药材及蛇床子素对照品鉴定标志性成分以及采用液相色谱仪测定独活中蛇床子素的含量。

There are more than 230 Chinese patent medicines containing Duhuo, of which more than 20 are contained in the *Pharmacopoeia of the*

People's Republic of China so far. Among them, prescriptions with Duhuo as a sovereign or main medicinal include Duhuo Jisheng Wan, and Duhuo Jisheng Heji, etc. In the quality control, TLC is often used to identify the marker components (osthole) by comparing of the reference material medica and Esthole-coutained references. Besides, the LC was also used to determine the content of osthole in Duhuo.

【制药】
[Pharmacy]

一、产地加工
I Processing in Production Area

采收后，除去杂质，洗净，润透后切薄片，晒干或低温烘干即可。

After being harvested and cleaned, Duhuo is cut into thin slices, and then dried in the sun or baked at a low temperature.

二、饮片炮制
II Processing of Decoction Pieces

独活的炮制方法曾有淫羊藿制、盐水浸焙、炒制、焙制、酒制等方法。目前，独活在临床上多生用。

Duhuo can be processed by Yinyanghuo (Epimedii Herba), salt water soaking and roasting, stir-frying, baking, and liquor. Now, the unprocessed Duhuo (raw Duhuo) is commonly used in clinical practice.

三、中成药制药
III Pharmacy of Chinese Patent Medicines

含独活的中成药剂型较多，有外用剂型和内服剂型。中成药制药中以生品独活入药，采用乙醇提取，打粉入药或提取挥发油后药渣再煎煮，如天和追风膏、天麻丸、天麻祛风补片等。

There are many pharmaceutical forms of Chinese patent medicines containing Duhuo for external and internal use. In traditional Chinese patent medicine such as Tianhe Zhuifeng Gao (Paste), Tianma Wan, Tianma Qufeng Bu Pian (Teblets) Shengduhuo is applied, or extracted with ethanol ,or then ground into powder ,or with the volatile oils extracted and residue decocted.

例如独活寄生丸，来源于孙思邈《备急千金要方》的独活寄生汤，为大蜜丸或水蜜丸。制成丸剂解决了汤剂需要长期反复煎煮的问题，使服用更为方便。

Duhuo Jisheng Wan are from Duhuo Jisheng Tang (Decoction) recorded in Sun Simiao's *Beiji Qianjin Yaofang* as the honey bolus, or water-honeyed pills. Making pills solves the problem that the decoction needs to be repeatedly cooked, making it more convenient to take.

【性能功效】
[Property and Efficacy]

一、性能
I Property

独活辛、苦，微温；归肾、膀胱经。
Duhuo is pungent, bitter in flavor, slightly warm in nature,and it enters the kidney and the bladder meridian.

二、功效
II Efficacy

1. **祛风除湿** 独活辛散苦燥，气香温通，善祛风湿，止痹痛。其功效的发挥与其抗炎、镇痛、镇静、抗骨质疏松等药理作用密切相关。独活抗炎、镇痛的有效物质基础主要是挥发油类、香豆素类、蛇床子素，通过抑制 COX-1、COX-2 发挥抗炎镇痛作用。

1 Dispelling Wind and Dampness
Duhuo is capable of dispelling the wind and dampness and alleviating pain due to

pungent-dispersing, bitter-drying and warm in property. This efficacy is closely related to the anti-inflammatory, analgesic, sedative, anti-osteoporosis effects. The effective material basis of Duhuo's anti-inflammatory and analgesic efficacy is mainly volatile oils, coumarins, and osthole, which work by inhibiting COX-1 and COX-2.

2. 通痹止痛　独活苦燥温通，善通痹止痛，为治风湿痹痛之要药。其功效的发挥与抗炎、镇痛、抗血栓等药理作用密切相关。独活抗血栓的物质基础主要是二氢欧山芹醇、二氢欧山芹醇乙酸酯、二氢欧山芹素、蛇床子素等。

此外，现代研究显示独活具有扩张血管、降血压、对抗实验性心律失常、解痉、抗肿瘤等作用。

2 Relieving Impediment to Alleviate Pain

Duhuo can effectively treat impediment by its bitter-drying and warming property, and is the main medicinal for treatment of impediment pain due to wind-dampness. Its efficacy is closely related to its pharmacological action in anti-inflammatory, analgesic, and antithrombotic effects. Its main substance basis of anti-thrombus ingredients are columbianetin, columbianetin acetate, columbianadin, and osthole, etc.

Modern studies also suggest that Duhuo has the angiectatic, hypotensive, antiarrhythmic, spasmolytic and antitumor effects.

【应用】
[Applications]

一、主治病证
I Indications

1. 风寒湿痹痛　独活可以其他药物配伍治疗风寒湿邪所致的腰痛、腿痛，方如《备急千金要方》独活寄生汤；治少阴伏风头痛，痛连齿颊，方如《症因脉治》独活细辛汤。

现代临床，独活配伍常用于治疗颞颌关节功能紊乱综合征、颈椎病、腰椎间盘突出症、骨折延迟愈合等属于风寒湿痹者。

1 Wind-cold-dampness Arthralgia Pain

Duhuo could be combined with other medicinal for treatment of the pain in lower extremities and waist caused by wind-cold-dampness pathogen, such as Duhuo Jisheng Tang (Decoction) recorded in *Beiji Qianjin Yaofang*, for treatment of the Shaoyin incubated wind headache which affects teeth and cheek, such as Duhuo Xixin Tang (Decoction) recorded in *Zhengyin Maizhi*.

In modern clinical research, Duhuo compatibility is often used to treat patients with temporomandibular joint dysfunction syndrome, cervical spondylosis, lumbar disc herniation, and delayed fracture healing caused by wind-cold-dampness arthralgia.

2. 风寒表证　治外感风寒表证夹湿者，常配伍羌活、防风、藁本等，如《内外伤辨惑论》羌活胜湿汤，增强发散风寒、胜湿止痛功效。

现代临床，独活配伍常用于治疗头痛头重、一身疼痛、肢节疼痛等属于风寒夹湿之表证者。

此外，以独活为主的复方（如独活寄生汤等）在现代亦常用于治疗出血证，相当于西医学的原发性血小板减少性紫癜。独活片剂配合长波紫外线照射治疗银屑病。

2 Wind Cold Exterior Syndrome

Duhuo can be used with Qianghuo, Fangfeng, Gaoben, etc. to treat the wind cold exterior syndrome mixed with dampness in order to enhance the effect of dispelling wind and cold, to alleviate dampness and inhibit pain, such as Qianghuo Shengshi Tang (Decoction) in *Neiwaishang Bianhuolun (Clarifying Doubts about Damage from Internal and External Causes)*.

In modern clinical research, Duhuo compatibility is often used to treat headache, carebaria, body pain, and joint pain in exterior syndrome of wind-cold mixed with dampness.

In addition, Duhuo-based formulae (such as Duhuo Jisheng Tang (Decoction) are also commonly used in the treatment of the bleeding syndrome which is equivalent to Western medicine's primary thrombocytopenic purpura now. Duhuo tablets combining with long-wave ultraviolet irradiation are used for psoriasis.

二、用法用量
II Administration and Dosage

3~10g。

3~10g.

三、注意事项
III Precautions

1. 阴虚血燥及实热内盛者慎用。

1 It should be used with caution in those with *yin* deficiency and blood dryness, or internal exuberance of excessive heat.

2. 内服过量时对胃肠道有刺激作用，不可过量服用。

2 Oral overdosage will cause a stimulating effect on the gastrointestinal tract, that's forbidden to take .

【知识拓展】
[Knowledge Extension]

古代本草对独活和羌活存在使用混淆的问题。陶弘景从形态、产地进行区分《本草经集注》云："羌活形细而多节，软润，气息极猛烈。出益州北部、西川者为独活，色微白，形虚大。"李时珍从植物来源和特征上予以区别。《本草纲目》载："独活、羌活乃一类二种，以他地者，为独活；西羌者，为羌活。羌活，须用紫色有蚕头鞭节者。独活，是极大羌活有臼如鬼眼者。"

There was confusion existing on the use of Duhuo and Qianghuo in the ancient Chinese materia medica literatures. In the Northern and Southern Dynasties, Tao Hongjing distinguished between Duhuo and Qianghuo from the shape and production area. *Bencaojing Jizhu* recorded that, Qianghuo is thin, knobby, and soft and moisten, with strong odour. Those from northern part of Yizhou and Xichuan are Duhuo, with a slight white color and a puffy large shape. Li Shizhen distinguished between Duhuo and Qianghuo from the source plant and of their characteristics. *Bencao Gangmu* described that Duhuo and Qianghuo were the same plant which were planted in two different places. Duhuo was planted in the other places except Xiqiang, while Qianghuo was only planted in Xiqiang. Qianghuo, purple in color, with silkworm-head like flagella is good for use. Duhuo is a big Qianghuo with joint like a ghost eye.

第十二章 化 湿 药
Chapter 12　Dampness-Resolving Medicinals

凡气味芳香，性偏温燥，具有化湿运脾作用的药物，称为化湿药。此类药物多辛香温燥，善芳化燥除湿浊，舒畅气机而健运脾胃，具有化湿健脾、和中开胃之功，适用于脾为湿困、运化失常所致的脘腹痞满、呕吐泛酸、大便溏薄、食少体倦、舌苔白腻，或湿热困脾之口甘多涎等，暑温、阴寒闭暑、湿温等证亦可选用。化湿药多属辛温香燥之品，易耗气伤阴，故阴虚血燥及气虚者宜慎用。现代研究表明，化湿药多具有调节胃肠运动功能、促进消化液分泌、抗溃疡、抗病原微生物等药理作用，部分还兼有抗炎、抗风湿、止痛作用，常见化湿药有广藿香、苍术、紫苏、厚朴等。

Medicinals eliminating dampness, aromatic in flavor and warm, dry in property, with actions of eliminating dampness and invigorating spleen are called dampness-resolving medicinals. Most of these kinds of herbs are pungent, aromatic, warm and dry, good at transforming dryness and eliminating dampness-turbidity, soothing qi and invigorating the spleen and stomach, and have the functions of dispelling dampness, strengthening the spleen, harmonizing the middle and promoting appetite. These medicinals are applicable to abdominal distension, vomiting, acid regurgitation, thinand loose stool, poor appetite and tiredness, white greasy tongue, sweet taste in mouth and polysialia due to dampness and heat obstructing spleen. They can also be used in the treatment of summer-heat febrile, closed-summer-heat due to the cold and dampness-warmth syndromes. Most of dampness-resovling medicinals are pungent, warm, aromatic and dry, so they can potentially consume qi and injure yin. Therefore, they must be used with caution in cases of yin deficiency, blood dryness or qi deficiency. Modern research shows that these medicinals can have the following pharmacological effects of regulating gastrointestinal movement, promoting digestive fluids secretion, antiulceration antipathogenic microorganisms. Some medicinals also have anti-inflammatory, anti-rheumatic and analgesic effects including Guanghuoxiang (Pogostemonis Herba), Cangzhu, Zisu (Perillae Folium), Houpo and so on.

广 藿 香

Guanghuoxiang
(Pogostemonis Herba)

广藿香是著名的广东道地药材。广藿香味辛，性微温，归脾、胃、肺经，有芳香化浊、和中止呕、发表解暑的功效，主治湿浊中阻，脘痞呕吐，暑湿表证，湿温初起，发热倦怠，胸闷不舒，寒湿闭阻，腹痛吐泻，鼻渊头痛。广藿香主要含挥发油（如广藿香醇与广藿香酮），有促进胃液分泌、调整胃肠运动、抗病原微生物、抗炎、对免疫的影响等药理作用，可用于治疗消化不良、胃肠功能低下、胃肠型感冒等属湿浊中阻、暑湿、湿温、呕吐、表证夹湿证者。

Guanghuoxiang is a noted genuine regional medicinal in Guangdong Province. The medicinal properties of Guanghuoxiang are pungent and slightly warm in nature, and it enters meridians of spleen, stomach and lung. It can remove dampness with aromatics, harmonize stomach and spleen, arrest vomit, release exterior syndromes and remove summer-heat. The medicinal can be used to treat the syndromes of dampness obstructing the middle energizer, vomiting and epigastrium stuffiness, exterior syndromes of summer-heat and dampness, beginning of dampnesswarm, fever and tired, tightness and discomfort of chest, obstruction of cold and dampness, abdominal pain, vomiting, diarrhea, nasosinusitis and headache. Guanghuoxiang mainly contains volatile oils (like patchoulic alcohol and pogostone) and possess various pharmacological effects, including promoting gastric juice secretion, regulating gastrointestinal movement and immunity, inhibiting pathogenic microorganisms, and anti-inflammation, influence of immunity. It can be used to treat indigestion, gastrointestinal dysfunction, gastrointestinal type cold belonging to dampness obstructing the middle energizer, summerheat dampness, dampnesswarm, vomiting, and exterior syndrome mixed with dampness.

【品种品质】
[Variety and Quality]

一、基原品种与品质
I Origin Varieties and Quality

1. 品种概况　来源于唇形科植物广藿香 *Pogostemon cablin* (Blanco) Benth. 的干燥地上部分。

1 Variety

Guanghuoxiang is the dry aerial parts of *Pogostemon cablin* (Blanco) Benth.

广藿香以"藿香"之名始载于东汉杨孚的《异物志》。《本草图经》载："……叶似桑而小薄并绘蒙州藿香为图。《证类本草》亦绘蒙州藿香。《本草纲目》为藿香释名："豆叶曰藿，其叶似之，故名"并详述其性状"叶微似茄叶"。各典籍关于"藿香"形态、繁殖方式、产地的描述印证古时记载的藿香是现在的广藿香。

Guanghuoxiang was first recorded as "Huoxiang" in the *Yiwu Zhi (Foreign Body Records)* written by Yangfu in the Eastern Han Dynasty. The *Bencao Tujing* recorded that the leaves are like mulberry but smaller and thinner and the drawing of Mengzhou Huoxiang was included. *Zhenglei Bencao (Classified Materia Medica)* also painted the figure of Mengzhou Huoxiang. *Bencao Gangmu* clarified the meaning of the name of Huoxiang: "Bean's leaves are called huo, and the leaves of huoxiang are similar, hence named it." It also described "the leaves are slightly like eggplant leaves". The morphology, breeding methods, and origins confirm that Huoxiang recorded in ancient books is Guanghuoxiang.

2. 种植采收　广藿香主产广东、海南、广西等地，多采用传统扦插繁殖，亦有组培育苗。广东广藿香根据种植时间的不同分秋冬季和翌年夏季采收，海南广藿香在夏季和秋冬季均采收。收时择晴天露水刚干后进行，将全株拔起或挖起。

2 Planting and Harvesting

Guanghuoxiang are majorly planted in Guangdong, Hainan and Guangxi Provinces. Most of Guanghuoxiang propagates by traditional cutting technique, and a few by tissue culture-originated seedling technique. Guanghuoxiang is harvested in autumn, winter or next summer according to the planting time. Guanghuoxiang in Hainan Province is harvested in summer, autumn or winter in the year. When being harvested, Guanghuoxiang were pulled up or dug up in a sunny day after the dew drying out.

3. **道地性和品质评价**　自古以来广东为广藿香的道地产区。以茎枝粗壮，色青绿色，叶多，肥厚柔软，香气浓郁者为佳。

3 Genuineness and Quality Evaluation

Since the ancient time, Guangdong province has been the genuine producing area of Guanghuoxiang. Good quality is characterized by thick and firm green stems and branches with many thick and soft leaves and an intense aroma.

广藿香主要含有挥发油，约占 1.5%，主要是广藿香醇（又称百秋李醇）以及广藿香酮。其他成分有苯甲醛、丁香油酚、桂皮醛、广藿香吡啶等。该类成分为广藿香的主要活性成分。此外，广藿香尚含有多种倍半萜及黄酮类成分。《中国药典》规定广藿香药材中百秋李醇含量不得少于 0.10%。

Guanghuoxiang mainly contains 1.5% volatile oils, which are patchouli alcohol (also known as patchoulol) and pogostone dominated. Other components of Guanghuoxiang include benzaldehyde, eugenol, cinnamaldehyde, and patchoulipyridine, which are the main active component of Guanghuoxiang. In addition, Guanghuoxiang contains components of sesquiterpenes and flavonoids. According to the *Pharmacopoeia of the People's Republic of China*, patchoulol content in Guanghuoxiang should not be less than 0.10 %.

二、炮制品种与品质
II Processed Varieties and Quality

广藿香的主要炮制品有饮片。广藿香饮片以茎略呈方柱形，表面有柔毛。切面有白色髓。叶两面均被灰白色绒毛；基部楔形或钝圆，边缘具大小不规则的钝齿；叶柄细，被柔毛。气香特异，味微苦为佳。饮片品质评价同药材。

Guanghuoxiang's main processed product is decoction pieces. The decoction pieces have a slightly columnar stem, and the surface is with pubescence. The cut surface has white medulla. Both sides of leaves are covered with gray-white tomentum. The base is wedge-shaped or blunt, and the edge is with irregular blunt teeth. The petiole is thin covering with pubescence. The aroma is unique intense and the flavor is slightly bitter. The quality evaluation of Guanghuoxiang decoction pieces is the same as that of the medicinal.

三、中成药品种与品质
III Varieties and Quality of Chinese Patent Medicines

含有广藿香的中成药有 200 余个，其中药典收载 40 余个。以广藿香为君药或主药的品种有藿香正气口服液、藿香正气水等。含广藿香的中成药在质量控制多采用薄层色谱法进行指标成分百秋李醇测定。

There are more than 200 Chinese patent medicines containing Guanghuoxiang, of which over 40 are included in the *Pharmacopoeia of the People's Republic of China*. Prescriptions with Guanghuoxiang as a sovereign or main medicinal include Huoxiang Zhengqi Koufuye, Huoxiang Zhengqi Shui and so on. The quantity control in preparations containing Guanghuoxiang is to detect the index of patchoulol by TLC.

【制药】
[Pharmacy]

一、产地加工
I Processing in Production Area

广藿香采收后，白天摊晒数小时，稻草覆盖发汗和发酵。重复以上步骤，直至全干。

After being harvested, it is exposed to the sun for several hours during the day, and then, they are covered by straw to induce sweating and fermenting. Repeat the above steps until it is completely dried.

二、饮片炮制
II Processing of Decoction Pieces

广藿香在古代记载的炮制方法有净制、切制、酒制、烘焙和油制等 5 种。现代以净制、润透、切段为炮制工艺，由此生产的生广藿香为商品规格中的主流。

There are five methods of Guanghuoxiang recorded in ancient times: cleansing, cutting, processing with liquor, baking and processing with oil. In modern times, the processing technology includes cleansing, moisturizing, and cutting into segments, and Shengguanghuoxiang (raw) produced from these methods is the mainstream of commodity specifications.

广藿香所含挥发油易散失。可减少水处理步骤，控制干燥的次数、温度和时间等，从而保证饮片的质量。

Volatile oils of Guanghuoxiang are easily lost. Through reducing water treatment steps, controlling the number of drying times, temperature and time, it can ensure the quality of decoction pieces.

三、中成药制药
III Pharmacy of Chinese Patent Medicines

含广藿香的中成药剂型十分丰富，涵盖固体、液体剂型。成药制药中多以生广藿香投料。由于广藿香的药用成分主要是挥发油，也有部分品种采用广藿香油（广藿香经水蒸气蒸馏提取的挥发油）代替广藿香作为生产原料，如藿香正气口服液、藿香正气软胶囊、藿香正气滴丸、藿香正气水等。

There are many pharmaceutical forms of Chinese patent medicines containing Guanghuoxiang, covering solid and liquid pharmaceutical forms. In the pharmaceutical industry, Shengguanghuoxiang (raw) is often used. Since volatile oils are mainly medicinal ingredients of Guanghuoxiang, some medicinals use Guanghuoxiang oil (volatile oils extracted from Guanghuoxiang by steam distillation) instead of Guanghuoxiang as a raw material, such as Huoxiang Zhengqi Koufuye (Mixture), Huoxiang Zhengqi Ruanjiaonang (Soft Capsules), Huoxiang Zhengqi Diwan, Huoxiang Zhengqi Shui and so on.

例如藿香正气口服液，源于《太平惠民和剂局方》藿香正气散，原方以广藿香与其他药味打粉为细末，与姜、枣一起煎汤服用，现采用广藿香油作原料投料，在方便生产操作的同时，可以减少加热过程对挥发油的损耗。

Huoxiang Zhengqi Koufuye is from Huoxiang Zhengqi San (Powder) recorded in the *Taiping Huimin Heji Ju Fang*. In the original presciption, Guanghuoxiang and other medicinals and is decocted together with ginger and jujube to take. Now, Guanghuoxiang oil is directly used as the raw material, which facilitating production operations and reducing the consumption of volatiles oil during the heating process.

【性能功效】
[Property and Efficacy]

一、性能
I Property

广藿香辛，微温；归脾、胃、肺经。
Guanghuoxiang is aromatic, pungent in flavor, slightly warm in nature, and enters the spleen, stomach and the lung meridians.

二、功效
II Efficacy

1. 芳香化浊　广藿香芳香化浊辟秽，通利九窍，能散邪气，辟恶毒，解时疫。其功效的发挥与抗病原微生物、止咳、化痰、增强免疫功能等药理作用密切相关。广藿香发挥该作用的主要药效物质基础是挥发油。

1 Eliminating Turbid Pathogen with Aroma

Guanghuoxiang can aromatically reduce filth, dredge nine orifices, dispersing pathogenic evils, and avoid vicious to xin, dispel time epidemic. Its efficacy is closely related to pharmacological effects, such as anti-pathogenic microorganisms, cough suppression, phlegm elimination, and immune function enhancement. The main material basis of Guanghuoxiang to exert these effects is volatile oil.

2. **和中止呕** 广藿香辛温芳香，化湿浊，运脾胃、调中焦，可和中止呕。其功效的发挥与调节胃肠道功能、促进消化液分泌、保护肠黏膜屏障等药理作用密切相关。主要物质基础为挥发油。其中，拮抗肠道钙离子是其抑制胃肠道平滑肌运动的机制之一。

2 Regulating Stomach and Stopping Vomiting

Guanghuoxiang is pungent, warm, aromatic, and it eliminates dampness-turbidity, promotes the spleen and stomach and coordinates middle energizer, which can regulate stomach and stop vomiting. This efficacy is closely related to pharmacological effects such as regulating gastrointestinal function, promoting digestive juice secretion, and protecting the intestinal mucosal barrier. The active components are volatile oils. Antagonizing intestinal calcium ions is one of mechanism that in hibiting gastrointestinal movement.

3. **发表解暑** 广藿香性温而不燥，既能散表寒又可化湿浊，对于暑月外感风寒、内伤生冷证甚为适宜。其功效的发挥与抗病原微生物、抗炎、镇痛、解热等药理作用密切相关。主要物质基础有挥发油。

3 Releasing Exterior and Clearing Summerheat

Guanghuoxiang is warm but not dry. It can disperse exterior cold and dampness-turbidity. It is very suitable for the syndromes of exogenous wind-cold in summer and endogenous cold. Its efficacy is closely related to pharmacological

effects such as defensing infection of pathogenic anti-microorganisms, anti-inflammation, analgesia, and antipyresis. The main active components are volatile oils.

【应用】
[Applications]

一、主治病证
I Indications

1. **湿阻中焦证** 广藿香可与他药配伍治疗湿阻中焦证，方如《太平惠民和剂局方》不换金正气散，《六科准绳》七味白术散。

1 The Syndrome of Dampness Obstructing the Middle Energizer

Guanghuoxiang can be combined with other medicinals to treat the syndrome of dampness obstructing the middle energizer, such as Buhuanjinzhengqi San (Powder) in *Taiping Huimin Heji Ju Fang*, Qiwei Baizhu San (Powder) in the *Liuke Zhunsheng (Six Principles)*.

在现代临床广藿香配伍常用于治疗慢性浅表性胃炎、急性胃肠炎、功能性消化不良、糖尿病性胃轻瘫、老年性腹胀、慢性乙型肝炎、化疗后胃肠道毒副作用、肠易激综合征、溃疡性结肠炎、抗生素致胃肠反应、手足口病、反流性食管炎、急性酒精中毒等消化系统疾病属于湿阻中焦证者，如藿香正气口服液、藿香正气软胶囊、藿香正气滴丸、藿香正气水等。

In modern clinical practice, Guanghuoxiang compatibility is often used to treat chronic superficial gastritis, acute gastroenteritis, functional dyspepsia, diabetes gastroparesis, senile abdominal distension, chronic hepatitis B, gastrointestinal side effects after chemotherapy, irritable bowel syndrome, ulcerative colitis, antibiotic-induced gastrointestinal reactions, hand-foot-mouth disease, reflux esophagitis, acute alcoholism and so on, which due to the syndrome of dampness obstructing the middle energizer. Huoxiang Zhengqi Koufuye (Mixture), Huoxiang

Zhengqi Ruanjiaonang (Soft Capsules), Huoxiang Zhengqi Diwan, Huoxiang Zhengqi Shui can be used for the above syndromes.

2. **呕吐、泄泻** 广藿香可与他药配伍治疗湿浊中阻所致的呕吐，方如《太平惠民和剂局方》藿香半夏汤，《中国医学大辞典》藿香和中汤，藿香安胃散等。在现代临床广藿香配伍（与丁香、半夏、黄连等）常用于治疗各种呕吐。

2 Vomiting and Diarrhea

Guanghuoxiang in combination with other medicinals can treat vomiting caused by dampness obstructing the middle energizer, such as Huoxiang Banxia Tang (Decoction) in *Taiping Huimin Heji Ju Fang*, Huoxiang Hezhong Tang (Decoction) and Huoxiang Anwei San (Powder) in the *Chinese Medical Dictionary*. In modern clinical practice, Guanghuoxiang combined with Dingxiang, Banxia, Huanglian is often used to treat various types of vomiting.

广藿香可与他药配伍治疗治寒湿或暑湿而致腹痛泄泻，方如《百一选方》回生散，《太平惠民和剂局方》藿香正气散，《温病条辨》茵陈白芷汤等。在现代临床广藿香配伍常用于治疗急性胃肠炎、功能性消化不良属于湿阻中焦证者，如藿香正气口服液、藿香正气软胶囊、藿香正气滴丸、藿香正气水等。

Guanghuoxiang can be combined with other medicinals to treat abdominal pain and diarrhea caused by cold-dampness or summer-dampness, such as Huisheng San (Powder) in the *Baiyi Xuanfang (Selected Prescriptions from the Praiseworthy Studio)*, Huoxiang Zhengqi San (Powder) in *Taiping Huimin Heji Ju Fang*, Yinchen Baizhi Tang (Decoction) in *Wenbing Tiaobian*. In modern clinical practice, Guanghuoxiang with other medicinals is often used to treat patients with acute gastroenteritis, functional dyspepsia, who have dampness obstructing the middle energizer syndrome, such as Huoxiang Zhengqi Koufuye, Huoxiang Zhengqi Ruanjiaonang (Soft Capsules), Huoxiang Zhengqi Diwan, Huoxiang Zhengqi Shui.

3. **外感、暑湿及湿温初起** 广藿香可与他药配伍治疗外感风寒兼内伤湿滞证，方如《太平惠民和剂局方》藿香正气散、《医原》藿朴苓夏汤、《温热经纬》甘露消毒丹等。

3 Exogenous Cold, Summer-dampness and Dampness-warmth Beginning

Guanghuoxiang can be combined with other medicinals to treat the syndromes of exogenous wind-cold with endogenous dampness stagnation, such as Huoxiang Zhengqi San (Powder) in *Taiping Huimin Heji Ju Fang*, Huopo Lingxia Tang (Decoction) in the *Yiyuan (Bases of Medicine)*, Ganlu Xiaodu Dan in *Wenre Jingwei*.

在现代临床广藿香配伍常用于治疗胃肠型感冒，如藿香正气口服液、藿香正气软胶囊、藿香正气滴丸、藿香正气水等。

In modern clinical practice, Guanghuoxiang often combined with others medicinals treats gastrointestinal type cold, such as Huoxiang Zhengqi Koufuye, Huoxiang Zhengqi Ruanjiaonang (Soft Capsules), Huoxiang Zhengqi Diwan, and Huoxiang Zhengqi Shui.

4. **寒湿疟疾** 广藿香可与他药配伍治疗寒湿内蕴之疟疾寒热往来，胸脘痞闷，神疲肢倦，口不渴，方如《鸡峰普济方》藿香散。

4 Cold-dampness and Malaria

Guanghuoxiang can be combined with other medicinals to treat alternate attacks of chill and fever of malaria, chest and epigastrium stuffiness discomfort, limbs weakness and spirit tiredness, lack of thirst due to internal cold-dampness, such as Huoxiang San (Powder) in *Jifeng Pujifang (Jifeng Prescription for Universal Relief)*.

此外，以广藿香为主的复方（如藿香正气口服液、藿香正气软胶囊、藿香正气滴丸、藿香正气水等）在现代亦用于支气管哮喘属于"寒哮"者、急性高山反应属于水湿内停证者以及偏头痛属于痰浊阻滞证者。

In addition, Guanghuoxiang-based formulas (such as Huoxiang Zhengqi Koufuye, Huoxiang

Zhengqi Ruanjiaonang, Huoxiang Zhengqi Diwan, Huoxiang Zhengqi Shui, etc.) are also used for bronchial asthma caused by cold wheezing, acute mountain sickness belongs to the syndrome of internal stagnation of fluid-dampness and migraine due to the syndrome of phlegm-turbidity stagnation now.

二、用法用量
II Administration and Dosage

3~10g。
3~10g.

三、注意事项
III Precautions

阴虚不宜应用。

It should not be used in the cases with yin deficiency.

【知识拓展】
[Knowledge Extension]

传统认为产于广州石牌的牌香品质最优，但现今石牌藿香产量极低；产于肇庆的肇香品质稍逊于石牌藿香，也较少。湛江和海南产的广藿香药材商品统称为南香，传统认为南香质次、不供药用；但由于牌香、肇香产量小，故南香被广泛用于配方与制剂生产。

Traditionally, Paixiang from Shipai Country in Guangzhou City is considered superior, and Zhaoxiang from Zhaoqing City is of secondary quality. The yields of Guanghuoxiang in both of them are very low at present. Guanghuoxiang from Zhanjiang City and Hainan Province are collectively called Nanxiang. Nanxiang is considered inferior and not for medicinal use traditionally, however, it is widely used in the production of medicinal preparations now, owing to the lack of Paixiang and Zhaoxiang.

苍 术
Cangzhu
(Atractylodis Rhizoma)

苍术的道地产区为江苏茅山地区。常用苍术、炒苍术和焦苍术。苍术味辛、苦，性温，归脾、胃、肝经，具燥湿健脾、祛风散寒、明目的功效，主治湿阻中焦证、风湿痹证、外感表证夹湿、痿证、夜盲症等。苍术主要含挥发油、多糖、黄酮等，有促进胃肠运动、保肝利胆、抗病原微生物、抗炎、增强免疫、利尿、降糖等药理作用，可用于治疗胃肠功能紊乱、消化道溃疡、类风湿性关节炎、痛风，并防治病毒性传染性疾病等。苍术温燥，阴虚内热或气虚多汗者忌服。

The genuine region of Cangzhu is the Maoshan area of Jiangsu Province. Common used Cangzhu are the Chaocangzhu (stir-frying) and Jiaocangzhu (charred). The flavor of Cangzhu is pungent, bitter, and the property is warm. Cangzhu enters the spleen, stomach and liver meridians. It has the effects of drying dampness and invigorating spleen, dispelling wind and cold, and improving eyesight. The indications are dampness obstructing the middle energizer syndrome, rheumatism arthralgia syndrome, exterior syndrome mixed with dampness, flaccidity syndrome, night blindness, etc. Cangzhu mainly contains volatile oil, polysaccharides, flavone etc. It has pharmacological effects such as promoting gastrointestinal motility, protecting liver and gallbladder, anti-pathogenic microorganism, anti-inflammation, enhancing immunity, diuretic and hypoglycemic functionsetc. It can be used to treat gastrointestinal dysfunction, digestive ulcer, rheumatoid arthritis, gout, and prevent and cure viral infectious diseases. Because Cangzhu is warm and dry, so it is contraindicated for the patients with yin deficiency and internal heat or qi deficiency and hyperhidrosis.

【品种品质】
[Variety and Quality]

一、基原品种与品质
I Origin Varieties and Quality

1. **品种概况**　来源于菊科植物茅苍术 *Atractylodes lancea* (Thunb.) DC. 或北苍术 *Atractylodes chinensis* (DC.) Koidz. 的干燥根茎。

1 Variety

Cangzhu is derived from the dried rhizome of chrysanthemum *Atractylodes lancea (Thunb.)* DC. (Maocangzhu). or *Atractylodes chinensis* (DC.) Koidz. (Beicangzhu).

《神农本草经》载术。《本草经集注》指出术有白术、赤术两种。《本草衍义》明确提出苍术。《本草纲目》记载"苗高二三尺，其叶抱茎而生，梢间叶似棠梨叶，其脚下叶有三五叉，皆有锯齿小刺。根如老姜之状，苍黑色，肉白有油膏"，其形态描述及附图均与现今所用茅苍术相类。

Shennong Bencao Jing contains the medicinal. In *Bencaojing Jizhu* it was pointed that there were 2 kinds as the white and the red one. *Bencao Yanyi (The Meaning of Materia Medica)* clearly put forward "the sapling is two or three feet high, its leaves embrace the stem, the tip of the leaves is like Tang pear leaves, its foot leaves have three or five forks, all are with sawtooth small thorns. The root is like ginger and has black, white pulp with ointment", and its morphological description and drawings are similar to those used today.

2. **种植采收**　现今茅苍术主产于河南、江苏、湖北、安徽、浙江、江西等省；北苍术主产于黑龙江、吉林、辽宁、内蒙古、河北、山西等省。多采用较高海拔田间育种栽培。茅苍术多在秋季采挖，北苍术分春、秋两季采挖。

2 Planting and Harvesting

Nowadays, the main production of Maocangzhu is in Henan, Jiangsu, Hubei, Anhui, Zhejiang, Jiangxi and other provinces; Beicangzhu mainly produced in Heilongjiang, Jilin, Liaoning, Inner Mongolia, Hebei, Shanxi and other provinces. More of higher altitude field breeding cultivation is adopted. Maocangzhu is mostly dug in autumn and Beicangzhu in spring and autumn.

3. **道地性及品质评价**　自陶弘景之后历代均认为茅山出产的苍术品质最优。苍术形态上"似姜"，颜色上是"黑而肉白且有油膏"，历来性状评价指标以有红色的"朱砂点"（即油室）和"白毛"（即白色针状结晶）为佳，且气香特异，味微甘、辛、苦。

3 Genuineness and Quality Evaluation

Since Tao Hongjing, the quality of Cangzhu from Maoshan has been considered to be the best. The shape of Cangzhu is "like ginger", and the color of pulp is "black and white with ointment". The evaluation index of traditional characters is red "cinnabar point" (that is, oil chamber) and "white hair" (that is, white needle crystal), and the aroma is special, the flavor is slightly sweet, pungent, and bitter.

苍术所含化学成分主要为挥发性成分和非挥发性成分。挥发性成分主要包括倍半萜类（如茅术醇、β-桉叶醇、苍术酮等）和聚乙烯炔类成分（如苍术素、苍术素醇等），非挥发性成分主要为倍半萜苷类（如苍术苷 A 等）和多糖类（如汉黄芩苷等），另外还含有氨基酸、脂肪酸及少量糠醛、黄酮和酚酸类等。挥发油是苍术的药效物质基础，其中倍半萜类成分是调节胃肠功能、保肝、抗炎、利尿、调节免疫等功能的主要物质基础。《中国药典》规定苍术药材中苍术素的含量不得少于 0.3%。

The chemical components of Cangzhu are mainly volatile and non-volatile components. Volatile components mainly include sesquiterpenoids (e.g., citronellol, β-eucalyptus alcohol, xanthone, etc.) and polyvinylidene compounds (e.g. atractylodes, xanthoprostol, etc.). The non-volatile components are mainly sesquiterpenoids (e.g. Atractylidin A) and polysaccharides (e.g. baicalin, etc.) and also the compoents contain amino acids, fatty acids and a small amount of furfural, flavonoids and phenolic acids. Volatile oil is the pharmacodynamic material basis of Cangzhu, among which sesquiterpenoids are the main material bases for regulating gastrointestinal function, protecting liver, anti-inflammation, diuretic, and regulating immunity etc. The *Pharmacopoeia of the People's Republic of China* stipulates that atractylodes in Cangzhu should not be less than 0.3%.

二、炮制品种与品质
II Processed Varieties and Quality

苍术的现代炮制品种有 8 个，临床常用品种 4 种，如苍术、土炒苍术、麸炒苍术、米泔水制苍术、焦苍术等。苍术以表皮灰棕色至黄棕色，有白色针状结晶析出为佳；土炒苍术以表面土黄色且挂一层土为佳；麸炒苍术以表面焦黄色且有浓郁香气为佳；焦苍术以表面焦褐色且有焦香气为佳。《中国药典》规定苍术炮制品中苍术素含量不得少于 0.2%。

There are 8 modern processed varieties of Cangzhu, and 4 are commonly used in clinics, such as Cangzhu, Tuchaocangzhu (stir-frying with earth), Fuchaocangzhu (stir-frying with bran), Miganshuizhicangzhu (processing with rice swill), Jiaocangzhu (charred), etc. Cangzhu is grayish brown or yellowish brown with white needle-like crystal precipitation as the best. The best Tuchaocangzhu (stir-frying with earth) has yellowish surface hanging a layer of soil. Fuchaocangzhu (stir-frying with bran) is the best with scorched yellow surface and rich aroma. The best Jiaocangzhu (charred) has scorched brown surface and scorched aroma. The *Pharmacopoeia of the People's Republic of China* stipulates that

the content of atractylodes in processed products of Cangzhu should not be less than 0.2% of the total.

三、中成药品种与品质
III Varieties and Quality of Chinese Patent Medicines

含有苍术或其炮制品的中成药有 120 余个，《中国药典》收载含苍术的中成药 63 个。以苍术为君药或主药的品种有香砂平胃丸、越鞠丸、二妙丸等。在中成药的品质控制中多采用显微鉴别及薄层色谱法确定苍术的存在。如香砂平胃丸，用薄层色谱法与苍术对照药材提取液对比鉴别苍术；越鞠丸、二妙丸等，用显微观察薄壁细胞中草酸钙针晶、用薄层色谱法与苍术对照药材提取液对比鉴别苍术。

There are more than 120 Chinese patent medicines containing Cangzhu or its processed products. The *Pharmacopoeia of the People's Republic of China* contains 63 Chinese patent medicines containing Cangzhu. The varieties of Cangzhu as sovereign medicinal or main medicinal include Xiangsha Pingwei Wan, Yueju Wan, Ermiao Wan etc. In the quality control of Chinese patent medicines, microscopic identification and TLC are used to determine the existence of Cangzhu. For example, Xiangsha Pingwei Wan were used to identify Cangzhu by TLC. For Yueju Wan, Ermiao Wan, etc., microscope is used for the observation of calcium oxalate needle crystals in parenchyma cells, and TLC and the Cangzhu control medicinal material extract were used to identify Cangzhu.

【制药】
[Pharmacy]

一、产地加工
I Processing in Production Area

苍术于采挖后除去茎叶和泥土，逐步晒干

并多次撞去须根及老皮。然后经浸泡、洗净、润透、切厚片、干燥，筛去碎屑，供加工成不同炮制品。

After digging out Cangzhu, remove stems and leaves and soil, gradually dry it and repeatedly hit the fibrous root and old skin. Then soaking, washing, moistening, cutting thick pieces, drying, sieving off debris, Cangzhu is processed into different processed products.

二、饮片炮制
II Processing of Decoction Pieces

自古苍术的炮制方法繁复。目前形成了"清炒、麸炒、土炒、炒焦、炒炭"等炮制工艺，由此加工的苍术、麸炒苍术、焦苍术、苍术炭成为了商品规格中的主流。其中，苍术偏于燥湿祛风散寒，麸炒苍术偏于燥湿健脾，焦苍术偏于固肠止泻。

The processing methods of Cangzhu have been complicated since ancient times. At present, the processing technology of "simple stir-frying, stir-frying with bran, stir-frying with earth, stir-frying to brown, stir-frying to scorch" has been formed and Cangzhu, Fuchaocangzhu (stir-frying with bran), Jiaocangzhu (charred), Cangzhutan (carbonized) which were processed through these methods have become the mainstream of commodity specifications. Among them, Cangzhu is for drying dampness, dispelling wind and dispersing cold, Fuchaocangzhu (stir-frying with bran) is for drying dampness and invigorating spleen and Jiaocangzhu (charred) is for the consolidation of intestines to stop diarrhea.

苍术挥发油具有利尿、增加全血粘度等作用，大剂量能使中枢神经抑制，导致呼吸麻痹。经炮制后的苍术饮片中挥发油含量比生苍术饮片挥发油含量低，相应作用亦减缓，这也与李时珍提出的"以制其燥去其油"内涵一致。传统的泔制、麸炒、炒焦等炮制工艺均能达到降低挥发油含量、缓和燥性的目的。

Volatile oil of Cangzhu has diuretic effect, and it can increase whole blood viscosity etc. High dose can inhibit central nervous system, and cause respiratory paralysis. The content of volatile oil in processed Cangzhu decoction pieces was lower than that in raw Cangzhu decoction pieces, and the corresponding effect is milder, which is consistent with Li Shizhen's connotation of "through processing moderating its dryness by removing its oil". Traditional processing techniques such as swill, stir-frying with bran and stir-frying to brown can reduce the content of volatile oil and reduce dryness.

三、中成药制药
III Pharmacy of Chinese Patent Medicines

含苍术的中成药，剂型十分丰富，涵盖固体、液体与半固体剂型。苍术所含成分种类较多，既有水溶性成分又有挥发性成分，因而其传统中成药制剂多制成散剂或丸剂，可以最大程度保留其挥发油而加强疗效。现今为服用和保存方便也常制成片剂、胶囊剂和颗粒剂等，多以苍术粉末，或分别提取挥发油与水溶性成分入制剂中。

For Chinese patent medicine containing Cangzhu, the pharmaceutical form is very rich, covering solid, liquid and semi-solid pharmaceutical forms. Cangzhu contains many kinds of components, both water-soluble and volatile components, so its Chinese patent pharmaceutical preparation is made into powder or pills, which can retain its volatile oil to the greatest extent and strengthen the curative effect. Nowadays, tablets, capsules and granules are often prepared for easy use and preservation, in which mostly Cangzhu powder, or extraction of volatile oil and water-soluble components are used into the preparation.

如以苍术为君药的现代制剂香砂平胃片，选用麸炒苍术研末入制剂以保证疗效，同时将其开发成为新剂型分散片，遇水迅速崩解而分散速度快，保留了"散者，散也"的特点。在颈复康颗粒制剂工艺中，苍术与其他部分药物提取挥发油后用 β - 环糊精包结，其药渣与余药加水煎煮，滤液浓缩干燥后，加入挥发油 β-环糊精包结物及适量乳糖、硬脂酸镁，制成颗粒，既保留了苍术的有效成分，又能掩盖其不良气味，改善药物的口感。

For example, the modern preparation of Xiangsha Pingwei Pian, which uses Cangzhu as the sovereign medicinal, uses Fuchaocangzhu (stir-frying with bran) that is ground into powder to ensure the curative effect. At the same time, it is developed into a new pharmaceutical form of dispersible tablets, which disintegrate quickly when exposed to water and disperse quickly and retains the characteristics of "San, means scattered". In the preparation process of Jingfukang Keli, after extracting volatile oil from Cangzhu and other medicines, it is clumped with β-cyclodextrin; the residue and residual medicine are boiled with water. After the filtrate is concentrated and dried, volatile oil β- cyclodextrin inclusion and appropriate amount of lactose and magnesium stearate are added to make granules. It not only retains the active ingredients of Cangzhu, but also can cover up its bad smell and improve the taste of the medicinal.

【性能功效】
[Property and Efficacy]

一、性能
I Property

苍术辛、苦，性温；归脾、胃、肝经。

Cangzhu is pungent, bitter in flavor and warm in nature, and enters to the spleen, stomach, liver meridians.

二、功效
II Efficacy

1. 燥湿健脾　苍术燥湿健脾，助脾健运。其功效的发挥与其调节胃肠运动、调节胃肠激素、抗溃疡、抗炎、保肝利胆、利尿等药理作用

密切相关。苍术的调节胃肠运动、抗溃疡、保肝、利尿作用的有效物质基础主要是 β-桉叶醇、苍术烯内酯、苍术酮及茅术醇等，通过抑制甾体激素释放、抗 H_2 受体发挥调节胃肠激素、抗溃疡作用；并通过抑制 Na^+, K^+-ATP 酶活性阻止 Na^+ 重吸收，增加排尿量发挥利尿作用。

1 Drying Dampness and Invigorating the Spleen

Cangzhu can dry dampness and invigorate spleen and help improve the function of spleen in transportation. Its effect is closely related to its pharmacological effects such as regulating gastrointestinal motility, regulating gastrointestinal hormones, anti-ulcer, anti-inflammatory, protecting liver and gallbladder, diuresis etc. The effective material basis of Cangzhu in regulating gastrointestinal motility, anti-ulcer, protecting liver and diuresis is mainly β- eucalyptus alcohol, atractylenolide, atractylon amd ainesol, etc. By inhibiting steroid hormone release, anti-H_2 receptors play a role in regulating gastrointestinal hormones and anti-ulcer. By inhibiting Na^+-K^+-ATP enzyme's activity and preventing Na^+ reabsorption, the urine outputcan be increased and the diuretic effect can be played.

2. 祛风散寒　苍术辛散温燥，能祛肌表风寒湿之邪。其功效的发挥与其抗炎、抗病原微生物、增强免疫等药理作用密切相关。苍术抗病原微生物、增强免疫作用的有效物质基础主要是挥发油、苍术多糖等，通过提升血清溶血素水平及免疫球蛋白、促进脾脏淋巴细胞增殖、增加胸腺质量、提高肠免疫系统功能等发挥增强免疫作用。

2 Dispelling Wind and Dispersing Cold

Cangzhu, which is pungent, warm and dry, can dispel the wind-cold-dampness pathogen of skin surface. Its efficacy is closely related to its anti-inflammatory, anti-pathogenic microorganisms, enhanced immunity and other pharmacological effects. The effective material basis of anti-pathogenic microorganism and enhanced immune effect of Cangzhu is mainly volatile oil, Cangzhu polysaccharides etc. It can enhance immune function by raising serum hemolysin level and immunoglobulin, promoting spleen lymphocyte proliferation, increasing thymus quality and improving intestinal immune system function.

3. 明目 苍术入肝经，明目。现代药理研究尚未明确报道苍术对视力的相关药理作用，但其调节免疫、抗炎、抗病原微生物等作用可能与明目有关。苍术中含有的维生素A原在肠道转换为维生素A，参与到视网膜感光物质视紫红质的合成，可能是其明目的机制之一。

3 Improving Eyesight

Cangzhu enters the liver meridian, and can improve eyesight. Modern pharmacological studies have not clearly reported the related pharmacological effects of Cangzhu on visual acuity, but its effects on regulating immunity, anti-inflammatory and anti-pathogenic microorganisms may be related to improving eyesight. The original vitamin A contained in Cangzhu converts to vitamin A in the intestine. Which involved in the synthesis of retinal photosensitive rhodopsin. This may be one of the mechanisms of improving eyesight.

此外，现代研究显示苍术还有抗肿瘤、促进成骨细胞增殖、降血糖、降尿酸、降血压以及保护心肌等作用。

In addition, modern studies have shown that Cangzhu has functions of anti-tumor, promoting osteoblast proliferation, lowering blood sugar, lowering blood uric acid, lowering blood pressure and protecting myocardium, etc..

【应用】
[Applications]

一、主治病证
I Indications

1. 湿阻中焦证 治湿阻中焦，脾失健运，常与厚朴、陈皮配伍以燥湿行气，如《太平惠民

和剂局方》平胃散和现代制剂香砂平胃片；若脾为湿困，清浊不分，大便溏泻，小便短少或水肿者，常与厚朴、茯苓、泽泻等配伍以祛湿运脾，如《丹溪心法》胃苓汤；治脾湿积久而成饮癖，胁痛，食减，吐酸者，可单用苍术为末、枣肉为丸服以燥湿健脾而化痰饮，如《普济本事方》苍术丸。

1 Syndrome of Dampness Obstructing the Middle Energizer

Treating dampness obstructing the middle energizer and dysfunction of spleen in transportation, Cangzhu is often used with Houpo combined with Chenpi to remove dryness and activating qi-flowing, such as Pingwei San (Powder) and modern preparation of Xiangsha Pingwei Pian (Tablets) in *Taiping Huimin Heji Ju Fang*. If there are patients with dampness encumbering spleen, no distinction between clear and turbid manifested by loose stool or diarrhea, scanty or short urine and edema, it is often used with Houpo, Fuling, Zexie to remove dampness and invigorate spleen, such as Weiling Tang (Decoction) form *Danxi Xinfa*. For the treatment of spleen dampness accumulation for a long time and becoming hyprochondrium retention of fluid, hypochondriac pain, food reduction, acid regurgitation, Cangzhu powder can be used alone, jujube meat are used as pills to dry dampness, invigorate spleen, in order to dissipatephlegm and fluid retention, such as Cangzhu Wan in *Puji Benshi Fang (Experiential Prescriptions for Universal Relief)*.

现代临床，苍术配伍常用于治疗功能性消化不良，急、慢性胃肠炎，消化道溃疡，胃下垂，胆囊炎，肠易激综合征等属湿阻中焦者，如平胃散、越鞠丸等。

In modern clinical practice, Cangzhu compatibility is often used for the treatment of patients with dampness obstructing the middle energizer such as functional dyspepsia, acute or chronic gastroenteritis, digestive tract ulcer, gastric prolapse, cholecystitis, irritable bowel syndrome and etc. For example, Pingwei San (Powder) and Yueju Wan are used for the syndromes above.

2. 风湿痹证　治疗风寒湿痹证，常与独活、薏苡仁等配伍以祛风散寒除湿，如《类证治裁》薏苡仁汤和现代制剂通痹胶囊；治风湿热痹或湿热痹证，多与知母、石膏、黄柏等配伍以清热燥湿，如《类证活人书》白虎加苍术汤、《丹溪心法》二妙散。

2 Wind-cold-dampness Arthralgia Syndrome

For the treatment of wind-cold-dampness arthralgia syndrome, Cangzhu often combined with Duhuo, Yiyiren to dispel wind and dissipate dampness, such as Yiyiren Tang (Decoction) from *Leizheng Zhicai (Syndrome Differentiation and Treatment)* and modern preparation Tongbi Jiaonang (Capsules). For the treatment of wind-dampness heat arthralgia or damp-heat arthralgia syndrome, Cangzhu often combined with Zhimu, Shigao, Huangbo and others to clear heat and dry dampness, such as Baihu plus Cangzhu Tang in *Leizheng Huorenshu (Class of the Living Book)*, and Ermiao San in *Danxi Xinfa*.

现代临床，苍术配伍常用于治疗类风湿性关节炎、风湿性关节炎、痛风、血栓闭塞性脉管炎等属风湿痹阻者，如薏苡仁汤、白虎加苍术汤、二妙丸等。

In modern clinical practice, Cangzhu compatibility is often used for the treatment of rheumatoid arthritis, rheumaticd arthritis, gout, thromboangiitis obliterans and others which belonging to rheumatism obstruction, such as Yiyiren Tang (Decoction), Baihu plus Cangzhu Tang (Decoction), Ermiao Wan (Pills), etc..

3. 外感表证夹湿　治疗外感风寒夹湿，寒热无汗，头身重痛者，常与羌活、川芎、白芷等配伍以解表除湿，如《太平惠民和剂局方》神术散、《此事难知》九味羌活汤；治疗太阴经头风头痛兼见脘腹胀痛，食欲不振者，常与白芷、生姜、川芎等同用，如《审视瑶涵》苍术汤。

3 The Exterior Syndrome Mixed With Dampness

For the treatment of patients with exogenous wind-cold mixed with dampness, cold heat without sweat, head and body heavy pain, Cangzhu is often combined with Qianghuo, Chuanxiong, Baizhi and other compatibility to relieve exterior and dissipate dampness, such as Shenzhu San (Powder) in *Taiping Huimin Heji Ju Fang,* Jiuwei Qianghuo Tang (Decoction) in *Cishi Nanzhi (This Matter is Difficult to Know)*. For the treatment of Taiyin meridian wind headache and epigastric distended pain, loss of appetite, it is often together with Baizhi, Shengjiang, Chuanxiong, such as Cangzhu Tang (Decoction) in *Shenshi Yaohan (Precious Book of Ophthalmology)*.

现代临床，苍术配伍常用于治疗各种上呼吸道感染合并腹泻、病毒性流行性感冒、乙型脑炎、慢性鼻炎或鼻息肉等属表证夹湿者，如藿香正气液、白虎加苍术汤等。

In Modern clinical practice, Cangzhu compatibility is often used for the treatment of all kinds of upper respiratory tract infections with diarrhea, viral influenza, encephalitis B, chronic rhinitis or nasal polyps and other symptoms of exterior syndrome mixed with dampness, such as Huoxiang Zhengqi Ye, Baihu plus Cangzhu Tang (Decoction).

4. 夜盲证　治疗夜盲证苍术可单味研末，纳入猪或羊肝煎服，如《太平圣惠方》抵圣散；《证治准绳·眼目集》以炒苍术伍白术、蝉蜕、黄连等为末，治疗睑硬睛痛、目生翳障；《幼幼新书》以苍术末入猪胆中，煎煮熏眼，并服煎汁，治疗婴儿目混涩不开或出血者。

4 Night Blindness

Treatment of night-blindness can grind Cangzhu alone, or mix it into the pig or sheep liver for decoction, such as Disheng San (Powder) in *Taiping Shenghui Fang*; In *Zhizheng Zhunsheng·Yanmu Ji* Chaocangzhu, Chantui, Huanglian, etc., are used as powder for the treatment of stiff eyelids and eye pain and cataract. In *Youyou Xinshu (New Book of Pediatrics)*, Cangzhu powder was put into the pig gallbladder, and was decocted for fumigating eyes.

Its decoction juice was taken for the treatment of infants with dry eyes which can't open or bleeding.

现代临床，苍术单用或配伍还常用于治疗角膜软化症、眼结膜干燥症、流行性角结膜炎等，如苍术粉、霍朴夏苓汤等。

In modern clinical practice, Cangzhu is singlely used or its compatibility is often used to treat corneal malacia, conjunctival dryness, epidemic keratitis, such as Cangzhu Powder, Huopu Xialing Tang (Decoction) etc.

5. 痿证　苍术常与黄柏相须为用，"除湿清热，为治痿要药"。治湿热痿证，常与黄柏、薏苡仁、牛膝等配伍，如《成方便读》四妙散；治气虚痿证，四君子汤加苍术、黄芩、黄柏；治血虚痿证，四物汤加苍术、黄柏。

5 Flaccidity Syndrome

Cangzhu often used together with Huangbo for mutual reinforcement. They were used for eliminating dampness and clearing heat, and for the treatment of flaccidity syndrome. For the treatment of flaccidity syndrome of dampness-heat, it often combined with Huangbo, Yiyiren, Niuxi and other compatibility, such as Simiao San (Powder) in *Chengfang Biandu (Convenient Reader of Established Prescriptions)*. For the treatment of flaccidity syndrome of qi deficiency, Sijunzi Tang (Decoction) is combined with Cangzhu, Huangqin, and Huangbo. For the treatment of flaccidity syndrome of blood deficiency, Siwu Tang (Decoction) is combined with Cangzhu and Huangbo.

现代临床，苍术配伍常用于治疗肌营养不良症、多发性神经炎、重症肌无力、运动神经元病等属湿热内蕴者，如加味四妙丸。

In modern clinical practice, Cangzhu compatibility is often used in the treatment of muscular dystrophy, multiple neuritis, myasthenia gravis, motor neurone disease and other syndromes of internal retention of dampness-heat, such as Jiawei Simiao Wan.

此外，苍术配伍还常用于治疗代谢性疾病、皮肤病、泌尿、生殖系统疾病，如糖尿病、湿疹、过敏性紫癜、非淋菌性尿道炎、尖锐湿疣、外阴瘙痒等病证。以苍术水煎剂口服或苍术注射液肌注治疗窦性心动过速，苍术挥发油制成软胶囊口服治疗佝偻病，亦有较好疗效。

In addition, Cangzhu compatibility is often used to treat metabolic diseases, skin diseases, urinary and reproductive system diseases, such as diabetes, eczema, allergic purpura, non-gonococcal urethritis, condyloma acuminatum, vulvar pruritus, etc. The treatment of sinus tachycardia by using Cangzhu decoction orally or intramuscular injection of Cangzhu Injection and the oral treatment of rickets by using volatile oil of Cangzhu in soft capsules also have a good effect.

二、用法与用量
II Administration and Dosage

3~9g，煎服。
3~9g, water decoction.

三、注意事项
III Precautions

苍术辛温燥烈，阴虚内热、气虚多汗者忌服。
Cangzhu is pungent, warm, dry and drastic, so patients with internal heat caused by yin deficiency and qi deficiency with hyperhidrosis should not take it.

【知识拓展】
[Knowledge Extension]

现代研究发现茅苍术与其他地区苍术在挥发油的含量及组成上明显不同，主要表现为茅苍术总挥发油含量低，含量较大的组分数目较多；茅苍术的水溶性浸出物、水溶性总糖、粗蛋白的总体水平亦较其他苍术高。此外，江苏句容和内蒙古等地所产苍术之苍术素含量较高。不同的炮制方法会使苍术的有效成分发生变化从而引起功效侧重的差异，须规范炮制、合理配伍、对证用药保证疗效。苍术烧烟熏蒸还有较好的净化空气、抑制病原微生物作用，自古就被用为防疫治疫的首选药物之一。

Modern studies have found that the content and composition of volatile oil in Mao Cangzhu and Cangzhu in other areas are obviously different. The main manifestations are that the total volatile oil content of Mao Cangzhu is low and the number of components with large content is more. The overall level of water soluble extract, water soluble total sugar and crude protein of Mao Cangzhu is also higher than that of other Cangzhu. In addition, the content of Cangzhu was higher in Jiangsu Jurong and Inner Mongolia. Different processing methods will change the effective components of Cangzhu and cause the difference of efficacy. It must be prepared in a standardized manner, reasonably compatible, and ensure the efficacy of the medicines used for syndromes. Cangzhu burnt smoke fumigation also has a better effect of purifying the air and inhibiting pathogenic microorganisms, and has been used as one of the first choice medicines for epidemic prevention and treatment since ancient times.

第十三章 利 湿 药
Chapter 13　Diuresis-Promoting Medicinals

　　凡以通利小便、排泄水湿为主要作用，治疗水湿病症的药物，称为利湿药，又叫利水渗湿药，分为利水消肿药、利湿退黄药和利尿通淋药三类。此类药物通过渗利之性，使水湿邪气化为尿液，达到治疗水湿病症的作用，故可用于水湿为患的多种病症。利湿药一般具有淡味，药性多平；部分药物具有清热作用，偏于寒凉，并有苦味；部分药物如香加皮、泽泻有毒。利湿药为渗湿通利之品，易耗损津液，又具降泄滑利之性，凡阴液亏虚者慎用，肾气不固者不宜使用。现代研究表明，利湿药具有利尿、调节免疫、抗肿瘤、增强心肌收缩及加快心率、降低胃液分泌及胃酸含量、延缓衰老、防结石、抗病原微生物、抗炎和镇静等作用。常见的利湿药有茯苓、猪苓、泽泻、茵陈、金钱草、虎杖、车前子、滑石和关木通等。

Diuresis-promoting medicinals, also named dampness-draining diuretics, refer to the medicinals that can treat dampness syndromes by promoting urination and draining dampness, which can be divided into edema-alleviating diuretic, dampness-excreting jaundice-resisting medicinal and stranguria-relieving diuretic. The medicinals transform dampness pathogens into urination with its draining and eliminating effects so as to play the role of treating dampness diseases and syndromes. The property of diuresis-promoting medicinals is generally bland and neutral, but some with heat-clearing effect are cold and bitter, and some medicinals such as Xiangjiapi and Zexie are toxic. With dampness-draining and diuretic effects, the diuresis-promoting medicinals can easily injure body fluids and since they also have purgation and relaxation-promoting effects, the medicinals must be used with caution for patients with syndrome of yin-fluid deficiency, and patients with insecurity of kidney qi should not use them. Modern researches show that the diuresis-promoting medicinals have many pharmacological effects, such as promoting urination, regulating immunity, resisting tumor, enhancing myocardial contraction, accelerating heart rate, reducing gastric secretion and gastric acid content, delaying aging process, preventing stone formation, resisting pathogenic microorganism and anti-inflammation and sedation. Common diuresis-promoting medicines include Fuling, Zhuling, Zexie, Yinchen, Jinqiancao, Huzhang, Cheqianzi, Huashi and Guanmutong.

茯 苓

Fuling
(Poria)

野生茯苓道地产区为云南，称"云苓"；栽培茯苓道地产区为安徽，称"安苓"。常用茯苓个、茯苓块和茯苓片，加工过程中削下的外皮，称为茯苓皮，可单独入药。茯苓味甘、淡，性平，归心、肺、脾、肾经，有利水渗湿，健脾，宁心安神的功效，主治水肿、淋浊、泄泻、痰证、痰饮证、脾虚、心悸、失眠和健忘等证。茯苓主要含多糖、三萜酸、甾醇类、蛋白质及衍生物等化学成分，有利尿、保护胃肠功能、抗胃溃疡、免疫调节、镇静等药理作用，可用于治疗浮肿严重的肾炎及心脏病、免疫功能低下、胃溃疡、肿瘤、病原微生物感染等属脾虚湿困者。

The genuine production place of wild Fuling, known as "Yunling", is Yunnan province. Anhui province for cultivated Fuling is known as "Anling". The common forms of Fuling used include the "intact Fuling", "Fuling masses" and "Fuling slices". Fuling cortex, the skin of Fuling cutting off during the processing, can be used alone as medicine. Fuling is neutral in property and sweet and bland in flavor, with the meridian tropism of the heart, lung, spleen and kidney meridians. It has the effects of promoting urination and draining dampness, invigorating the spleen, and calming the heart to tranquilize mind. Fuling can be used to treat edema, strangury disease, diarrhea, phlegm related syndromes, phlegm-fluid related syndromes, spleen deficiency syndrome, palpitations, insomnia and amnesia, etc. Fuling mainly contains polysaccharides, triterpenic acid, sterols, proteins and their derivatives, which possess various pharmacological effects, such as promoting urination, protecting gastrointestinal functions, resisting gastric ulcer, regulating immunity, sedating, etc. It can be used to treat diseases with the syndrome of spleen deficiency and dampness retention, including nephritis and cardiac disease with severe edemas, low immunity, gastric ulcer, tumor, pathogenic microorganism infectious diseases and so on.

【品种品质】
[Variety and Quality]

一、基原品种与品质
I Origin Varieties and Quality

1. 品种概况 多孔菌科真菌茯苓 *Poria cocos* (Schw.) Wholf 的干燥菌核。

1 Variety

Fuling is the dried sclerotium of *Poriacocos* (Schw.) Wholf derived from Polyporaceae.

茯苓始载于《神农本草经》。《名医别录》《新修本草》《蜀本草》和《本草图经》等记载"茯苓"生泰山、华山、嵩山，出大松下，附根而生，形块无定。《增订伪药条辨》云："云南产者，天然生者为多，亦皮薄起皱纹，肉带玉色，体糯质重为佳"。梁代陶弘景《本草经集注》有栽培记载。

Fuling is first recorded in the book *Shennong Bencao Jing*. According to the records in *Mingyi Bielu, Xinxiu Bencao, Shu Bencao, Bencao Tujing*, Fuling grows in Mount Tai, Huashan Mountain, Songshan Mountain, usually growing together with the roots of the big pine without definite shape. In *Zengding Weiyao Tiaobian (Revision and Supplementation on 'Systematic Differentiation of Erroneous Medicinals')*, "there are mainly wild Fuling from Yunnan province, in which good Fuling had the characteristics of thin skin with wrinkles, meat with jade color, being glutionous with heavy weighteight and glutinous. According to *Bencaojing Jizhu* written by Tao Hongjing in Liang Dynasty, it recorded the artificial cultivation of Fuling.

2. 种植采收　现茯苓已在多省广泛栽培，以云南、安徽、湖北等地最为适宜。在栽培技术上除了原有的椴木栽培之外，还有树兜栽培、活立木培育、伐根栽培等新方式。野生茯苓常在7月至次年3月到松林中采挖；人工栽培的茯苓一般是在第二年7~9月采挖。

2 Planting and Harvesting

Now Fuling is widely planted in many provinces, and the best producing areas include Yunnan, Anhui and Hubei. In addition to the original basswood cultivation, there are new cultivation methods, such as tree pocket cultivation, standing live tree cultivation and stump cultivation. Wild Fuling is generally harvested in the pinewoods from July this year to March in the next year, while the planted Fuling is mainly harvested in the next year from July to September.

3. 道地性及品质评价　《药物出产辨》记载，云南是野生茯苓的道地产区，安徽是人工栽培茯苓的道地产区。古人提出了以形、色、味等方面的茯苓性状评价指标，现代增加了"重量"评价指标，以"人形，龟形""外皮褐色或黑褐色，内部白色""粘牙力强"和"体重者"为佳。

3 Genuineness and Quality Evaluation

According to the records in *Yaowu Chuchan Bian (Differentiation on Materia Medica and Their Producing Areas)*, Yunnan Province is the genuine production place of wild Fuling, and Anhui is the genuine production place of planted Fuling. The ancients proposed the evaluation indexes of characters of Fuling from the aspects of shape, color and taste, while the weight is added for the evaluation in modern times. It is of good quality to have "human-like" or "tortoise-like" shape, the scarfskin with "brown" or "dark brown" and "interior white" color, "strong sticky" taste, and "heavy weight".

茯苓主要含有多糖、茯苓素、三萜、脂肪酸和其它成分。一般认为，茯苓素和多糖是茯苓的药效物质基础，其中茯苓素是利尿的主要物质基础，多糖是茯苓增强免疫功能、镇静、保肝、抗炎的主要物质基础，茯苓素和多糖是茯苓抗肿瘤的物质基础。《中国药典》规定茯苓药材及饮片浸出物含量不得少于2.5%。

Fuling mainly contains polysaccharides, poriatin, triterpene, fatty acids and other components. It is generally believed that polysaccharides and poriatin are the therapeutic material basis of Fuling. The latter is the major material basis for diuretic effect, and the former is the major material basis for the effects such as enhancing immunity, sedation, protecting liver functions, and resisting inflammation. Polysaccharides and poriatin are both the major material bases for anti-tumor effect of Fuling. According to the *Pharmacopoeia of the People's Republic of China*, the content of extract from Fuling and its decocting pieces should not be less than 2.5%.

二、炮制品种与品质
II Processed Varieties and Quality

茯苓的炮制品种有1个。饮片的品质评价同药材。

There is one processed product of Fuling. The quality evaluation of Fuling decoction pieces is the same as that of Fuling medicinal material.

三、中成药品种与品质
III Varieties and Quality of Chinese Patent Medicines

含有茯苓或其炮制品的中成药有229种，其中药典收载219个。以茯苓为君药或主药的品种有桂枝茯苓（胶囊、片、丸）、四君子汤、五苓散等，非以茯苓为君药的制剂，三九胃泰颗粒、小儿泻痢片、小儿速泻停颗粒等，在中成药的品质控制中多采用显微镜观察或薄层色谱法鉴别确定茯苓的存在，其中显微观察呈"颗粒状团块或不规则分枝状团块无色；菌丝无色或淡棕色，细长，稍弯曲，有分枝，直径4~6μm"。薄层色谱法以"对照药材为标准，在色谱相应的位置上显相同颜色的荧光斑点"。

At present, there are 229 Chinese patent medicines containing Fuling or its processed product, and 219 are recorded in the *Pharmacopoeia of the People's Republic of China*. Among them, prescriptions with Fuling as sovereign or major medicinal are as follows: Guizhi Fuling (Capsules, Tablets or Pills), Sijunzi Tang (Decoction), Wuling San (Powder), etc. In the preparations without taking Fuling as sovereign medicinal are as follows: Sanjiu Weitai Keli, Xiao'er Xieli Pian (Tablets) and Xiao'er Suxieting Keli. In the process of quality control of Chinese patent medicines, microscopic identification and TLC are mostly used to determine whether there is Fuling. Under microscope, Fuling shows as "colorless granular or irregular branched block mass, and colorless or light brown mycelium which is long and thin, slight winding with branches, 4~6μm in diameter". TLC is based on control medicinal materials as the standard, showing fluorescent spots of the same color on the corresponding position of the chromatogram.

【制药】
[Pharmacy]

一、产地加工
I Processing in Production Area

挖出后除去泥沙，针对不同的炮制品，采取不同的产地工艺。堆置"发汗"后，摊开晾至表面干燥，再"发汗"，反复数次至现皱纹、内部水分大部散失后，阴干，称为"茯苓个"；或将鲜茯苓按不同部位切制，阴干，分别称为"茯苓块"和"茯苓片"。

The mud and sand should be removed after digging out Fuling. For different processed products of Fuling, different processing technologies in producing area are used. The "intact Fuling" is usually prepared as follow: Fuling is firstly stacked for "sweating", spread out untill surface dry, and then "sweating" again. Keep repeating the same method several times until most of the water inside is dried and wrinkles appear. Lastly, it is dried in shade, which was called Fuling Ge（singleton）. While "Fuling masses" and "Fuling slices" are usually prepared by cutting the Xianfuling (fresh) according to different parts, and drying it without sunlight.

二、饮片炮制
II Processing of Decoction Pieces

从古至今茯苓逐渐形成了"浸泡-润透-切片"工艺的炮制方法，由此加工的茯苓块和茯苓片为商品规格中的主流。茯苓中间夹有松木的，称为"茯神"。将茯苓片加一定量的朱砂细粉拌匀，即为"朱茯苓"。

Since ancient times, the "soaking-moisturizing-slicing" processing technics of Fuling have been gradually formed, and Fuling masses and Fuling slices processed by such technics have become the popular commodity specifications of Fuling. Fushen refers to the Fuling sandwiched with pine, while Zhufuling is the Fuling slices well mixed with a certain amount of the Zhusha fine powder.

三、中成药制药
III Pharmacy of Chinese Patent Medicines

含茯苓的中成药，剂型十分丰富，涵盖了固体、液体剂型。传统中药制剂中根据临床病症对炮制品加以区分利用。现代中药制剂中多选用生品，其中朱茯苓只宜作丸散剂服用，不宜做汤剂。

There are various kinds of Chinese patent medicines containing Fuling with rich pharmaceutical forms, covering solid and liquid forms.

According to different clinical syndromes, the processed products of Fuling are used respectively in Chinese pharmaceutical preparations. In modern Chinese pharmaceutical preparations, Shengfuling (raw) are usually chosen. Zhufuling can only be used for pills and powder, and it is not suitable in decoction.

如以茯苓为君药的桂枝茯苓胶囊，其制备过程采用部分茯苓粉碎成细粉，部分茯苓乙醇提取浓缩，制成的胶囊保留制剂中茯苓所含的多糖类、脂肪酸类和少部分脂溶性成分，达到活血、化瘀、消癥目的，又减少服用剂量，提高患者顺应性。如在肾炎舒片制备工艺中，茯苓通过水煎煮，保留茯苓素的利尿作用，达到益肾健脾，利水消肿之功效。

For example, in the preparation process of the Chinese patent medicine Guizhi Fuling Jiaonang (Capsules), Fuling as the sovereign medicinal, some Fuling is ground into fine powder, the other are extracted with ethanol and concentrated. The capsules prepared with the method above mentioned retain the components of Fuling such as the polysaccharide, fatty acids and some liposoluble constituents, which can activate blood, resolve stasis and mass. Furthermore, for the dose of the capsule, patients need to take is less, thereby raising patient's compliance. In the preparation of Shenyanshu Pian (Tablets), in order to retain the diuretic effect of poriatin, Fuling is decocted with water. In this way, the tablets achieve the effects of tonifying kidney and invigorating spleen, and inducing diuresis for removing edema.

【性能功效】
[Property and Efficacy]

一、性能
I Property

茯苓甘、淡、平。归心、肺、脾、肾经。

Fuling is sweet and bland in flavor, neutral in nature, and enters the heart, lung, spleen and kidney meridians.

二、功效
II Efficacy

1. **利水渗湿**　茯苓甘淡，淡能渗湿利水，药性平和，适用于寒热虚实各种水肿，故为利水渗湿之要药。其功效的发挥与利尿等药理作用密切相关。茯苓的有效物质基础是茯苓素，可调节机体水盐代谢，通过拮抗醛固酮活性，提高尿中 Na^+/K^+ 比值，激活机体对 Na^+-K^+-ATP 酶和细胞总 ATP 酶活性发挥作用。

1 Promoting Urination and Draining Dampness

Fuling is sweet and bland in flavor, and medicinals with bland flavor often can promote urination and drain dampness. Furthermore, it is neutral in property, so it can be used for all kinds of edema, no matter owing to cold or heat, deficiency or excess. Therefore, it is regarded as "the first medicinal to promote urination and drain dampness". The function of Fuling is closely related to its diuretic effect. Poriatin is the effective material basis for its diuretic effect, which works by regulating the metabolism of water and salt in the body, antagonizing aldosterone activity, increasing the ratio of Na^+/K^+ in the urine, and activating the activities of Na^+-K^+-ATP enzyme and total cellular ATPase.

2. **健脾**　茯苓甘淡，淡能利水渗湿以健脾，甘能补中健脾。其功效的发挥与其保护胃肠功能、抗胃溃疡、保肝、增强免疫、抗炎等药理作用密切相关。茯苓保护胃肠、增强免疫的有效物质基础主要是茯苓多糖和茯苓素，通过松弛胃肠平滑肌，抑制胃液分泌，改善代谢障碍，增强体液免疫和细胞免疫能力等发挥作用。

2 Invigorating Spleen

Fuling is sweet and bland in flavor. The medicinals with bland flavor can often promote urination and drain dampness to invigorate spleen, and those with sweet flavor can tonify the middle energizer and invigorate spleen. The function of Fuling is closely related to its pharmacological effects such as protecting gastrointestinal functions, resisting gastric ulcer, protecting liver functions, improving immunity, resisting inflammation, etc. Polysaccharides and poriatin are the effective material bases for the effects such as protecting gastrointestinal functions and enhancing immunity, which work through relaxing gastrointestinal smooth muscle, inhibiting gastric juice secretion, improving metabolic disorders, enhancing humoral immunity and cellular immunity.

3. **宁心安神** 茯苓性甘淡，甘能补，入心脾、益心脾而宁心安神；味淡能渗湿，水湿不能上凌于心。功效的发挥与其镇静等药理作用密切相关。茯苓镇静的有效物质基础主要是多糖类成分，通过抑制神经中枢，抑制机体自发活动和过度兴奋发挥作用。

3 Tranquilizing the Mind

Fuling is sweet and bland in flavor. With sweet flavor, it has tonifying functions and by entering heart and spleen, it can tonify them so as to tranquilize the mind. While with bland flavor, it can drain dampness and avoid it to interfere upward the heart. The function of Fuling is closely related to its sedative effect. Polysaccharides are the effective material bases for its sedation effect, which work through inhibiting the nerve center so as to inhibit the spontaneous activity and excessive excitation of the body.

此外，现代研究显示茯苓具有延缓衰老、抗肿瘤、抗炎、抗菌、抗诱变等作用。

Besides, modern research shows that Fuling also has anti-aging, anti-tumor, anti-inflammatory, anti-bacterial, and anti-mutagenesis effects, etc.

【应用】
[Applications]

一、主治病证
I Indications

1. **小便不利、水肿、泄泻、痰饮、带下证** 治疗水湿所致的小便不利、水肿、泄泻、痰饮、带下证，茯苓常与猪苓、泽泻、白术等配伍，以增强利水消肿之效。若水湿壅滞，水肿、小便不利，可配伍猪苓、泽泻、白术，如《伤寒论》五苓散和现代制剂肾炎消肿片；若寒湿停滞，脾肾阳虚水肿，可配伍附子、干姜、桂枝等温里助阳药，以温阳利水，如《医学心悟》茯苓升麻汤；若脾虚湿盛的泄泻、水肿、带下等，可配伍人参、白术、薏苡仁，如《太平惠民和剂局方》参苓白术散；若湿热带下，可配伍黄柏、车前子、泽泻以清利湿热；若湿痰咳嗽，可配伍半夏、天南星、橘皮以除湿化痰。

1 Dysuria, Edema, Diarrhea, Phlegm and Fluid Retention and Leukorrheal Syndromes

When Fuling is used in the treatment of dysuria, edema, diarrhea, phlegm and fluid retention and leukorrheal syndomes which originate from dampness, it can be combined with Zhuling, Zexie and Baizhu to enhance the function of inducing diuresis for removing edema. For the edema and dysuria caused by dampness stagnation, Fuling can be combined with Zhuling, Zexie and Baizhu, such as Wuling San (Powder) in *Shanghan Zabing Lun*, and Shenyan Xiaozhong Pian (Tablets) as a modern Chinese pharmaceutical preparation. Used in the treatment of edema caused by cold-dampness retention and spleen-kidney yang deficiency, Fuling can be combined with Fuzi, Ganjiang, Guizhi and other interior-warming and yang-assisting medicinals to warm yang and excrete water, such as Fuling Shengma Tang (Decoction) in *Yixue Xinwu*. Fuling can be combined with Renshen, Baizhu and Yiyiren for the treatment of diarrhea, edema and leukorrheal diseases due to spleen deficiency and dampness exuberance, such as Shenling Baizhu San (Powder) in *Taiping Huimin Heji Ju Fang*. Fuling can be combined with Huangbo, Cheqianzi, and Zexie to treat dampness-heat leukorrhea by clearing heat-dampness. Fuling can be combined with Banxia, Tiannanxing, Jupi to treat cough due to dampness-phlegm by eliminating dampness and dissolving phlegm.

现代临床，茯苓配伍常用于治疗心源性水肿、肾炎水肿、非特异性水肿，如胃苓丸、苓桂阿胶汤、四君子汤。

In modern clinical practice, Fuling compatibility is often used to treat cardiogenic edema, nephritis edema and non-specific edema, such as in Weiling Wan, Linggui Ejiao Tang (Decoction) and Sijunzi Tang (Decoction).

2. 脾虚证　治疗脾虚证，茯苓常与人参、桂枝、白术、山楂配伍，以治疗脾气虚弱、运化失调之证。若脾胃虚弱，食少纳差，倦怠乏力，可配伍人参、白术，如《太平惠民和剂局方》四君子汤；若脾阳不运，水湿停蓄，痰饮咳嗽，可配伍桂枝、白术，如《伤寒论》苓桂术甘汤；若脾胃虚弱，食不消化，腹胀便溏，可配伍人参、白术、山楂、神曲以补脾胃。

2 Spleen Deficiency Syndrome

When Fuling is used in the treatment of spleen deficiency with disharmony of transportation and transformation, it is usually combined with Renshen, Guizhi, Baizhu and Shanzha. Fuling can be combined with Renshen and Baizhu for the treatment of deficiency of spleen and stomach related with poor appetite, lassitude and lack of strength, such as in Sijunzi Tang (Decoction) in *Taiping Huimin Heji Ju Fang*. Fuling can also be combined with Guizhi and Baizhu for the treatment of phlegm-fluid cough due to water-dampness retention caused by spleen yang failing in transportation, such as in Linggui Zhugan Tang (Decoction) in *Shanghan Lun*. Fuling can be combined with Renshen, Baizhu, Shanzha and Shenqu to treat indigestion, abdominal distension and loose stool due to spleen-stomach deficiency by invigorating spleen and stomach.

现代临床，茯苓配伍常用于治疗脾胃虚弱而食欲不振、阳虚衰而食滞、脾胃阳虚有寒而运化受阻等的消化系统疾病，如异功散、理苓汤、理中散。

In modern clinical practice, Fuling compatibility is often used to treat digestive system diseases which include poor appetite due to deficiency of spleen and stomach, food retention due to yang deficiency, inhibited transportation and transformation due to spleen-stomach yang deficiency with cold, such as in Yigong San (Powder), Liling Tang (Decoction) and Lizhong San (Powder).

3. 心神不宁证　治疗心神不宁，茯苓常与人参、当归、酸枣仁等配伍，以治疗心悸、失眠、多梦、健忘等证。若心肝血虚，虚烦不寐，可配伍酸枣仁、柏子仁，如《世医得效方》天王补心丹；若心脾两虚，气血不足，心神不宁，心悸，健忘，可配伍人参、当归、酸枣仁，如《医学心悟》安神定志丸。

3 Syndrome of the Heart-mind Restlessness

Fuling is used in the treatment for the heart-mind restlessness usually by combining with Renshen, Danggui and Suanzaoren, manifesting as palpitations, insomnia, dreaminess and amnesia. Fuling can also be combined with Suanzaoren and Baiziren for the treatment of dysphoric insomnia due to heart-liver blood deficiency, such as Tianwang Buxin Dan (Pills) in *Shiyi Dexiaofang (Effective Prescriptions Handed Down for Generations of Physicians)*. Besides, used in the treatment of heart-mind restlessness, palpitation and amnesia due to deficiency of qi and blood caused by heart-spleen deficiency, Fuling can be combined with Renshen, Danggui and Suanzaoren, such as in Anshen Dingzhi Wan in *Yixue Xinwu*.

现代临床，茯苓配伍常用于治疗心悸气短、眩晕虚烦等，如铁砂汤。

In modern clinical practice, Fuling compatibility is often used to treat palpitation, short breath, vertigo and restlessness, such as Tiesha Tang (Decoction).

二、用法与用量
II Administration and Dosage

9~15g，煎服。
9~15g, water decoction.

三、注意事项
III Precautions

阴虚无湿热、虚寒滑精、气虚下陷者慎用。

The patients with syndrome of yin deficiency who have no manifestations of dampness-heat, deficiency-cold spontaneous seminal emission, and those with qi deficiency and sinking should use Fuling with cautions.

茵　陈

Yinchen
(Artemisiae Scopariae Herba)

茵陈以陕西为道地产区。茵陈味苦、辛，性微寒，归脾、胃、肝、胆经，具清利湿热、利胆退黄功效，主治湿热黄疸、寒湿阴黄、湿热疮疹证。茵陈主要含香豆精、挥发油、黄酮、有机酸类等成分，有利胆、保肝、利尿、解热、镇痛、抗炎、降血压、降血脂、抗动脉粥样硬化、抗病原微生物、抗肿瘤、兴奋平滑肌等药理作用，可用于治疗黄疸、皮肤感染性疾病、感冒、高脂蛋白血症、胆绞痛、中暑、胸闷、腹痛、消化不良、水肿、月经不调和白带异常等属湿热内蕴或温热下注者。

The genuine region of Yinchen is Shanxi province. Yinchen is slight cold in property, bitter and pungent in flavor, it enters the spleen, stomach, liver and gallbladder meridians. It has the effects of clearing and draining dampness-heat, draining-bile and resisting jaudice. Yinchen can be mainly used to treat the syndromes of jaundice due to dampness-heat, yin jaundice due to cold-dampness, sore and eruption due to dampness-heat. Yinchen mainly contains coumarins, essential oils, flavones, organic acids, which possess various pharmacological effects, such as draining gallbladder, protecting liver, diuresis, resisting fever, analgesia, resisting inflammatory, decreasing blood pressure and blood lipids, resisting atherosclerosis, resisting pathogen microorganism, resisting tumor, exciting smooth muscle, etc. It can be used to treat syndrome of internal retention of dampness-heat or warm-heat in lower energizer such as jaundice, skin infectious, common cold, hyperlipoprotememia, gallbladder pain, summerheat stroke, oppression in the chest, abdominal pain, indigestion, edema, irregular menstruation and abnormal leucorrhea, etc..

【品种品质】
[Variety and Quality]

一、基原品种与品质
I Origin Varieties and Quality

1. 品种概况　来源于菊科植物滨蒿 *Artemisia scoparia* Waldst. et Kit. 或茵陈蒿 *Artemisiacapillaris* Thunb. 的干燥地上部分。

1 Variety

Yinchen is the dried ground portion of *Artemisia scoparia* Waldst. et Kit. or *Artemisia. Capillaries* Thunb. from Asteraceae.

茵陈首载于《神农本草经》。《名医别录》、《本草经集注》和《本草拾遗》等记载茵陈与菊科的两个近缘品种滨蒿和茵陈蒿相似。

Yinchen is first recorded in the book of *Shennong Bencao Jing*. According to the records in *Mingyi Bielu*, *Bencaojing Jizhu* and *Bencao Shiyi*, there is a similarity between Yinchen and two allied species of *Artemisia scoparia* Waldst.

et Kit. and *Artemisia. Capillaries* Thunb. from Asteraceae.

2. **种植采收**　茵陈以野生型为主，主产于陕西、山西、安徽等地。茵陈一年可采收2次，春季采收的习称"绵茵陈"，秋季采割的称"花茵陈"或"茵陈蒿"。采收时除去杂质及老茎，晒干生用。

2 Planting and Harvesting

Wild type is the main species of Yinchen in market, which mainly produced in Shaanxi, Shanxi, Anhui, etc. Yinchen is harvested twice a year. The one harvested in the spring is called "Mianyinchen", while "Yinchenhao" or "Huayinchen" harvested in the autumn. As soon as it is harvested, its impurities and old stems should be removed, dried for raw using.

3. **道地性及品质评价**　历代本草记载，陕西为茵陈的道地产区。绵茵陈形态上"多卷曲呈团状，茎细小"，颜色上"灰绿色，全体密被白色茸毛"，质"脆易折断，绵软如绒"，气"清香"，味"微苦"者为佳；花茵陈形态上"瘦果长圆形"，颜色上"黄棕色"，质"脆"体"轻"，气"芳香"，味"微苦"者为佳。现代还增加了绵茵陈以绿原酸、花茵陈以滨蒿内酯的含量测定等化学评价。

3 Genuineness and Quality Evaluation

According to historical records, Shaanxi province is the genuine producing area of Yinchen. Mianyinchen is better to have "most curl into lumps" and "small stem" in shape, "grey-green" and "the whole body covered with fine hair" in color, "fragile and easily broke" and "soft and like-velvet" in texture, "delicate fragrance" in smell and "slightly bitter" in flavor. While Huayinchen is better to have "achenium" and "long circular" in shape, "yellow-brown" in color, "fragile" in texture, "slight" in weight, "delicate fragrance" in smell and "slightly bitter" in flavor. Currently, the chemical character indexes evaluation adds the chlorogenic acid content of Mianyinchen and the escoparone content of Huayinchen.

茵陈主要含有香豆精、挥发油、黄酮、多肽、有机酸类、微量元素和维生素等成分，因其药材来源、生长期、部位等不同存在明显差异，幼苗至花前期的主要有效成分为绿原酸，花穗期的主要有效成分为6,7-二甲基香豆素。一般认为绿原酸、6,7-二甲基香豆素和挥发油是茵陈的主要药效物质基础，其中6,7-二甲基香豆素是利胆保肝、解热、镇痛、抗炎、降血脂、抗动脉粥样硬化的主要物质基础，绿原酸、黄酮和挥发油是抗病原微生物感染的主要物质基础，挥发油是降血压的主要物质基础。《中华人民共和国药典》2020年版规定绵茵陈药材含绿原酸（$C_{16}H_{18}O_9$）不得少于0.50%，花茵陈含滨蒿内酯（$C_{11}H_{10}O_4$）不得少于0.20%。

Yinchen mainly contains coumarin, volatile oil, flavonoids, polypeptide, organic acids, trace elements and vitamins, etc. The chemical compositions of Yinchen vary due to different origins, periods of growth and positions. The main active ingredient from seedling to pre-flower stage is chlorogenic acid, while 6,7-dimethyl coumarin during flower sprouting. It is generally believed that chlorogenic acid and 6,7-dimethyl coumarin are the therapeutic material basis of Yinchen, among which 6,7-dimethyl coumarin is the major material basis for draining bile, protecting liver, antipyretic, analgesia, anti-inflammatory, reducing blood lipids, and anti-atherosclerosis effects. And organic acids, flavonoids and volatile oil are the major material basis for anti-pathogen microorganism effect. However, the volatile oil is the major material basis for reducing blood pressure. According to the *Pharmacopoeia of the People's Republic of China*, the total amount of chlorogenic acid ($C_{16}H_{18}O_9$) in Mianyinchen materials should not be less than 0.50%, and the content of escoparone ($C_{11}H_{10}O_4$) in Huayinchen materials should not be less than 0.20%.

二、炮制品种与品质
II Processed Varieties and Quality

茵陈炮制品种有1种，流通品种有2种。饮

片的品质评价同药材。

There is one processed product of Yinchen, and 2 varieties are available in market. The quality evaluation of Yinchen decoction pieces is the same as that of Yinchen medicinal materials.

三、中成药品种与品质
III Varieties and Quality of Chinese Patent Medicines

含茵陈（包括茵陈提取物）或其炮制品的中成药共计30余个，其中药典收载31个。以茵陈为主药或君药的品种有茵芪肝复颗粒、茵栀黄（颗粒、口服液、软胶囊、胶囊、泡腾片），非以茵陈为君药的制剂如桑葛降脂丸、养正消积胶囊、痔炎消颗粒等。在中成药的品质控制中，若为茵陈药材，多采用薄层色谱法以"对照药材为标准，在色谱相应的位置上显相同颜色的荧光斑点"鉴定茵陈的存在。若为茵陈提取物，以茵陈药材为对照，采用薄层色谱法和含量测定法进行指标成分限量，其中薄层色谱法通过鉴别蓝色荧光斑点确定茵陈的存在，含量测定法采用高效液相色谱法测定对羟基苯乙酮或绿原酸含量限定每个最小规格（粒）中有效成分的下限以保证作用。

At present, there are more than 30 Chinese patent medicines containing Yinchen and its extracts or its processed products, and 31 are recorded in the *Pharmacopoeia of the People's Republic of China*. Among which, prescriptions with Yinchen as sovereign medicinal are as follows: Yinqi Ganfu Keli, Yinzhihuang [Keli, Koufuye, Ruanjiaonang (Soft Capsules), Jiaonang (Capsules) or Paotengpian (Effervescent Tablets)], etc. In the preparations not taking Yinchen as sovereign medicinal, there are Sangge Jiangzhi Wan, Yangzheng Xiaoji Jiaonang (Capsules) and Zhiyanxiao Keli, and so on. In the quality control of Chinese patent medicines, if it is Yinchen medicinal materials, TLC is often used to identify the existence of Yinchen with "reference medicinal materials as the standard, showing the same color

fluorescent spots on the corresponding positions of the chromatogram". If it is an extract of Yinchen, take Yinchen medicinal materials as the control, and use TCL and content determination method to limit the index components, in which TLC determines the existence of Yinchen by identifying blue fluorescent spots, and the content determination method adopts HPLC to determine the content of p-hydroxyacetophenone or chlorogenic acid to limit the lower limit of the effective ingredients in each minimum size (grain) to ensure the effect.

【制药】
[Pharmacy]

一、产地加工
I Processing in Production Area

茵陈收割后净制，拣去残根、老梗和杂质，晾晒，切制。应"抢水洗、抢天晒、抢瓷藏"，以防腐烂；忌大火炮制，以防挥发油成分丢失。

After being harvested, Yinchen is cleansed by removing residual root, old stem and impurity. Then cleansed Yinchen is dried and cut. Yinchen should be timely washed, dried in the sun and preserved in porcelain jar to prevent rot. To prevent loss of essential oil, strong fire should not be used when Yinchen is processed.

二、饮片炮制
II Processing of Decoction Pieces

古代茵陈的炮制方法较多，如南朝有去根细剉法，宋代增加了焙制、酒制，元代又有酒炒和去枝，叶手搓碎用，明代有酒浸制、酒洗法、醋制。现代饮片主要通过除去残根和杂质，搓碎和切碎，绵茵陈筛去灰屑。

In ancient times, there are more processing methods such as removing root by filing in Southern dynasty, processing with baking or liquor in Song dynasty, stir-frying with liquor, getting rid of branch and triturating leaves by hand in Yuan dynasty, soaking with liquor, washing with liquor and processing with vinegar in Ming dynasty. In modern times, Yinchen decoction pieces are also processed by removing residual root and impurity, triturating and cutting, screening out dust and crumbs of Mianyinchen.

三、中成药制药
III Pharmacy of Chinese Patent Medicines

含茵陈的中成药，剂型十分丰富，涵盖了固体、液体和半固体剂型。传统中药制剂中多选用茵陈及其炮制品。现代中药制剂多选用生茵陈或茵陈提取物。

There are various kinds of Chinese patent medicine containing Yinchen, covering preparations of solid, liquid and semi-solid. Yinchen and its processed products can be often used in the application of Chinese pharmaceutical preparations. However, Shengyinchen or its extracts are mostly chosen in modern Chinese pharmaceutical preparations.

如以茵陈为君药的黄疸肝炎丸，其制备过程采用茵陈粉碎成细粉而入药，将含有茵陈和其他中药细粉加工制成蜜丸，制成的蜜丸在体内溶散缓慢，使茵陈有效成分发挥缓慢而持久的舒肝理气、利胆退黄作用。在茵栀黄口服液制剂工艺中，取茵陈的水煎液和70%乙醇提取物制备的混合提取物，保留水溶性和部分脂溶性成分，达到口服液制剂要求。

For example, as sovereign medicinal used in the Chinese patent Medicine - Huangdan Ganyan Wan, Yinchen is crushed into fine powder in the preparation processing. Because honey pills can slowly dissolve in the body, the fine powder of Yinchen and other medicinals are processed into honey pills, and the active components of Yinchen play a slow and lasting role in soothing the liver and regulating qi, draining bile, resisting icterus. To meet the requirements of oral liquid preparation, the mixture extracts of Yinchen decoction and 70% ethanol was prepared to retain water-soluble and partially fat-soluble components in Yinzhihuang Koufuye.

【性能功效】
[Property and Efficacy]

一、性能
I Property

茵陈苦、辛，微寒。归脾、胃、肝、胆经。

Yinchen is bitter and pungent in flavor, slight cold in nature, and enters the spleen, stomach, liver and gallbladder meridians.

二、功效
II Efficacy

1. **清利湿热**　茵陈苦寒清热，尤善清理肝胆湿热。其功效的发挥与解热、镇痛、抗炎、抗病原微生物、杀虫和增强免疫等药理作用相关。茵陈解热、镇痛、抗炎、抗病原微生物、增强免疫的有效物质基础主要是6,7-二甲氧基香豆精、黄酮、挥发油和绿原酸，通过抑制或杀灭细菌和病毒发挥抗病原微生物作用；并通过降低 IL-2 水平，升高 IL-4 水平，使 Th1/Th2 平衡状态向 Th2 细胞因子转化发挥增强免疫功能作用。

1 Clearing and Draining Dampness-heat

Yinchen is bitter and cold, which can clear heat especially in liver- gallbladder dampness-heat. The function of Yinchen is closely related to its pharmacological effects such as antipyretic, analgesic, anti-inflammatory, anti-pathogen microorganism, insecticidal activity and enhancing immune function etc. 6,7-dimethoxy coumarin, flavonoids, essential oils and chlorogenic acids are the effective material basis for antipyretic, analgesic, anti-inflammatory, anti-pathogenic microorganisms and enhancing immune action. Yinchen appears the effects of anti-pathogenic microorganisms through inhibiting or killing microorganisms, enhancing immune function through reducing IL-2 level and increasing IL-4 level which make Thl/Th2 balance transform to Th2 cytokines.

2. **利胆退黄** 茵陈苦寒降泄, 利胆退黄, 为治黄疸之要药。其功效的发挥与保肝、利胆、利尿、降血脂等药理作用密切相关。茵陈利胆退黄的有效物质基础主要是 6,7- 二甲氧基香豆素、茵陈色原酮、绿原酸、咖啡酸, 通过抗肝细胞氧化损伤和促进肝细胞再生发挥保肝利胆作用。

2 Draining Bile to Eliminate Jaudice

Yinchen is bitter and cold which can rush down, draining bile to eliminate jaudice, so it has been honored as "the first medicinal for treating jaundice". The function of Yinchen is closely related to its pharmacological effects such as liver-protecting, bile-draining, diuresis and blood-lipid-reducing etc. The effective material basis for draining bile to eliminate jaudice is 6,7-dimethoxy coumarin, capillarisin, chlorogenic acids and caffeic acid, which can prevent oxidative damage of hepatocyte and promote hepatocyte regeneration to protect liver and drain bile.

此外, 现代研究显示茵陈具有抗肿瘤、降血压、降血脂、兴奋子宫等作用。

Besides, modern research showed that Yinchen has the effects of anti-tumor, lowering blood pressure, decreasing blood lipid, and exciting uterus, etc.

【应用】
[Applications]

一、主治病证
I Indications

1. **黄疸** 治疗黄疸, 茵陈常与大黄、栀子等配伍, 以增强清热利湿之功, 如《伤寒论》茵陈蒿汤; 若湿邪偏盛, 小便不利, 可配伍茯苓、猪苓、泽泻, 如《金匮要略》茵陈五苓散; 若寒湿郁滞, 黄色晦暗, 畏寒腹胀之阴黄, 可与干姜、附子同用以温阳祛湿利黄疸, 如《卫生宝

鉴·补遗》茵陈四逆汤和现代制剂茵陈术附汤; 若阳黄可配伍石膏、栀子, 如《外台秘要》三物茵陈蒿汤; 若血黄, 可配伍桃仁; 若食积发黄, 可配伍枳实、山楂。

1 Jaundice

To enhance the effects of clearing heat and draining dampness, Yinchen can be often combined with Dahuang or Zhizi for the treatment of jaundice, such as Yinchenhao Tang (Decoction) recorded in *Shanghan Lun*. Yinchen can be combined with Fuling, Zhuling and Zexie for the treatment of syndromes of dampness pathogen exuberance and dysuria, such as Yinchen Wuling San (Power) in *Jinkui Yaolue (Synopsis of the Golden Chamber)*. If the patients with syndrome of yin jaundice due to cold-dampness stagnation, dim complexion and abdominal distension with fear of cold, Yinchen can be combined with Ganjiang and Fuzi to drain jaundice by warming yang and dispelling dampness, such as Yinchen Sini Tang (Decoction) in *Weishengbaojianbuyi (Supplement to the Precious Mirror of Health)* and Yinchen Zhufu Tang (Decoction) in modern Chinese pharmaceutical preparations. For the patients with syndrome of yang jaundice, Yinchen can be combined with Shigao and Zhizi such as Sanwu Yinchenhao Tang (Decoction) in *Waitai Miyao*. And for the patients with syndrome of blood jaundice, Yinchen can be combined with Taoren. While combined with Zhishi and Shanzha, yinchen can treat jaundice due to food accumulation.

现代临床, 茵陈配伍常用于治疗急性传染性黄疸型肝炎、新生儿黄疸、肝胆结石、胆囊炎、病毒性肝炎、急慢性肝炎等属于肝胆湿热蕴结者, 如清肝利胆口服液、茵莲清肝合剂; 治疗高血脂、高胆固醇、痰瘀互结等属于脾虚湿停者, 如茵栀降脂片、降脂减肥胶囊。

In modern clinical practice, Yinchen compatibility is commonly applied to treat syndromes of accumulated dampness-heat of liver and gallbladder, which refers to acute infectious jaundice hepatitis, jaundice in the new born infant, stone of liver and gallbladder, cholecystitis, viral hepatitis, acute and chronic hepatitis, such as in Qinggan Lidan Koufuye, Yinlian Qinggan Heji. Yinchen compatibility is also commonly applied to treat syndromes of spleen deficiency with dampness retention, which refers to hyperlipidemia, and hypercholesterolemia, and intermingled phlegm and stasis, such as Yinzhi Jiangzhi Pian (Tablets) and Jiangzhi Jianfei Jiaonang (Capsules).

2. 风瘙隐疹、湿疹、湿疮　治疗湿热蕴结之疮疹瘙痒，可单味煎水外用，如《千金方》茵陈煎汤，洗遍身风痒生疮疥；亦可与黄柏、土茯苓配伍成方内服。因内蕴湿热，复感风寒，郁于皮腠而发的风瘙隐疹，可配伍黄芩、栀子，如《圣济总录》茵陈蒿散；风湿热邪郁于皮肤，接触传染所致的风痒疥疮，与黄柏、苦参、地肤子等同用，煎汤外洗。

2 Syndromes on Urticaria, Dampnesseruption and Dampness-sore

Water Decoction of Yinchen can be applied alone for external application to treat sore, eruption and pruritus due to accumulated dampness-heat, such as Yinchen decoction in *Qianjinfang (Essential Prescriptions Worth a Thousand Gold for Emergencies)* which can be used for patients with pruritus and scabies by washing the whole body, while it can also be combined with Huangbo and Tufuling for oral administration. It can be combined with Huangqin and Zhizi for patients with urticaria due to myocutaneous junction accumulation with internal retention of dampness-heat and recurrence of wind-cold, such as Yinchenhao San (Powder) in *Sheng Ji Zonglu*. However, for patients with pruritus and scabies due to wind-dampness-heat accumulation on the skin or contagious infection, Yinchen combined with Huangbo, Kushen and Difuzi can be decocted for external washing.

现代临床，茵陈配伍可治疗接触传染所致的风痒疥疮、婴儿湿疹、体癣和足癣，如用茵陈配伍青黛、冰片制成散剂，外敷；配合苍黄止痒汤外洗，治疗难治性婴儿湿疹；此外，茵陈挥发油可用于治疗体癣和足癣。

In modern clinical practice, the powder of Yinchen combined with Qingdai and Bingpian can be applied externally to treat contagious infection diseases such as pruritus and scabies, infant eczema, tineacorporis and tineapedis. Yinchen combined with Canghuang Zhiyang Tang (Decoction) can be used to treat refractory infant eczema by external washing. Besides, the volatile oil of Yinchen is also used to treat tinea corporis and tinea pedis.

二、用法用量
II Administration and Dosage

6~15g，外用适量，煎汤熏洗。

6~15g, reasonable dosage for external application, decoction for fumigating and washing.

三、注意事项
III Precautions

1. 脾虚未有湿盛者慎用。

1. The patients with syndrome of spleen deficiency without dampness exuberance should use Yinchen with cautions.

2. 无湿热而发黄由于蓄血者禁用。

2. For those have jaundice without dampness-heat caused by blood-retention, Yinchen should be forbidden to use.

第十四章 温里药
Chapter 14　Warming Interior Medicinals

凡以温里祛寒、治疗里寒证为主要作用的药物，称为温里药，又叫祛寒药。此类药物多味辛性温热，辛散温通，行于脏腑而能温里散寒、温经止痛，某些药物还有回阳救逆、温阳通脉，故可用于治疗里寒证，体现了《黄帝内经》之"寒者热之"和《神农本草经》"疗寒以热药"的中医治则。温里药多辛热燥烈，易耗阴助火，凡实热证、阴虚火旺、津血亏虚者忌用，孕妇及气候炎热时慎用。现代研究表明，温里药多具有强心、抗心律失常、扩张血管、改善血液循环、抗休克、增加交感-肾上腺皮质系统功能、促进胃肠运动、促消化、止吐、抗溃疡、镇痛、抗炎等药理作用。常见的温里药有附子、干姜、肉桂、吴茱萸等。

Warming interior medicinals, also called cold-dispelling medicinals refer to medicinals that can warm the interior to dissipate cold and treat internal cold syndromes. The medicinal properties of warming interior medicinals are normally pungent and warm. The pungent flavor can disperse cold and the warm property helps to pass through the meridian. Thus, warming interior medicinals can warm the internal organs to disperse cold and warm the meridians to relieve pain. Besides, some of the medicinals have the effect of restoring yang to save from collapse and warming yang to promote pulse, and they can be used to treat interior cold syndromes, which reflect the Chinese medicine treatment principle of "treating cold syndrome with heat methods" in *Huangdi Neijing (Huangdi's Internal Classic)* and "treat coldness with hot medicinals" in *Shennong Bencao Jing*. Generally, the interior-warming medicinals have pungent, warm, fiery properties and may easily consume *yin* and tonify fire. Therefore, patients with excessive heat syndrome, syndrome of *yin* deficiency with effulgence fire and blood deficiency should not use it. Medicinals should be used with caution for pregnant women and in hot climate. Modern researches show that the interior-warming medicinals have many pharmacological effects, such as strengthening heart, anti-arrhythmia, expanding blood vessel, improving blood circulation, anti-shock, increasing sympathetic adrenocortical system function, promoting gastrointestinal movement, promoting digestion, resisting vomit, resisting ulcer, relieving pain and anti-inflammation. Fuzi, Ganjiang, Rougui, Wuzhuyu, etc. are commonly-used interior-warming medicinals.

附 子

Fuzi
(Aconiti Lateralis Radix Preparata)

附子是著名的川产道地药材。生附子毒性大，内服时需炮制入药，常用炮制品为黑顺片、白附片，生附子主要用于外用制剂。附子辛甘大热，归心、脾、肾经，具回阳救逆、补火助阳、散寒止痛功效，主治亡阳证、诸阳亏虚证、寒凝诸痛证。附子主要含生物碱、多糖等成分，有强心、抗心律失常、镇痛、抗炎等药理作用，可用于治疗心力衰竭、心律失常、慢性肾功能衰竭、类风湿性关节炎等属寒证者。附子毒性靶器官有心脏、神经、胚胎、胃肠等，可通过依法炮制、对证用药、合理配伍、控制剂量等控毒增效。

Fuzi is a noted genuine regional medicinal in Sichuan. The Shengfuzi is toxic and needs to be processed for oral-taking. The commonly used processed products are Heishun Pian and Baifu Pian and the Shengfuzi is mainly used for external use preparations. Fuzi is pungent and hot in property and sweet in flavor, it enters the heart, lung and kidney meridians. It has the effects of restoring yang and rescuing to save from collapse, tonifying fire to assist yang, dispelling cold and relieving pain. Its indications are syndromes of *yang* collapse, *yang* depletion and cold coagulation and pain. Fuzi mainly contains alkaloid and polysaccharide components, which possess various pharmacological effects, such as strengthening heart, anti-arrhythmia, relieving pain and anti-inflammation etc. It can be used for the treatment of heart failure, arrhythmia, chronic renal failure, rheumatoid arthritis and so on. Target organs of Fuzi toxicity mainly involve the heart, nerve, embryo and gastrointestinal tract. The toxicity can be controlled after processing according to prescribed methods, syndrome differentiation, rational compatibility and controlled dosage.

【品种品质】
[Variety and Quality]

一、基原品种与品质
I Origin Varieties and Quality

1. 品种概况 来源于毛茛科植物乌头 *Aconitum carmichaelii* Debx. 的子根。

附子首载于《神农本草经》称"乌头"，宋代苏颂《图经本草》和杨天惠《彰明附子记》所载"乌头"原植物实为乌头属多种植物的总称，李时珍在《本草纲目》中记载乌头植物可生七品，如乌头、附子、鬲子、天雄、天锥、侧子、漏篮子等，其中附乌头而旁生者为附子。今将乌头的子根统称为附子，而主根称川乌。

1 Variety

Fuzi is derived from the daughter roots of *Aconitum carmichaelii* Debx. (Fam. Ranunculaceae). Fuzi was first recorded in the book of *Shennong Bencao Jing*. According to *Tujing Bencao (Illustration of Meteria Medica)* written by Susong in Song Dynasty and *Zhangming Fuzi Ji (Zhangming's Aconite Biography)* written by Yang Tianhui in Song Dynasty, the original plant of Wutou is actually the general term of various plants of aconitum plants. In *Bencao Gangmu*, Li Shizhen recorded that there were seven kinds of products of aconitum plants, such as Wutou, Fuzi, Gezi, Tianxiong, Tianzhui, Cczi, Loulanzi etc. Among them, Fuzi is the daughter root of aconitum, while the axial root is called Chuanwu.

2. 种植采收 附子以栽培为主，主产于四川青川、北川、布拖等地。一般采用"高山引种、平坝栽培"，种源称乌药。附子种植采收季节随地理、气候不同有明显差异。江油一般冬至下种，夏至采收；其余产地多霜降下种，立秋后采收。刚采挖的附子除去母根、须根及泥沙，习称"泥附子"。

2 Planting and Harvesting

Fuzi is mainly cultivated and produced in Qingchuan, Beichuan, and Butuo in Sichuan province. Generally, the rule of "introducing from high mountains and cultivating in plain" is adopted for the planting of Fuzi. The provenance of Fuzi is called Wuyao (Linderae Radix). The time of planting and harvest of Fuzi vary due to different geography and climate features. It is generally planted in the winter solstice and harvested in the summer solstice in Jiangyou. In other areas, it is planted in the Frost's Descent and harvested after the autumn begins. As soon as Fuzi is harvested, its parent root, fibrous roots and sediment shall be removed, and the Fuzi at that situation is often called "Nifuzi".

3. 道地性及品质评价　自古以来四川江油地区是附子的道地产区。古人从形、色、气、味等方面提出了泥附子性状评价指标，形态上以"底平"、"体圆"者为佳，颜色上以"皮黑"、"肉花白"为佳，重量上认为"一个重一两，即是气全，堪用"。附子主要含有生物碱类，其中双酯型生物碱（如乌头碱）和单酯型生物碱（如苯甲酰乌头碱）为脂溶性生物碱，醇胺型生物碱（如乌头原碱）具有一定的水溶性，生物碱盐和小分子的生物碱苷为水溶性生物碱，如盐酸去甲乌药碱。一般认为，总生物碱是附子的药效物质基础，其中水溶性生物碱是强心的主要物质基础、脂溶性生物碱既是镇痛的主要物质基础，也是导致毒性的主要物质基础。此外，附子还含有多糖、甾醇、微量元素等。按药典规定，附子中含双酯型生物碱以新乌头碱、次乌头碱和乌头碱计总量不得过0.020%，含苯甲酰新乌头原碱、苯甲酰乌头原碱、苯甲酰次乌头原碱总量不得少于0.010%。

3 Genuineness and Quality Evaluation

According to historical records, Jiangyou in Sichuan province is the genuine production place of Fuzi. The ancients proposed the evaluation indexes of characters of Nifuzi from the aspects of shape, color, flavor and taste. It is better to have "flat bottom" and "round body" in shape, and "black skin" and "white flesh" in color. In terms of weight, more than 50g is considered as having enough qi and can be used. Fuzi mainly contains alkaloids. Among them, diester alkaloids (such as aconitine) and monoester alkaloids (such as benzoylaconitine) are liposoluble alkaloids. Alcohol amine alkaloids (such as aconine) possess certain water solubility. Alkaloid salts and small molecule alkaloid glycosides are water-soluble alkaloids, such as demethylaconitine hydrochloride. It is generally believed that total alkaloids are the therapeutic material basis of Fuzi. Water-soluble alkaloids are the major material basis for cardiotonic effect. Diester alkaloids are the major material basis for the analgesic effect and the main toxic material basis of Fuzi as well. In addition, Fuzi also contains polysaccharides, sterols and trace elements etc. According to *Pharmacopoeia of the People's Republic of China*, the total contents of neoaconitine, aconitine, hypaconitine in Fuzi shall not be higher than 0.020%. The total contents of benzoylneoaconine, benzoylaconine and benzoylhypaconine shall not be lower than 0.01%.

二、炮制品种与品质
II Processed Varieties and Quality

附子的炮制品种有30多个，临床常用有20余种，如中间体盐附子，以及黑顺片、白附片、淡附片、熟附片、蒸附片、炒附片、炮附片、炮附子、刨附片、配方颗粒等。盐附子以个大、体重、色灰黑、表面起盐霜者为佳；黑顺片以皮黑褐、切面油润有光泽者为佳；白附片以片大、色黄白、油润半透明者为佳；炮附片以片大、油润者为佳；淡附片以切面油润有光泽者为佳。不同炮制品的含量测定要求同附子药材。

There are more than 30 processed products of Fuzi, in which nearly 20 kinds of products are commonly used, such as the processing intermediate-Yanfuzi (processed with salt), Heishunpian, Baifupian, Danfupian, Shufupian, Zhengfupian, Chaofupian, Paofupian, Paofuzi (processed), Baofupian and dispensing granules etc. Yanfuzi with a big size, heavy weight, greyish black color and salty efflorescence surface are considered to have better quality. Heishunpian with dark brown skin, oily and glossy section are considered to have better quality. Baifupian with yellow and white color, oily and translucent large flakes are considered to have better quality. Paofupian with large flakes and oily and glossy section are considered to have better quality. Danfupian with oily and glossy sections are considered to have better quality. The content determination requirement for the processed products is the same as required for the raw medicinal above.

三、中成药品种与品质
III Varieties and Quality of Chinese Patent Medicines

含有附子或其炮制品的中成药有 250 余个，其中药典收载 16 个。以附子为君药或主药的品种有参附注射液、附子理中丸、附桂骨痛片（胶囊、颗粒）等。在中成药的品质控制中多采用显微鉴别确定附子的存在，采用薄层色谱法和含量测定法进行指标成分限量。如附桂骨痛片（胶囊、颗粒）中以附子（制）和制川乌为君药，薄层色谱法限定双酯型生物碱的含量，含量测定法限定每个最小规格（片、粒）中有效成分苯甲酰新乌头原碱、苯甲酰乌头原碱和苯甲酰次乌头原碱总量的下限以保证作用；参附注射液中限定每 1ml 含乌头类生物碱以乌头碱计的高限以保证安全性。非以附子为君药的制剂如乌梅丸、济生肾气丸、桂附地黄丸等，通过显微鉴别"糊化淀粉粒团块类白色"确定含有附子。

At present, there are more than 250 Chinese patent medicines containing Fuzi or its processed products and 16 are recorded in *Pharmacopoeia of the People's Republic of China*. Among them, prescriptions with Fuzi as the sovereign medicinal are as follows: Shenfu Zhusheye, Fuzi Lizhong Wan, Fugui Gutong Pian (Tablets), [Jiaonang (Capsules) and Keli], etc. Presently, the existence of Fuzi is mainly determined by microscopic identification, and the content of aconitine in the above Chinese patent medicines is limited by TLC and content determination. For example, in Fugui Gutong Pian (Tablets), Jiaonang (Capsules) and Keli, Fuzi (processed) and Zhichuanwu (processed) are used as sovereign medicinals. The content of diester alkaloids is determined by TLC, and the lower limit of the total amount of benzoylneoaconitine, benzoylaconitine and benzoylhypaconitine in each minimum size (tablet and granule) is determined by content determination method to ensure the effect. The content of alkaloids in Shenfu Zhusheye is limited every 1ml for safety. In the preparations not taking Fuzi as sovereign medicinal, such as Wumei Wan, Jisheng Shenqi Wan and Guifu Dihuang Wan, microscopic identification is applied to identify gelatinized starch granules to confirm the the existence of Fuzi.

【制药】
[Pharmacy]

一、产地加工
I Processing in Production Area

泥附子一般于收获后 24 小时内洗净泥沙、胆巴浸渍，以防腐烂，并降低毒性。然后经浸泡、切片、煮蒸等工序，加工成不同规格的附片。

Within 24 hours after being harvested, Nifuzi should be removed its soil and washed, then soaked in Danba (bittern), to prevent corrosion and reduce toxicity. Then the procedures of soaking, slicing, boiling and steaming will be carried out to produce different specifications of slices.

二、饮片炮制
II Processing of Decoction Pieces

从古至今附子炮制方法繁复。明清以来，江油地区逐渐形成了"泡胆→退胆→煮制→剥皮→切片→蒸制（火烤）"工艺，由此加工的黑顺片、白附片成为商品规格中的主流。

Since ancient times, the processing methods for Fuzi have been complex. The processing technology of "soaking in Danba → removing Danba → boiling → peeling → slicing → steaming (roasting)" has been used in Jiangyou since the Ming Dynasty and Qing Dynasty. Heishunpian and Baifupian processed by this technology have become the mainstream of commodity specifications.

炮制是对有毒中药附子"减毒"的重要手段，其减毒原理是：附子中主要毒性物质双酯型生物碱遇水加热极易水解，先脱去 C_8 乙酰基变为单酯型生物碱，其毒性仅为双酯型生物碱的 1/50~1/500。继续加热水解，脱去 C_{14} 苯甲酰基，转化为水溶性的醇胺类原碱，其毒性仅为双酯型生物碱的 1/2000~1/4000。因此，炮制中的蒸、煮、烘、炒、炮、煨、微波等方法均可降低毒性。

Processing is an important mean to reduce the toxicity of Fuzi and the principle of detoxification of Fuzi is to remove the main toxic substance, diester alkaloid, which is easily hydrolyzed when heated in water. When heated, the C_8 acetyl group of diester alkaloid is removed firstly and converted into monoester alkaloid, remaining only 1/50-1/500 toxicity of that of diester alkaloids. Then, remained heating for longer time, the monoester alkaloids are hydrolyzed to remove C_{14} benzoyl and converted to water-soluble alkanolamine, with only 1/2000-1/4000 toxicity of that of diester alkaloids. Therefore, the toxicity of Fuzi can be reduced by steaming, boiling, baking, stir-frying, blast-frying, roasting and microwaving etc.

三、中成药制药
III Pharmacy of Chinese Patent Medicines

含附子的中成药，剂型十分丰富，涵盖了固体、液体与半固体剂型。传统中药制剂中遵循"丸散炮，惟汤生用"的用药原则。现代中药制剂中内服均选用炮制品，生品不可流通。含附子的传统中成药制剂多制成蜜丸而非水丸。现今为满足现代制剂处方成形性及减少服用剂量，一般制剂如片剂和胶囊剂等多以附子（制）水提取物入制剂中。

There are various kinds of Chinese patent medicines containing Fuzi, covering preparations of solid, liquid and semi-solid types. The principle of "processed products for pills and powder preparations, raw material for decoction only" is considered in the application of Chinese pharmaceutical preparations. In modern Chinese pharmaceutical preparations, processed products are chosen for oral-taking preparations and patent medicine containing raw medicinal of Fuzi is prohibited. The Chinese patent medicines containing Fuzi are mostly made into honey pills instead of water pills. However, to meet the modern prescription forms and reduce the dose in Chinese patent medicines, in general preparations such as tablets and capsules, the water extract of Fuzi (prepared) is usually added into the preparation.

如以附子为君药的附子理中丸，其制备过程采用制附子入药，制成的蜜丸在体内溶散缓慢，确保了安全性。在参附注射液制剂工艺中，因附子中的生物碱类强心成分具有亲水性，故附子多采用水煎法提取；随后对附子液与人参液混合后得到的提取物，采用95%乙醇逐级沉淀和冷藏的方法除去水不溶性成分，同时保留水溶成分，达到注射剂制剂要求。

For example, Fuzi Lizhong Wan, which takes Fuzi as the sovereign medicinal, is prepared by using Zhifuzi as medicinal. Furthermore, it is produced into honey pill which slowly dissolves in the body to ensure security. While in Shenfu Zhusheye, the alkaloids with cardiotonic effect are hydrophillic, so Fuzi in this injection is extracted by water decocting. Then the mixed extracts of Fuzi decoction and Renshen decoction, is processed by 95% ethanol step by step precipitation and refrigeration method to remove water-insoluble ingredients and reserve water soluble matters, so as to meet the requirements of injection preparation.

【性能功效】
[Property and Efficacy]

一、性能
I Property

附子辛、甘、大热；有毒，归心、肾、脾经。

Fuzi is pungent, sweet in flavor, extremely hot in nature, and toxic, and enters the heart, kidney and spleen meridians.

二、功效
II Efficacy

1. 回阳救逆 附子大辛大热，能峻补元阳、驱散阴寒，力挽厥脱，被历代医家尊为"回阳救逆第一品药"。其功效的发挥与强心、抗心律失常、升压、抗休克、抗心肌缺血等药理作用密切相关。附子的强心、抗心律失常作用的有效物质基础主要是水溶性生物碱和多糖类成分，通过作用于心肌细胞上钙、钾等离子通道和α、β受体，调节细胞内外环境稳态，细胞能量代谢等发挥作用。

1 Restoring *Yang* to Save from Collapse

Fuzi, extremely pungent and hot, which is capable of greatly tonifying the original *yang*, dissipating cold, and saving from collapse, has been honored as "the first medicine to restore yang to save from collapse". The function of Fuzi

is closely related to its pharmacological effects such as cardiotonic effect, anti-arrhythmia, blood pressure rising, anti-shock and anti-myocardial ischemia effects, etc. Water-soluble alkaloids and polysaccharides of Fuzi are the active constituents for cardiotonic and anti-arrhythmia effects, with mechanisms of acting on Ca^{2+}, K^+ and other ion channels and α, β receptors on cardiomyocytes, regulating homeostasis of intracellular and extracellular environment, celluar energy metabolism, etc.

2. 补火助阳 附子纯阳辛热，归心、肾、脾经，上助心阳而复脉、中温脾阳而止吐泻、下补肾阳而补真火，加之走而不守，故能助心、脾、肾之阳。其功效的发挥与抗寒冷、耐缺氧、增强免疫功能等药理作用有关，有效物质基础主要是生物碱、多糖。

2 Assisting *Yang* to Tonify Fire

Fuzi is pure yang, pungent and hot in nature. The meridian entries of Fuzi are the heart, lung and kidney. Fuzi can go upward to assist heart yang to restore the pulse, go to the middle to warm the spleen yang to stop vomiting and diarrhea, and go downward to tonify the kidney yang and fill the true fire. For the nature of moving not staticit, Fuzi can assist the heart, spleen and kidney yang. The effect of Fuzi is related to its pharmacological effects, such as, anti-cold, anti-oxidation and enhancing immune functions. Alkaloids and polysaccharides are the active ingredients.

3. 散寒止痛 附子性大热可祛寒，温通经脉，甘可益元阳，益火消阴，故能温通经脉，逐经络寒湿之邪。其功效的发挥与抗炎、镇痛等药理作用密切相关。附子抗炎、镇痛作用的有效物质基础主要是双酯型生物碱，可通过调节炎症因子、兴奋下丘脑-垂体-肾上腺皮质系统和作用于神经系统而发挥作用。

3 Dissipating Cold to Relieve the Pain

Fuzi, with the hot property, can dissipate cold to relieve pain and warmly dredge the meridians. It is sweet in flavor so it can replenish the original yang and fire to disperse yin. Fuzi can also dispel the cold and dampness of meridians. Its effects are closely related to its anti-inflammatory and analgesic effects. The related active constituents are diester alkaloids, which work by regulating inflammatory factors, and activating hypothalamic pituitary adrenocortical system and the nervous system.

此外，现代研究显示附子具有调节血管、抑制胃肠运动、抗肿瘤等作用。

Besides, modern research shows that Fuzi has the effects of regulating blood vessel, inhibiting gastrointestinal motility, and anti-tumor effects, etc.

【应用】
[Applications]

一、主治病证
I Indications

1. 亡阳证 治疗亡阳证，附子常与干姜配伍以回阳救逆，如《伤寒论》四逆汤和现代制剂四逆汤口服液；若元气大亏，阳气暴脱，汗出肢冷、脉微欲绝者，可配伍人参以大补元气，如《严氏济生方》参附汤和现代制剂参附注射液；若阴盛格阳、浮阳上越者，可与干姜、葱白同用以破阴回阳，宣通阳气，如《伤寒论》白通汤。

1 *Yang* Collapse Syndrome

Fuzi can be combined with Ganjiang in compatibility for treatment of *yang* collapse syndrome by restoring yang to save from collapse, such as Sini Tang (Decoction) recorded in *Shanghan Lun* and its mixture of modern preparation. If the patient suffers from the loss of original qi, sudden collapse of *yang* qi, sweat with cold limbs and extremely weak pulse, Fuzi can be combined with Renshen to replenish original qi, such as Shenfu Tang (Decoction) in *Yanshi Jisheng Fang (Yan's Saving Prescription)* and Shenfu Zhusheye in modern times. Patients with symptoms of exuberance yin repelling yang and yang with upper manifestation are suggested to take Fuzi with Ganjiang and Congbai (the white part of Green onion) to break yin to restore yang and invigorate yang qi, such as Baitong Tang (Decoction) in *Shanghan Lun*.

现代临床，附子配伍常用于治疗慢性心功能不全、缓慢型心律失常、冠状动脉心脏病、休克等临床慢性病、危急症属于心阳衰微或亡阳证者，如四逆汤、参附汤。

In modern clinical practice, Fuzi compatibility is often used to treat chronic cardiac insufficiency, slow arrhythmia, coronary heart disease, shock and other clinical chronic diseases, critical symptoms with the heart *yang* decline or *yang* collapse syndrome, such as in Sini Tang (Decoction), Shenfu Tang (Decoction).

2. 心脾肾阳虚证 对心阳虚证见心悸气短者，可与桂枝、甘草等配伍；对脾阳虚证见脘腹冷痛，大便溏泄者，附子可与干姜、白术等配伍以温中补脾，如《阎氏小儿方论》附子理中汤；对肾阳虚证见阳痿滑精、肢冷畏寒、小便自遗者，常与肉桂、熟地等配伍以补肾阳，如《景岳全书》右归丸；对脾肾阳虚证见脘腹冷痛，大便溏泄者，可与白术茯苓等配伍，如《伤寒论》真武汤。

2 Syndrome of Yang Deficiency of Heart, Spleen and Kidney

Fuzi can be combined with Guizhi, Gancao to treat patients with palpation due to *yang* deficiency of heart. For abdominal cold pain, loose stools due to yang deficiency of spleen, Fuzi can be combined with Ganjiang, Baizhu to warm the spleen such as in Fuzi Lizhong Tang (Decoction) in *Yanshi Xiaoer Fanglun (Yanshi Children's Prescription)*. For impotence, night emission, cold limbs, aversion to cold, enuresis due to yang deficiency of kidney, Fuzi can be used in combination of Rougui, Shudi and others to tonify kidney yang, such as Yougui Wan in *Jingyue Quanshu*. For abdominal cold pain, loose stools due to yang deficiency of spleen and kidney, Fuzi can be combined with Baizhu, Fuling, such as Zhenwu Tang (Decoction) in *Shanghan Lun* and etc.

现代临床，附子配伍常用于治疗慢性肾功能

衰竭属于阳虚水泛证者及慢性胃肠炎属于脾肾虚寒证者，前者如真武汤，后者如附子理中丸、大黄附子汤等。

In modern clinical practice, Fuzi compatibility is often applied to treat chronic renal failure of syndrome of water overflowing due to yang deficiency, and chronic gastroenteritis of syndrome of deficient cold of spleen and kidney, such as Zhenwu Tang (Decoction) for the former disease and Fuzi Lizhong Wan, and Dahuang Fuzi Tang (Decoction), etc. for the latter disease.

3. **寒凝疼痛证** 对寒凝心脉之胸痹痛证，可与桂枝配伍，如《伤寒论》桂枝附子汤；对寒湿内结致胁腹疼痛便秘者，可与大黄、细辛等配伍，如《金匮要略》大黄附子汤；对寒凝气滞之痛经，可配伍当归，如《简易方议》小温经汤；对湿痹见阳虚阴盛者，可配川乌、官桂等，如《宣明论方》附子丸等；对寒性疮疽漫肿不溃者，可与黄芪、当归等配伍，扶正托毒，如《外科正宗》回阳三建汤。

3 Syndrome of Coagulated Cold and Pain

The compatibility of Fuzi with Guizhi can be used to treat heart and chest discomfort and pain caused by yang deficiency and cold congelation as shown in Guizhi Fuzi Tang (Decoction) in *Shanghan Lun*. The compatibility of Fuzi with Dahuang and Xixin can be used to treat abdominal pain and constipation caused by internal cold and dampness as in Dahuang Fuzi Tang (Decoction) in *Jinkui Yaolue (Synopsis of the Golden Chamber)*. Fuzi combined with Danggui for treating dysmenorrhea caused by cold congelation and *qi* stagnation as in Xiaowenjing Tang (Decoction) in *Jianyi Fangyi (A Brief Prescription of Discussion)* and with Chuanwu and Guangui for fixed arthralgia with yang deficiency and yin excessiveness as in Fuzi Wan in *Xuan Ming Lun Fang*. For patients with sores due to cold and gangrene, Fuzi can be combined with Huangqi and Danggui to strengthen vital qi and eliminate the toxins as in Huiyang Sanjian Tang (Decoction) in *Waike Zhengzong (Orthodox Manual of External Diseases)*.

现代临床，附子配伍常用于治疗疼痛性疾病（如偏头痛、风湿性关节炎、神经痛、腰腿痛等）属于风寒湿外袭证者，如甘草附子汤。

In modern clinical practice, Fuzi compatibility is applied to treat migraine, rheumatic arthritis, neuralgia, lumbocrural pain and other painful diseases of syndroms of external assault by wind, cold and dampness, such as Gancao Fuzi Tang (Decoction).

二、用法用量
II Administration and Dosage

3~15g，先煎，久煎。
3~15g, decoct first and for a long time.

三、注意事项
III Precautions

1. 附子不宜与半夏、瓜蒌、瓜蒌子、瓜蒌皮、天花粉、川贝母、浙贝母、平贝母、伊贝母、湖北贝母、白蔹、白及及含以上药物的中成药同用。

1 It should not be used with Banxia, Gualou, Gualouzi, Gualoupi, Tianhuafen, Chuanbeimu, Zhebeimu, Pingbeimu, Yibeimu, Hubeibeimu, Bailian, Baiji and Chinese patent medicines containing the above medicinals.

2. 附子为辛热之品，实热证、阴虚火旺、津血亏虚者忌用。

2 As Fuzi is pungent in flavor and hot in property, it should be avoided for patients with syndromes of excessive heat, *yin* deficiency with effulgent fire, fluid and blood deficiency.

3. 附子有生殖、胚胎毒性，故孕妇和哺乳期女性应慎用甚至禁用。

3 Due to the reproductive toxicity and embryotoxicity of Fuzi, women in pregnant and lactation period should use it with cautions or even be forbidden to use.

【知识拓展】
[Knowledge Extension]

附子具有悠久的炮制历史，但炮制不当会导致药效物质的丢失，需规范炮制。现代研究表明，附子具有心脏、神经、胚胎、消化系统等多系统毒性，临床应用可通过选用正品药材、规范炮制、合理配伍、对证用药、延长煎煮时间等控毒方法控制毒性和保证疗效。附子是毛茛科植物乌头的子根，其主根称"川乌"，是临床常用的祛风湿药。

Fuzi has a long history of producing and processing. However, it is necessary to standardize the processing methods; otherwise, therapeutic substances can be lost due to improper processing. Modern research shows that Fuzi is toxic to multiple systems, such as heart, nerve, embryo and digestive systems. In clinical applications, the toxicity of Fuzi can be controlled and its efficacy can be guaranteed by selecting the authentic medicinal materials, standardizing the processing procedure, reasonable compatibility of medicinals, syndrome and syptom-targeted medications and prolonging the decocting time. Fuzi is the root of aconitum, and its main root is called "Chuanwu" and commonly used as wind-dampness dispelling medicinal in clinic.

干 姜

Ganjiang
(Zingiberis Rhizoma)

干姜是川产道地药材。常用的炮制品为干姜、炮姜和姜炭。干姜味辛，热。归脾、胃、肾、心、肺经。有温中散寒，回阳通脉，温肺化饮的功效。可配伍人参、白术、炙甘草、附子、半夏、五味子、麻黄等，治疗脾胃虚寒、亡阳虚脱、寒疝腹痛、肺寒咳嗽诸证。干姜主要含挥发油、姜辣素、二苯基庚烷成分，有镇痛抗炎、抑制血小板聚集、抗菌、抗腹泻、利胆、抗肿瘤等活性。可用于治疗肠炎、腹泻、呕吐、冠心病、心肌梗死、手足龟裂等属于寒证者。

Ganjiang is a famous genuine regional medicinal of Sichuan Province. The main processed products used in clinic are Ganjiang, Paojiang and Jiangtan. The property and flavor of Ganjiang is hot and pungent and it enters the spleen, stomach, kidney, heart and lung meridians. It has the actions of warming spleen and stomach for dispelling cold, restoring yang and promoting blood circulation, warming the lung to resolve fluid retention. It can be combined with Renshen, Baizhu, Zhigancao (processed), Fuzi, Banxia, Wuweizi, Mahuang, etc, to treat deficient cold of spleen and stomach, collapse due to yang depletion, cold hernia, abdominal pain, cough due to cold invading lung. The main chemical compounds of Ganjiang are volatile oil, gingerol, diphenylheptane, and have pharmacological effects including anti-platelet aggregation, anti-inflammation, and analgesic, anti-bacterial, anti-diarrhea, choleretic, anti-tumor and other effects. It can be used to treat the diseases of cold syndrome, such as enteritis, diarrhea, vomiting, coronary heart disease, myocardial infarction, hand and foot crazing, etc.

【品种品质】
[Variety and Quality]

一、基原品种与品质
I Origin Varieties and Quality

1. 品种概况　来源于姜科植物 *Zingiber offcinale* Rosc. 的干燥根茎。

1 Variety

Ganjiang is the dried rhizome of *Zingiber offcinale* Rosc.

干姜首载于《神农本草经》,《本草图经》载:"苗高二、三尺,叶似箭竹而长,两两相对,苗青,根黄,无花实。秋采根,于长流水洗过,日晒为干姜,"与今生姜形态相符。

Ganjiang is first recorded in the book of *Shennong Bencao Jing. Bencao Tujing* states the height of seedling is 2 or 3 feet, leaves are like arrow bamboo and long ,and opposite each other. Its seedling is cyan and root is yellow, with no flower and fruit. Its root is harvested in autumn, washed in the flowing water, and dried in the sun, and thus gets Ganjiang. It is consistent with Shengjiang used currently.

2. 种植采收　四川乐山犍为、山东莱芜等地有种植。姜的种植是无性繁殖,栽培技术用根茎(种姜)繁殖,穴栽或条栽。每年4月份前后种植,10月下旬至12月下旬茎叶枯萎时挖取根茎。

2 Planting and Harvesting

Ganjiang is cultivated in Qianwei county, Leshan city of Sichuan Province, Laiwu of Shandong Province and other places. Ginger (Jiang) planting is asexual propagation, and the cultivation technology is to propagate with rhizome (seed ginger), hole planting or strip planting. It is planted around April every year, and dig out the rhizomes from late October to late December when the stems and leaves wither.

3. 道地性评价及品质评价　历代本草记载,四川乐山市犍为县、湖北荆州、江苏扬州为道地产区。干姜以质坚实、断面色黄白、粉性足、气味浓者为佳。

3 Genuineness and Quality Evaluation

According to historical records, Qianwei County, Leshan city of Sichuan province, Jingzhou city of Hubei province, and Yangzhou city of Jiangsu province are the genuine production places of Ganjiang. The good quality of Ganjiang is characterized of compact texture, yellowish-white section, enough powdering and strong smell.

干姜化学成分主要有三类,挥发油(α- 姜烯)、姜辣素(6- 姜酚、8- 姜酚、6- 姜稀酚)、二苯基庚烷(姜稀酮类)三大类成分。姜酚类成分是干姜辣味的主要物质基础,也是干姜扩张血管,促进血液循环,强心的主要成分。二苯基庚烷是镇吐、抗炎、抗血栓主要药效物质基础。此外干姜还含有少量黄酮类,糖苷类,氨基酸,多种维生素和多种微量元素。《中国药典》规定干姜含挥发油不得少于 0.8%(ml/g),6- 姜辣素($C_{17}H_{26}O_4$)不得少于 0.60%。

There are three main types of chemical constituents of Ganjiang: volatile oils (α-zingerene), gingerol (6-gingerol, 8-gingol, 6-shogaol), diphenylheptane (Gingerenone). Gingerol is not only the main material basis of the pungent flavor of Ganjiang, but also the main component to expand blood vessel, promote blood circulation and strengthen heart. Diphenylheptane is the main material basis of antiemetic, anti-inflammatory and anti-thrombotic effects. In addition, it also contains a small amount of flavonoids, glycosides, amino acids, a variety of vitamins and trace elements. *Pharmacopoeia of the People's Republic of China* records that the content of essential oil should not be less than 0.8% (ml/g), and 6-gingerol ($C_{17}H_{26}O_4$) should not be less than 0.60% in Ganjiang.

二、炮制品种与品质
II Processed Varieties and Quality

干姜的炮制品主要有干姜、炮姜、姜炭,炮姜以鼓起,表面棕褐色,内部深黄色,质地疏松为佳；姜炭以表面焦黑色，内部棕褐色，体轻，质松脆为佳。《中国药典》规定干姜含量测定同药材，炮姜中 6- 姜辣素不得少于 0.30%，姜炭含 6- 姜辣素不得少于 0.05%。

The processed products of Ganjiang mainly include Ganjiang, Paojiang, and Jiangtan. Good quality of Paojiang is characterized by bulging, brown on the surface, dark yellow in the interior, and loose in texture; the Jiangtan has good quality with focal black on the surface, brown inside, light in weight, and crisp in texture. According to the *Pharmacopoeia of the People's Republic of China*, the content determination of Ganjiang is same as required for the medicinal. The content of 6-gingerol ($C_{17}H_{26}O_4$) in Paojiang should not be less than 0.30%, and should not be less than 0.05% in Jiangtan.

三、中成药品种与品质
III Varieties and Quality of Chinese Patent Medicines

含干姜的中成药品种有 280 余个，《中国药典》收载有 37 个，以干姜为君药或主药的有小青龙合剂（颗粒）、附子理中片、理中丸等，在质量控制多采用薄层色谱法以对照药材进行定性鉴别。非以干姜君药的制剂，如健步丸、催汤丸等通过显微鉴别，以"淀粉粒"特征确定含有干姜。

There are more than 280 Chinese patent medicines containing Ganjiang and 37 of them are recorded in *Pharmacopoeia of the People's Republic of China*. Among them, prescriptions with Ganjiang as the sovereign medicinal are as follows: Xiaoqinglong Heji, Fuzilizhong Pian (Tablets), Lizhong Wan, etc. In quality control, TLC is often used for qualitative identification with the contrast of the raw medicinal. Microscopic identification is used for identifying preparations with Ganjiang not as the sovereign medicinal, such as Jianbu Wan, Cuitang Wan. The characteristics of "starch granules" are used to determine the content of Ganjiang.

【制药】
[Pharmacy]

一、产地加工
I Processing in Production Area

干姜采挖后，去掉茎叶、须根，烘干。干燥后去掉泥沙、粗皮，扬净即成。

Remove the stems, leaves, fibrous roots after digging and drying the Ganjiang, then remove the soil and coarse cortex, and winnow for cleaning after it is totally dried.

二、饮片炮制
II Processing of Decoction Pieces

干姜以润透、切片、砂烫、炒炭为主要工序，由此生产出来的干姜、炮姜、姜炭为临床及成药选用的品种。

The main process of Ganjiang is moistening, slicing, heating with sand and stir-frying to scorch. Ganjiang, Paojiang and Jiangtan produced by these processes are selected for clinical and patent medicines.

干姜的辛燥之性主要成分为挥发油及姜辣素类成分，在炮制过程中随着炮制程度的加深，挥发油、姜酚类成分逐渐减低甚至消失，同时产生一些极性大的化合物。干姜的辛燥之性也随着炮制程度的降低、消失，炒炭后姜炭性味苦涩，而偏于温经止血作用。

The pungency and dryness of Ganjiang is due to the existence of volatile oil and gingerol. During the processing of Ganjiang, with the deepening of processing, the volatile oil and gingerol gradually decrease or even disappear, and some compounds with large polarity are randomly produced. The pungency and dryness of Ganjiang also decrease or even disappear. After stir-frying to scorch, the flavor of Jiangtan is bitter and the property is astringent, and it is better at warming the channel for stopping bleeding.

三、中成药制药
III Pharmacy of Chinese Patent Medicines

含干姜及炮制品的中成药，剂型十分丰富，涵盖了固体、液体与半固体剂型。在含干姜的中成药制剂中多制成丸剂，同时为满足现代制剂处方成型性及减少服用剂量，一般制剂如片剂、口服液和颗粒剂等多以干姜挥发油加入制剂中。

Chinese patent medicines containing Ganjiang are rich in preparations, covering solid, liquid and semi-solid types. Chinese patent medicines containing Ganjiang are mostly made into pills. Meanwhile, in order to meet the requirements of prescription molding of modern preparations and reduce the dosage, volatile oil of Ganjiang is used in general preparations, such as tablets, mixture and granules.

如在四逆汤（口服液）制备工艺中，干姜用水蒸气蒸馏提取挥发油，再与其它提取液醇沉后的滤液合并制备口服液，能最大程度保留干姜挥发油的含量，发挥其协同附子增效的作用。

For example, in the preparation process of Sini Tang (Decoction), the volatile oil is extracted by steam distillation of Ganjiang, and then combined with the filtrate after alcohol precipitation of other extracts to prepare mixture, which can retain the content of the volatile oil of Ganjiang to the greatest extent and have a synergistic effect with Fuzi.

【性能功效】
[Property and Efficacy]

一、性能
I Property

干姜味辛，热。归脾、胃、心、肺经。

Ganjiang is pungent in flavor, hot in nature, and it enters the spleen, stomach, heart and lung meridians.

二、功效
II Efficacy

1. 温中散寒　干姜辛热，主入脾胃，长于温脾胃之阳，祛脾胃之寒，为温中散寒之要药。其功效的发挥与抗炎镇痛、抗溃疡、止泻、调节胃肠功能、止吐等药理作用密切相关。干姜抗炎镇痛、调节胃肠功能、止吐的有效物质基础主要是干姜挥发油，通过下调花生四烯酸代谢相关基因表达，发挥抗炎镇痛作用。

1 Warming Spleen and Stomach for Dispelling Cold

Ganjiang, pungent and hot, which mainly enters the meridians of the spleen and stomach, is capable of warming the yang of spleen and stomach, dissipating the cold of spleen and stomach. It is the most important medicinal to dissipate cold. The function of Ganjiang is closely related to its pharmacological effects such as anti-inflammation and analgesia, anti-ulcer, anti-diarrhea, regulating gastrointestinal and antiemetic function. Volatile oils in Ganjiang are the main effective components for anti-inflammatory, analgesic and antiemetic effect, and regulating gastrointestinal function. Through down-regulating the expression of arachidonic acid metabolism related gene, it has anti-inflammatory and analgesic effect.

2. 回阳通脉　干姜入心肾经，有温阳守中，回阳通脉的功效。其功效的发挥与强心、抗缺氧、扩张血管、增加血流量、抗血栓等药理作用密切相关。干姜强心、扩张血管、抗血栓的有效物质基础主要是 8-姜辣素、姜酚和姜烯酚。

2 Restoring *Yang* to Promote Blood Circulation

Ganjiang enterings the meridians of the heart and kidney, is capable of warming yang to keep it in the middle, restoring yang to promote the blood circulation. The function of Ganjiang is closely related to its pharmacological effects of cardiotonic function, anti-hypoxia and antithrombus effects, expanding blood vessel and promoting blood circulation. The effective material basis of Ganjiang (dried) for strengthening the heart, dilating blood vessels and anti-thrombosis is mainly 8-gingerol, gingerol and gingerol.

3. **温肺化饮** 干姜兼入肺经，上能温肺散寒以化寒痰，中能温脾运水以消痰，亦为寒饮喘咳之良药。其功效与抗炎、镇静、抗病原微生物、提高免疫力有关。干姜抗病原微生物的有效物质基础主要是姜酮和姜烯酮。

3 Warming the Lung to Resolve Fluid Retention

Ganjiang also enters the lung meridian. It can warm the lung and dissipate cold to resolve cold retained fluid in the upper body, warm the spleen and move water to resolve phlegm in the middle body. And it is also a good medicinal for dyspneic cough due to cold fluid. Its function is related with anti-inflammation, sedation, resisting pathogenic microorganism and enhancing immune functions.

现代研究还发现，干姜具有对肝损伤的保护作用、抗肿瘤作用。

Besides, modern research shows that Ganjiang has protective effect on liver injury and anti-tumor.

【应用】
[Applications]

一、主治病证
I Indications

1. **脾胃寒证** 对脾胃虚寒证之脘腹冷痛，呕吐泄泻，干姜可与人参配伍以温中散寒，如《伤寒论》理中丸、《金匮要略》大建中汤；若外寒直中脾胃之实寒证，可与炮姜配伍，以养脾温胃，去冷消痰，宽胸下气，如《太平惠民和剂局方》二姜丸。

1 Cold Syndrome of Spleen and Stomach

Ganjiang can be combined with Renshen to warm the middle and dissipate cold for treatment of epigastric cold pain, vomiting and diarrhea, such as in Lizhong Wan recorded in *Shanghan*

Lun, Dajianzhong Tang (Decoction) in *Jinkui Yaolue (Synopsis of the Golden Chamber)*. For the patients with excessive cold syndrome of external cold attacking spleen and stomach, it can be combined with Paojiang to nourish the spleen and warm the stomach, to dissipate cold and resolve phlegm, to broad chest and lower qi, such as Erjiang Wan in *Taiping Huimin Heji Ju Fang*.

现代临床，干姜配伍常用于肠炎、腹痛，腹泻、呕吐等脾胃虚寒证，如理中汤、大建中汤。

In modern clinical practice, Ganjiang compatibility is often used to treat enteritis, abdominal pain, diarrhea and vomiting, such as Lizhong Tang (Decoction), and Dajianzhong Tang (Decoction).

2. **亡阳证** 治疗亡阳证，附子常与干姜配伍以回阳救逆，如《伤寒论》之四逆汤、干姜附子汤。若亡阳暴脱，下利，亡血，四肢厥逆，脉微者，可配伍人参以益气生津，回阳复脉，如《伤寒论》四逆加人参汤。

2 Yang Collapse Syndrome

To treat yang collapse syndrome, Ganjiang is often combined with Fuzi to restore *yang* to save from collapse, such as in Sini Tang (Decoction) and Ganjiang Fuzi Tang (Decoction) in *Shanghan Lun*. For the patients with syndromes of sudden yang collapse, diarrhea, blood collapse, reversal of cold limbs and faint pulse, it can be combined with Renshen to replenish qi and produce fluid, to restore yang and restore the vessels, such as in Sini Jia Renshen Tang (Decoction) in *Shanghan Lun*.

在现代临床干姜配伍常用于治疗冠心病、心肌梗死、急性心肌梗死并发低血压危重症和心源性休克亡阳证患者的临床治疗等，如四逆汤。

In modern clinical practice, Ganjiang compatibility is commonly applied to treat coronary heart disease, myocardial infarct, acute myocardial infarction complicated with hypotension and cardiogenic shock of the yang collapse syndrome, such as in Sini Tang (Decoction).

3. **寒饮喘咳** 对于寒饮伏肺之咳喘、痰多清稀，形寒背冷，干姜与半夏、五味子、麻黄等配伍以温肺止咳，如《伤寒论》小青龙汤。若肺寒停饮，咳嗽胸满，痰涎清稀，舌苔白滑，可配伍细辛、茯苓、五味子以温肺化饮，如《金匮要略》苓甘五味姜辛汤。

3 Coughing and Panting with Cold Fluid

For the syndromes of coughing and panting, copious watery phlegm, body and back cold caused by cold fluid retained in the lung, Ganjiang can be combined with Banxia, Wuweizi, Mahuang, etc. such as Xiaoqinglong Tang (Decoction) in *Shanghan Lun*. For patients with syndromes of lung cold and fluid retention, coughing and fullness in the chest, clear phlegm and saliva, and white and slippery tongue coating, Ganjiang can be combined with Xixin, Fuling, Wuweizi, such as Ling Gan Wuwei Jiang Xin Tang (Decoction) in *Jinkui Yaolue (Synopsis of the Golden Chamber)*.

在现代临床干姜配伍常用于治疗哮喘性、过敏性支气管炎、过敏性鼻炎和风寒咳嗽等寒饮喘咳证，如小青龙汤。

In modern clinical practice, Ganjiang compatibility is commonly applied to treat asthmatic and allergic bronchitis, allergic rhinitis, and wind-cold cough, such as Xiaoqinglong Tang (Decoction).

此外干姜配伍还可用于对抗中枢兴奋药、解热、利胆保肝和促进免疫功能等作用。

Besides, Ganjiang compatibility with other medicinals can also be used as anti-central stimulant ,has antipyretic, choleretic, liver protection and immune functions .

二、用法用量
II Administration and Dosage

3~10g，煎服。
3~10g, water decoction.

三、注意事项
III Precautions

血热妄行、阴虚内热者忌用。孕妇慎用。
Patients with syndromes of bleeding due to blood heat or internal heat due to yin deficiency should not take Ganjiang. Pregnant women should use it with great caution.

第十五章 行 气 药
Chapter 15　Qi-activating Medicinals

　　凡以疏理气机、治疗气滞或气逆证为主要作用的药物，称为行气药，又叫理气药。其中行气力强者，又称破气药。此类药物多味辛香苦温，主归脾、肝、肺等经。因其辛香行散、苦能降泄、温能通行，故有疏理气机的作用，某些药物还有燥湿化痰、破气散结、降逆止呕等作用，故可用于治疗气滞、气逆等证，体现了《黄帝内经》"结者散之"、"逸者行之"的中医治则。行气药多辛温香燥，易耗气伤阴，凡阴亏气虚者慎用。作用峻猛的破气药孕妇慎用。现代研究表明，行气药多具有调节胃肠运动、调节消化液分泌、解痉止痛、抗炎、利胆、松弛支气管平滑肌等药理作用。常见的行气药有陈皮、枳实、木香、香附等。理气药多含挥发油成分，入汤剂一般不宜久煎。

Qi-activating medicinals, also called qi-regulating medicinals, refer to the medicinals that can regulate qi movement to treat syndromes of qi stagnation or reversed qi. Those that can drive qi flow furiously are called qi-breaking medicinals. Qi-regulating medicinals are usually aromatic in smell, pungent and bitter in flavor and warm in nature, mainly entering meridians of the spleen, liver and lungs. They can regulate qi-movement because the pungent flavor and aromatic smell can drive qi flow and disperse stagnation, the bitter flavor can direct rebellious qi downward, and the warm nature can activate qi. Some of them can also dry dampness and resolve phlegm, break qi stagnation to dissipate mass, as well as descend adverse qi to relieve vomiting. Thus they can be used to treat qi stagnation or reversed qi, which demonstrate the Chinese medicine treatment principle of dispersing the stasis, and activating the over-leisure in *Huangdi Neijing (Huangdi's Internal Classic)*. Because they are often pungent, aromatic, warm and dry, which easily exhaust qi and harm yin, patients with deficiency of yin and qi should take them carefully. Those severe qi-breaking medicinals should be used especially cautiously with pregnant women. Modern researches show that qi-regulating medicinals have pharmacological effects of regulating gastrointestinal motility and the secretion of digestive juice, relieving spasm to stop pain, resisting against inflammation, being cholagogic effects, and relaxing bronchial smooth muscle. Commonly used qi-regulating medicinals involve Chenpi, Zhishi, Muxiang, Xiangfu, etc. Most qi-regulating medicinals have volatile oils so that they should not be boiled for long time.

陈 皮

Chenpi
(Citri Reticulatae Pericarpium)

陈皮的道地产区为广东新会。常用陈皮和炒陈皮。陈皮味辛、苦，性温，归脾、胃、肺经，具理气健脾，燥湿化痰功效，主治脾胃气滞证、肺胃气逆证及痰湿咳嗽。陈皮主要含挥发油、黄酮苷、生物碱等成分，有调节胃肠平滑肌、促进消化液分泌、祛痰平喘、抗炎等药理作用，可用于治疗急慢性胃肠炎、呼吸道感染等属脾肺气滞、痰湿壅遏者。

Chenpi's genuine production place is Xinhui in Guangdong Province. Chenpi and Chaochenpi (stir-frying) are commonly used. Chenpi is pungent and bitter in flavor, warm in nature, entering the meridians of the spleen, stomach and lungs, with the effect of regulating qi and strengthening the spleen, drying dampness and resolving phlegm, mainly treating syndromes of stagnation of spleen and stomach qi, lung and stomach reversed qi and cough of phlegm-dampness. Chenpi mainly contains volatile oils, flavone glycosides, alkaloids and other components, showing the pharmacological effects of regulating gastrointestinal smooth muscle, promoting the secretion of digestive fluid, expectorating, anti-asthmatic, and anti-inflammatory functions, etc. It can be used to treat acute and chronic gastroenteritis, respiratory tract infection, etc., pertaining to stagnation of spleen and lung qi, and abundant phlegm-dampness.

【品种品质】
[Variety and Quality]

一、基原品种与品质
I Origin Varieties and Quality

1. 品种概况 来源于芸香科植物橘 *Citrus reticulata* Blanco 及其栽培变种的干燥成熟果皮。

1 Variety

Chenpi is the dried pericarp of the ripe fruit of *Citrus reticulata Blanco* or its cultivars varieties of Fam Rutaceae.

陈皮首载于《神农本草经》。《本草经集注》载"以东橘为好……以陈者为良"，《食疗本草》首次明确提出"陈皮"。《开宝本草》新增"橙子皮"，始确定陈皮来源为橘及其栽培变种。《本草图经》载"橘柚……木高一、二丈，叶与枳无辨，刺出于茎间。夏初生白花，六月、七月而成实，至冬黄熟，乃可啖"，与今陈皮基原品种相类。

Chenpi is first recorded in *Shennong Bencao Jing*. *Bencaojing Jizhu* records "The east oranges are of a good quality...... and the preserved are also good". Chenpi is first clearly stated in *Shiliao Bencao*. *Kaibao Bencao (Kaibao Materia Medica)* adds "orange peel" to determine the origin and its cultivated varieties. *Bencao Tujing* states "height of the orange tree is one or two *zhang*s, leaves and indistinguishable with trifoliate orange, and the thorns grow from the stems. White flowers appear in early summer, the fruits initiately come out in June or July, and are mature in winter when the peels turned yellow, and then Chenpi can be eatable". These Chenpi stated in the book are similar in the original varieties of Chenpi used today.

2. 种植采收 陈皮主产于广东、福建、浙江、广西、江西、四川等地，多在山地、丘陵坡地人工栽培。于秋末冬初果实成熟时采收。

2 Planting and Harvesting

Chenpi is mainly produced in Guangdong, Fujian, Zhejiang, Guangxi, Jiangxi, Sichuan provinces and other places, mostly cultivated in mountainous and hilly slopes. Chenpi is harvested in late autumn and early winter when the fruit matures.

3. 道地性及品质评价 宋元以后历代均认为陈皮以广东产者佳，尤以新会品质最优，称新会陈皮。陈皮性状评价一般以形态上瓣大、整齐，颜色鲜艳、油润，质地柔软，且香气浓者为佳。

3 Genuineness and Quality Evaluation

After Song Dynasty and Yuan Dynasty, Chenpi was of good quality in Guangdong, especially in Xinhui, which was called Xinhui Chenpi. The evaluation for the Chenpi with good qualify is generally characterized by large and unified shape, bright color, oily skin, soft texture, and strong aroma.

陈皮主要含有挥发油（如柠檬烯）、黄酮苷（如新橙皮苷、橙皮苷、川陈皮素）、生物碱（如对羟福林、N-甲基酪胺）等，为其药效物质基础，其中挥发油是抗炎、祛痰、平喘的主要物质基础。此外，陈皮还含有多糖、微量元素、柠檬苦素、甾醇等。《中国药典》规定陈皮药材中橙皮苷含量不得少于3.5%。

Chenpi mainly contains volatile oils (such as limonene), flavone glycosides (such as neohesperetin, hesperidin, and nobiletin), alkaloids (such as p-hydroxoflorin, N-methyl tyramine) and so on, which are the material basis of its efficacy. Among them, volatile oils are the main material basis of anti-inflammation, dissipating phlegm and antiasthma effects. In addition, Chenpi also contains polysaccharides, trace elements, limonin, sterols and so on. *Pharmacopoeia of the People's Republic of China* stipulates that the content of hesperidin in the raw medicinal of Chenpi should not be less than 3.5%.

二、炮制品种与品质
II Processed Varieties and Quality

陈皮的炮制品种及临床常用品种有2个，为陈皮与炒陈皮。陈皮以外表面橙红色或红棕色，有细皱纹和凹下的点状油室，内表面浅黄白色且粗糙，香气浓郁者为佳；炒陈皮以外表面颜色加深带火色，内表面黄色，质脆气香为佳。《中国药典》规定陈皮炮制品中橙皮苷含量不得少于2.5%。

There are two processed varieties and commonly used clinical varieties of Chenpi, which are Chenpi and Chaochenpi. The outer surface of Chenpi is orange-red or reddish brown, with fine wrinkles and concave dot oil chamber, the inner surface is yellowish-white and rough, and the aroma is strong. *Pharmacopoeia of the People's Republic of China* stipulates that the content of hesperidin in the processed products of Chenpi shall not be less than 2.5%.

三、中成药品种与品质
III Varieties and Quality of Chinese Patent Medicines

含有陈皮或炒陈皮的中成药有300余个，《中国药典》收载含陈皮的中成药168个。以陈皮为主药的品种有二陈丸（浓缩丸、合剂）、参贝陈皮、蛇胆陈皮散（片、胶囊、口服液）、加味蛇胆陈皮片等。在中成药的品质控制中多采用显微鉴别确定陈皮的存在，采用薄层色谱法和含量测定法进行指标成分限量。如二陈丸、蛇胆陈皮散等，均采用显微鉴别及薄层色谱法鉴定陈皮及其有效成分橙皮苷，用HPLC法限定橙皮苷的含量下限以保证药品质量。

There are more than 300 Chinese patent medicines containing Chenpi or Chaochenpi and 168 Chinese patent medicines containing Chenpi are included in *Pharmacopoeia of the People's Republic of China*. As the sovereign medicinal, Chenpi is used in Erchen Wan , Heji, Shenbei Chenpi, Shedan Chenpi San (Powder) [Pian (Tablets), Jiaonang (Capsules), Koufuye], Jiawei Shedan Chenpi Pian (Tablets) and so on. In the quality control of Chinese patent medicine, the existence of Chenpi is determined by microscopic identification, and the index component limit was determined by TLC and content determination.

For example, Erchen Wan and Shedan Chenpi San (Powder) are identified by microscopic identification and TLC, and the lower limit of hesperidin content is defined by HPLC method to ensure the quality of medicinals.

【制药】
[Pharmacy]

一、产地加工
I Processing in Production Area

剥取成熟果实的果皮，晒干或低温干燥。

Peel the pericarp of the mature fruit, and dry in the sun or at low temperature.

二、饮片炮制
II Processing of Decoction Pieces

自古以来陈皮的炮制方法繁复，多达20余种，宋代以来形成了切条切丝的工艺。目前炮制以润后切丝为主要加工工序，由此形成的陈皮成为商品规格中的主流。陈皮以燥湿化痰为主，炒陈皮（清炒）以理气和中为主。

Since ancient times, the processing methods of Chenpi have been complicated with over 20 kinds, and the process of slices has been formed since Song Dynasty. At present, the main processing process is slicing after soaking, and the sliced Chenpi is the mainstream of commodity specifications. Chenpi has the main function of drying dampness to remove phlegm, and Chaochenpi is mainly to regulate qi and to harmonize the middle.

陈皮素有"陈久者良"之说，其贮藏年限从一年至十余年不等，道地药材"新会陈皮"贮藏长达数十年。陈化过程中挥发油不断降低，燥性得以缓和，而黄酮类物质不断增加，可能与陈皮表面的黑曲霉等真菌产生的酶类促进黄酮苷转化为黄酮苷元有关。现代采用炒制或蒸制方法，能快速去除部分挥发油，降低陈皮的辛燥之性。

There is a saying all along that the preserved Chenpi is better. Its storage life ranges from 1 years to more than 10 years, and the genuine regional medicinal, Xinhui Chenpi, has been stored for even several decades. In the process of aging, the volatile oil is decreasing, the dry property of Chenpi gradually reduces or disappears, and the flavonoids are increasing, which may be related to the enzymes produced by fungi such as aspergillus niger on the surface of Chenpi to promote the conversion of flavonoid glycosides into flavonoid aglucone. In modern times, the method of stir-frying or steaming can quickly remove some volatile oils and reduce the dry and pungent nature of Chenpi.

三、中成药制药
III Pharmacy of Chinese Patent Medicines

含陈皮的中成药，剂型十分丰富，涵盖固体、液体等剂型。陈皮中的主要活性成分挥发油与黄酮类具有一定的脂溶性，现今多采用打粉或醇提的方法入制剂，挥发油亦可单独提取。

The pharmaceutical forms of Chinese patent medicine containing Chenpi are very rich, covering solid, liquid type and other pharmaceutical forms. The volatile oils and flavonoids, the main active components in the Chenpi are certain liposoluble. Nowadays, Chenpi is usually used in powder of extracted by alcohol, and its volatile oil can be extracted separately for use.

如以陈皮为君药的二陈汤，先后发展为二陈丸（水丸）、二陈浓缩丸及二陈合剂3种不同剂型，陈皮的制法亦不同。二陈丸中陈皮与它药粉碎成细粉，以生姜汁泛丸；二陈浓缩丸中，用70%乙醇为溶剂渗漉提取陈皮中的黄酮与挥发油，以降低服用量、实现精制；二陈合剂中，先采用水蒸气蒸馏法提取陈皮中的挥发油，药渣再进一步水提，以保证各类成分的提取率。

For example, Erchen Tang (Decoction), with Chenpi as the sovereign medicinal, has developed three different pharmaceutical forms, including Erchen Wan [Shuiwan (Water Pills)], Erchen Nongsuowan and Erchen Heji and the process of

Chenpi in the three forms are different. In Erchen Wan, Chenpi and other medicinals are made into fine powder and then into pills with ginger juice; and in Erchen Nongsuowan, flavonoids and essential oils are extracted with 70% ethanol as solvent to reduce the dosage and realize refining; in Erchen Heji, the volatile oil is extracted by steam distillation, and the residue was further extracted to ensure the extraction rate of all kinds of components.

【性能功效】
[Property and Efficacy]

一、性能
I Property

陈皮味辛、苦，性温，归脾、胃、肺经。

Chenpi is pungent and bitter in flavor, warm in nature, and enters the spleen, stomach and lung meridians.

二、功效
II Efficacy

1. **理气健脾**　陈皮辛香，能行脾肺之滞气、降肺胃之逆气，而健脾和中，为治脾胃气滞之要药。其功效的发挥与调节胃肠平滑肌、促进消化液分泌、利胆及缓解气管平滑肌痉挛等药理作用密切相关。陈皮调节胃肠平滑肌、促进消化液分泌、利胆作用的有效物质基础主要是挥发油。

1 Regulating Qi-flowing for Strengthening the Spleen

Pungent and fragrant in flavor, Chenpi can move the stagnation qi of the spleen and lung, reduce the inverse qi of the lung and stomach, and strengthen the spleen to regulate stomach. Chenpi is the key medicinal for the treatment of stagnation of the spleen and stomach qi. Its effect is closely related to regulating gastrointestinal smooth muscle, promoting digestive fluid

secretion, cholagogic function and relieving tracheal smooth muscle spasm. The volatile oil is the effective material base of Chenpi in regulating gastrointestinal smooth muscles, promoting digestive fluid secretion and promoting gallbladder action.

2. **燥湿化痰**　陈皮辛散温通、入肺走胸，长于理气调中，燥湿化痰。其功效的发挥与祛痰、平喘、抗炎等药理作用密切相关。陈皮的祛痰、平喘、抗炎作用的有效物质基础主要是川陈皮素、橙皮苷和挥发油中的柠檬烯，通过松弛气管平滑肌和解除痉挛，降低支气管肺泡灌洗液中嗜酸性粒细胞数等发挥祛痰平喘作用；并通过降低毛细血管的通透性，防止微血管出血发挥抗炎作用。

2 Eliminating Dampness and Phlegm

Chenpi, pungent in taste to disperse and warm in nature to smooth, enters the lung and goes to the chest and is good at regulating qi to harmonize the middle and eliminating dampness and phlegm. Its effect is closely related to the expectorating, antiasthmatic, anti-inflammatory and other pharmacological effects. The effective material basis of expectorant, antiasthmatic and anti-inflammatory effects of Chenpi is mainly nobiletin, hesperidin and limonene in volatile oil. By relaxing tracheal smooth muscle and relieving spasm, the reduction of eosinophils in bronchoalveolar lavage fluid can play the role of expectorant and anti-asthmatic effect, and the anti-inflammation is performed by preventing microvascular bleeding through reducing capillary permeability and so on.

此外，现代研究显示陈皮中的黄酮类成分还有抗氧化、抗肿瘤、抗动脉粥样硬化、降低血清胆固醇等作用。

In addition, modern studies have shown that flavonoids in Chenpi also have antioxidate, anti-tumor, anti-atherosclerosis effect, and has the functions of reducing serum cholesterol and so on.

【应用】

[Applications]

一、主治病证
I Indications

1. **脾胃气滞证** 治疗脾胃气滞证，陈皮常与木香、白术配伍以行气止痛、健脾和中，如《鸡峰普济方》宽中丸和现代制剂胃立康片等；若脾虚气滞者，可配伍人参、白术等以益气健脾和胃，如《小儿药证直诀》异功散和现代制剂启脾口服液等；治湿阻中焦兼气滞者，可与苍术、厚朴等配伍，如《太平惠民和剂局方》平胃散和香砂平胃丸等；治肝气乘脾、腹痛泄泻，可与白芍、白术、防风配伍，如《丹溪心法》痛泻要方。

1 Syndrome of Qi Stagnation of Spleen and Stomach

Chenpi often is combined with Muxiang, Baizhu to regulating qi-flowing for relieving pain and strengthening the spleen for regulating stomach for the treatment of qi stagnation of the spleen and stomach, such as in Kuanzhong Wan recorded in *Jifeng Pujifang* and modern preparation of Weilikang Pian (Tablets); for patients with qi stagnation due to spleen deficiency, Chenpi can be combined with Renshen and Baizhu and other medicinals to invigorate the spleen and stomach, such as in Yigong San (Powder) recorded in *Xiaoer Yaozheng Zhijue* and modern preparation Qipi Koufuye, etc.; for the treatment of dampness obstructing in the middle energizer combined with qi stagnation, Chenpi can be combined with Cangzhu and Houpo, such as in Pingwei San (Powder) and Xiangsha Pingwei Wan in *Taiping Huimin Heji Ju Fang*, etc.; for the treatment of abdominal pain or diarrhea due to liver qi over-restricting spleen, Chenpi can be combined with Baishao, Baizhu and Fangfeng, such as in Tongxie Prescription in *Danxi Xinfa*.

现代临床，陈皮配伍常用于治疗急慢性胃肠炎、功能性消化不良、肠易激综合征等属脾胃气滞者，如平胃散、痛泻要方等。

In modern clinical practice, Chenpi compatibility is often used in the treatment of acute and chronic gastroenteritis, functional dyspepsia, irritable bowel syndrome and others belonging to qi stagnation of the spleen and stomach, such as in Pingwei San (Powder), Tongxie Yaofang (Formula).

2. **肺胃气逆证** 治胃寒气逆，恶心呕吐或呃逆者，常与生姜等配伍，如《金匮要略》橘皮汤；治胃虚有热，呕吐呃逆者，多与人参、竹茹等配伍，如《金匮要略》橘皮竹茹汤；治痰湿中阻，胃失和降，恶心呕吐，宜与半夏、茯苓等配伍，如《太平惠民和剂局方》二陈汤；治外感风寒、内伤湿滞之呕吐、泄泻，可与藿香、紫苏等配伍，如《太平惠民和剂局方》藿香正气散和现代制剂藿香正气口服液。

2 Syndrome of Reversed Qi of the Lung and Stomach

For the treatment of nausea due to stomach cold, vomiting or hiccup, Chenpi often can be used with Shengjiang and other compatibility, such as in Jupi Tang (Decoction) in *Jinkui Yaolue (Synopsis of the Golden Chamber)*; for the treatment of vomiting and hiccup due to stomach deficiency with heat, Chenpi is used usually with Renshen and Zhuru, as Jupi Zhuru Tang (Decoction) in *Jinkui Yaolue (Synopsis of the Golden Chamber)*; for the treatment of nausea and vomiting due to phlegm and dampness obstruction and failure of stomach qi to descend, Chenpi is applied with Banxia, Fuling and other compatibility, such as in Erchen Tang (Decoction) in *Taiping Huimin Heji Ju Fang*; for the treatment of vomiting, diarrhea due to encountering external wind-cold and suffering from dampness obstruction can be combined with Huoxiang, Zisu, such as in Huoxiang Zhengqi San (Powder) in *Taiping Huimin Heji Ju Fang* and its modern preparations.

现代临床，陈皮配伍常用于治疗内耳眩晕综合征、胃肠型感冒等属于痰湿中阻、肺胃气逆者，前者如二陈汤，后者如藿香正气散。

In modern clinical practice, Chenpi compatibility is often used in the treatment of internal ear dizziness syndrome or gastrointestinal common cold, etc. The previous one belongs to phlegm dampness obstruction as in Erchen Tang (Decoction) and the latter one belongs to the inversion of lung and stomach qi as in Huoxiang Zhengqi San (Powder).

3. **痰湿咳嗽** 治湿痰壅滞，肺失宣降，咳嗽痰多，常与半夏、茯苓等配伍，如《太平惠民和剂局方》二陈汤；治寒痰咳嗽，痰多清稀，多与干姜、甘草等配伍，如《圣济总录》四顺散和现代制剂风寒咳嗽丸等。

3 Cough Due to Phlegm-dampness

For the treatment of stagnation of phlegm-dampness, lung qi failing in dispersing with cough and too much phlegm, Chenpi is often combined with Banxia, Fuling and other compatibility as shown in Erchen Tang (Decoction) in *Taiping Huimin Heji Ju Fang*; for the treatment of cold phlegm cough, too much clear phlegm, Chenpi is likely to be used with Shengjiang, Gancao and other compatibility, as in Sishun San (Powder) in *Sheng Ji Zonglu* and modern preparation of Fenghan Kesou Wan.

现代临床，陈皮配伍常用于治疗急、慢性支气管炎、哮喘等属于痰浊阻肺者，如二陈汤、杏仁止咳合剂、五味陈皮合剂等。此外，陈皮还常用于治疗各种代谢疾病，如高脂血症属痰湿中阻者。

In modern clinical practice, Chenpi compatibility is often used to treat acute, chronic bronchitis, asthma and other diseases belonging to phlegm turbid obstruction in the lung, such as Erchen Tang (Decoction), Xingren Zhike Heji, Wuwei Chenpi Heji and so on. In addition, Chenpi is often used to treat various metabolic diseases, such as hyperlipidemia due to phlegm-dampness obstruction.

二、用法用量
II Administration and Dosage

3~10g，水煎。

3-10g, water decoction.

三、注意事项
III Precautions

陈皮辛温苦燥，实热津伤、阴虚燥咳、咯血、吐血者慎用。

Chenpi is pungent, warm and bitter with dryness, and patients with excessive heat injury, dry cough, hemoptysis, vomiting blood due to yin deficiency should use it with great caution.

【知识拓展】
[Knowledge Extension]

陈皮是常用大宗药材，临床用量大、用途广。古人认为陈皮须陈置方可入药，尤其是道地药材"新会陈皮"陈置时间更长，讲究"天然生晒，自然陈化"。但陈皮陈化受地理气候及储存条件等多重因素影响，难以控制，品质不稳定，不利于大规模标准化生产。现代研究发现微生物生长代谢是陈皮陈化过程中的一个要素，因而尝试研究人工接种如黑曲霉来加速陈皮陈化的工艺，以期缩短陈化时间，提高经济效益与产量。

Chenpi is commonly and widely used medicinal material clinically in large quantities. The ancients believed that only the long time preserved Chenpi can be used in medicine, especially for the regional genuine medicinal, "Xinhui Chenpi", preserving for longer time. The process of Xinhui Chenpi pays attention to "drying under the sun naturally for aging". However, aging of Chenpi is affected by many factors, such as geographical climate and storage conditions, which is difficult to control and unstable in quality and also is not conducive to large-scale standardized production. Modern studies have found that microbial growth and metabolism are key elements in the aging process of Chenpi, so manufacturers try to study the process of artificial inoculation such as aspergillus niger to accelerate the aging process, in order to shorten the aging time and improve the economic benefit and yield.

木　香

Muxiang

(Aucklandiae Radix)

木香原产于印度、缅甸等地，经广州进口，称广木香；现在云南等地种植，称云木香。常用木香和煨木香。木香味辛、苦，性温，归脾、胃、大肠、肝、胆经，具行气止痛、健脾消食功效，主治脾胃气滞证、痢疾、肝胆气滞证等。木香主要含挥发油、生物碱、有机酸、多糖等成分，可用于治疗胃肠炎、胆囊炎、胆结石、功能性消化不良、肠易激综合征、细菌性痢疾、心绞痛等属气滞者。

Muxiang originated in India, Myanmar and other places, imported through Guangzhou, called Guangmuxiang; now those planted in Yunnan province are called Yunmuxiang. Muxiang and Weimuxiang (Roasted) are commonly used. Muxiang is pungent and bitter in flavor, warm in nature, entering the spleen, stomach, large intestine, liver, gallbladder meridians, with the effect of regulating qi to relieve pain, strengthening the spleen to digest food, for the treatment of qi stagnation of spleen and stomach, dysentery, qi stagnation of liver and gallbladder. Muxiang mainly contains volatile oils, alkaloids, organic acids, polysaccharides and other components, and can be used to treat gastroenteritis, cholecystitis, gallstones, functional dyspepsia, irritable bowel syndrome, bacillary dysentery, angina pectoris and other diseases pertaining to qi stagnation.

【品种品质】
[Variety and Quality]

一、基原品种与品质
I Origin Varieties and Quality

1. 品种概况　来源于菊科植物木香 *Aucklandia lappa* Decne. 的干燥根。

1 Variety

Muxiang is the dried roots of *Aucklandia lappa Decne.*

木香始载于《神农本草经》。《新修本草》云："此有二种，当以昆仑来者为佳，出西胡来者不善。叶似羊蹄而长大，花如菊花，其实黄黑，所在亦有之。"直到唐代，木香仍然依赖进口，有两个来源地，以昆仑（可能为东南亚地区的某个国家）所产质量为优，而西胡大约指今阿富汗、伊朗一带，从分布来看，这两种进口木香都有可能是现在的正品木香。《本草品汇精要》认为木香指菊科木香，一直沿用至今。

Muxiang was first recorded in *Shennong Bencao Jing*. *Xinxiu Bencao* states that "There are two kinds, those from Kunlun are the best, and those from the West Hu are not good. Leaves grow up like sheep's hoofs, flowers similar to those of the chrysanthemum, but dark yellow for differentiation." Until the Tang Dynasty, Muxiang still relied on imports, with two sources. The quality of those from Kunlun (may be a certain Country in Southeast Asia) are the best, and West Hu possibly refers to area around Afghanistan and Iran. From the distribution point of view, these two imported Muxiang may be the regional genuine Muxiang at present. *Bencao Pinhui Jingyao (Compendium of Materia Medica)* states that Muxiang, the part of *Aucklandia lappa Decne.*, has been used today.

2. 种植采收　木香主产于云南，四川、贵州及湖北等地亦有栽培。多采用种子繁殖，春季或秋季用种子直播，2~3 年后可收获，9 月下旬至 10 月下旬于晴天收获。

2 Planting and Harvesting

It is mainly produced in Yunnan, Sichuan, Guizhou and Hubei provinces. Seeds are often used for propagation, and seeds are sowed in spring or autumn and it can be harvested after 2~3 years' growing, in late September to late October in sunny days.

3. 道地性及品质评价　古代药用之木香，来源复杂，既有国产，亦有进口。国内种木香，主产于云南丽江、鲁甸等地，以云南产者为道地。木香性状评价以重量为核心，根粗壮均匀、体重坚实、香气浓郁、油性足、无须根者为佳。

3 Genuineness and Quality Evaluation

The sources Muxiang in ancient times are complex, with both domestic and imported ones. Domestic species of Muxiang are mainly produced in Lijiang, Ludian and other places in Yunnan province, as the regional genuine medicinals. The quality of Muxiang is mainly evaluated by its weight as the key indicator, and characterized by strong and even root, heavy weight, rich aroma, sufficient oil, and without fibrous root.

木香主要含有挥发油（主要为倍半萜及其内酯，如去氢木香内酯、木香烃内酯、木香内酯、二氢木香内酯、木香酸、α-木香烯等）及生物碱（如木香碱），为其药效物质基础，其中去氢木香内酯、木香烃内酯是调节胃肠运动、保护胃黏膜、利胆、解痉、抗炎的主要物质基础。此

外，木香还含有树脂、菊糖、氨基酸及甾醇等成分。《中国药典》规定木香药材中木香烃内酯和去氢木香内酯的总量不得少于 1.8%。

Muxiang mainly contains volatile oils (mainly sesquiterpenes and their lactones, such as dehydrocostus lactone, costunolactone, costuslactone, dihydrowoody lactone, costusic acid, α-costen, etc.) and alkaloids (such as xylacrine), which are the main material basis for regulating gastrointestinal motility, protecting gastric mucosa, promoting function of gallbladder, anti-spasm and anti-inflammation effects. In addition, Muxiang also contains resin, inulin, amino acids and sterols and other components. *The Pharmacopoeia of the People's Republic of China* stipulates that the total amounts of olefin lactone and dehydrocein lactone in the raw material of Muxiang shall not be less than 1.8%.

二、炮制品种与品质
II Processed Varieties and Quality

木香的炮制品种及临床常用品种有 2 个，即木香和煨木香。木香以切面中部有明显菊花心状放射纹理，形成层环棕色，褐色油点（油室）散在，气香特异为佳；煨木香以气微香为佳。《中国药典》规定木香炮制品中木香烃内酯和去氢木香内酯的总量不得少于 1.5%。

There are 2 commonly used processed varieties of Muxiang in clinical practice, namely Muxiang and Weimuxiang (roasted). For Muxiang, those with obvious radial texture of chrysanthemum-shape in center in the middle of the section to form the brown cambium ring with the scattered brown oil point (oil chamber) and special fragrance are of great quality, while those with mild fragrance of Weimuxiang (roasted) are better. *The Pharmacopoeia of the People's Republic of China* stipulates that the total amount of costunolactone and dehydrocostus lactone in the processed Muxiang products shall not be less than 1.5%.

三、中成药品种与品质
III Varieties and Quality of Chinese Patent Medicines

含有木香或煨木香的中成药有 250 余个。《中国药典》收载含有木香的中成药 139 个。以木香为君药或主药的品种有木香顺气丸、木香槟榔丸等。在中成药的品质控制中多采用显微鉴别和薄层色谱法确定木香的存在，采用含量测定法进行指标成分限量。如调经活血片（胶囊），用显微观察木香木纤维束、薄层色谱法与木香对照药材提取液相鉴别以确定木香的存在，用 HPLC 法限定每个最小规格（片、粒）中有效成分木香烃内酯和去氢木香内酯总量的下限，以保证药品质量。

There are more than 250 Chinese patent medicines containing Muxiang or Weimuxiang (roasted). *The Pharmacopoeia of the People's Republic of China* collects 139 Chinese patent medicines containing Muxiang. Muxiang as the sovereign medicinal or main medicinal can be seen in Muxiang Shunqi Wan, Muxiang Binglang Wan and so on. In the quality control of Chinese patent medicine, microscopic identification and TLC are used to determine the existence of Muxiang, and the content determination method is usually used to test the limits of the indicator components. For example, microscope is used to observe fiber bundle of Muxiang and TLC is to identify with the extract of the control medicinal materials of Muxiang for detecting the existence of Muxiang in Tiaojing Huoxue Pian (Tablets) [Jiaonang (Capsules)]. The lower limit of the total amount of active components in Muxiang, lactone and dehydroxylofen lactone, in each minimum specification (slice, grain) is defined by HPLC method to ensure the quality of the medicine.

【制药】
[Pharmacy]

一、产地加工
I Processing in Production Area

收获后除去泥沙和须根，切段，大的再纵剖成瓣，干燥后撞去粗皮。

After harvest, remove sediment and fibrous root, Muxiang is cut into section. Large ones then cut laterally into flap. Remove the rough skin after totally died.

二、饮片炮制
II Processing of Decoction Pieces

从古至今木香有多种炮制方法，并逐渐形成了"闷润 - 切片 - 煨制"工艺，由此加工的木香、煨木香成为商品规格中的主流。其中，木香偏于行气止痛，煨木香偏于固肠止泻。

Since ancient times, there have been many processing methods, and gradually the process of "soaking for moisture-section-roasting" has been formed. The Muxiang and Weimuxiang (roasted) processed in this way have become the mainstream of commodity specifications. Among them, Muxiang is better for activating qi to relieve the pain, and Weimuxiang (roasted) is better for astringing intestine to stop diarrhea.

木香煨制后挥发油含量降低约 20%，同时挥发油组成发生改变，α - 水芹烯等成分消失，新生成多种挥发性组分，如 α - 紫罗兰酮、α - 石竹烯、β - 倍半水芹烯及 α - 长叶松烯等，从而使其功效发生改变。此外，在传统煨法的基础上，出现了麦麸炒煨和麦麸蒸煨、滑石粉烫煨及隔纸煨等一些改进方法，较面裹煨或湿纸煨法操作简便、适于批量生产。

The content of volatile oils is reduced after

roasting by about 20%, and the composition of volatile oils changes, and the components such as α- water celene disappears, and many volatile components are newly generated, such as α-ionone, α-caryophyllene, β-hemicellulene and α-long leaf pinene, which changes the efficacy. In addition, on the basis of the traditional roasting methods, some improved methods emerge, such as stir-frying and roasting with wheat bran, steaming and roasting with wheat bran, roasting with talc powder and paper-separating roasting. These improvements in operation are simple and suitable for scale production compared with traditional processing methods.

三、中成药制药
III Pharmacy of Chinese Patent Medicines

含木香的中成药, 剂型十分丰富, 涵盖固体、液体与半固体剂型。木香的主要成分为挥发油, 因而多以研粉或提取挥发油入制剂, 以保证有效成分与疗效。含木香的传统中成药制剂多制成水丸。现今为满足现代制剂处方成形性及减少服用剂量, 一般制剂如片剂、胶囊剂、合剂等多以木香挥发油及水提取物入制剂中。

The pharmaceutical forms of Chinese patent medicine containing Muxiang are very rich, covering solid, liquid and semi-solid pharmaceutical forms. The main components of Muxiang are volatile oils, so it is mostly used by grinding into powder or extracting volatile oils into preparation to ensure effective compositions and curative effects. Chinese patent medicine preparations containing Muxiang are mostly made into water pills. Nowadays, in order to satisfy the formability of modern preparations and reduce the dosage, the general preparations such as tablets, capsules, mixtures and so on are mostly put into the preparation with essential oil and water extract.

如木香槟榔丸制剂工艺中, 木香与它药打

粉, 制成水泛丸, 以提高疗效、发挥持久的作用。在活血通脉片制剂工艺中, 提取木香挥发油入制剂以精简药量。在正骨水制剂工艺中, 木香在乙醇溶液中加热回流提取并蒸馏, 收集蒸馏液入制剂, 以形成外用药液。

For example, in the preparation process of Muxiang Binglang Wan, Muxiang and other medicinals are powdered to make water pan pill to improve the curative effect and play a lasting effect. In the preparation process of Huoxue Tongmai Pian (Tablets), the volatile oils of Muxiang are extracted and then put together with other medicinals into the preparation to reduce the dosage. In the process of Zhenggushui preparation, Muxiang is extracted and distilled by heating reflux in ethanol solution, and the distilled liquid is applied into the preparation to form external medicine solution.

【性能功效】
[Property and Efficacy]

一、性能
I Property

木香味辛、苦, 性温, 归脾、胃、大肠、肝、胆经。

Muxiang is pungent and bitter in flavor, warm in nature, enters the spleen, stomach, large intestine, liver, and gallbladder meridians.

二、功效
II Efficacy

1. **行气止痛** 木香味辛而芳香气厚, 为治脾胃气滞、脘腹胀痛之要药。其功效的发挥与调节胃肠运动、保护胃黏膜、止泻、利胆、抗炎、解痉镇痛等药理作用密切相关。木香调节胃肠运动、保护胃黏膜、利胆、解痉作用的有效物质基础主要是去氢木香内酯、木香烃内酯等挥发油成分及木香总生物碱, 通过增加血清胃动素含量、促进缩胆囊素分泌等发挥作用。

1 Activating Qi to Relieve Pain

Muxiang, pungent in flavor with strong fragrance, is the key medicinal for the treatment of qi stagnation of the spleen and stomach and abdominal distension and pain. Its effect is closely related to regulating gastrointestinal motility, protecting gastric mucosa, stopping diarrhea, promoting gallbladder, anti-inflammation and analgesia effect, antispasmodic effect and so on. The effective material base of the functions of regulating gastrointestinal motility, protecting gastric mucosa, gallbladder and antispasmodic effect is mainly the volatile oils, such as dehydrocostus lactone and lactone, as well as the total alkaloids of Muxiang.

2. **健脾消食** 木香味辛性温，归脾、胃、大肠、肝、胆经，可行脾胃之气而健脾消食。其功效的发挥与调节胃肠运动、保护胃黏膜、利胆等药理作用密切相关。

2 Invigorating the Spleen to Promote Digestion

Muxiang, pungent in flavor and entering the spleen, stomach, large intestine, liver, gallbladder meridians, can activate the spleen and stomach qi to strengthen the spleen for digestion. Its effect is closely related to regulating gastrointestinal motility, protecting gastric mucosa and promoting function of gallbladder.

此外，现代研究显示木香具有调节心血管、松弛支气管平滑肌、抑制血小板聚集等作用。

In addition, modern studies have shown that Muxiang can regulate cardiovascular function, relax bronchial smooth muscle and inhibit platelet aggregation and so on.

【应用】
[Applications]

一、主治病证
I Indications

1. **脾胃气滞证** 治疗脾胃气滞证，木香常与陈皮、厚朴配伍以行气止痛，如《医学发明》木香顺气汤、《证治准绳》木香顺气丸；若脾虚气滞，脘腹胀满、食少便溏，可配伍人参、白术、陈皮，如《古今名医方论》香砂六君子汤；若脾虚食少，兼食积气滞，可配伍砂仁、枳实、白术，如《景岳全书》香砂枳术丸。

1 Syndrome of Qi Stagnation of the Spleen and Stomach

For the treatment of qi stagnation of the spleen and stomach, Muxiang is often used with Chenpi and Houpo to activating qi to relieve pain, such as used in Muxiang Shunqi Tang (Decoction) in *Yixue Faming*, Muxiang Shunqi Wan from *Zhengzhi Zhunsheng*; for the treatment of qi stagnation due to spleen deficiency, abdominal distention, poor appetite, loose stool, Muxiang can be combined with Renshen, Baizhu and Chenpi, as in Xiangsha Liujunzi Tang (Decoction) in *Gujin Mingyi Fanglun*; for the treatment of poor appetite due to spleen deficiency with food retention and qi stagnation, Muxiang can be combined with Sharen, Zhishi and Baizhu, as in Xiangsha Zhizhu Wan from *Jingyue Quanshu*.

现代临床，木香配伍常用于治疗食管炎、功能性消化不良、慢性胃炎、慢性结肠炎、肠易激综合征、胆结石、消化系统肿瘤等属脾胃气滞者，如香砂六君子汤、木香槟榔丸、厚朴温中汤等。

In modern clinical practice, Muxiang compatibility is often used to treat esophagitis, functional dyspepsia, chronic gastritis, chronic colitis, irritable bowel syndrome, gallstones, and digestive system tumors, etc., pertaining to qi stagnation of the spleen and stomach, as in Xiangsha Liujunzi Tang (Decoction), Muxiang Binglang Wan, and Houpo Wenzhong Tang (Decoction).

2. **痢疾** 木香为治泻痢见里急后重之要药。治疗湿热痢疾，木香常与黄连、黄芩配伍，如《太平惠民和剂局方》大香连丸、《素问病机气宜保命集》芍药汤；若脾元不足，有痢无积，久不愈者，可与人参、白术、陈皮、诃子等配伍，如

《症因脉治》钱氏异功散；若饮食积滞之脘腹胀满、大便秘结或泻而不爽，可与槟榔、青皮、大黄配伍，如《儒门事亲》木香槟榔丸。

2 Dysentery

Muxiang is the key medicinal for the treatment of dysentery and tenesmus. For the treatment of dampness-heat dysentery, Muxiang is often used with Huanglian and Huangqin as in Daxianglian Wan from *Taiping Huimin Heji Ju Fang* and Shaoyao Tang (Decoction) from *Suwen Bingji Qiyi Baomingji (Collection of Writings on the Mechanism of Disease, Suitability of Qi and Safeguarding of life Discussed in Plain Questions)*; for the treatment of deficiency of the original qi of spleen with dysentery but no retention, lasting for a long-term, Muxiang can be combined with Renshen, Baizhu, Chenpi, Hezi (Chebulae Fructus) as in Qianshi Yigong San (Powder) from *Zhengyin Maizhi*; for the treatment of epigastric fullness, constipation or diarrhea due to the food retention, Muxiang can be combined with Binglang, Qingpi and Dahuang as Muxiang Binglang Wan from *Rumen Shiqin (Confucian Family Affairs)*.

现代临床，木香配伍常用于治疗细菌性痢疾、慢性结直肠炎、溃疡性结肠炎等属中医痢疾者。

In the clinics of modern times, Muxiang compatibility is often used to treat bacillary dysentery, chronic colorectal enteritis, ulcerative colitis, pertaining to Liji in Chinese medicine.

3. 肝胆气滞证　治疗脾失运化、肝失疏泄而致湿热郁蒸、气机阻滞之脘腹胀痛、胁痛、黄疸，可与郁金、大黄、茵陈等配伍，如现代制剂利胆排石颗粒、利胆丸；若治寒疝腹痛及睾丸偏坠疼痛，可与川楝子、小茴香等配伍，如《圣济总录》天台乌药散、《医方集解》导气汤。

3 Syndrome of Qi Stagnation of Liver and Gallbladder

For the treatment of dampness-heat steaming, abdominal distension and pain, hypochondriac pain, jaundice due to qi blockage caused by spleen failure in transportation and transformation and liver failure in controlling conveyance and dispersion, Muxiang can be combined with Yujin, Dahuang, Yinchen, etc., as in modern preparations of Lidan Paishi Keli, Lidan Wan; for the treatment of abdominal pain due to cold hernia and testicular partial dropping pain, Muxiang can be combined with Chuanlianzi (Toosendan Fructus) and Xiaohuixiang (Foeniculi Fructus) as in Tiantai Wuyao San (Powder) recorded in *Sheng Ji Zonglu* and Daoqi Tang (Decoction) in *Yifang Jijie (Collected Exegesis of Prescriptions)*.

现代临床，木香配伍常用于治疗肝炎、胆囊炎、胆结石、肠疝气等属肝胆气滞者，如利胆排石颗粒、导气汤等。

In modern clinical practice, Muxiang compatibility is often used in the treatment of hepatitis, cholecystitis, gallstones, intestinal hernia and others belonging to the syndrome of the qi stagnation of liver and gallbladder, such as Lidan Paishi Keli, Daoqi Tang (Decoction) and so on.

4. 胸痹心痛　治疗寒凝气滞心痛，可与赤芍、姜黄、丁香等配伍，如《经验良方》二香散；若治气滞血瘀之胸痛，可配伍郁金，如《医宗金鉴》颠倒木金散。

4 Chest Painful Impediment and Heart Pain

For the treatment of heart pain due to cold coagulation and qi stagnation, Muxiang can be combined with Chishao, Jianghuang, Dingxiang and so on, as in Erxiang San (Powder) from *Jingyan Liangfang (Good Experience)*; for the treatment of chest pain due to qi stagnation and blood stasis, Muxiang can be combined with Yujin, as in Diandao Mujin San (Powder) in *Yizong Jinjian*.

现代临床，木香配伍常用于治疗冠心病、心绞痛、高血压等属气滞者，如顺气活血汤、活血通脉片等。

In the clinics of modern times, Muxiang compatibility is often used to treat coronary heart diseases, angina pectoris, hypertension and other diseases belonging to the syndrome of qi stagnation, such as in Shunqi Huoxue Tang

(Decoction), Huoxue Tongmai Pain (Tablets).

二、用法用量
II Administration and Dosage

3~6g，水煎。
3~6g, water decoction.

三、注意事项
III Precautions

1. 木香辛温，易耗气伤阴，故阴虚津亏者慎用。

1 Muxiang is pungent and warm, easy to consume qi and lead to yin damage, so it should be carefully used for patients with yin deficiency and body fluid deficiency.

2. 木香含有挥发性成分，故入汤剂一般不宜久煎，以免有效成分耗散，影响疗效。

2 Muxiang contains volatile components, so it should not be decocted for a long time, in case of dissipation of the active components, thus affecting the curative effects.

【知识拓展】
[Knowledge Extension]

木香具有悠久的药用历史，但由于本土资源十分有限，自南朝时就主要依赖进口，且一度与其它药用植物相混。历史上地方习用的木香品种中尚有一种"川木香"，主产于四川、西藏交界，来源于菊科植物川木香 *Vladimiria souliei* (Franch.) Ling 或灰毛川木香 *Vladimiria souliei* (Franch.) Ling var. *cinerea* Ling 的干燥根。其性味同木香，归脾、胃、大肠、胆经，功能行气止痛。研究表明木香与川木香所含化学成分相近但有所区别，尤其是挥发油成分及含量有较大差异。现行药典将川木香单列，以与木香区分。

Muxiang has a long history for medicinal use and, it has mainly relied on imports since the Southern Dynasty because of the limited domestic resources. It once was used with mixture of other similar medicinal plants. There is still a kind of "Chuanmuxiang (Vladimiriae Radix)" in the local varieties used in history, which is mainly produced at the junction of Sichuan and Tibet. It is derived from the dry roots of the *Vladimiria souliei* (French.) Ling or *Vladimiria souliei* (Franch.) Ling var. *cinerea* Ling. Its nature and taste are similar with Muxiang, entering the spleen, stomach, large intestine and gallbladder meridians, with the function of activating qi to relieve pain. Study results show that the chemical compositions of these two medicinals are similar but different from components of the volatile oils and their contents. The current *Pharmacopoeia of People's Republic of China* separates these two medicinals for differentiation.

第十六章 消 食 药
Chapter 16　Food Stagnation Relieving Medicinals

凡以消积导滞、促进消化，治疗饮食积滞为主要作用的药物称为消食药，又叫消导药。此类药多性味甘平或甘温，主归脾胃二经。功能消食化积，开胃和中。主要用治饮食积滞，脘腹胀满，嗳腐吞酸，恶心呕吐，不思饮食，大便失常等脾胃虚弱的消化不良症。气虚无积滞者慎用消食药。现代研究表明，消食药多具有调节胃肠运动、促消化、促进胃蛋白酶活性和胃液分泌、排除肠道积气、降血脂的作用，有些还有抗菌、强心、降压、增加冠脉流量、抗心肌缺血及心律失常等作用。常见的消食药有山楂、神曲、莱菔子、鸡内金等。哺乳期妇女不宜使用麦芽，服用人参时忌用莱菔子。

Food stagnation relieving medicinals are the medicinals of eliminating indigestion, promoting digestion and removing food retention, which are also called medicinals of promoting digestion. Most of them are placid and warm in nature and sweet in flavor, enter the spleen and stomach meridians. The main actions are dissolving or relieving food accumulation and stagnation, appetizing and regulating middle energizer. And it is mainly used to treat indigestion caused by weakness or deficiency of spleen and stomach such as food stagnation, abdominal distention, putrid belching and acid swallowing, nausea and vomiting, poor appetite, stool movement (defecating) disorders and soon. For patients with qi deficiency but without food accumulation stagnation, it should be used cautiously. Modern research shows that the relieving food stagnation medicinals have the functions of regulating gastrointestinal movement, promoting digestion, promoting pepsin activity and gastric juice secretion, eliminating intestinal gas, reducing blood lipid. Apart from that, some of them also have the functions of antibacteria, heart-strengthening, antihypertension, coronary flow increasing, anti-myocardial ischemia, anti-arrhythmia and so on. Common food stagnation relieving medicinals involve Shanzha, Shenqu, Laifuzi, Jineijin and so on. Nursing women should not use Maiya. When taking Renshen, the use of Laifuzi should be avoided.

山　楂

Shanzha
(Crataegi Fructus)

山楂为临床常用消食药。常用炮制品有净山楂（生山楂）、炒山楂、焦山楂、山楂炭。山楂味酸、甘，性微温，归脾、胃、肝经，具有消食健胃，行气散瘀，化浊降脂的功效，主治于肉食积滞，胃脘胀满，泻痢腹痛，瘀血经闭，产后瘀阻，心腹刺痛，胸痹心痛，疝气疼痛，高脂血症。山楂中主要含黄酮类、有机酸类等活性物质，有促进胃液分泌、促进蛋白质和脂肪消化、调节胃肠运动功能、降血脂、抗动脉粥样硬化、抗凝血、抗血栓、抗心肌缺血、降压、强心、抗氧化、抑菌、免疫促进等药理作用，可用于治疗消化不良、冠心病、心绞痛、高脂血症等。

Shanzha is the most commonly used food stagnation relieving medicinals in clinical practice. The main clinical processing varieties of Shanzha are Jingshanzha (Jing means clean raw products), Chaoshanzha (stir-frying), Jiaoshanzha (charred), Shanzhatan (carbonized), etc. Shanzha is sour and sweet in flavor, slightly warm in nature, enters the spleen, stomach and liver meridians. It has main actions of promoting digestion and invigorating stomach, promoting the circulation of qi and dissipating stasis, dissolve the turbidity in vivo and reducing blood lipid. Shanzha is mainly used to treat food stagnation caused by intaking meat excessively, abdominal distention, and diarrhea with abdominal pain, amenorrhea caused by blood stasis, postpartum blood stasis, thoracoabdominal sting, chest painful impediment, heart pain, and hyperlipemia. Shanzha mainly contains flavonoids, organic acids and other active constituents. It has the pharmacological functions of promoting gastric juice secretion, promoting protein and fat digestion, regulating gastrointestinal movement, reducing blood lipid, anti-atherosclerosis, anti-coagulation, anti-thrombosis, anti-myocardial ischemia, reducing blood press, cardiac function, anti-oxidation, bacteriostasis, and immune promotion and so on. It is often used to treat indigestion, coronary heart disease, angina pectoris and hyperlipidemia.

【品种品质】
[Variety and Quality]

一、基原品种与品质
I Origin Varieties and Quality

1. 品种概况　来源于蔷薇科植物山里红 *Crataegus pinnatifida* Bge. var. *major* N. E. Br. 或山楂 *Crataegus pinnatifida* Bge. 的干燥成熟果实。

1 Variety

Shanzha is the dried ripe fruit derived from the *Rosaceous* plant of *Crataegus pinnatifida* Bge. var. *major* N.E.Br. or *Crataegus pinnatifida* Bge.

山楂始载于《本草衍义补遗》。《新修本草》载有赤爪木，《本草纲目》曰："赤爪、棠梂、山楂，一物也"。上述与今作山楂用之多种山楂属植物一致。

Shanzha was first recorded in *Bencao Yanyi Buyi (Addendum of Materia Medica)*. And it is recorded in *Xinxiu Bencao* with name of Chizhaomu. *Bencao Gangmu* recorded: "Chizhao, Tangqiu and Shanzha are the same plant." The morphological characteristics of plant above-mentioned are consistent with the variety of Shanzha plants used today.

2. 种植采收　山楂主产于河北、河南、山东、辽宁、黑龙江、内蒙古等省。山里红或山楂为正品山楂的来源，其中山里红均为栽培，而山楂多野生。生产上常采用嫁接繁殖，春、夏、秋季均可进行嫁接。9~10月间果实皮色显露，果点明显时即可采收。

2 Planting and Harvesting

Shanzha produces mainly in Hebei, Henan, Shandong, Liaoning, Heilongjiang, Neimengu and other provinces. *Crataegus pinnatifida* Bge.var. *major* N.E.Br. and *Crataegus pinnatifida* Bge are the sources of authentic Shanzha. But *Crataegus pinnatifida* Bge.var.*major* is mainly cultivated, and *Crataegus pinnatifida* Bge is mostly wild. In production, grafting is often used in spring, summer and autumn. From September to October, when the fruit color is most beautiful and the spots on the fruit skin are obviously, that's the time to make a harvest.

3. 道地性及品质评价　山楂道地性不明显，以"个大、核少、肉厚，皮红，气味浓厚"者为佳。

3 Genuineness and Quality Evaluation

The genuineness of Shanzha is not obviously. The one with high quality should be bigger, kernel less, pulp thick, skin red, and smell fruitier.

黄酮类及有机酸类是山楂的主要活性物质基础，黄酮类化合物主要有牡荆素、槲皮素、槲皮苷、金丝桃苷、7，4'，5，7- 四羟基黄酮 -7- 葡萄糖苷和芦丁等；有机酸主要有山楂酸、柠檬酸、熊果酸等。有机酸是其助消化、调节胃肠运动功能的主要物质基础，黄酮是降血脂、抗凝血、抗血栓的主要物质基础。另外尚含有糖类、鞣质、磷脂、维生素 C、维生素 B$_2$ 与微量元素等化学成分。《中国药典》规定山楂药材中含有机酸以枸橼酸计，不得少于 5.0%。

The flavonoids and organic acids are the main active substances of Shanzha. The main flavonoids in Shanzha mainly include vitexin, quercetin, quercitrin, hyperin, 7,4',5,7-tetrahydroxy flavonoid-7-glucoside and rutin etc. The main organic acids in Shanzha mainly include maslinic acid, citric acid, ursolic acid and so on. The organic acids are the main active material basis for its effects of promoting digestion and regulation of gastrointestinal movement; flavonoids are the main active material basis for reducing blood lipid, anticoagulation and antithrombotic effect. Shanzha

also contains carbohydrate, tannin, phospholipid, vitamin C, vitamin B$_2$ and microelement additionally. *Pharmacopoeia of the People's Republic of China* regulates that the concentration of organic acid, citrate determined in Shanzha medicinal material shall not be less than 5.0 %.

二、炮制品种与品质
II Processed Varieties and Quality

山楂的现代炮制品种有 4 个，临床常用品种有净山楂、炒山楂、焦山楂、山楂炭等。净山楂以果肉深黄色至浅棕色，气清香，味酸、微甜者为佳；炒山楂以果肉黄褐色，偶见焦斑，气清香，味酸、微甜者为佳；焦山楂以表面焦褐色，内部黄褐色，有焦香气者为佳。净山楂饮片的品质评价同药材。

There are four modern processing varieties of Shanzha available, clinically often used including Jingshanzha, Chaoshanzha (stir-frying), Jiaoshanzha (charred), Shanzhatan (carbonized), etc. The better one of Jingshanzha should have its pulp in deep yellow to light brown color, fruitier fragrance, sour taste and slightly sweet. Chaoshanzha (stir-frying) in better quality should have yellow pulp, occasionally brown coke spots, fragrance, sour taste, slightly sweet. Jiaoshanzha (charred) should have the black and brown surface, yellow and brown interior, and scorched incense smelling. The quality evaluation for Jingshanzha should be taken the same as that for medicinal materials.

三、中成药品种与品质
III Varieties and Quality of Chinese Patent Medicines

据统计，现行版《中国药典》收载含有山楂的中成药 90 余个。以山楂为君药或主药的品种有乐脉颗粒、大山楂丸、山菊降压片、山楂化滞丸、小儿七星茶口服液（颗粒）、小儿化食口服液等。

According to statistics, *Pharmacopoeia of the*

People's Republic of China records more than 90 Chinese patent medicine which contains Shanzha. Many varieties collecte Shanzha as the sovereign medicinal or main medicinal, such as Lemai Keli, Dashanzha Wan, Shanju Jiangya Pian (Tablets), Shanzha Huazhi Wan, Xiaoer Qixingcha Koufuye, Xiaoer Huashi Koufuye.

在含山楂的中成药品质控制中，多采用薄层色谱法确定山楂的存在；采用薄层色谱扫描法对山楂中熊果酸进行含量测定；另在山楂粉碎成细粉入药的中成药中，如大山楂丸、山楂化滞丸等，还可同时采用显微鉴别"果皮石细胞淡紫色、红色或黄棕色，类圆形或多角形"确定山楂的存在。

In the quality control process of Chinese patent medicines containing Shanzha, TCL and TLCS can be used to identify Shanzha and determine content of ursolic acid of Shanzha respectively. In some formula like Dashanzha Wan, Shanzha Huazhi Wan, for Shanzha is pulverized into fine powder for medicines; the presence of "pericarp stone cells mauve, red or yellowish brown, rounded or polygonal" can be identified by microscopy.

【制药】
[Pharmacy]

一、产地加工
I Processing in Production Area

山楂以净制、切制、炒制为主要加工工序，果实采收后，去核、切片、干燥，加工生产成不同规格品种。

The processing in producing area of Shanzha is cleansing, cutting, stir-frying. After harvesting, removing the kernels, cutting into slices and drying, it is processed into different specifications.

二、饮片炮制
II Processing of Decoction Pieces

在古代，山楂的炮制方法就有10余种。元

代以来，主要以净山楂、炒山楂、焦山楂、山楂炭为商品规格中的主流。

In ancient times, the processing methods of Shanzha have more than 10 kinds. Since the Yuan dynasty, main commercial specifications were Jingshanzha, Chaoshanzha (stir-frying), Jiaoshanzha (charred), Shanzhatan (carbonized).

研究表明，山楂受热时间越长，温度越高，被破坏的总黄酮越多，总黄酮含量：净山楂＞炒山楂＞焦山楂＞山楂炭；高温炮制还会导致山楂中枸橼酸的含量和总磷脂含量均下降，尤其是山楂炭中下降更加明显。

The study showed that the more damaged of total flavonoids with the longer heating time and higher temperature, total flavonoids content in Shanzha: Jingshanzha ＞ Chaoshanzha (stir-frying) ＞ Jiaoshanzha (charred) ＞ Shanzhatan (carbonized). The citric acid content and total phospholipid content in Shanzha all will be reduced with being processed in high temperature especially for Shanzhatan (carbonized).

生山楂长于活血化瘀，常用于血瘀经闭，产后瘀阻，心腹刺痛，以及高脂血症、高血压、冠心病，如乐脉颗粒、山菊降压片等中的配伍使用，但因生山楂有克伐正气之弊，脾胃虚弱而无积滞者或胃酸分泌过多者均应慎服；炒山楂酸味减弱，可缓和对胃的刺激性，善于消食化积，用于脾虚食滞，食欲不振，神疲乏力，如健胃片、小儿化滞健脾丸等中的配伍使用；焦山楂不仅酸味减弱，而且苦味增加，消食导滞作用增强，长于消食止泻，尤善于消肉食积滞，泻痢不爽，如保和丸、小儿厌食颗粒等中的配伍使用；山楂炭其性收涩，偏于止血止泻，用于胃肠出血或脾虚腹泻兼食滞者。

Main efficacy of Jingshanzha is activating blood circulation to dissipate blood stasis, and often used for blood stasis menstrual closure, postpartum stasis, sting of heart and stomach, hyperlipidemia, hypertension and coronary heart disease treatment. It is often be used in compatibility of medicinals, such as Lemai Keli, Shanju Jiangya Pian (Tablets), etc. But

Shengshanzha (raw) should be taken cautiously for the patients with deficiency of spleen and stomach but without food accumulation stagnation or gastric acid secretion bulls, because its antagonism for vital qi. The sour of Chaoshanzha (stir-frying) is reduced, and the stimulation of stomach is eased. Chaoshanzha (stir-frying) is good at relieving food stagnation and transforms accumulation, and mainly make treatment for food stagnation with spleen deficiency, poor appetite, fatigue and weak. Such as Jianwei Pian (Tablets), Xiaoer Huazhi Jianpi Wan, etc. The peculiarity of Jiaoshanzha (charred) is sour abated and bitter increasesed, good at dissolving food accumulation and antidiarrheal, especially from meat and greasy foods stagnation, diarrhoea and sticky loose stools. Such as Baohe Wan, Xiaoer Yanshi Keli, etc. Shanzhatan (carbonized) is astringent and good at hemostasis, stop diarrhea, used for gastrointestinal bleeding or spleen deficiency diarrhea with food stagnation.

三、中成药制药
III Pharmacy of Chinese Patent Medicines

含山楂的中成药剂型主要以固体和液体剂型为主，如丸剂、片剂、颗粒剂、胶囊、散剂、口服液等。山楂可粉末入药，也可水提、醇提入药。如在大山楂丸、山楂化滞丸等中成药中，山楂直接粉碎成细粉入药，即可全面利用原料药材，又保留了山楂原本的酸甜口感。又如乐脉颗粒，由生山楂与丹参、川芎、红花等多种活血行气药配伍，以金丝桃苷为代表的黄酮类成分是山楂活血化瘀的主要活性物质基础，具有一定的水溶性，因此，全方采用水提法制备，浓缩后直接制粒成型，减少有效物质的损失，确保原方疗效。

The Chinese patent medicines pharmacy pharmaceutical forms containing Shanzha are mainly solid and liquid, such as pills, tablets, granules, capsules, powder, mixture, etc. Medicines powder, water extraction, alcohol extraction all can be uesd according to pharmaceutical process requirements. In some formula like Dashanzha Wan, Shanzha Huazhi Wan, Shanzha is pulverized into fine powder for medicines; the process can make full use of raw materials, and retain the original sweet and sour taste of Shanzha. For the other example, Lemai Keli is combined with Shengshanzha (raw), Danshen, Chuanxiong, Honghua and other medicinals that promoting circulation of blood and qi. The flavonoids represented by hyperoside in Shanzha are the main active constituent to promote blood circulation and remove stasis. And they are water-soluble, so can be extracted by water, then concentrated and made granules directly to reduce the loss of effective material and ensure the efficacy of the original prescription.

【性能功效】
[Property and Efficacy]

一、性能
I Property

山楂酸、甘，微温；归脾、胃、肝经。
Shanzha is sour and sweet in flavor, slightly warm in nature, enters the spleen, stomach and liver meridians.

二、功效
II Efficacy

1. 消食健胃　山楂味酸而甘，微温不热，主入脾、胃经，功善消食化积健胃，尤为消化油腻肉食积滞之要药。其功效的发挥与助消化、促进胃肠运动等药理作用密切相关。山楂助消化、促进胃肠运动作用的有效物质基础主要是有机酸及维生素 C、维生素 B_2，通过刺激胃黏膜分泌胃液，增强胃液酸度，提高胃蛋白酶活性，促进胰液的分泌和增加胰淀粉酶、胰脂肪酶活性发挥作用。

1 Promoting Digestion and Invigorating Stomach

Shanzha tastes sour and sweet, slightly warm but not hot, and enters the spleen and stomach meridians. The main effects are promoting digestion, dissolving relieving food accumulation and invigorating stomach, and be good at eliminating meat accumulates stagnation especially. Its effect is closely related to helping digestion and promoting gastrointestinal movement. And the active substances are organic acids, vitamin C, vitamin B_2 and so on. They can stimulate gastric mucosa secretion of gastric juice, enhance gastric juice acidity, improve pepsin activity, also can promote the secretion of pancreatic juice and increase the activity of pancreatic amylase, pancreatic lipase, and thereby promoting digestion.

2. 行气散瘀 山楂入肝经，通行气血，故能行气散瘀。其功效的发挥与抗凝血、抗血栓、抗缺血再灌注损伤等药理作用密切相关。山楂抗血栓、抗缺血再灌注损伤的有效物质基础主要是总黄酮、黄烷醇及其聚合物，通过降低血液黏度、延长特征性血栓形成时间（CTFT）和纤维蛋白血栓形成时间（TFT）发挥抗血栓作用，并通过抗氧化损伤和减轻炎症反应发挥抗缺血再灌注损伤作用。

2 Promoting the Circulation of Qi and Dissipating Stasis

Shanzha also enters the liver meridian to drive qi and blood, so can promote the circulation of qi and dissipate stasis. Its effect and efficacy are closely related to anticoagulation, antithrombus, anti-ischemia-reperfusion injury and other pharmacological effects. Total flavonoids, flavanols and their polymers of Shanzha are effective substances of the antithrombotic and antiischemia-reperfusion injury. The effects of anticoagulant and antithrombotic exert themselves through reducing blood viscosity, prolonging the time of characteristic thrombus formation (CTFT) and fibrin thrombus formation (TFT). It can show a protective effect on cerebral ischemia injury through antioxidative damage and reducing inflammatory response.

3. 化浊降脂 山楂化浊降脂的功效与降血糖、降血脂和抗动脉粥样硬化作用有关。山楂降血糖、降血脂和抗动脉粥样硬化作用的有效物质基础主要是山楂黄酮，通过抑制肝糖原分解和促进其合成发挥降血糖作用；并通过抑制内源性胆固醇合成，加快胆固醇代谢，促进胆汁酸排出和脂质代谢发挥降血脂作用。

3 Resolving Turbidity and Reducing Blood Lipid

The efficacy of dissolving turbidity in vivo and reducing blood lipid is related to lowering blood glucose, reducing blood lipid, anti-atherosclerosis of Shanzha. The total flavonoids contained in Shanzha are effective substances of lowering blood glucose, reducing blood lipid and anti-atherosclerosis. It can lower blood glucose by inhibiting hepatic glycogen decomposition and promoting its synthesis. And it can reducing blood lipid by inhibiting the endogenous cholesterol synthesis, accelerating the metabolism of cholesterol, promoting bile acid discharge and lipid metabolism.

【应用】
[Applications]

一、主治病证
I Indications

1. 肉食积滞 治肉食积滞之脘腹胀满，嗳气吞酸，腹痛便溏者，单味应用即有效，如《简便方》用一味山楂水煎服；或配莱菔子、神曲等同用，如山楂化滞丸；治食积发热者，可配伍连翘等，如《丹溪心法》保和丸；治食积气滞脘腹胀痛者，可配伍木香、青皮、枳实、莪术等同用，如《证治准绳》匀气散。

1 Indigestion and Stagnation from Meat and Greasy Foods

Shanzha can be used alone to treat abdominal

distention, putrid belching and acid swallowing, abdominal pain with loose stools caused by meat and greasy foods accumulation, such as *Jianbianfang* recorded; or combined with Laifuzi, Shenqu, such as Shanzha Huazhi Wan. Treatment of food accumulation with fever can be combined with Lianqiao, such as Baohe Wan recorded in *Danxi Xinfa*. Treatment of food accumulation and qi stagnation with abdominal distention pain can be combined with Muxiang, Qingpi, Zhishi, Ezhu, such as Yunqi San (Powder) recorded in *Zhengzhi Zhunsheng*.

现代临床，山楂配伍常用于治疗消化不良、小儿厌食症、高血脂症、高血压病，如大山楂丸、小儿化滞健脾丸、复方山楂口服液、山菊降压片、化降脂乐片等。

In modern clinical practice, Shanzha compatibility is often used to treat dyspepsia, infantile anorexia, hyperlipidemia, and hypertension. Such as Dashanzha Wan, Xiaoer Huazhi Jianpi Wan, Fufang Shanzha Koufuye, Shanju Jiangya Pian (Tablets), Huajiangzhile Pian (Tablets) and so on.

2. 泻痢腹痛 治泻痢腹痛，可单用焦山楂水煎服，或用山楂炭研末服，亦可配伍木香、槟榔、枳壳等；治湿热食滞互结，痢下赤白，腹痛后重者，可配伍黄连、苦参等。

2 Diarrhea and Abdominal Pain

To treat diarrhea and abdominal pain, we can use Jiaoshanzha (charred) water decoction, or Shanzhatan (carbonized) powder, also can combined with Muxiang, Binglang, Zhiqiao, etc. To treat intermingled dampness-heat and food stagnation, red and white dysentery, abdominal pain and sticky loose stools, it can be combined with Huanglian, Kushen, etc.

现代临床，山楂配伍常用于治疗婴幼儿腹泻、急性菌痢肠炎、慢性胃炎，如山楂糖浆、养胃活血汤等。

In modern clinical practice, Shanzha compatibility is often used in the treatment of infant diarrhea, acute bacterial dysentery enteritis, and chronic gastritis, such as Shanzha Tangjiang, Yangwei Huoxue Tang (Decoction), etc..

3. 瘀阻胸腹痛、痛经 本品性温，能通行气血，有活血祛瘀止痛之功。治瘀滞胸胁痛者，可配伍川芎、桃仁、红花；治产后瘀阻腹痛、恶露不尽、或瘀阻经行腹痛，可单用本品水煎服，或配伍当归、川芎、益母草、香附、红花等，如《景岳全书》通瘀煎；治瘀血阻滞、崩漏下血，常配伍蒲黄炭、茜草炭等。

3 Thoracoabdominal Pain and Dysmenorrhea Caused by Stasis Resistance

Shanzha is warm in nature with the effects of activating qi and blood, and the effects of activating blood circulation, removing stasis and relieving pain. For treatment of stasis chest pain, it can be combined with Chuanxiong, Taoren, and Honghua. In the treatment of postpartum stasis abdominal pain, lochia or dysmenorrhea, Shanzha water decoction can be only used, or combined with Danggui, Chuanxiong, Yimucao (Leonuri Herba), Xiangfu, Honghua and so on, such as Tongyu Jian (Decoction) recorded in *Jingyue Quanshu*. It could be used for the treatment of blood stasis block, lochia endless, often combined with Puhuangtan (carbonized), Qiancaotan (Rubiae Radix Et Rhizoma, carbonized), etc.

现代临床，山楂配伍常用于治疗冠心病、心绞痛、如乐脉颗粒、益心酮胶囊、心血宁片等。

In the modern clinical practice, Shanzha compatibility is often used in the treatment of coronary heart disease, angina pectoris. Such as Lemai Keli, Yixintong Jiaonang (Capsules), Xinxuening Pian (Tablets).

二、用法用量
II　Administration and Dosage

9~12g，煎汤。
9~12g, decoct to drink.

三、注意事项
III　Precautions

1. 生山楂因有克伐正气之弊，脾胃虚弱而无积滞者或胃酸分泌过多者均应慎服。

1 Shengshanzha (raw) has antagonism for vital qi, so should be taken cautiously for the patients with deficicency of spleen and stomach but without food accumulation stagnation or excess gastric acid secretion.

2. 因山楂中含有多种有机酸、鞣质，有机酸可与重金属相结合，鞣质可与胃酸中的蛋白相结合，均可生成不溶于水的聚合物沉积，形成硬块即结石，因此不可多用或久用。

2 Shanzha contains a variety of organic acid and tannin, and organic acid can combine with heavy metals, tannin can combine with the protein in stomach acid, so all could produce insoluble polymer deposition to be lithiasis. So do not use Shengshanzha (raw) for large dose or a long time.

第十七章 止 血 药
Chapter 17　Bleeding-Arresting Medicinals

凡以制止体内或体外出血为主要作用的药物，称为止血药。此类药药性有寒、温、散、敛之异。止血药主要适用于内外出血症，如咯血、咳血、衄血、吐血、便血、尿血、崩漏、紫癜以及外伤出血等。根据其具体作用分为止血凉血药、化瘀止血药、收敛止血药、温经止血药四类。三七等化瘀止血药的活血之力强，孕妇慎用。现代研究表明，止血药可通过收缩小动脉及毛细血管，或增强血小板功能，或加速、加强血液凝固过程，或抑制血块溶解过程等，起到止血作用。常见的止血药有止血凉血药（大蓟、地榆、槐花等）、化瘀止血药（三七、茜草、花蕊石等）、收敛止血药（白芨、仙鹤草、血余炭等）、温经止血药（炮姜、艾叶等）。

These medicinals that mainly used to stop internal and external bleeding are called bleeding-arresting medicinals, which are mainly used for internal and external bleeding, such as hemoptysis, epistaxis, hematemesis, hematochezia, hematuria, uterine bleeding, metrorrhagia, purpura and traumatic bleeding. According to their specific functions, bleeding-arresting medicinals can be divided into four categories: stopping and cooling blood hemostatic medicinals, removing stasis hemostatic medicinals, astringent hemostatic medicinals and warm-meridian hemostatic medicinals. Sanqi and other removing stasis hemostatic medicinals have a strong effect on promoting blood circulation, so pregnant women should use them with caution. Modern studies have shown that bleeding-arresting medicinal effect can be played by narrowing the arteries and capillaries, or enhancing the function of platelets, or accelerating and strengthening the coagulation process of blood, or inhibiting the process of clot dissolution. The frequently-used bleeding-arresting medicinals are cooling blood hemostatic medicinals (Daji, Diyu, Huaihua, etc.), removing stasis hemostatic medicinals (Sanqi, Qiancao, Huaruishi, etc.), astringent hemostatic medicinals [Baiji, Xianhecao (Agrimoniae Herba), Xueyutan, etc.], warm-meridian hemostatic medicinals (Paojiang, Aiye, etc.).

三 七

Sanqi
(Notoginseng Radix et Rhizoma)

三七是一味化瘀止血的名贵中药材，云南和广西为其道地产区。临床常用炮制品主要为生三七粉与熟三七粉。三七味甘、微苦，性温，归肝、胃经，有散瘀止血、消肿定痛的功效，用于治疗咯血，吐血，衄血，便血，崩漏，外伤出血，胸腹刺痛，跌扑肿痛。三七中主要含皂苷、黄酮、挥发油、糖类、氨基酸等成分，有止血、促进造血、抗血栓、抗动脉粥样硬化、扩血管、降血压、抗心肌梗死、抗心律失常、抗炎、镇痛、保肝利胆、抗肿瘤等药理作用。可用于治疗颅内出血、上消化道出血等各种出血症，属出血而兼有瘀血阻滞证者，及瘀血肿痛、跌打损伤、冠心病、高血压、偏头痛、急性脑梗死、慢性萎缩性胃炎、化脓性阑尾炎等，属瘀血阻滞证者。

Sanqi is a valuable Chinese medicinal material for bleeding-arresting medicinal, and Yunnan and Guangxi are the genuine producing areas. Clinical commonly used processed products are Shengsanqi (raw) powder and Shusanqi (prepared) powder. Sanqi is sweet and slightly bitter in flavor, and warm in nature, entering the liver and stomach meridians. The main effects are dispersing blood stasis and stoping bleeding, reducing swelling and relieving pain. And Sanqi is used to treat hemoptysis, hematemesis, epistaxis, hematochezia, uterine bleeding, traumatic bleeding, thoracoabdominal pricking, swelling and pain caused by tumble fell. Sanqi mainly contains saponins, flavonoids, volatile oils, saccharides and amino acids, etc. Sanqi has broader pharmacological effects such as hemostasis, promotion of hematopoietic, anti-thrombotic effect, anti-atherosclerosis, vasodilator effect, lowering blood pressure, anti-myocardial infarction, anti-arrhythmia, anti-inflammatory effect, relieving pain, protecting liver and gallbladder, anti-tumor effect and so on. Sanqi can be used to treat intracranial hemorrhage, cerebral hemorrhage, upper gastrointestinal hemorrhage and other haemorrhage, which belongs to bleeding with syndrome of static blood obstruction and stagnation. And it also can be used to treat stasis swelling pain, injury, coronary heart disease, hypertension, migraine, acute cerebral infarction, chronic atrophic gastritis, suppurative appendicitis, etc., which belongs to static blood obstruction and stagnation syndrome.

【品种品质】
[Variety and Quality]

一、基原品种与品质
I Origin Varieties and Quality

1. **品种概况**　来源于五加科植物三七 *Panax notoginseng* (Burk.) F. H. Chen 的干燥根和根茎。

1 Variety

Sanqi is the dried root and rhizome derived from the *Araliaceae* plant of *Panax notoginseng* (Burk.) F.H. Chen.

三七始载于《本草纲目》，李时珍云"生广西南丹诸州番恫深山中，采根曝干，黄黑色，团结者，状略似白及；长者如老干地黄有节"。《本草纲目拾遗》按以上三七形态及生长环境的记述，其原植物与现用五加科三七一致。

Sanqi was first recorded in *Bencao Gangmu*. Li shizhen recorded that Sanqi was born in the Fantong Mountains of Guanxi Nandan states, harvested the root on the field under the blazing sun, showed yellow and black block mass, the shape was similar to Baiji; elder root was like dry Dihuang with knob. *Bencao Gangmu Shiyi (Supplement to the Compendium of Materia Medica)* recorded the morphology and growth environment of Sanqi according to description mentioned above, its original plant was consistent with *Panax notoginseng* (Burk.) F.H. Chen that used now.

2. **种植采收**　三七主产于云南文山，广西田阳、靖西，现以栽培品为主，通常以大棚遮阴的方式进行栽培。一般于种后第三至第四年采收，采收期分秋、冬两季。秋季花开前采挖的三七，叫做"春七"，其根饱满、质优、产量高；冬季种子结实后采挖的三七，叫做"冬七"，其根松泡、质次、产量低。

2 Planting and Harvesting

Sanqi is mainly produced in Wenshan of Yunnan, Tianyang and Jingxi of Guangxi. It is mainly cultivated now and usually be cultivated in the way of greenhouse shading. Generally Sanqi is harvested in the third to fourth year after cultivating, and the harvest period is divided into autumn and winter. Sanqi which harvested before blooming in autumn is called Chunqi with full roots, superior quality and high yield. Sanqi, harvested after seeding in winter, is called Dongqi with flabby roots, poor quality and low yield.

3. 道地性及品质评价 三七原产广西，称之为广三七、田七，云南产者后来居上，称滇三七，成为继广西之后三七新道地产区，其中以云南文山产者质量最好。现云南和广西均为三七的道地产区。以 "蓝皮蓝肉者为佳，黄皮黄肉者略差。暑天收成者佳，冬天收成者次之"。实际流通中，一般以外观及体质特征、个头大小为性状评价指标。

3 Genuineness and Quality Evaluation

Sanqi was produced originally from Guangxi that known as Guangsanqi and Tianqi. Later Sanqi produce from Yunnan surpassed and was called Diansanqi. Yunnan and Guangxi are the genuine production area now. Sanqi with the blue skin and blue interior is better, and the one with yellow skin and yellow interior is slightly worse. Sanqi that be harvested in hot summer is superior quality, while in winter is poor quality. In market circulation, the general evaluation indexes of Sanqi are appearance, physical characteristics and size.

三七中主含皂苷、黄酮类成分，其中皂苷是三七的主要有效成分，和人参所含皂苷类似，但主要为达玛脂烷系皂苷，有人参皂苷 Rb_1、Rb_2、Rc、Rd、Re、Rg_1、Rg_2、Rh_1 及三七皂苷 $R_{1\sim4}$、R_6 等。三七总皂苷是其补血、抗血栓、调节心血管系统功能、抗炎、镇痛的主要物质基础。尚含有止血活性成分田七氨酸。此外，三七还含有少量黄酮、挥发油、氨基酸、甾醇、聚炔醇、有机酸类、无机元素等。《中国药典》规定三七中人参皂苷 Rg_1、人参皂苷 Rb_1 和三七皂苷 R_1 三者的总量不得少于 5.0%。

Sanqi mainly contains saponins and flavonoids, among which saponins are the main effective components of it. The saponins of Sanqi are similar to the saponins contained in Renshen, but mainly contains the damalidine saponins such as ginsenosides Rb_1, Rb_2, Rc, Rd, Re, Rg_1, Rg_2, Rh_1 and sanchinoside $R_{1\sim4}$, R_6, etc. Total saponins of Sanqi are the main material basis of enriching the blood, anti-thrombotic, cardiovascular system function regulation, anti-inflammatory and analgesic effects. In addition, it also contains the hemostatic active components dencichine and a few inorganic elements, etc. *Pharmacopoeia of the People's Republic of China* stipulates that the total amount of ginsenoside Rg_1, ginsenoside Rb_1 and notoginsenoside R_1 in Sanqi should not be less than 5.0%.

二、炮制品种与品质
II Processed Varieties and Quality

三七的炮制品种和临床常用品种均主要有 3 个，生三七、三七粉、熟三七等。三七以体重，质坚实，断面为灰绿色、黄绿色或灰白色（俗称 "铜皮铁骨"），气微，味苦回甜者为佳；三七粉以灰黄色粉末，气微，味苦回甜者为佳。三七饮片的品质评价同药材。

There are 3 main processing varieties of Sanqi in market, Shengsanqi (raw), Sanqifen (Powder), Shusanqi (prepared) etc. The good quality of Sanqi should show the follow characteristics as heavy weight, solid, gray green cross section, yellow green or gray white, that commonly known as "copper skin and iron bone", and with slightly smelling, taste bitter and sweet later. The quality evaluation of Sanqi decoction pieces is the same as that of medicinal materials.

三、中成药品种与品质
III Varieties and Quality of Chinese Patent Medicines

据统计，《中国药典》收载含有三七的中成药共计 90 余个。以三七为君药或主药的品种有三七片、丹七片、三七血伤宁胶囊、三七通舒胶囊等。在含三七的中成药品质控制中，多采用薄层色谱法和高效液相色谱法对三七中人参皂苷 Rg_1、人参皂苷 Rb_1 和三七皂苷 R_1 进行鉴别和含量测定。对三七直接粉碎成细粉入药的，还可采用显微鉴别"树脂道碎片含黄色分泌物"确定其存在。

According to the statistics, *Pharmacopoeia of the People's Republic of China* records that Chinese patent medicines containing Sanqi are totally more than 90. Many varieties make Sanqi as the sovereign medicinal or main medicinal, such as Sanqi Pian (Tablets), Danqi Pian (Tablets), Sanqi Xueshangning Jiaonang (Capsules), Sanqi Tongshu Jiaonang (Capsules), etc. In the quality control of Chinese patent medicines containing Sanqi, TLC and HPLC were used to identify and determine the content of ginsenoside Rg_1, ginsenoside Rb_1 and notoginsenoside R_1 in Sanqi. When Sanqi is pulverized into fine powder for medicine, the presence of "resin channel debris containing yellow secretions" can be identified by microscopy.

【制药】
[Pharmacy]

一、产地加工
I Processing in Production Are

采挖后，洗净，除去杂质，剪去残茎和须根，须根晒干即得商品"绒根"。把摘下须根的三七根曝晒至根开始变软时，剪下支根和羊肠头（根茎），分别晒干即得商品"筋条"和"剪口"。剩下的三七头需每日曝晒至其全干，质坚实为止，最后将其置于麻袋中，反复相互碰撞摩擦，使其外表皮棕黑发亮即得商品。

Sanqi should be washed and removed impurities after harvesting, cut residual stems and fibres, dried in the sun, and then fibres can be made into commodity Ronggen. When the Sanqi root without fibres have been dried soft in the sun, to cut the rootlets and "head of sheep intestine

(which means rhizome)", then dry them in sun separately to get the product Jingtiao and Jiankou. The remaining Sanqi heads shall be exposed to the sun every day until dry and solid. Finally, they will be placed in gunny bags and repeatedly collided with each other to make the skin show shiny brown and black, ready for commercial use.

二、饮片炮制
II Processing of Decoction Pieces

在古代，三七的炮制方法有为末、研、焙等。现代，三七以净制、捣碎、研粉为工艺，由此加工生产的生三七、三七粉、熟三七等成为市场中的主流商品。

In ancient times, processing methods of Sanqi were mainly crumbling, broken to pieces powder, roasting and so on. In modern times, the main processing of Sanqi is cleansing, smashing, pounding to pieces, grinding powder, and then to be products of different specifications such as Shengsanqi (raw), Sanqifen (Powder), Shusanqi (prepared), as the mainstream commodities in markets.

三七碾成细粉有利于有效成分的溶出，促进药效的发挥。三七经油炸或蒸制后，人参皂苷 Rh_1、Rg_2、$20R$-Rg_2、Rg_3、Rh_4、Rh_2 和 Rk_1 等皂苷类成分含量增加，这些成分大多具有补血、提高免疫、抗肿瘤活性的功能，从而使熟三七补益功效增强。三七生用以散瘀止血，消肿定痛更胜，用于各种出血证及跌打损伤，瘀滞肿痛，如三七伤药片等中的配伍使用；熟三七滋补作用更胜，用于身体虚弱、气血不足的患者，如熟三七丸等中的配伍使用。

Grinding fine powder promotes the dissolution of the effective constituents of Sanqi and promotes the exertion of pharmacodynamics. After being fried or steamed, the contents of saponins in Sanqi such as ginsenosides Rh_1, Rg_2, $20R$-Rg_2, Rg_3, Rh_4, Rh_2 and Rk_1 increased. And most of these constituents have the functions of nourishing blood, immunity enhancement and anti-tumor activity, so as to enhance the tonic effect of Shusanqi (prepared). Shengsanqi (raw) is used for dispersing blood stasis and stopping bleeding, reducing swelling and relieving pain, and for all kinds of bleeding and traumatic injury, swelling and pain caused by stasis, such as Sanqi Shangyao Pian (Tablets). The tonic effect of Shusanqi (prepared) is enhanced, which can treat the patients with weak body, insufficient of qi and blood, such as Shusanqi Wan.

三、中成药制药
III Pharmacy of Chinese Patent Medicines

含三七的中成药剂型主要有固体、液体与气体制剂，可供内服或外用。成药制剂中，为提高三七的利用率，常粉碎成细粉应用，如三七片、三七伤药片等，因为三七氨酸被认为是三七止血的活性成分，但受热后易被破坏。现多将三七粉碎成微粉入药，可缩短药物的崩解时限，加速药物的释放，更利于疗效的发挥。也有制剂以三七的乙醇提取物三七三醇皂苷或三七总皂苷为原料入药，如三七通舒胶囊就是以三七三醇皂苷提取物为原料制备的，是具有严格质量控制标准的中间提取物，保证了制剂质量的稳定性。

The pharmaceutical forms of Chinese patent medicine containing Sanqi are mainly solid, liquid and gas, for oral administration or external use. In order to improve the utilization rate, Sanqi is pulverized into fine powder for application generally, such as Sanqi Pian (Tablets), Sanqi Shangyao Pian (Tablets) and so on. Because dencichine is considered to be the active ingredient for hemostasis of Sanqi, while it is easy to be destroyed after heat. Now Sanqi is also be broken into micro powder, that can shorten the disintegrating time limit of medicinals, accelerate the release of medicinals and more conducive to treatment. Some preparations are made with ethanol extract of Sanqi such as notoginseng triol saponins or notoginseng total saponins as raw materials. For example, Sanqi Tongshu Jiaonang (Capsules) is prepared with notoginseng triol saponins. The quality of the compound preparation can ensure the stability with strict quality control standards of the intermediate extract.

【性能功效】
[Property and Efficacy]

一、性能
I Property

三七甘、微苦，温；归肝、胃经。

Sanqi is sweet and slightly bitter in flavor, warm in nature, entering the liver and stomach meridians.

二、功效
II Efficacy

1. 散瘀止血　三七甘缓，苦泄，温通，入肝经血分，长于止血妄行，活血散瘀，清泄血热和化瘀血以止血，有"止血不留瘀、化瘀不伤正"的特点。其功效的发挥与止血、促进造血功能、抗血栓和抗心肌缺血等药理作用密切相关。三七止血的作用与收缩局部血管、增加血小板数量、促进血小板脱颗粒、增加血液中凝血酶含量等有关，三七氨酸被认为是三七止血的活性成分之一，但其受热后易被破坏，故止血宜生用。

1 Dispersing Stasis and Bleeding-arresting
Sanqi is sweet and mild, bitter and discharging, warmly dredging and entering the liver meridian blood aspect, and be good at stopping blood travelling disorder, promoting blood circulation and dissipating blood stasis, stopping bleeding by clearing blood heat and dissipating blood stasis. Sanqi has the characteristics of stopping bleeding without leaving blood stasis, dispersing blood stasis without damage of the vital qi. Its effect is closely related to multiple pharmacologic actions such as hemostasis, promoting hematopoietic function, antithrombosis,

anti-myocardial ischemia and so on. The hemostatic mechanism of Sanqi is related to constricting local blood vessels, increasing platelet count, promoting platelet degranulation and increasing thrombin content in blood. As an active component of Sanqi for hemostasis, dencichine is easy to be destroyed by heat, so Sanqi is suitable in raw for stopping bleeding.

2. 消肿定痛　三七散瘀活血，可使血脉通利，瘀血消散，故能消肿定痛。其功效的发挥与抗心肌缺血、抗炎、镇痛、调节代谢等药理作用密切相关。三七总皂苷是其抗心肌缺血的主要有效物质，能促进骨髓多能造血干细胞增殖、分化，对胶原、ADP 等不同因素诱导的体内或体外血小板聚集有抑制作用，可增加缺血区血流量、降低心肌耗氧量、抗心肌缺血和氧化损伤。以人参二醇皂苷为主的三七总皂苷是其抗炎镇痛的主要有效物质，其抗炎作用可能与垂体 - 肾上腺素系统有关。三七可调节物质代谢，有降脂作用，对糖代谢有双向调节作用，三七皂苷 C_1 能拮抗胰高血糖素的升血糖作用，而三七总皂苷则有协同胰高血糖素的升血糖作用。

2 Reducing Swelling and Relieving Pain

Sanqi can dissipate blood stasis and promote blood circulation to make blood circulation unobstructed and blood stasis dissipated, so as to reduce swelling and relieve pain. Its effect is closely related to the pharmacological action of anti-myocardial ischemia, anti-inflammation, relieving pain and metabolism regulation and so on. Total saponins of Sanqi are the main effective substances against myocardial ischemia, which can promote the proliferation and differentiation of bone marrow multipotent hematopoietic stem cells, inhibit platelet aggregation *in vivo* or *in vitro* induced by different factors such as collagen and ADP and so on, increase blood flow in the ischemic area, reduce myocardial oxygen consumption, and resist myocardial ischemia and oxidative damage. Total saponins mainly contained with ginsenodiol saponins of Sanqi are the effective substances for its anti-inflammatory

and analgesic effects, which may be related to the pituitary-adrenalin system. Sanqi can regulate the metabolism of substances, lower lipid and make bidirectional regulation of glucose metabolism. Notoginsenoside C_1 can antagonize the effect of glucagon on raising blood glucose while the total saponins of Sanqi have a synergistic effect on glucagon to increase blood sugar.

【应用】
[Applications]

一、主治病证
I Indications

1. 各种出血证　广泛用于体内外各种出血，不论有无瘀滞，均可配伍使用，尤宜于出血兼有瘀滞肿痛者。治吐血、衄血、崩漏、外伤出血等，可用三七粉米汤调服或外敷。或与其他温经止血、收敛止血药配伍，既助止血之效，又防留瘀之弊。如治咳血，吐血，衄血，二便下血，可配伍花蕊石、血余炭研粉吞服，如《医学衷中参西录》化血丹；治痢久，脓血腥臭，肠中欲腐，兼下焦虚惫，气虚滑脱者，配伍生山药、鸭蛋子，如《医学衷中参西录》三宝粥；治妇人肝气郁结，致患血崩，口干舌渴，呕吐吞酸者，配伍白芍、白术，如《傅青主女科》平肝开郁止血汤。

1 All Kinds of Bleeding

Sanqi is widely used in all kinds of bleeding *in vivo and in vitro*, and combining with other medicinals no matter whether with stasis, especially for bleeding with stasis and swelling and pain. Sanqifen (Powder) mixed with rice soup or external application can treat hematemesis, epistaxis, uterine bleeding, and traumatic bleeding and so on. Or it can be combined with other medicinals such as warm-meridian hemostatic medicinals and astringent hemostatic medicinals, to help the effect of hemostasis and prevent the remaining of stasis at the same time. To treat hemoptysis, hematemesis, epistaxis, hematochezia and hematuria, Sanqi can be combined with Huaruishi and Xueyutan (Crinis Carbonisatus) to grind powder for swallowing, such as Huaxue Dan (Pills) recorded in *Yixue Zhongzhong Canxi Lu*. To treat long-term dysentery, pus and blood with stench, intestinal decay, and lower energizer deficiency exhausted, qi deficiency slithered, it can be combined with Shengshanyao (Dioscoreae Rhizoma, raw), Yadanzi (Bruceae Fructus), such as Sanbao Zhou (Gruel) recorded in *Yixue Zhongzhong Canxi Lu*. To treat liver qi stagnation of woman, which causes suffering from metrorrhagia, dry mouth tongue thirst, vomiting and stomach acid regurgitation, it can be combined with Baishao, Baizhu, such as Pinggan Kaiyu Zhixue Tang (Decoction) recorded in *Fuqingzhu Nvke (Fu Qing Zhu's Obstetrics and Gynecology)*.

现代临床，三七配伍后常用于血液系统、心脑血管系统等方面的疾病治疗，尤其是各种损伤性出血和内出血，如消化道出血、脑出血等。如用参三七注射液、三七粉治疗胃溃疡、十二指肠球部溃疡出血及慢性胃炎等消化道出血，三七也常被加在牙膏里用于治牙龈出血。

In modern clinical practice, Sanqi compatibility is often used in the blood system, cardiovascular system and other aspects of the disease treatment. Especially all kinds of traumatic bleeding and internal bleeding, such as gastrointestinal bleeding, cerebral hemorrhage and so on. For example, Shensanqi Zhusheye and Sanqifen (Powder) are used in the treatment of gastric ulcer, duodenal bulb ulcer bleeding and chronic gastritis and other gastrointestinal bleeding, etc. Sanqi is often added in toothpaste to treat gingival bleeding.

2. 跌打损伤、瘀血肿痛　适宜于跌打损伤、瘀血肿痛，或胸腹刺痛，可单味内服或外敷，或与其他活血疗伤止痛药配伍。如治疮疡初起肿痛者，敷之可消；而痛疽疮疖，破烂不敛者，可配伍儿茶、乳香，如《医宗金鉴》腐尽生肌散；治外伤骨折，配伍乳香、没药，如《伤科大成》止痛接骨散；治闪挫胁痛，瘀凝于络者，配伍郁

金、青皮、赤芍、桃仁，如《马培之医案》清肝活瘀汤；治瘀滞疼痛及伤痛，可与当归配伍，如《伤科大成》活血止痛汤；治疗跌打损伤，风湿瘀阻，关节痹痛，可配伍草乌、红花，如三七伤药片；治血瘀上焦，肝区刺痛者，常配伍丹参、当归，如《临证医案医方》活血祛瘀汤。

2 Traumatic Injury, Blood Stasis, Swelling and Pain

Sanqi can be swallowed alone or externally used to treat traumatic injury, swelling and pain caused by stasis, chest pain, and also can be combined with other medicinals of promoting blood circulation, curing injury, and relieving pain. The swelling and pain caused by sore and ulcer at the beginning, can be eliminated by applying with Sanqi. And treatment of the ulcer, sore, boil and wound won't heal, Sanqi can be combined with Ercha, Ruxiang, such as Fujin Shengji San (Powder) recorded in *Yizong Jinjian*. To treat traumatic fractures it shall be combined with Ruxiang and Moyao, such as Zhitong Jiegu San (Powder) recorded in *Shangke Dacheng*. Treatment of sprain, contusion, hypochondriac pain and stasis in meridians, it can be combined with Yujin, Qingpi, Chishao (Paeoniae Radix Rubra), Taoren, etc., such as Qinggan Huoyu Tang (Decoction) recorded in *Mapeizhi Yian (Ma Peizhi Medical Case)*. Treatment of stasis pain or injury pain, it can be combined with Danggui, such as Huoxue Zhitong Tang (Decoction) recorded in *Shangke Dacheng (Traumatology Department Recording)*. Treatment of traumatic injury, rheumatism and stasis, joint pain, it can be combined with Caowu, Honghua, etc, such as Sanqi Shangyao Pian (Tablets). To treat blood stasis in upper warmer, liver pricking, it is often combined with Danshen, Danggui, such as Huoxue Quyu Tang (Decoction) recorded in *Linzheng Yian Yifang (Medical Prescription of Clinical Cases)*.

现代临床，三七配伍常用于治疗各种血瘀、血栓类疾病，如心肌缺血、心绞痛、脑血栓、脑缺血等。如丹七片、三七通舒胶囊、羊藿三七胶

囊。治疗开放性骨折，消肿止痛，如田七正骨水。此外，本品尚能补虚，多用于产后血虚或久病体虚者。常与人参配伍，如《辨证录》中完肤续命汤、肺肾两益汤。

In modern clinical practice, Sanqi compatibility is often used to treat various blood stasis and thrombotic diseases, such as myocardial ischemia, angina pectoris, cerebral thrombosis, cerebral ischemia, etc. Such as Danqi Pian (Tablets), Sanqi Tongshu Jiaonang (Capsules), Yanghuo Sanqi Jiaonang (Capsules). For the treatment of open fractures, detumescence pain, such as Tianqizhenggu Shui (Oral liquid) could be used. In addition, Sanqi also can tonify deficiency, to be used for postpartum blood deficiency or body deficiency for chronic illness. It is often combined with Renshen, such as Wanfu Xuming Tang (Decoction) and Feishen Liangyi Tang (Decoction)

recorded in *Bianzhenglu (Syndrome Differentiation to Record)*.

二、用法用量
II Administration and Dosage

3~9g；研粉吞服，一次 1~3g。外用适量。

3~9g. Grinding powder to swallow, 1~3 g each time. Moderate amount for external application.

三、注意事项
III Precautions

孕妇慎用。

The pregnant woman should be cautiously when take it.

第十八章 活血化瘀药

Chapter 18 Blood-activating and Stasis-removing Medicinals

凡以改善瘀阻、通畅血脉为主要作用的药物，称为活血化瘀药，简称活血药、或化瘀药。此类药物性味多辛、苦，主归肝、心经，擅入血分，辛散通行，功能活血化瘀，主治瘀血证。活血药通过化瘀通络作用，又可产生止痛、通经、消癥、疗伤等作用。活血化瘀药散瘀导滞作用强，易耗血动血，凡月经过多或有出血倾向者当忌用，孕妇慎用或忌用。现代研究表明，活血化瘀药多具有抗血栓、抑制血小板聚集、改善微循环、改善血液流变学、镇痛等药理作用。常见的活血化瘀药有丹参、川芎、莪术等。

Medicinals improving the blood stasis, blood vessels as the main role are known as blood-activating and stasis-removing medicinals, blood-activating medicinals, or stasis-removing medicinals for short. Blood-activating and stasis-removing medicinals taste much bitter and pungent, entering liver and heart meridian, breaking and entering the blood, with the functions of promoting blood circulation and removing blood stasis, mainly treating blood stasis syndrome. Blood-activating medicinals can remove blood stasis and dredge collaterals, and can relieve pain and menstruation, eliminate symptoms, and heal wounds, etc. The effect of blood-activating and stasis-removing medicinals in dispersing blood stasis and leading stagnation is strong, so it is easy to consume blood and stir blood, therefore patients with excessive menstruation or bleeding tendency should not use them, and pregnant women should use them with caution or avoid them. Modern research shows that most of the medicinals for promoting blood circulation and removing blood stasis have pharmacological effects in anti-thrombotic properties, inhibiting platelet aggregation, improving microcirculation and hemorheology, analgesic. Common blood-activating and stasis-removing medicinals are Danshen, Chuanxiong, and Ezhu etc.

川 芎

Chuanxiong
(Chuanxiong Rhizoma)

川芎是著名的川产道地药材。川芎辛温，归肝、胆、心包经，具活血行气、祛风止痛的功效，主治血瘀气滞诸痛证、风湿痹痛证、妇科经产血瘀诸证。川芎主要含挥发油、生物碱、酚性成分、内酯、有机酸等成分，有抗血栓、扩张血管、降血压、抗动脉粥样硬化、镇静镇痛等药理作用，可用于治疗冠心病、心绞痛、头痛、肢体疼痛、闭经痛经、月经量少、月经后期、跌扑伤痛等属血瘀气滞证者。川芎辛燥，活血作用强，孕妇、月经过多者慎用，有出血倾向者忌用。

Chuanxiong, which is warm in nature and pungent in flavor, enters liver, gallbladder and pericardium meridians, is a famous genuine regional medicinal from Sichuan province. The functions of Chuanxiong are promoting blood circulation to dissipate blood stasis, promoting qi to activate blood and dispelling wind and relieving pain. The indications of Chuanxiong are to treat the syndromes of stagnation of qi, due to blood stasis, arthralgia due to rheumatism and blood stasis in gynecologic delivery, etc. Chuanxiong mainly contains volatile oil, alkaloids, lipid compounds and organic acid components, which have pharmacological effects such as anti-thrombosis, dilation of blood vessels, lowering blood pressure, anti-atherosclerosis, sedation and analgesia. It can be used for the treatment of the blood stasis and qi stagnation syndromes, such as coronary heart disease angina, headache, limb pain, amenorrhea, dysmenorrhea, low menstrual flow, late menstruation, falling thrashing pain, etc. Because Chuanxiong is pungent and has a strong blood-activating effect, it should be used with caution for pregnant women and menorrhagic patients, and be avoided for patients with bleeding tendency.

【品种品质】
[Variety and Quality]

一、基源品种与品质
I Origin Varieties and Quality

1. **品种概况**　来源于伞形科植物川芎 *Ligusticum chuanxiong* Hort. 的干燥根茎。

1 Variety

Chuanxiong is the dried rhizomes of umbelliefrae (*Ligusticum chuanxiong* Hort.)

川芎首载于《神农本草经》。《救荒本草》云："叶似芹而微细窄，有丫叉，又似白芷，叶亦细，又似胡荽叶而微壮，一种似蛇床叶而亦粗。"历代本草对川芎形态及生长环境的描述与现代伞形科植物川芎一致。

Chuanxiong was first recorded in the book of *Shennong Bencao Jing*. It is recorded in *Jiuhuang Bencao* that: "leaves are a little narrow like celery, and have a crotch, also like root of Baizhi, leaves are also skinny, also like Husuiye (coriander leaf), which are a little strong, and another kind of leaves are also like shechuangye, which are broad." The description of morphology and growing environment of Chuanxiong in all the past dynasties is also consistent with that of Chuanxiong in modern umbelliferae.

2. **种植采收**　川芎以人工种植为主。主产于四川都江堰、彭州、崇州等地，主要采用高山育种和平坝轮作或间套作栽培。山区培育苓子（川芎的繁殖材料）一般在 12 月底至次年 1 月中旬。8 月上中旬在平坝区栽种川芎苓子。栽种次年 5 月下旬至 6 月，当茎上节盘显著突出，并略带紫色时采挖。

2 Planting and Harvesting

Chuanxiong is mainly cultivated-planted, mainly grown in Dujiangyan, Pengzhou, Chongzhou and other places in Sichuan province and it mainly adopts alpine breeding and flat areas rotation or intercropping cultivation. The cultivation of Lingzi (the propagating material of Chuanxiong) in mountainous areas generally takes place from the end of December to mid-January. Chuanxiong is planted in flat areas in early and mid-August. Plant from late May to June of the following year, and excavate when the upper section of the stem is prominent and slightly purple.

3. **道地性及品质评价**　自宋代起四川成为川芎的道地产区，并以四川彭州、都江堰产者为优。川芎性状评价以个大、质坚实、断面黄白色、心似菊花、油性大、香气浓者为佳。

3 Genuineness and Quality Evaluation

According to historical records, from Dynasty

Song, Sichuan province has become the genuine producing area of Chuanxiong, and Chuanxiong planted Pengzhou in Sichuan and Dujiangyan is regarded as the best. For the evaluation of Chuanxiong, Chuanxiong with big size, solid quality, and yellow white section, chrysanthemum like heart, rich oil and strong aroma is preferred.

川芎主要含挥发油、生物碱、酚性成分、内酯、有机酸等成分。一般认为，川芎嗪、川芎总生物碱、藁本内酯及阿魏酸是川芎活血行气止痛的药效物质基础。现代主要以阿魏酸、欧当归内酯对其进行质量评价。《中国药典》规定川芎药材中含阿魏酸（$C_{10}H_{10}O_4$）不得少于 0.10%。

Chuanxiong mainly contains volatile oils, alkaloids, lipid compounds and organic acid components. It is generally believed that ligustrazine, total alkaloids, ligusticum officinale and ferulic acid are the material basis of Chuanxiong for promoting blood circulation and promoting qi circulation and relieving pain. Nowadays, ferulic acid and Angelica lactone are mainly used to evaluate the quality of Chuanxiong. The *Pharmacopoeia of the People's Republic of China* stipulates that the quantity of Ferulic acid ($C_{10}H_{10}O_4$) in Chuanxiong should not be less than 0.10%.

二、炮制品种与品质
II Processed Varieties and Quality

川芎的炮制品种有 20 多个，临床常用品种主要有 2 种，包括川芎和酒川芎。川芎以片大、质坚实、切面黄白或灰白、油性大、香气浓者为佳。酒川芎形如川芎片，以色泽加深、偶见焦斑、质坚脆、略具酒气为佳。《中国药典》规定，川芎饮片的含量测定同药材，含阿魏酸（$C_{10}H_{10}O_4$）不得少于 0.10%。

There are more than 20 processed products of Chuanxiong, 2 specials often used in clinic, which involves the Chuanxiong and Jiuchuanxiong (liquor processed), etc. Chuanxiong with big size, solid quality, yellow or gray section, rich oil, strong aroma is considered as good quality. Jiuchuanxiong (liquor processed) is shaped like Chuanxiong Pian (Tablets), which is regarded as the best with dark color, occasionally seeing focal spot, texture crisp, slightly with the smell of liquor. According to *Pharmacopoeia of the People's Republic of China*, the ferulic acid ($C_{10}H_{10}O_4$) in Chuanxiong decoction pieces should not be less than 0.10%.

三、中成药品种与品质
III Varieties and Quality of Chinese Patent Medicines

含有川芎或其炮制品的中成药有 1000 多个，其中《中国药典》收载 20 多个，以川芎为君药或主药的品种有川芎茶调袋泡茶、复方川芎片等。在中成药的品质控制中多采用显微鉴别与薄层色谱法确定川芎的存在，采用高效液相色谱法测定指标成分阿魏酸含量，并限定阿魏酸下限以保证疗效。如川芎茶调袋泡茶以川芎为君药，用显微鉴别"网状螺纹导管"特征及薄层色谱法确定制剂中含有川芎；复方川芎片含川芎、当归两味药，用薄层色谱法确定川芎药材的存在，用高效液相色谱法测定阿魏酸含量并限定其下限以保证疗效。

At present, there are more than 1000 Chinese patent medicines containing Chuanxiong or its processed products and 20 are recorded in *Pharmacopoeia of the People's Republic of China*. Among which, prescriptions with Chuanxiong as the sovereign medicinal or main medicinal is as follow: Chuanxiong Chatiao tea-bag and compound Chuanxiong tablets. In the quality control of Chinese patent medicines, microscopic identification and TLC are often used to determine the existence of Chuanxiong, and the content of the index component ferulic acid is determined by HPLC, and the minimum quantity of ferulic acid is limited to ensure the efficacy. For example, Chuanxiong Chatiao tea-bag uses Chuanxiong as the sovereign medicinal. The characteristic of "reticular thread catheter" is identified by micrography and the existence of Chuanxiong is determined by TLC. Compound Chuanxiong Pian contain Chuanxiong and Danggui. The existence of Chuanxiong is determined by TLC, and the content of ferulic acid was determined by HPLC and its lower limit was determined to ensure the curative effect.

【制药】
[Pharmacy]

一、产地加工
I Processing in Production Area

采挖后除去茎叶及泥土，晒后烘干，再置竹制容器内，来回抖撞，除去须根。通常用柴火烘炕，现代也有用远红外干燥和微波干燥等方式进行干燥处理。

After harvesting, usually Chuanxiong should be removed the leaves, stems and soil and dried in sun when knocking off the tendrils. In modern times, Chuanxiong is also dried with far-infrared and microwave.

二、饮片炮制
II Processing of Decoction Pieces

自唐代以来，川芎的炮制方法有醋炒、酒炒、焙、煅、蒸等20余种。逐步形成了"润透-蒸煮-切片-酒制"工艺，由此加工的川芎与酒川芎成为商品规格的主流品种。《中国药典》规定将药材除去杂质，分开大小，洗净，润透，切厚片即得饮片。

Since the Tang Dynasty, there have been more than 20 kinds of processing methods of Chuanxiong, such as Cuzhi (stir-frying with vinegar), Jiuzhi (liquor stir-frying), Wei (roasting), Duan (calcining) and Zheng (steaming). The process of "moisturizing-steaming-slicing-liquor making" has gradually formed, and the Zhichuanxiong (processed) and Jiuchuanxiong (liquor processed) have become the mainstream

varieties of commodity specifications. The *Pharmacopoeia of the People's Republic of China* stipulates that the medicinal materials should be removed from impurities, divided into different sizes, washed, thoroughly moisturized, and cut into thick slices to obtain decoction pieces.

传统认为酒炙后可引药上行，并加强活血行气止痛的作用。酒制后总生物碱及阿魏酸含量增加，而川芎嗪与挥发油含量降低。一般认为，酒川芎较川芎活血止痛作用更好。

The traditional view thinks that Jiuchuanxiong (liquor processed) can lead medicinal's action up and strengthen blood circulation, promote qi and relieve pain. Content of alkaloids and ferulic acid increase and ligustrazine and volatile oil decrease in Jiuchuanxiong (liquor processed). The Jiuchuanxiong (liquor processed) has better effects of promoting blood circulation and relieving pain.

三、中成药制药
III Pharmacy of Chinese Patent Medicines

含川芎的中成药剂型比较丰富，涵盖固体、液体和气体制剂。川芎大多以生品入药，如川芎茶调丸、复方川芎片等，少部分以酒制川芎入药，如中风回春丸，以增强其活血化瘀的作用。含川芎的中成药主要以饮片粉碎入药，其次以乙醇提取物和水溶性提取物入药，个别也有以盐酸川芎嗪或磷酸川芎嗪入药。

There are various kinds of Chinese patent medicines containing Chuanxiong, covering solid, liquid and gas dosages. Chuanxiong is mostly used as medicine, such as Chuanxiong Chatiao Wan, Fufang Chuanxiong Pian (Tablets), etc. A small number of Jiuchuanxiong (liquor processed), such as Zhongfeng Huichun Wan, can enhance its effect in promoting blood circulation. The major preparations apply the crushed Chuanxiong pieces; the others put the alcohol extraction and the water boiling into the medicine. Some of them also use Chuanxiong extract as medicine, Such as tetramethylpyrazine hydrochloride, and ligustrazine phosphate Chuanxiong crop.

如以川芎为主药的复方川芎片，制剂采用乙醇回流提取和水提醇沉的方式结合，既保留了醇溶性成分，又除去了水溶性分，达到片剂制剂要求。

For example, with Chuanxiong as the sovereign medicinal, Fufang Chuanxiong Pian (Tablets), were extracted by ethanol and boiled in water, which keep the alcohol soluble ingredient, remove the water soluble component and meet the requirements of tablet preparation.

【性能功效】
[Property and Efficacy]

一、性能
II Efficacy

川芎辛、温，归肝、胆、心包经。

Chuanxiong is pungent in flavor, warm in in nature and enters liver, gallbladder and heart meridians.

二、功效
II Efficacy

1. **活血行气** 川芎辛散温通，既能入心包经活血化瘀通络，又能入肝经调疏泄、畅气机，历来被称为血中之气药。其功效的发挥与抗血栓、抗心脑缺血、扩张冠状动脉、改善微循环等药理作用密切相关。川芎抗血栓、抗心脑缺血等作用的有效物质基础主要是阿魏酸和川芎嗪，通过抑制血小板聚集、减少血小板 TXA_2 生成等发挥作用。

1 Moving Qi and Activating Blood

Chuanxiong is pungent in flavor, and warm in nature, entering into the pericardium through promoting blood circulation and regulating qi movement, and go into the liver. Chuanxiong is known as the qi medicinal working on blood in the Chinese medicine. Its efficacy is closely related with the pharmacological effect of anti-thrombotic, resisiting cardio-cerebral ischemia, dilating

coronary artery and improving microcirculation. Effective material basis on anti-thrombosis and resisiting cardio-cerebral ischemia are ferulic acid and ligustrazine, and they play the role by inhibiting platelet aggregation and reducing platelet TAX_2 formation.

2. **祛风止痛** 川芎辛以散之，上行头目，下行血海，能祛风化瘀止痛。其功效的发挥与镇静、镇痛、抗炎等药理作用相关。川芎镇静、镇痛、抗炎作用的有效物质基础主要是川芎嗪等成分，通过作用于大脑皮层等发挥作用。

2 Eliminating Wind and Relieving Pain

Chuanxiong is pungent to disperse, which can act up to head, down to blood and good at dispelling pathogentic wind, removing blood stasis and relieving pain. The full play of efficacy is associated with sedation, analgesia, anti-inflammatory and other pharmacological effects. Chuanxiong's mainly effective material basis of sedation, analgesia, anti-inflammatory are ligustrazine and other components,which work through cerebral cortex, etc.

【应用】
[Applications]

一、主治病证
I Indications

1. **血瘀气滞诸证** 治胸痹心痛，胸胁刺痛，常配伍桃仁、红花，如《医林改错》血府逐瘀汤；治跌扑损伤，瘀肿疼痛，如《医林改错》身痛逐瘀汤；治癥瘕积聚，配伍没药、赤药，如《医林改错》少腹逐瘀汤；治中风后遗症，气虚血瘀致半身不遂、肢体麻木，配伍黄芪、地龙，如《医林改错》补阳还五汤；治瘀血所致的痛经、闭经、月经后期，配伍当归、桃仁，如《医宗金鉴》桃红四物汤；治产后瘀阻腹痛，如《傅青主女科》生化汤。

1 Syndromes of Stagnation of Qi Due to Blood Stasis

To treat chest obstruction and pain or sting, it

is often combined with Taoren and Honghua, such as Xuefu Zhuyu Tang (Decoction) in *Yilin Gaicuo (Correction on Errors in Medical Works)*; it can be used for treating the traumatic injury caused falling and flapping, with blood stasis, swelling and pain, such as Shentong Zhuyu Tang (Decoction) in *Yilin Gaicuo*; combined with Moyao and Chishao to treat mass accumulation of abdominal mass, such as Shaofu Zhuyu Tang (Decoction); combined with Huangqi and Dilong to treat qi deficiency and blood stasis lead to hemiplegia and numbness of limbs caused by stroking, such as Buyang Huanwu Tang (Decoction) in Yilin Gaicuo; treating dysmenorrhea, amenorrhea, late period of menstruation caused by blood stasis, it is often combined with Danggui, Taoren, such as Taohongsiwu Tang (Decoction) in *Yizong Jingjian*; treatment of abdominal pain due to postpartum stasis, such as Shenghua Tang (Decoction) in *Fuqingzhu Nvke* .

现代临床，川芎配伍常用于冠心病，心绞痛，心肌梗死，脑动脉硬化，脑梗死及脑出血后遗症，脑供血不足等属于瘀血证者，如速效救心丸、复方川芎片等。

In modern clinical practice, Chuanxiong com patibility is often used for treating coronary heart disease, myocardial infarction, and arteriosclerosis, cerebral infarction and cerebral hemorrhage sequela, cerebral insufficiency of blood supply belonging to blood stasis syndrome, such as Suxiao Jiuxing Wan and Fufang Chuanxiong Pian (Tablets), etc.

2. **头痛，风湿痹痛**　川芎擅于祛风止痛，无论风寒、风热、风湿、血虚、血瘀所致头痛，均可配伍应用，故有"头痛不离川芎"之说。治风寒头痛，配伍细辛、白芷，如《太平惠民和剂局方》川芎茶调散；治风湿头痛，配伍羌活、藁本，如《内外伤辨惑论》羌活胜湿汤；治血瘀头痛，配伍麝香、葱白，如《医林改错》通窍活血汤。治风湿痹痛，配伍独活、桑寄生，如《千金方》独活寄生汤。

2 Headache, Rheumatism and Arthralgia

Chuanxiong is good at dispelling wind and relieving pain. It can be used in compatibility to treat headaches no matter caused by wind-cold, wind-heat, wind-dampness, blood deficiency, and blood stasis. Therefore, it is said that "headache can not leave off Chuanxiong". To treat wind-cold headache, compatible with Xixin and Baizhi, it could be used with Xixin, Baizhi, such as Chuanxiong Chatiao San (Porder) in *Taiping Huimin Heji Ju Fang*; for wind-dampness headache, compatible with Qianghuo and Gaoben such as Qianghuo Shengshi Tang (Decoction) in *Neiwaishang Bianhuolun*; for blood stasis and headache, compatible with Shexiang and Congbai (Allii Fistulosi Bulbus), such as Tongqiaohuaoxue Tang (Decotion) in *Yilin Gaicuo (Correction on Errors in Medical Works)*; treating arthralgia due to rheumatism, compatible with Duhuo and Sangjisheng, such as Duhuojisheng Tang (Decoction) in *Qianjin Fang*.

现代临床常配伍用于三叉神经痛、血管神经性头痛等属于瘀血证者，如通天口服液；用于高血压头痛、眩晕，如大川芎口服液、天舒片；用于风热头晕目眩，偏正头痛，鼻塞牙痛，如清眩片；用于感冒头痛，偏正头痛，鼻炎头痛、鼻塞不通等，如依据民间验方研制的中成药都梁丸，由川芎、白芷二药组成。

Modern clinical application like rigeminal nueralgia, angioneurotic headache belongs to blood stasis syndrome, Chuanxiong compatibility is often used, for example, Tongtian Koufuye. Its compatibility can also be used for treating hypertension headache, dizziness, such as Dachuanxiong Koufuye, Tianshu Pian (Tablets); for treating wind-heat dizziness, migraine headache, nasal toothache, such as Qingxuan Pian (Tablets); for treating cold headache, partial headache, rhinitis headache, nasal obstruction, etc., for example, Liang Wan, which is developed according to folk prescription, is composed of Chuanxiong and Baizhi.

此外，现代临床又有以川芎为主的复方治疗哮喘属于痰瘀互结证者，如川芎平喘合剂。

In addition, in modern clinical practice, Chuanxiong-based compound formula such as Chuanxiong Pingchuan Heji is used to treat asthma belonging to the binding of phlegm and blood stasis syndrome.

三、用法用量
II Administration and Dosage

3~10g，煎服，或入丸散。

3~10g, decoct, or made into pills or powder.

四、注意事项
III Precautions

孕妇，月经过多者慎用；有出血倾向者忌用。

Pregnant women and patients with profuse menstruation should use Chuanxiong with cautions. The patients have bleeding tendency should not use it.

【知识拓展】
[Knowledge Extension]

江西产的抚芎 *Ligusticum chuanxiong Hort. cv.Fuxiong*，因江西民间常用之和茶叶一起泡水饮用，故名茶芎，可治疗感冒头痛。

Ligusticum chuanxiong Hort. cv. Fuxiong produced in Jiangxi Province is commonly used in Jiangxi folks to drink with tea, so it is named Chaxiong, which can treat colds and headaches.

丹 参

Danshen
(Salviae Miltiorrhizae Radix et Rhizoma)

丹参是著名的川产道地药材。临床常用炮制品有丹参和酒丹参。丹参苦、微寒，归心、肝经，具活血祛瘀，清心除烦，凉血消痈，通经止痛的功效，主治瘀血证，瘀热证及热扰心神证。丹参主要含脂溶性二萜醌（如丹参酮类、丹参内酯类等）和水溶性酚性酸（如丹酚酸类、丹参素等）两大类成分，有抗血栓、改善血液流变学、改善微循环、镇静、抗心律失常、抗炎、镇痛、抑菌等药理作用，可用于治疗冠心病、心绞痛、心律失常、脑梗死、失眠、月经稀发、闭经、痛经、痤疮、乳腺炎、蜂窝组织炎等属瘀血证或瘀热证者。丹参不宜与藜芦及含有藜芦的中成药同用。丹参活血作用强，孕妇及月经过多者慎用；有出血倾向者忌用。

Danshen, a noted genuine regional medicinal in Sichuan, Clinically, the commonlyused processed products are Shengdanshen and Jiudanshen . Danshen is bitter in flavor, slightly cold in nature, entering the heart and liver meridians. It has the effect of promoting blood circulation and removing blood stasis, clearing heart and relieving vexation, cooling blood and eliminating carbuncle, regulating menstruation and relieving pain. Danshen can be used to treat the syndromes of blood stasis and heat as well as syndrome of heat disturbing mind. Danshen mainly contains liposoluble diterpenoid quinones salviae miltiorrhizae, (such as tanshinones, lactones of salviae milyiorrhizae) and water-soluble phenolic acids (such as salvianolic acid, salvianolic acid), etc. which possess various pharmacological effects, such as the anti-thrombotic, anti-coagulant, improving micro-circulation, anti-arteriosclerosis, sedation, anti-arrhythmia, anti-inflammation, analgesia, anti-bacteria. It can be used for the treatment of coronary heart disease, angina, arrhythmia, insomnia, oligomenstruation, postponed period, amenorrhoea, dysmenorrhea, sore carbuncle and swelling belonging to blood stasis or stagnant heat. Danshen should not be used with Lilu (Veratrum Nigrum) and Chinese patent medicines containing Lilu. Danshen is strong in promoting blood circulation. Therefore, it should be used cautiously in pregnant women and females with menorrhagia and should not be used for people with bleeding tendency.

【品种品质】
[Variety and Quality]

一、基原品种与品质
I Origin Varieties and Quality

1. **品种概况** 来源于唇形科植物丹参 *Salvia miltiorrhiza* Bge. 的根及根茎。

1 Variety

Danshen is the roots and rhizomes of *Salvia miltiorrhiia Bge.* (Fam. Labiatae).

丹参首载于《神农本草经》,《本草经集注》、《本草纲目》等历代本草对丹参的生长环境、植物形态、颜色、生长习性等作了详细的描述,如《本草纲目》云:"一枝五叶,叶如野苏而尖,青色皱毛。小花成穗如蛾形,中有细子。其根皮丹而肉紫。"诸家本草所言丹参的主要形态特征与今用唇形科植物丹参一致。

Danshen was first recorded in the book of *Shennong Bencao Jing*. In *Bencaojing Jizhu (Variorum of Shennong's Classic of Materia Medica)*, and *Bencao Gangmu* it described the growing environment, planting form and color, and growing habits of Danshen, like *Bencao Gangmu* stating that: "A branch has 5 leaves, shape of leaves is sharp like wild Zishu, its color is green and shrink. Its flower is like moths ,and in shape of spike . The color of velamen is red and the fruit is purple." The main morphological characteristics of Danshen suggested by various herbages are consistent with those of Salvia Miltiorrhiza.

2. **种植采收** 丹参以人工种植为主。在全国各地广有种植,以四川中江县为道地产区。丹参传统栽培多用根扦插繁殖,四川多在立春前后栽种,春分时结束。一般在栽种当年11月至次年3月未萌发前采收,除去茎叶、芦头、泥沙,晒干。

2 Planting and Harvesting

Mainly planted artificially, Danshen is cultivated and distributed all over the country. Zhongjiang County in Sichuan province is its genuine production area. Root cutting propagation is the traditional cultivation method of it. In Sichuan, Danshen is often planted around the beginning of spring and ends at the Spring Equinox. Generally, it is harvested before germination from November of the planting year to march of the second year, with the stems and leaves, rhizomes and mud being removed and the medicinal parts being dried in the sun.

3. **道地性及品质评价** 自清代以来,四川中江县就以盛产丹参闻名,并逐渐发展为道地产区。传统认为丹参以 "皮色红,肉紫有纹,质燥体松,头大无芦" 为最佳。现代一般以条粗壮、色紫红、质坚实、无芦头、无须根者为优。丹参主要含有脂溶性二萜醌(如丹参酮类、丹参内酯类等)和水溶性酚性酸(如丹酚酸类、丹参素等)两大类成分,质量上主要以丹参酮 II$_A$、隐丹参酮、丹参酮 I 和丹酚酸 B 作为化学评价指标。一般认为,丹参酮类与丹酚酸类是丹参的主要药效物质基础,其中丹参酮是抗血栓、改善微循环、抗炎、抗菌的主要物质基础,丹酚酸是增加冠脉流量、抗心肌缺血的主要物质基础。现代主要以丹参酮与丹酚酸对其进行质量评价。《中国药典》规定丹参药材中含丹参酮 II$_A$、隐丹参酮和丹参酮 I 的总量不得少于 0.25%;含丹酚酸 B 不得少于 3.0%。

3 Genuineness and Quality Evaluation

Since the Qing Dynasty, Zhongjiang County in Sichuan Province is famous for its abundant Danshen, and gradually developed into genuine production areas. The ancients put forward the evaluation index of Danshen including shape, color and so on, and it is considered that "the best is red skin, purple flesh with veins, loose body and large head without rhizomes". In modern times it is generally believed those with thick stem, purple-red color, solid quality, no rhizomes and no fibrous roots are best in quality. Danshen mainly contains two major components, lipid-soluble diterpenoid quinones (such as tanshinones, salvia lactones, etc.), and water-soluble phenolic acids (such as salvianolic acid, salviol, etc.). Tanshinone II_A, cryptotanshinone, tanshinone I and salvianolic acid B were used as chemical evaluation indexes. It is generally believed that tanshinone and salvianolic acids are the material basis of Salvia miltiorrhiza, among which tanshinone is the main material basis for antithrombotic, microcirculation improving, anti-inflammatory and antibacterial, and salvianolic acid is the main material basis for increasing coronary flow and anti-myocardial ischemia. In the *Pharmacopoeia of the People's Republic of China*, the total contents of tanshinone II_A, cryptotanshinone and tanshinone I should not be less than 0.25%; and salvianolic acid B should not be less than 3.0%.

二、炮制品种与品质
II Processed Varieties and Quality

丹参的炮制品种有 10 多个，临床常用品种主要有 2 种，包括丹参和酒丹参。丹参以片大、片面红黄色至黄棕色，外皮暗红棕色，味微苦涩为佳。酒丹参以形如丹参片，表面红褐色，略具酒香气为佳。饮片的品质评价同药材。

There are more than 10 processed products of Danshen, among them; mainly 2 varieties are available in the clinical, which involve Danshen and Jiudanshen (liquor-processed). Danshen with a big size, red yellow to yellow brown in color, dark red brown in skin, slightly bitter astringent in taste is considered to have better quality. The Jiudanshen is the same as Danshen slices in shape, reddish brown in skin, slightly liquor in aroma

are considered to have better quality. The quality evaluation of decoction pieces is the same as that of medicinal materials.

三、中成药品种与品质
III Varieties and Quality of Chinese Patent Medicines

含有丹参或其炮制品的中成药有 700 多个，其中 2015 版药典收载 28 个。以丹参为君药或主药的品种有复方丹参喷雾剂、复方丹参片等。在中成药的品质控制中多采用薄层色谱法确定丹参的存在，采用高效液相色谱法测定指标成分的含量，并限定其下限以保证疗效。如复方丹参喷雾剂，用薄层色谱法确定制剂中含有丹参酮II_A；用高效液相色谱法测定丹参酮II_A含量并限定其下限以保证疗效。

At present, there are more than 700 Chinese patent medicines containing Danshen or its processed products and 28 are recorded in *Pharmacopoeia of the People's Republic of China*. Among which, prescriptions with Danshen as sovereign are: Fufang Danshen Penwuji and Fufang Danshen Pian (Tablets), etc. The existence of Danshen is mainly determined by TLC and fingerprint. HPLC are used to determine the contents of the target components, and define its lower limit in order to guarantee the curative effect. Taking Fufang Danshen Penwuji as example, TLC is used to confirm the quantity of tanshinone II_A in the preparation and the lowest limit of the content of tanshinone II_A was determined by HPLC to ensure the therapeutic effects.

【制药】
[Pharmacy]

一、产地加工
I Processing in Production Area

采挖后除去茎叶及泥土，晒至六七成干时，把每株丹参的根捏拢，再晒至八九成干，又捏 1

次，把须根全部捏断，晒干即得。

Remove leaves, stems and soil after harvesting. When it's 60 to 70 percent dry, compact the roots of Danshen, and sun it to 80% to 90% dry and pinch again, snap off all the roots and let them dry.

二、饮片炮制
II Processing of Decoction Pieces

从古至今，丹参形成了炒、猪血炒、酒制、醋制、炒炭等多种炮制方法，逐渐形成了"润透-切片-液体辅料炙"的炮制工艺，由此加工的酒丹参与切片后即干燥制成的丹参成为商品规格中的主流品种。

There has been many processing methods forming since the ancient time, such as Chao (stir-frying), Zhuxuechao (stir-frying with pig's blood), Jiuzhi (liquor processed), Cuzhi (vinegar processed), Chaotan (stir-frying to scorch) and so on. The processing technique of "moistening - slicing - liquid excipients" was formed gradually. Thus, the Jiudanshen (liquor-processed) and Danshen pieces dried after being sliced became the mainstream varieties in the commodity specification.

丹参生用性微寒，凉血消痈、清心除烦、安神多生用；酒炙后，寒性得以缓和，活血化瘀之力增强，血瘀疼痛及痛经、闭经多用酒丹参。现代研究发现，丹参酒制或醋制后，水溶性总酚浸出量显著增加，活血、镇痛作用也增强。

The ShengDanshen (raw), slightly cold, it is commonly used in cooling blood and eliminating carbuncle, clearing heart and mind, calming the spirit; after processed by liquor, the cold nature can be alleviated, and the effect is strengthened in promoting blood circulation and removing blood stasis. Jiudanshen (liquor-processed) is used for blood stasis, pain, dysmenorrhea and amenorrhea. Modern research found that when Danshen was processed with liquor or vinegar, the amount of water-soluble total phenols increased significantly, and the effects of promoting blood circulation and analgesic effect also strengthened.

三、中成药制药
III Pharmacy of Chinese Patent Medicines

在中成药中，丹参常与其他活血化瘀药配伍应用，也有以单味饮片或提取物入药制成的制剂。含丹参的中成药，剂型十分丰富，涵盖了固体、液体剂型，具体包括丸剂、片剂、颗粒剂、胶囊剂、注射剂、口服液等，大多是以生丹参入药。丹酚酸与丹参酮均是丹参活血作用的物质基础。丹酚酸含量较高，极性较好，既可水提，也可醇提；丹参酮含量较低，脂溶性强，以醇提为主。

There are various kinds of Chinese patent medicines containing Danshen, compatibility of Danshen with other medicinals for promoting blood circulation and removing blood stasis. There are also medicine preparations made from only medicinal slices or extract of Danshen. Chinese patent medicines containing Danshen are very rich in dosage, covering solid, liquid form of dosage, specifically, pills, tablets, granules, capsules, injections, mixture, etc.; most of them are made of raw Danshen. Salvianolic acid and tanshinone are the material basis for the effect of promoting blood circulation of Danshen. The content of salvianolic acid is higher and the polarity is better, it can be extracted either by water or by ethanol; tanshinone content is low, strongly lipid-soluble, and alcohol-based, it should be mainly extracted by ethanol.

中成药制药中，以丹参粉碎为细粉直接入药的，如天王补心丸；以水溶性提取物入药的，如丹七片、消栓通络胶囊等；以乙醇提取物入药的，如复方丹参片、丹膝颗粒等；以水溶性提取物和乙醇提取物合并入药的，如丹参片；以有效成分入药的，如丹参酮ⅡA磺酸钠注射液、丹参酮胶囊等；多数是以水提醇沉处理的提取物入药，如复方丹参滴丸、丹参注射液等。

In Chinese Patent Medicines, the preparation

method of Danshen is quite diverse. Danshen is crushed as a powder directly applying into the medicine, for example, Tianwang Buxing Wan; water-soluble extracts used as medicines, for example, Danqi Pian (Tablets), Xiaoshuan Tongluo Jiaonang (Capsules); ethanol extracts used as medicine, for example, Compound Danshen Pian (Tablets), Danxi Jiaonang (Granules) etc; water-soluble extract and ethanol extract combined into medicines, for example, Danshen Pian (Tablets); active ingredients used in medicines, such as sodium tanshinone II_A sulfonate Injection, Tanshinone Jiaonang etc.; most of the extracts were extracted by water and then precipitated by alcohol, such as Fufang Danshen Diwan, Danshen Zhusheye, etc.

【性能功效】
[Property and Efficacy]

一、性能
I Property

丹参苦，微寒；归心、肝经。

Danshen is bitter in flavor, slightly cold in nature, and entries the heart and liver meridians.

二、功效
II Efficacy

1. 活血祛瘀 丹参色赤入血，能破宿血，化瘀滞。其功效的发挥与抗血栓、改善微循环、调节血脂、抗动脉硬化等药理作用密切相关。丹参抗血栓、改善微循环的主要物质基础是丹酚酸和丹参素等成分；增加冠脉流量、抗心肌缺血的主要物质基础是丹酚酸。通过作用于 P-selectin、TXB_2、抑制血小板聚集等发挥作用。

1 Promoting Blood Circulation and Removing Blood Stasis

Danshen is red in color and enters into the blood; it can activate the blood flow and remove the stasis. Its effects extertion are

closely related to the following effects like anti-thrombotic, anti-coagulant, improving microcirculation, regulating lipids, and resisting arteriosclerosis actions. Salvianolic acid and danshensu are the main material basis for anti-thrombosis and microcirculation improvement of Danshen, and salvianolic acid is the main material basis for increasing coronary flow and preventing myocardial ischemia. It works by acting on P-selectin, TXB_2, and inhibiting platelet aggregation.

2. 通经止痛 丹参活血通经，逐瘀止痛。其功效的发挥与雌激素样作用、镇痛等药理作用密切相关。雌激素样作用与镇痛作用的主要物质基础是丹参酮，通过作用于子宫、调节血清 E_2 水平等发挥雌激素样作用。

2 Regulating Menstruation and Relieving Pain

Danshen can invigorate the blood and meridians, expel blood stasis and relieve pain. Its effect is closely related to estrogenic action, analgesic action and so on. The main material basis of estrogen-like effect and analgesia is tanshinone, which exerts estrogen-like effect by acting on the uterus and regulating the level of serum E_2.

3. 清心除烦 丹参味苦入心经，性寒清心火，除烦安神。其功效的发挥与抑制中枢神经系统、抗心律失常等药理作用密切相关。抗心律失常的主要物质基础是丹参素和丹参酮，通过清除自由基、抑制钙超载等发挥作用。

3 Clearing the Mind and Relieving Anxiousness

Danshen tastes bitter and enters the heart meridian, cold in nature and clears the heat of heart, calms the mind and relieves anxiousness. Its efficacy is closely related to inhibiting central nervous system and anti-arrhythmic. The main material basis for anti-arrhythmia is Danshensu and Tanshinone, which play a role by scavenging free radicals and inhibiting calcium overload.

4. 凉血消痈 丹参性寒，入血分，凉血消痈。其功效的发挥与抗炎、抑菌、促进组织修复等药理作用密切相关，主要物质基础是丹参酮和丹参素，通过减少血管活性物质释放，抑制炎症细胞聚集等发挥作用。

4 Cooling Blood and Resolving Carbuncle

Danshen is cold in nature and enters into the blood, cools the blood and resolves carbuncle. Its function is closely related to anti-inflammation, bacteriostasis, tissue repairing and so on. Its efficacy is closely related to the pharmacological effects such as anti-inflammatory, antibacterial, and promotion of tissue repair. The main material basis of the effect is tanshinone and danshensu, which play a role by reducing the release of vasoactive substances and inhibiting the aggregation of inflammatory cells.

【应用】
[Applications]

一、主治病证
I Indications

1. 瘀血证　治胸痹心痛，配伍三七、冰片，如复方丹参滴丸；治心腹诸痛，配伍檀香、砂仁，如《医学金针》丹参饮；治痛经闭经，月经后期、量少色暗，产后瘀滞腹痛，可单味为末，温酒调服，如《妇人良方》丹参散，或配伍川芎、当归等，如《卫生鸿宝》宁坤至宝丹；治跌打损伤，瘀血作痛，配伍乳香、没药等，如《医学衷中参西录》活血通络丹。

1 Blood Stasis Syndrome

To treat chest pain and heartache, Danshen is compatible with Sanqi, Bingpian, such as Fufang Danshen Diwan . To treat various pains in the heart and abdomen, compatible with sandalwood and Amomum, such as Danshen Yin (Decoction) from *Yixue Jinzhen (Medical Golden Needle)*; to treat dysmenorrhea, amenorrhea, late menstruation, less volume, dark color, postpartum stasis and abdominal pain, the single medicinal can be powdered and mixed with warm liquor, such as Danshen San (Powder) in *Furen Liangfang (Women's Recipe)*. Danshen could be compatible with Chuanxiong (Ligutici Rhizoma), and Danggui (Angelicae Sinensis Radix) etc., such as Ningkun Zhibao Dan (Pellets) in *Weisheng Hongbao (Health Hongbao)*; for treatment of bruises, blood stasis and pain, compatibility with frankincense, myrrh, etc., such as Huoxue Tongluo Dan (Pills) from *Yixue Zhongzhong Canxi Lu.*

现代临床，丹参配伍常用于治疗冠心病、心绞痛、脑梗死等心脑血管疾病属瘀血证者，如丹参注射液、香丹注射液等。此外，丹参现代也广泛用于慢性肝炎、肝纤维化等伴见瘀阻胁痛者，如丹参注射液、复方丹参注射液等。

In modern clinical practice, Danshen Zhusheye, Xiangdan Zhusheye and other Chinese patent medicines can treat coronary heart disease, angina pectoris, cerebral infarction and other cardiovascular and cerebrovascular diseases induced by blood stasis syndrome. Moreover, in modern times, Danshen can treat chronic hepatitis and hepatic fibrosis with blood stasis resistance and hypochondriac pain such as Danshen injections and compound Danshen injections, etc..

2. 热扰心神证　治热病邪入心营，热扰心神之心烦不眠，甚或神昏，配伍生地、竹叶等，如《温病条辨》清营汤；治心血不足、心火扰神之心悸怔忡，健忘不眠，配伍酸枣仁、柏子仁等，如《世医得效方》天王补心丹。治癫狂惊痫，妄言妄动，可单味醋炒研末，淡盐汤调服，如《本草汇言》引杨石林方。

2 Syndrome of Heat Disturbing the Mind

Danshen can be used to treat fever and disease into the heart, heat disturbing the mind, upset, sleepless, or even dizzy, compatible with the Shengdi, Zhuye (Lophatheri Herba), etc., such as Qingying Tang (Decoction) in *Wenbing Tiaobian*; for treating blood deficiency, palpitations caused by and heart fire disturbing mind, forgetfulness, Sleepless, compatible with Suanzaoren, Baiziren, etc., such as Tianwang Buxin Dan (Pill) in *Shiyi Dexiaofang;For treating insane,* madness, convulsions, epilepsy with uncontrolled talking and acting, take the stir-fried Danshen powder by vinegar with light salt soup, such as Yin Yang Shilin Fang in *Bencao Huiyan*.

现代临床，丹参配伍常用于治疗失眠属瘀热证者，如枣仁安神颗粒。

In modern clinical practice, Danshen compatibility is often used for the treatment of insomnia with stasis-heat syndrome, such as Zaoren Anshen Jiaonang.

3. **瘀热证疮疡痈肿** 治瘀热证乳痈初起或一切疮疡红肿疼痛者，配伍金银花，连翘，如《医学衷中参西录》消乳汤；治妇人乳痈肿痛，配伍赤芍、白芷，如《刘涓子鬼遗方》丹参膏。

3 Swelling of Sore and Ulcer with Blood Stasis-heat Syndrome

For treating breast carbuncle with blood stasis and heat syndrome or all sores with redness, swelling and pain, it is compatible with Jinyinhua (Lonicerae Japonicae Flos) and Lianqiao (Forsythiae Fructus), such as Xiaoru Tang (Decoction) from *Yixue Zhongzhong Canxi Lu*. It could be also used to treat breast carbuncle swelling and pain, compatible with Chishao (Paeoniae Radix Rubra) and Baizhi (Angelicae Dahuricae Radix), such as Danshen Gao (Ointment) from *Liu Juanzi Guiyi Fomula (Liu Juanzi's Ghost-Bequeathed Prescriptions)*.

现代临床，丹参提取物常用于治疗痤疮、扁桃腺炎、外耳道炎、疖、痈、外伤感染、烧伤感染、乳腺炎、蜂窝组织炎、骨髓炎等属于瘀热证者，如丹参酮胶囊。

In modern clinical practice, Danshen extract is often used to treat acne, tonsillitis, otitis externa, furuncle, carbuncle, trauma infection, burn infection, mastitis, cellulitis, osteomyelitis, etc., which belong to the syndrome of stasis and heat, such as Tanshinone Capsules.

二、用法用量
II Administration and Dosage

10~15g，煎服，或入丸散。

10~15g, decoction, or pill powder.

三、注意事项
III Precautions

1. 丹参不宜与藜芦及含有藜芦的中成药同用。

1 It should not be used with Lilu and Chinese patent medicines containing Lilu.

2. 孕妇，月经过多者慎用；有出血倾向者忌用。

2 It should be used cautiously for pregnant women and females with menorrhagia or for people with bleeding tendency.

3. 丹参及其复方制剂，仅少数病例有口干、头晕、乏力、手胀麻、气短、胸闷，稍有心慌、心前区痛、心跳加快、恶心、呕吐及胃肠道症状等，但不影响治疗，继续用药可自行缓解或消失。曾有使用丹参和复方丹参注射液引起皮肤过敏和肝损害各1例，休克2例的报道。另有报道，口服、静脉滴注复方丹参制剂偶可引起头痛。

3 Danshen and its compound preparation may cause symptoms like dry mouth, dizziness, fatigue, hand swelling numbness, shortness of breath, chest tightness, slightly flustered, precordial pain, increasing heart rate, nausea, vomiting, gastrointestinal, but they do not affect the treatment, and will be relieved or disappeared spontaneously. There were 1 case of skin allergy and 1 case of liver injury caused by Danshen and 1 case of compound Danshen injection, a report of 2 cases of shock. In addition, oral and intravenous infusion of compound Danshen can cause headache.

【知识拓展】
[Knowledge Extension]

《本草纲目》及《本草备要》皆谓丹参可"生新血，补新血"，这说明丹参既能活血，又可补血，所以历来被用作妇科调经要药，李时珍甚至赞誉其功效称"其功大类当归、地黄、川芎、苟药。"《本草化义》也谓：古人以此一味代四物汤，通主调经胎产！后人更将丹参的功效特点总结为：一味丹参，功同四物！

Both the *Bencao Gangmu* and the Bencao Beiyao (*Compendium of Materia Medica*) claim that Danshen "can promote blood production and replenish it", this shows that Danshen can not only invigorate the blood, but also enrich the blood. Therefore, it has been used as the main medicine for regulating menstruation in gynecology. Li Shizhen even praised its efficacy "its great effects are comparable to Danggui, Dihuang, Chuanxiong and Shaoyao." In *Bencao Huayi*, the ancients used the single Danshen to substitute Siwu Tang (Decoction), it can overall regulate the course of "menstruation, fetal period and birth period". Descendants regard the effect of single Danshen is as that of Siwu Tang (Decoction).

延 胡 索

Yanhusuo
(Corydalis Rhizoma)

延胡索是著名的浙江道地药材。临床常用炮制品主要为生延胡索、醋延胡索。延胡索味辛、苦，性温，归肝、脾经，有活血、行气、止痛的功效，主治胸胁、脘腹疼痛，胸痹心痛，经闭痛经，产后瘀阻，跌扑肿痛等。延胡索主要含生物碱、挥发油等，有镇痛、镇静、催眠、抗心肌缺血、抗脑缺血、抑制血小板聚集等药理作用，可用于急性胃炎、慢性浅表性胃炎、慢性胆囊炎、功能性子宫出血等属气血瘀滞者。

Yanhusuo is a famous genuine regional medicinal in Zhejiang Province. The main processed products used in clinical are Shengyanhusuo (raw) and Cuyanhusuo (vinegar-processed). The flavour of Yanhusuo is pungent, and bitter the nature of Yanhusuo is warm, and it enters the liver and spleen meridians. It can invigorate blood, promote movement of qi and relieve pain, which is applied for the treatment of abdominal pain, chest pain, precordial pain, amenorrhea, dysmenorrhea, postpartum stasis, swelling and pain, etc. The main contents of Yanhusuo are alkaloids and volatile oils, which have pharmacological effects including analgesia, sedation, hypnosis, anti-myocardial ischemia, cerebral ischemia inhibition, and anti-platelet aggregation inhibition. It can be used in treatment of acute gastritis, chronic superficial gastritis, chronic cholecystitis and functional menoxenia which belong to the syndromes of blood stasis and qi stagnation.

【品种品质】
[Variety and Quality]

一、基原品种与品质
I Origin Varieties and Quality

1. **品种概况**　来源于为罂粟科植物延胡索 *Corydalis yanhusuo* W. T. Wang 的干燥块茎。

1 Variety

Yanhusuo is the dried tuber of Papaveraceae plant, Corydalis yanhusuo W. T. Wang.

延胡索首载于《雷公炮炙论》。明朝《本草述》载延胡索"状如半夏，但色黄耳"。《本草纲目》谓："……每年寒露后栽，立春后生苗，叶如竹叶样……根丛生如芋卵样，立夏掘起。"按以上植物形态及生长环境的记述，与现用延胡索一致。

Yanhusuo was first recorded in the book of *Leigong Paozhi Lun*. *Bencao Shu* in Ming Dynasty described that the shape of Yanhusuo was like Banxia, but with yellow color. *Bencao Gangmu*

stated it is planted after the Cold Dew, and seedling appeared after the beginning of spring and the leaves were like those of bamboo. The roots were like small taros which were dug up at the beginning of summer. According to the above description of plant morphology and growth environment, it is consistent with Yanhusuo used currently.

2. 种植采收　延胡索主产于浙江、湖北、湖南等地，多为栽培，忌连作，一般隔3~4年再种。通常于栽种第2年夏初茎叶枯萎时采挖。

2 Planting and Harvesting

Yanhusuo is mainly produced in Zhejiang, Hubei, Hunan and other places Provinces. It is usually cultivated and avoids the continuous cropping, and usually replant after 3 to 4 years. They are usually excavated at the beginning of summer when the stems and leaves are withered in the second year of planting.

3. 道地性及品质评价　明朝时期，江苏为延胡索道地产区。现今，浙江产延胡索品质最优。延胡索形态上以个大饱满，颜色上以断面色黄，质地以坚实为佳。由于延胡索与其混淆品在性状上差别不大，故多用化学评价方法去鉴别其真伪。

3 Genuineness and Quality Evaluation

During the Ming Dynasty, Jiangsu Province is the genuine producing area of Yanhusuo. Nowadays, Yanhusuo cultivated in Zhejiang Province has the best quality. The good quality of Yanhusuo is characterized of full in shape, yellow in color of section and hard in texture. Because there is little difference between Yanhusuo and its adulterant, chemical evaluation methods are often used to identify its authenticity.

延胡索主要含有生物碱类，分为叔胺碱类和季胺碱类，主要为延胡索乙素（消旋四氢巴马汀）、甲素、丑素和去氢延胡索甲素。该类成分为延胡素的主要活性成分。此外，延胡索还含有三萜类、蒽醌类、酚酸类、甾醇和有机酸等非生物碱类成分。《中国药典》规定延胡索药材中延胡索乙素含量不得少于0.050%。

Yanhusuo mainly contains alkaloids, which are divided into tertiary aminetype alkaloids and quaternary aminetype alkaloids including tetrahydropalmatine, corydaline, tetrahydrocolumbamine and dehydrocoryd aline, which are major active components of Yanhusuo. In addition, it contains triterpenes, anthraquinones, phenolic acids, sterols and organic acids. The *Pharmacopoeia of the People's Republic of China* recorded that the content of tetrahydropalmatine in Yanhusuo should not be less than 0.050%.

二、炮制品种与品质
II Processed Varieties and Quality

延胡索的炮制品种有炒制、盐制、酒制、醋制等。目前，临床常用为延胡索饮片、醋炙延胡索、酒炙延胡索。延胡索以呈不规则的圆形厚片，具蜡样光泽，气微，味苦为佳；醋延胡索以形如胡索或片，表面和切面黄褐色，质较硬，微具醋香气为佳。饮片的品质评价方法同药材，且延胡索乙素含量不得少于0.050%。

Yanhusuo can be processed by stir-frying, stir-frying with salt, stir-frying with liquor, stir-frying with vinegar and so on. At present, Cuzhi Yanhusuo (stir-frying with vinegar), Jiuzhi Yanhusuo (stir-frying with liquor), and Yanhusuo decoction pieces are most frequently used in clinic. Good quality of Yanhusuo holds the characteristic of irregular thick piece, candle-like gloss, slight smell and bitter taste. Cuyanhusuo has good quality with the similar shape like Yanhusuo or its pieces, yellow brown surface, hard texture and slight smell of vinegar. The quality evaluation of Yanhusuo decoction pieces is the same as that of the medicinal and the content of tetrahydropalmatine in Yanhusuo should not be less than 0.050%.

三、中成药品种与品质
III Varieties and Quality of Chinese Patent Medicines

含有延胡索或其炮制品的中成药有400余个，其中药典收载70余个。以延胡索为君药或主药的品种主要为各类止痛药，有元胡止痛片（口服液、分散片、胶囊、软胶囊、滴丸）、可打灵片、安胃片（胶囊、颗粒）等。为确保制剂有效性，以延胡索为君药的中成药主要以有效成分延胡索乙素为质量控制指标。质量控制多采用薄层色谱法和液相色谱含量测定法进行指标成分检测。

There are more than 400 Chinese patent medicines containing Yanhusuo or its processed products, of which over 70 are concluded in the *Pharmacopoeia of the People's Republic of China*. Most of prescriptions with Yanhusuo as a sovereign or main medicinal are analgesics including Yuanhu Zhitong Tablets / Mixture / Dispersible Tablets / Capsules / Soft capsules / Droping pills, Kedaling Tablet, Anwei Tablet / Capsule / Granule and so on. In order to ensure the effectiveness of the preparations, Chinese patent medicines that mainly contain Yanhusuo usually use the active ingredient tetrahydropalmatine as the quality control marker. TLC and LC are most commonly used to measure the marker component.

【制药】
[Pharmacy]

一、产地加工
I Processing in Production Area

采收后除去须根，按块茎分为大、中、小三档，洗净，除杂，置沸水中煮至内无白心时捞出，晒干或低温干燥。

After harvested and cleaned by removing the fibrous roots, Yanhusuo is divided into 3 grades, large, medium and small according to the size of tubers. Then wash it, remove impurities, and boil it until white core disappears. After that, dry it in the sun or at low temperature.

二、饮片炮制
II Processing of Decoction Pieces

延胡索从古至今形成了系列的炮制方法。以"润透 - 切片 - 液体辅料炙"工艺加工的延胡索、醋炙延胡索成为商品规格中的主流。

There have been a series of processing methods of Yanhusuo since ancient times. Nowadays, Yanhusuo、and Chuzhiyanhusuo, which were processed by "moistening – slicing – liquid excipients have become the mainstream in commodity.

延胡索的炮制机理较为清楚，其游离生物碱难溶于水，醋制可使生物碱生成盐，易溶于水，提高煎出率，增强疗效。酒制也能提高延胡索生物碱与延胡索乙素的煎出量，增强镇痛与镇静效果。

The processing mechanism of Yanhusuo is relatively clear. Because its free alkaloids are difficult to dissolve in water, stir frying with vinegar can make alkaloids generate salts, which are easily soluble in water, improving the dissolution rate in water to increase the curative effects. Stir frying with liquor can also increase the dissolution rate of alkaloids including tetrahydropalmatine, therefore enhancing analgesic and sedative effects.

三、中成药制药
III Pharmacy of Chinese Patent Medicines

含延胡索的中成药剂型丰富，涵盖口服与外用制剂。中成药中，延胡索生品与醋品投料均较普遍。若用于行气止痛，多选用醋延胡索，如金铃子散；若用于活血、祛瘀、止痛，多选用酒炙延胡索，如瓜蒌薤白汤加减。

They are many kinds of Chinese patent medicines preparations containing Yanhusuo , covering oral and external preparations. ShengYanhusuo and Cuyanhusuo are commonly used in patent Chinese medicines. Cuyanhusuo is often used to promote the movement of qi and relieve pain such as Jinlingzi San (Powder). Jiuzhiyanhusuo is often used to invigorate blood, remove stasis such as Modified Gualou Xiebai Tang (Decoction).

例如基于元胡止痛方研制出的元胡止痛口服液、软胶囊、硬胶囊、滴丸、分散片等，不仅保留了其口服给药的服药方式，还能加速药物释放，提高临床疗效。

The new pharmaceutical forms of Yuanhu Zhitong San (Powder) have been developed, such as Yuanhu Zhitong Mixture / Soft Capsule / Hard Capsule / Dropping Pill / Dispersion Tablets. These new preparations not only retain the way of oral administration, but also accelerate effect releasing and improve clinical efficacy.

【性能功效】
[Property and Efficacy]

一、性能
I Property

延胡索辛、苦，归肝、脾经。

Yanhusuo are pungent and bitter in flavor, warm in nature, and enters the liver and spleen meridians.

二、功效
II Efficacy

1. **活血** 延胡索入血分，活血化瘀。其功效的发挥与抗心肌缺血、抗脑缺血、抑制血小板聚集等药理作用密切相关。延胡索发挥以上作用的主要物质基础为生物碱类。延胡索抗脑缺血的作用与降低脑组织中钙离子浓度、抑制氧化损伤有关。

1 Invigorating Blood

Yanhusuo invigorates the blood and alleviate blood stasis. Its efficacy is closely related to the pharmacological effects such as anti-myocardial ischemia, anti-brain ischemia, and inhibition of platelet aggregation. The active components are alkaloids. The anti-brain ischemia effect of Yanhusuo is related to reducing the concentration of calcium ion concentration and inhibiting antioxidant damage inhibition.

2. **行气，止痛** 延胡索具行气、止痛之功效，历来作为止痛要药，被誉为中药中的"吗啡"。其功效的发挥与镇痛、镇静、催眠等药理作用密切相关。延胡索镇痛的主要活性物质为生物碱，其中以延胡索乙素作用最强。延胡索的镇痛作用机制主要包括抑制网状结构的激活系统；阻滞纹状体、伏膈核、前额皮层等脑区的 D_2 受体，加强脑干下行痛觉调制系统的抗痛功能；剂量依赖性抑制神经元异位自发放电。延胡索镇静、催眠的主要物质基础是延胡索乙素，主要通过阻滞脑内多巴胺受体的功能发挥作用。

2 Activating Qi and Relieving Pain

Yanhusuo has the effect of activating qi and relieving pain, so it has always been used as an important analgesic and is known as "morphine" in Chinese medicine. Its efficacy is closely related to analgesia, sedation and hypnosis. The main anabgesic active components are alkaloids, among which tetrahydropalmatine has the strongest effect. The analgesic mechanism of Yanhusuo mainly includes inhibiting the activation system of the reticular structure, blocking D_2 receptors in the brain regions such as the striatum, the nucleus accumbens and the prefrontal cortex, strengthening the anti-pain function of the brain stem downward pain modulation system and dose-dependently inhibiting ectopic spontaneous firing of neurons. The sedative and hypnotic effects of tetrahydropalmatine are mainly related to the block of dopamine receptor function in the brain.

此外，现代研究显示延胡索具有抗溃疡、抑制胃酸分泌、调节内分泌、抗肿瘤等作用。

In addition, modern research shows that Yanhusuo has the effects of anti-ulcer, inhibiting gastric acid secretion, regulating endocrine, and anti-tumor, etc.

【应用】
[Applications]

一、主治病证
I Indications

血瘀气滞诸痛证
Pain Syndromes Due to Blood Stasis and Qi Stagnation

延胡索是行气止痛的要药，可与他药配伍治疗气滞血瘀之胸痹心痛，方如《素庵医案》桃仁红花煎；治肝郁气滞，胸胁胀痛者，可与郁金、柴胡配伍；治寒证胃痛，如《太平惠民和剂局方》安中散；治胃痛，可配伍红花、五灵脂，如《医林改错》膈下逐瘀汤；治肝脾血瘀所痛者，如《证治准绳》调营饮；治气滞血瘀，脘腹疼痛者，如《素问·病机气宜保命集》金铃子散；治妇女痛经，如《医林改错》少腹逐瘀汤；治小儿寒疝腹痛者，常与小茴香、吴茱萸等配伍；治肠痈腹痛者，如《中医内科学》清胆汤；治风湿痹痛者，常与当归、桂枝、秦艽等配伍；治跌打损伤者，如《中医伤科学讲义》新伤续断汤。

Yanhusuo is an essential medicinal that promotes the movement of qi, and strongly stops pain. It can be combined with other medicines to treat chest pain and heartache due to qi stagnation and blood stasis, such as Taoren Honghua Tang (Decoction) in *Su'an Yian (Su'an Medical Records)*. It can alleviate the syndromes of liver depression, qi stagnation and chest pain in combination with Yujin and Chaihu. It can also relieve stomach pain caused by cold syndrome, such as Anzhong San (Podwer) in *Taiping Huimin Heji Ju Fang*; treating stomach pain in combination with Honghua and Wulingzhi, such as Gexia Zhuyu Tang (Decoction) in *Yilin Gaicuo*; pain caused by blood stasis in liver and spleen, such as Tiaoying Yin (Decoction) in *Zhengzhi Zhunsheng (Standards of Diagnosis and Treatment)*, abdominal pain caused by qi stagnation and blood stasis, such as Jinlingzi San (Powder) in *Suwen Bingji Qiyi Baomingji*,

dysmenorrhea, such as Shaofu Zhuyu Tang (Decoction) in *Yilin Gaicuo*, children's cold hernia and abdominal pain in the combination with Xiaohuixiang and Wuzhuyu; abdominal pain caused periappendicular abscess, such as Qingdan Tang (Decoction) in *Zhongyi Neikexue (Internal Medicine of Traditional Chinese Medicine)*, wind-dampness pain in the combination with Danggui, Guizhi and Qinjiao. In addition, it can be used to treat people with bruises, such as Xinshang Xuduan Tang (Decoction) in *Zhongyi Shangkexue Jiangyi (Lectures on Traditional Chinese Traumatology)*.

现代临床，延胡索配伍常用于治疗多种以疼痛为主要症状的疾病，如治疗冠心病心绞痛属于气滞血瘀、痰阻心络者，如可达灵片；功能性子宫出血属于气血凝滞者，如妇女痛经丸；急性胃炎、慢性浅表性胃炎、消化性溃疡、慢性胆囊炎等属于气血瘀滞者，如九气拈痛散。

In modern clinical practice, Yanhusuo compatibility is often used to treat pain syndrome-based disease. It can treat coronary heart disease caused by qi stagnation and blood stasis, and phlegm obstructing heart collaterals, such as Kedaling Pian (Tablets). It can treat functional menstruation, which originates from qi and blood stagnation, such as Funv Tongjing Wan. It can treat acute gastritis, chronic superficial gastritis peptic ulcer, and chronic cholecystitis causing by qi and blood stasis, such as Jiuqi Niantong San (Powder).

二、用法用量
II Administration and Dosage

煎汤，3~10g；研末吞服，每次 1.5~3 g。
Decoction, 3~10g. Pulverized into powder to swallow, 1.5~3g each time.

三、注意事项
III Precautions

1. 孕妇禁用。

1 It's forbidden to be used during pregnancy.

2. 体虚者慎用。

2 Those who are physically weak should take it with cautions.

【知识拓展】
[Knowledge Extension]

延胡索是最早采用现代科学技术方法进行研究的中药之一。早在二十世纪二三十年代，我国化学家赵承嘏和中药药理学家陈克恢分别对延胡索的化学成分和药理作用进行研究。

Yanhusuo is one of the earliest Chinese medicinals studied by modern science and technology. In the 1920s and 1930s, Prof. Zhao Chenggu, a Chinese chemist, and Prof. Chen Kehui, a pharmacologist of Chinese medicines, respectively studied the chemical constituents and pharmacological effects of Yanhusuo.

莪 术

Ezhu
(Curcumae Rhizoma)

莪术因基原品种的不同，历来是分属于四川、广西、温州、福建多地的道地药材。临床常用炮制品有莪术和醋莪术。莪术辛、苦、温，归肝、脾经，有行气破血、消积止痛的功效，主治气滞血瘀证、疼痛证、食积证等。莪术主要含挥发油、姜黄素类及酚性物质等成分，有抗血栓、镇痛、兴奋胃肠平滑肌、抗肝纤维化、抗肿瘤等药理作用，可用于月经不调、冠心病心绞痛、肿瘤、慢性肝炎、慢性胃炎等属气滞血瘀证者。莪术破气逐瘀作用强，有耗气伤血之弊，应中病即止，体虚者慎用，月经过多者及孕妇忌用。

Due to the genetic diversity, the genuine regional place of Ezhu has always been distributed in Sichuan, Guangxi, Wenzhou and Fujian provinces since ancient times. The commonly used processed products in clinic are Ezhu and CuEzhu. Ezhu are pungent and bitter inflavour, and warm in nature, enters the liver and spleen meridians. It has the effects of promoting qi and breaking the blood, relieving food retention and stopping pain. It is mainly used for qi stagnation and blood stasis syndrome, pain syndrome, food accumulation syndrome, etc. Ezhu mainly contains volatile oil, curcumin and phenolic substances, which have the effects of improving blood circulation, anti-thrombosus, anti-hepatofibrosis and exciting the gastrointestinal smooth muscle. Ezhu can be used for patients with qi stagnation and blood stasis syndrome, such as irregular menstruation, coronary heart disease, angina, tumor, chronic hepatitis, and chronic gastritis. Ezhu has a strong effect of dispelling qi and expelling blood stasis. Because it has the disadvantages of consuming qi and blood, it should be discontinued as soon as the condition improve and used with caution for those who are weak, and it should not be used for menorrhagia and pregnant women.

【品种品质】
[Variety and Quality]

一、基原品种与品质
I Origin Varieties and Quality

1. **品种概况** 来源于姜科植物蓬莪术 *Curcuma phaeocaulis* Val.、广西莪术 *Curcuma kwangsiensis* S. G. Lee et C. F. Liang 或温郁金 *Curcuma wenyujin* Y. H. Chen et C. Ling 的干燥

根茎。

1 Variety

Ezhu is from dried rhizome and root of the Ginger Plant *Curcuma phaeocaulis* Val., *Curcuma kwangsiensis* S. G. Lee et C. F. Liang, and *Curcuma wenyujin* Y.H. Chen et C. Ling.

莪术古名蓬莪术，出自《药性论》，其原植物古籍记载有三种，《图经本草》曰："蓬莪术生西戎及广南诸州，今江浙或有之。"《本草图经》所载宜州姜黄与广西莪术相似，所载温州蓬莪术与温郁金近乎一致。因此，蓬莪术、广西莪术、温郁金三种莪术品种作药用已有较长的历史，与现代莪术商品的主流品种一致。

Ezhu, an ancient name is Peng Ezhu from *Yaoxing Lun*（*Theory of Property*）, its original plants have been recorded in 3 species, in *Bencao Tujing*: "Peng Ezhu (Curcuma zedoaria) grows in the western regions and in the states of Guangnan, there may be some ones in Jiangsu and Zhejiang today". The Yizhou Jianghuang (Curcumae Radix) contained in *Bencao Tujing* is similar to Ezhu in Guangxi, and the Wenzhou Ezhu recorded is almost the same with Wenyujin. Therefore, the three Ezhu varieties of Peng Ezhu, Guangxi Ezhu (Guangxi Curcuma), and Wenyujin have a long history of medicinal use, which are consistent with the mainstream varieties of modern Ezhu products.

2. 种植采收　莪术以人工种植为主。蓬莪术主产于福建、四川、广东、广西等地。广西莪术（桂莪术）主产于广西、云南、广东等地。温莪术主产于浙江、福建等地。莪术栽培采用根茎繁殖，以夏至前后几天为宜；在栽种当年12月下旬（冬至后），茎叶枯萎后采挖，抖落泥土，将根茎和块根分开，洗净即得。

2 Planting and Harvesting

Ezhu is mainly artificially planted. Peng Ezhu is mainly produced in Fujian, Sichuan, Guangdong, Guangxi provinces and other places. Guangxi Ezhu is mainly produced in Guangxi, Yunnan, Guangdong and other places. Wen Ezhu is mainly produced in Zhejiang, Fujian and other places. Rhizome propagation is used in the cultivation of Ezhu, and it is suitable for a few days before and after the summer solstice, at the end of December of the year of planting (after the winter solstice), the stems and leaves are withered and excavated, which will be available after shaking off the soil, separating the rhizomes and tubers, and washing out.

3. 道地性及品质评价　莪术因基原品种的不同，历来有多个道地产区。据历代本草记载，福建、四川、广东、广西是蓬莪术的道地产区，云南、广西、广东是广西莪术的道地产区，温州是温莪术的道地产区。莪术性状评价以个大、质坚实、断面灰绿色、气香者为佳。

3 Genuineness and Quality Evaluation

Because of the different species of Ezhu, there have always been many genuine production areas. According to historical records of Materia Medica, Fujian, Sichuan, Guangdong, and Guangxi are the genuine production areas of Peng Ezhu. Yunnan, Guangxi, and Guangdong are the genuine production areas of Guangxi Ezhu. Wenzhou is the genuine production area of Wen Ezhu. The evaluation of Ezhu regards the large, firm, gray-green in cross-section, and fragrant as the better one.

莪术主要含挥发油、姜黄素类及酚性物质等成分，一般认为，挥发油与姜黄素是其主要活性成分，现代研究主要以挥发油对其进行质量评价。莪术品质受品种、产地因素影响较大。《中国药典》规定莪术药材中含挥发油不得少于1.5%（ml/g）。

Ezhu mainly contains volatile oil, curcumin and of phenolic substances. It is generally believed that volatile oil and curcumin are the main active components. In modern researches, the quality of Ezhu is evaluated mainly by the quantity of volatile oil. However, the quality of Ezhu is affected by variety and producing area. *The Pharmacopoeia of the People's Republic of China* stipulates that volatile oil in Ezhu should not be less than 1.5% (ml/g).

二、炮制品种与品质
II Processed Varieties and Quality

莪术的炮制品种有 10 多个，临床常用品种主要有 2 种，包括莪术和醋莪术。莪术以切面黄绿色或棕褐色，内皮层散在"筋脉"小点，气微香，味微苦而辛为佳。醋莪术以形如莪术片，色泽加深，角质样，微有醋香气为佳。《中国药典》规定，莪术与醋莪术的含量测定同药材，含挥发油不得少于 1.0%（ml/g）。

There are more than 10 kinds of Ezhu, among which Ezhu and Cuezhu (stri frying with vinegar) are commonly used in clinical practice. Ezhu is considered as the best with yellow green and brown in section, endothelial layer scattered with small spots of the "tendons and veins", slightly fragrant, slightly bitter and pungent taste, Cuezhu (vinegar processed) which is like Ezhu pills in shape, with dark color, cutin-like appearance, slightly vinegar aroma is considered superior. *The Pharmacopoeia of the People's Republic of China* stipulates both Ezhu and Cuezhu (vinegar processed) containing volatile oil should be no less than 1.0% (ml/g).

三、中成药品种与品质
III Varieties and Quality of Chinese Patent Medicines

含有莪术或其炮制品的中成药有 200 余个，其中《中国药典》收载 5 个。以莪术为君药或主药的品种丹香清脂颗粒，乳康丸、灵泽片等。在中成药的品质控制中多采用薄层色谱法确定莪术的存在，采用高效液相色谱法或气相色谱法测定指标成分含量，并限定指标成分下限以保证疗效。如灵泽片，用薄层色谱法确定莪术醇的存在；用高效液相色谱法测定蒎牛儿酮及呋喃二烯的含量并限定其下限。如保妇康栓用薄层色谱法确定莪术对照药材的存在，用气相色谱法测定莪术油（以莪术二酮计）含量并限定其下限。

There were more than 200 Chinese patent medicines containing Ezhu or its processed products and 5 are recorded in *the Pharmacopoeia of the People's Republic of China*. Among them, prescriptions with Ezhu as sovereign are as follows: Danxiang Qingzhi keli, Rukang Wan, Lingze Pian (Tablets), etc. Presently, the quality control for the existence of Ezhu is mainly determined by TLC, the content of target components is determined by HPLC or GC, and the lower limit of the index component is defined to ensure the curative effect. For example, Lingze Pian (Tablets), use TLC to determine the presence of curcumol, use HPLC to determine the content of geranone and furandiene and define the lower limit. For example, Baofukang Shuan (Suppository) uses TLC to determine the existence of turmeric control medicinal materials, and uses GC to determine the content of turmeric oil (calculated as turmeric dione) and define its lower limit.

【制药】
[Pharmacy]

一、产地加工
I Processing in Production Area

采挖后洗净，略浸泡，再蒸或煮至透心，晒干或低温干燥后，除去须根和杂质。

After being dug up, wash and remove impurities, soak briefly, then steam or boil throughout the core; dry in sun or by low temperature, remove the fibril and impurities.

二、饮片炮制
II Processing of Decoction Pieces

从古至今形成了煨制、醋炒、酒炒、酒醋制、油制等 10 多种炮制方法。宋代以来，逐步形成了"净制 - 润制 - 切制 - 醋炙"的工艺，由此加工的莪术、醋莪术成为商品规格中的主流品种。

From ancient times to the present, more than

10 kinds of processing methods have been formed, including roasting, stir-frying with vinegar, stir-frying with liquor, liquor and vinegar processing, and processing with oil. Since the Song Dynasty, the process of "cleaning - moistening - cutting - vinegar broiling" has gradually formed, and the processed Ezhu and Cuezhu have become the mainstream varieties in commodity specifications.

莪术炮制品中以醋莪术的抗血栓作用最明显。莪术生用破气消积力强，多用于食积胀痛、闭经、癥瘕痞块；醋莪术重在入肝经血分，增强止痛作用，多用于瘀阻腹痛、痛经。

Among the processed Ezhu products, Cuezhu (stri frying with vinegar) has the most obvious antithrombotic effect. Ezhu has a strong ability to disperse qi and eliminate stagnation. It is mostly used for treating food accumulation, pain, amenorrhea, and lumps. Cuezhu (vinegar processed) focuses on entering the liver and blood to enhance analgesic effect. It is mostly used for stasis to block abdominal pain and dysmenorrhea.

三、中成药制药
III Pharmacy of Chinese Patent Medicines

含莪术的中成药，剂型较丰富，涵盖固体、液体与半固体剂型，具体包括丸剂、片剂、胶囊、口服液、药酒、黑膏药、栓剂等。成方制剂中可选用莪术或醋莪术，打粉、提取挥发油后，药渣与其他药味再水提，或直接水提、醇提入药。也有以莪术油入药的。

Chinese patent medicines containing Ezhu are rich in pharmaceutical forms, covering solid, liquid and semisolid pharmaceutical forms, specifically including pills, tablets, capsules, mixture, liquor, black plaster, suppository and so on. Ezhu or Cuezhu (vinegar processed) can be used in the preparation. After powdering and volatile oil extraction, the dregs and other medicinal flavors are then water-extracted, or directly water-

extracted or alcohol-extracted into the medicine. There is also turmeric oil used as medicine.

如以莪术为主药的灵泽片，在制剂中以莪术入药，采用水蒸气蒸馏法提取莪术挥发油，其他药味与提取挥发油后的药液药渣合并煎煮，采用水提醇沉法收膏干燥，再与莪术挥发油包合物等混合制片，如此，既除去了水不溶性成分，又保留了莪术挥发油与水溶性成分。

For example, Lingze Pian (Tablets) with Ezhu as the main medicine in the preparation, and the volatile oil of Ezhu is extracted by steam distillation. Other medicinal herbs are combined with the liquid medicine residue after the extraction of the volatile oil, and the ointment is collected by water extraction and alcohol precipitation. After drying, it is mixed with the zedoary turmeric oil inclusion compound to make tablets. In this way, the water-insoluble components are removed while retaining the zedoary volatile oil and water-soluble components.

【性能功效】
[Property and Efficacy]

一、性能
I Property

莪术辛、苦，温；归肝、脾经。
Ezhu is pungent and bitter in flavor, warm in nature, and enters liver and spleen meridians.

二、功效
II Efficacy

1. **行气破血** 莪术辛、温，归肝经，兼入气分与血分，擅行气破血。其功效的发挥与抑制血小板聚集、抗血栓等药理作用有关。莪术抗血栓作用的有效物质基础主要是莪术油和姜黄素类成分，通过作用于血小板、影响花生四烯酸的代谢途径等发挥作用。

1 Promoting Qi and Breaking Blood
Ezhu is pungent and bitter in flavor, warm

in nature, enters liver meridian and enter qi and blood to promote qi circulation and break the blood. Its efficacy is related to its pharmacological effects such as inhibition of platelet aggregation and anti-thrombosis. The effective material basis of the antithrombotic effect of Ezhu is mainly zedoary turmeric oil and curcumin, which act on platelets and affect the metabolic pathway of arachidonic acid.

2. 消积止痛　莪术入脾经，有较强的消食化积作用；入肝经，又擅行气止痛。其功效的发挥与促进胃肠运动、抗肿瘤、抗肝纤维化等作用有关。莪术抗肿瘤、抗肝纤维化等作用的有效物质基础是挥发油和榄香烯、莪术二酮等单体成分，通过作用于凋亡诱导因子、IL-1、TNF-α，促进细胞和体液免疫等发挥作用。

2 Relieving Food Retention and Relieving Pain

Ezhu, entering spleen meridian, has a strong effect of relieving food retention, it also enters liver meridian to promote qi and relieve pain. Its function is related to the promotion of gastrointestinal movement, anti-tumor, anti-liver fibrosis and other effects. The effective material bases of the anti-tumor and anti-liver fibrosis effects of Ezhu are volatile oil and monomer components such as elemene and turmeric dione. By acting on apoptosis-inducing factor, IL-1, TNF-α, it promotes cells and humoral immunity.

【应用】
[Applications]

一、主治病证
I Indications

1. 气滞血瘀证　治胸痹心痛，《圣济总录》单用莪术煎服或醋煎服；治寒凝血瘀、心腹疼痛，配伍木香，如《卫生家宝》蓬莪术散；治跌打损伤、瘀肿疼痛，配伍三棱、苏木等，如《救伤秘旨》十三味总方；治瘀阻日久而成癥瘕痞块，或经闭腹痛，配伍三棱、香附等，如《寿世

保元》莪术散。

1 Syndrome of Qi Stagnation and Blood Stasis

Ezhu is singly decocted or with vinegar to treat chest blockage and pain, recorded in *Sheng Ji Zonglu*. To treat cold congealing blood stasis, heart abdominal pain, Ezhu is combined with Muxiang, such as Peng Ezhu San in *Weisheng Jiabao,* to treat bruising, stagnant swelling and pain, it is combined with Sumu and Sanleng, such as 13 medicinals Fomula from the *Jiushang Mizhi*（*Secret Purpose of Rescuing Injuries*）, to treat the mass in the abdomen due to long-time obstruction, or abdominal pain due to amenorrhea, Sanleng and Xiangfu is combine, such as Ezhu San (Powder) in *Shoushi Baoyuan.*

现代临床，莪术常配伍用于月经不调、冠心病心绞痛、肿瘤、慢性肝炎等属气滞血瘀证者。

In modern clinical practice, Ezhu compatibility is often used for treating irregular menstruation, coronary heart disease angina, tumor and chronic hepatitis belong to syndrome of qi stagnation and blood stasis.

2. 食积气滞证　治食积气滞，脘痞腹痛，大便闭结，配伍三棱、香附等，如《证治准绳》莪术丸；治脾虚不运，脘腹胀痛，常配伍党参、白术、山药等。

2 Syndrome of Qi Stagnation Due to Food Retention

Ezhu is used to treat food retention and qi stagnation, swelling, abdominal pain, stool closure, compatibility with Sanleng and Xiangfu, etc., such as Ezhu Wan in *Zhengzhi Zhunsheng (Standards of Diagnosis and Treatmentk)*; to treat spleen deficiency, abdominal distension and pain, it is often compatible with Dangshen, Baizhu and Shanyao, etc.

现代临床，莪术常配伍用于消化不良、慢性胃炎等消化系统疾病属于食积气滞证者。

In modern clinical practice, Ezhu is often used for digestive system diseases such as dyspepsia and chronic gastritis, which belong to the syndrome of stagnation of qi and food stagnation.

此外，以莪术油为主的新制剂常用于肝癌、宫颈癌等恶性肿瘤属于气滞血瘀证的治疗。

In addition, new preparations based on zedoary turmeric oil are often used in the treatment of liver cancer, cervical cancer and other malignant tumors that belong to the syndrome of qi stagnation and blood stasis.

二、用法用量
II　Administration and Dosage

6~9g, 煎服，或入丸散。

6~9g, decoction, or used in pill and powder.

三、注意事项
III　Precautions

1. 本品为破气攻积之品，有耗气伤血之弊，应中病即止，不宜过量、久服。

1　It is liable to break qi and relieve stagnation, with the disadvantages of consuming qi and blood, thus it should not be taken overdose and overcourse, and should be discontinued as soon as the condition improves.

2. 体虚而有癥瘕积聚者，须佐人参、黄芪、白术等补虚药同用，使祛邪不伤正。

2　For the patients of deficiency and symptomatic accumulation of the mass, it should be combined with Renshen, Huangqi and Baizhu to dispel pathogen without destroying the vital qi.

3. 曾有报道，部分患者服用莪术后出现头晕、恶心、面色潮红、呼吸困难、胸闷，个别有发热、发绀、心慌、乏力等症状，或一过性谷丙转氨酶升高，临床使用中应注意剂量、疗程与辨证使用。

3　There have been reported that after taking Ezuh, some patients could have symptoms of dizziness, nausea and flushing, breathing difficulty, chest tightness, a few patients may have fever, cyanosis, palpitation and fatigue, or excessive alanine transaminase. Pay attention to the dosage, course of treatment and differentiation of symptoms and signs in clinical application.

4. 孕妇、月经过多者忌用。

4　It is taboo for the pregnant women and those with hypermenorrhea.

【知识拓展】
[Knowledge Extension]

莪术、郁金、姜黄三者皆为姜科植物，且原植物有交叉的情况，又都具活血、行气、止痛之效，但其药性不同，功效主治也有所区别，郁金性寒，又能清心凉血利胆，可用于热病神昏、癫痫、湿热黄疸证。姜黄与莪术性温，但姜黄长于散寒止痛，可用于风寒湿痹痛；莪术擅于攻坚消积，常用于食积、癥瘕痞块、肿瘤的治疗。

Ezhu, Yujin and Jianghuang are all plants of the ginger family, and the original plants have crossover conditions. They all have the effects of promoting blood circulation, promoting qi, and relieving pain, but their medicinal properties are different, and the efficacy and indications are also different. Yujin is cold and can clear the heart, cool blood and promote bile flow, and can be used for fever, faint, epilepsy, dampness-heat jaundice. Jianghuang and Ezhu are warm in nature, but Jianghuang is better in dispelling cold and relieving pain, and can be used for wind-cold dampness and arthralgia. Ezhu is good at attacking toughness and eliminating food retention, and is often used for the treatment of food accumulation, mass and unstable gathering in the abdomen and tumors.

第十九章　化痰止咳平喘药

Chapter 19　Dissipating Phlegm, Relieving Cough and Anti-asthmatic Medicinals

凡能祛痰或消痰，治疗"痰证"为主的药物，称化痰药。以制止或减轻咳嗽和喘息为主要作用的药物，称止咳平喘药。根据药性、功能及临床应用的不同，化痰止咳平喘药可分为温化寒痰药、清化热痰药及止咳平喘药三类。温化寒痰药多味辛苦性温燥，有温肺祛寒，燥湿化痰之功，部分药物外用有消肿止痛的作用，主治寒痰、湿痰证。清化热痰药多寒凉，有清化热痰之功，部分药物质润，兼能润燥，部分药物味咸，兼能软坚散结，故主治热痰证。止咳平喘药其味或辛或苦或甘，其性或温或寒，有的药物偏于止咳，有的偏于平喘，有的则兼而有之，主治咳喘。化痰止咳平喘药中某些温燥之性强烈的刺激性化痰药，凡痰中带血等有出血倾向者，宜慎用；麻疹初起有表邪之咳嗽，应忌单投止咳药。现代研究证明，化痰止咳平喘药一般具有祛痰、镇咳、平喘，抑菌、抗病毒、消炎利尿等作用，部分药物还有镇静、镇痛、抗惊厥、改善血液循环、调节免疫作用。常见的化痰止咳平喘药有半夏、天南星、禹白附、川贝母、浙贝母、瓜蒌、苦杏仁、紫苏子、紫菀等。

Medicinals that can eliminate phlegm or diffuse phlegm to treat "phlegm syndrome" are called phlegm-resolving medicinals. While the medicinals with the main functions of inhibiting or relieving cough and asthma are considered as medicinals of relieving cough and asthma. According to the difference of property, function and clinical application, cough and asthma-relieving medicines can be divided into three categories: warming cold phlegm, clearing heat phlegm and relieving cough and asthma. Warming cold phlegm medicines, which are mainly applied for the syndromes of cold and wet phlegm, are mostly pungent and bitter in taste as well as warm and dry in nature with the functions of warming lung and dispelling cold, removing dampness and phlegm. And some medicines have the effect of reducing swelling and relieving pain for external use. Clearing heat phlegm medicines are mostly cold and cool in nature with the function of clearing heat phlegm, and some of medicines are moist in nature so that they can moisturize dryness syndrome, while some are salty in taste so that they can soften hardness to dissipate masses. Therefore, they are the main treatment of heat phlegm syndrome. Cough-relieving and asthma-relieving medicines are pungent, bitter or sweet in taste, warm or cold in nature, among which some medicines tend to relieve cough, some tend to relieve asthma, and some have both functions, mainly used for the treatment of cough and asthma. Among phlegm-resolving and cough and asthma-relieving medicines, some irritating phlegm-resolving medicines with strong warm and dry nature should be used with caution if there is bloody sputum. At the beginning stage of measles disease, it often shows cough with exterior evil, so it should be avoided to administer cough medicine alone. Modern research has proved that phlegm-resolving, cough-relieving and asthma-relieving medicines generally have expectorant, antitussive, antiasthmatic, antibacterial, antiviral, and anti-inflammatory effects, and some medicinals also have sedative, analgesic, anticonvulsant, blood circulation improvement and immune regulation effects. Commonly-used medicines for eliminating phlegm, relieving cough and asthma include Banxia, Tiannanxing, Yubaifu, Chuanbeimu, Zhebeimu, Gualou, Kuxingren, Zisuzi, Ziwan and so on.

半 夏

Banxia
(Pinelliae Rhizoma)

半夏为四川的道地药材。生半夏有毒，麻舌而刺喉，一般内服以炮制品入药，临床常用的炮制品有法半夏、姜半夏和清半夏；半夏味辛，性温，有毒，归脾、胃、肺经，有降逆止呕、燥湿化痰、消痞散结的功效，主治湿痰、寒痰证。半夏主要含生物碱、β-谷甾醇、葡萄糖苷、β-氨基酸、胆碱、挥发油等成分，有抗肿瘤、祛痰镇咳、镇吐、镇痛、抗溃疡的药理作用，可用于治疗咳嗽、恶心呕吐、甲状腺肿大、淋巴结核等痰证。根据"十八反"，半夏不宜与川乌、制川乌、草乌、制草乌、附子同用。

Banxia is a genuine regional medicinal in Sichuan、Henan and Gansu. The raw material of Banxia is toxic and can cause "stinging tongue and throat", so processed material is mainly used for internal preparations. Clinically, the processed products like Fabanxia (Gancao-processed), Jiangbanxia (ginger-processed) and Qingbanxia (alumine-processed) are commonly used. Banxia is pungent in flavor, warm in nature, toxic and enters to the spleen, stomach and lung meridians. It has the effect of lowering the rebellious qi to stop vomiting, drying dampness and eliminating phlegm and dispersing stagnation and lumps. It is always used for dampness or cold phlegm syndrome. Banxia mainly contains alkaloids, β-sitosterol, glucosides, β-amino acids, choline and volatile oil, which possesses various pharmacological effects, such as anti-tumor, expectorant, antitussive, antiemetic, analgesic and antiulcerative functions, so it is applied to treat cough, nausea and vomiting, goiter, lymphatic tuberculosis and other phlegm syndromes. According to the "eighteen antagonisms", Banxia can not be used with Chuanwu (*Aconiti Radix*), Zhichuanwu (*Aconiti Radix Cocta*), Caowu (*Aconiti Kusnezoffii Radix*), Zhicaowu (*Aconiti Kusnezoffii Radix Cocta*) and Fuzi (*Aconiti Lateralis Radix Praeparata*) together.

【品种品质】
[Variety and Quality]

一、基原品种与品质
I Origin Varieties and Quality

1. **品种概况** 来源于天南星科植物半夏 *Pinellia ternata* (Thunb.) Breit. 的干燥块茎。

1 Variety

Banxia is from the dried rhizome of *Pinellia ternata (Thunb.) Breit,* of Araceae family.

半夏之名始载于《礼记·月令》："仲夏之月半夏生"；半夏入药始载于《五十二病方》第 376 号方；《蜀本草》及《本草图经》对半夏的形态特征进行了描述，《蜀本草》谓："苗一茎，茎端三，有二根相重，上小下大，五月采则虚小，八月采实大"；《本草图经》补充说："二月生苗一茎，茎端出三叶，浅绿色，颇似竹叶而光，江南者似芍药叶"。参照《证类本草》、《本草品汇精要》、《本草纲目》及《植物名实图考》等的附图，可以确证古籍记载的半夏与今用半夏的原植物是一致的。

It was first recorded in *Liji Yueling (The Book of Rites on order)* as "Banxia is born in midsummer"; the medicinal use of Banxia was first recorded in *Wushier Bing Fang (Prescriptions for Fifty-two Diseases)* No. 376. In *ShuBencao (Shu Meteria Medica)* and *Bencao Tujing,* the morphological characteristic of Banxia was described. *ShuBencao* stated that "the seedling has one stem and there are three leaves at the end of the stem. It has two stalks and the upper part is small while the lower part is big. When picked in May, it is small, while in August, it is large." In *Bencao Tujing,* the morphological features of Banxia was described as "the seedling is born in February, with three light green leaves at the end of the stem, which resemble bamboo leaves, while those from the south of the Yangtze River resemble peony leaves." And with reference to the drawings such as *Zhenglei Bencao (Essential Materia Medica)*, *Bencao Pinhui Jingyao (Collected Essentials of Species of Materia Medica)*, *Bencao Gangmu* and *Zhiwu Mingshi Tukao*, we can confirm that the Banxia recorded in ancient books is consistent with the current used one.

2. 种植采收　半夏药材一般以人工种植为主，在甘肃、四川、湖北、河南、贵州等地均有种植，一般采用块茎直播、珠芽直播和种子播种育苗移栽等方式进行种植。生产上，通常以块茎繁殖为主，并于当年或第2年的夏季5、6两月或秋季9、10两月采收。

2 Planting and Harvesting

Banxia is generally planted artifically in Gansu, Sichuan, Hubei, Henan and Guizhou provinces and its planting methods include tuber direct seeding, bulb bud direct seeding, and seed sowing and transplanting. In production, tuber propagation is mainly used and it is harvested in May and June in summer or September and October in autumn of the same year or the second year.

3. 道地性及品质评价　历代本草记载，甘肃、四川、河南是半夏的道地产区。形态上以呈"类球形"或者"扁球形"，下端"钝圆"，颜色上以"皮净、色白、质坚实、粉性足，无花、麻、油子"者为佳。现代半夏建立了以颜色、断面质地为主的性状评价方法，以及水溶性浸提物、总酸含量测定的化学评价方法。

半夏中主要含生物碱、β-谷甾醇、葡萄糖苷、β-氨基酸、胆碱、挥发油、有机酸等，其中，草酸钙针晶及其毒蛋白是其主要毒性物质，总游离有机酸是其止咳祛痰的主要物质基础，水溶性葡萄糖醛酸衍生物和水溶性苷是其镇吐的主要物质基础，总生物碱是其抗肿瘤的主要物质基础。《中国药典》规定半夏药材中含总酸以琥珀酸含量不得少于0.25%。

3 Genuineness and Quality Evaluation

According to the historical records, Gansu, Sichuan and Henan provinces are the genuine producing areas of Banxia. Banxia is considered superior should be "quasi-spherical" or "flat spherical" and "blunt-round bottom" in shape, "clean skin, white color, solid quality, powdery enough, no flowers, hemp, oil seeds" in color. In modern society, the character evaluation method based on color and cross-sectional texture, as well as a chemical evaluation method for the determination of water-soluble extracts and total acid contents have been established for Banxia.

Banxia mainly contains alkaloids, β-sitosterol, glucosides, β-amino acids, choline, volatile oil, organic acids, etc. Among them, needle crystal of calcium oxalate and its toxic protein are the main toxic substances of Banxia. The total free organic acids are the main therapeutic substances for relieving cough and expectoration. Water-soluble glucuronic acid derivatives and water-soluble glycosides are the main antiemetic substance basis, and the total alkaloids are the major material basis for its anti-tumor. According to the chemical index evaluation in the *Pharmacopoeia of the People's*

Republic of China, the total acid content in Banxia is calculated as succinic acid, which should not be less than 0.25%.

二、炮制品种与品质
II Processed Varieties and Quality

半夏的炮制品种有 5 种，临床常用品种，如清半夏、姜半夏、法半夏等。生半夏以色白、质坚实、粉性足者为佳；法半夏以表面淡白色、黄色或棕黄色，质较松脆，微有麻舌感者为佳；姜半夏以表面棕褐色，常呈角质样光泽，微有麻舌感，嚼之略粘牙者为佳；清半夏以切面淡灰色至灰白色，质脆，断面略呈角质样，味微涩、微有麻舌感者为佳。《中国药典》规定清半夏含总酸以琥珀酸含量不得少于 0.30%，而对法半夏和姜半夏无具体要求。

There are more than 5 processed products of Banxia. Different products are commonly used clinically, such as the processing Qingbanxia (alumine-processed), Jiangbanxia (ginger-processed), Fabanxia (Gancao-processed), etc. Shengbanxia (raw), the one with white color and solid texture, powdery root is considered to have better quality. Fabanxia (Gancao-processed) with pale white skin, crisp texture and slightly numbing-tongue sense is considered to have better quality. Jiangbanxia (ginger-processed) with brown color, keratinous with a slight tingling sensation is considered to have better quality. Qingbanxia (alumine-processed) with "light gray to off-white, crisp, and the section is slightly keratinous" is considered to have better quality. According to *the Pharmacopoeia of the People's Republic of China)*, the total acid content in Qingbanxia (alumine-processed) is calculated as the quantity of succinic acid, which should not be less than 0.30%, while there is no specific requirements about Fabanxia (Gancao-processed) and Jiangbanxia (ginger-processed).

三、中成药品种与品质
III Varieties and Quality of Chinese Patent Medicines

含有半夏或其炮制品的中成药有 200 余个，《中药药典》收载 80 余个。以半夏为君药或主药的品种有二陈丸、半夏止咳糖浆、半夏天麻丸、保宁半夏颗粒、川贝半夏液等。在中成药的品质控制中，多采用显微鉴别确定半夏的存在。如二陈丸以半夏为君药，通过显微鉴别"草酸钙针晶成束，存在于黏液细胞中或散在"确定含有半夏。

At present, there are more than 200 Chinese patent medicines containing Banxia or its processed products, 80 of which are contained in *the Pharmacopoeia of the People's Republic of China*. Among them, prescriptions with Banxia as sovereign medicinal are as follows: Er Chen Wan, Banxia Zhike Tangjiang, Banxia Tianma Wan, Baoning Banxia Keli and Chuanbei Banxia Ye (Mixture), etc. In the quality control of Chinese patent medicines, the existence of Banxia was determined by microscopic identification. Erchen Wan with Banxia as sovereign medicinal, the existence of Banxia in it was determined through the microscopic identification that "calcium oxalate needle crystal bundle, exist in the mucous cells or scattered".

【制药】
[Pharmacy]

一、产地加工
I Processing in Production Area

生半夏一般于夏至或秋分采收后洗净泥土，及时去皮且干燥，以防止药材腐烂。

Shengbanxia (raw) is usually collected after the summer solstice or autumn equinox, washed, peeled and dried in time to prevent corrosion.

二、饮片炮制
II Processing of Decoction Pieces

仅在古代，半夏的炮制方法就多达70余种。宋代以来，逐渐形成了"浸泡（加甘草汁、生姜汁或白矾溶液）、拌匀、煎煮"工艺，法半夏、姜半夏、清半夏成为商品规格中的主流。

Even in ancient times, there were more than 70 methods which can process Banxia. Since the Song Dynasty, the process of "soaking (adding licorice juice, ginger juice or alum solution), mixing well, and boiling" has gradually formed, and the Fabanxia (Gancao-processed), Jiangbanxia (ginger-processed), and Qingbanxia (alumine-processed) have become the mainstream of commodity specifications.

炮制是半夏减毒的重要减毒手段，其减毒原理是：半夏刺激性毒性成分是由尿黑酸（2，5-二羟基苯乙酸）及其葡萄糖苷、3，4-二羟基苯甲醛及其苷、草酸钙针晶三类成分引起的。刺激性毒性成分主要是蛋白和草酸钙结合形成的针晶复合物，即"毒针晶"。电镜下可见该毒针晶极细长、两头尖锐、质地坚韧，具有倒刺、凹槽。炮制所用辅料白矾及石灰具有确切的破坏生半夏刺激性毒性成分的作用。8%明矾水或pH > 12的碱水炮制可以使毒针晶晶体破坏，毒蛋白溶解变性，使其刺激毒性降低。

Processing is an important method for dealing with the poisonous Chinese medicine Banxia. Its attenuation principle is: the irritating and toxic component of Banxia (Pinellia) is composed of 3 kinds of substences, homogentisic acid (2,5-dihydroxyphenylacetic acid) and its glucoside, 3,4-dihydroxybenzaldehyde and its glycosides and calcium oxalate needle crystals. The irritating and toxic ingredients are mainly the needle crystal complex formed by the combination of protein and calcium oxalate, that is "poison needle crystal". Under the electron microscope, it can be seen that the poison needle is extremely slender, sharp at both ends, tough in texture, with barbeds and grooves. Alum and lime, the auxiliary materials used in the preparation, have the exact effect of destroying the irritating and toxic components of Shengbanxia (raw). The processing of 8% alum water or alkaline water with pH>12 can destroy the poisonous needle crystal crystals, dissolve and denature the poisonous protein, and reduce its stimulation and toxicity.

三、中成药制药
III Pharmacy of Chinese Patent Medicines

含半夏的中成药，具体包括丸剂、胶囊剂、口服液等。由于半夏具有刺激性毒性，故为保证用药安全，生半夏直接入中成药者少，如藿香正气口服液、暑湿感冒颗粒等；其余多以炮制品（如姜半夏、清半夏、法半夏等）入药，如二陈丸、乙肝益气解郁颗粒、小青龙合剂等。

There are various kinds of Chinese patent medicines containing Banxia, including pills, capsules, mixtures, etc. Because Banxia has irritating toxicity, in order to ensure the safety of the medication, fewer Chinese patent medicines directly use Shengbanxia (raw), such as Huoxiang Zhengqi Koufuye, Shushi Ganmao Keli, etc., the rest medicines are mostly made of processed products (such as Jiangbanxia, Qingbanxia, Fabanxia, etc.), such as Erchen Wan, Yigan Yiqi Jieyu Keli, Xiaoqinglong Heji, etc.

如以半夏为君药的二陈丸，其制备过程采用制半夏入药，制成的剂丸服用方便，容易储存，又保存了药效，其中的主要有效成分中含有挥发油，制成丸剂可减少饮片储存过程中药效挥发过快。在藿香正气口服液制剂工艺中，因使用的是生半夏，需与干姜同煮，以除去半夏的毒性，增加了制剂的安全性。

For example, Erchen Wan with Banxia as sovereign medicinals are prepared by making Banxia into medicine, which is convenient to take a store, and also keeps the efficacy. The main active ingredients of Banxia contain volatile oil, and making it into pills can reduce the rapid volatilization of the efficacy in the storage process of decocting pieces. In the preparation process of Huoxiang Zhengqi Koufuye, Shengbanxia (raw) was used, so it was boiled with dried ginger to remove the toxicity of Banxia and increase the safety of the preparation.

【性能功效】
[Property and Efficacy]

一、性能
I Property

半夏辛、温，有毒；归脾、胃、肺经。

Banxia is pungent in flavor, warm in nature, toxic, and enters the spleen, stomach and lung meridians.

二、功效
II Efficacy

1. 燥湿化痰　半夏味辛、性温燥，具有行气燥湿化痰功效。其功效的发挥与镇咳、祛痰等药理作用密切相关。半夏镇咳、祛痰的有效物质基础主要是总游离有机酸，通过抑制咳嗽中枢，降低呼吸道感受器敏感性等发挥作用。

1 Dry Dampness and Resolve Phlegm

Banxia, pungent in flavor and warm-dry in nature, can promote flow of qi, dry dampness and resolve phlegm. Its efficacy is closely related to its pharmacological effects such as being antitussive and expectorant. The effective material basis of its efficacy is the total free organic acids, which play a role by inhibiting cough center and reducing the sensitivity of respiratory tract receptors.

2. 降逆止呕　半夏味辛，归脾、胃、肺经，能散逆气，和胃降逆而止呕。其功效的发挥与镇吐、抗溃疡、调节胃肠运动等药理作用密切相关。主要的物质基础是水溶性葡萄糖醛酸衍生物和水溶性苷。

2 Lower the Adverse Rising Qi to Stop Vomiting

Banxia is pungent in nature and enters to the spleen, stomach and lung meridians. It can disperse qi, harmonize stomach and lower the adverse rising qi to stop vomiting. Its efficacy is closely related to pharmacological effects such as antiemetics, antiulcer, and regulation of gastrointestinal movement. The main material bases are the water-soluble glucuronic acid derivatives and water-soluble glycosides.

3. 消痞散结　半夏辛散消痞，化痰散结。其功效的发挥与抗肿瘤、抗菌、抗炎等药理作用密切相关。半夏抗肿瘤、抗菌、抗炎的主要物质基础是多糖、总生物碱。

3 Disperse Stagnation and Eliminate Lumps

Banxia can disperse stagnation and eliminating lumps, resolve phlegm and dissipate mass. Its efficacy is closely related to pharmacological effects of antitumor, antibacteria and anti-inflammation. The main material bases of its efficacy of anti-tumor, anti-bacteria and anti-inflammation are polysaccharides and total alkaloids.

4. 消肿止痛　半夏外用消肿止痛。其功效的发挥与抗炎、抗菌、镇痛等药理作用密切相关。主要的物质基础是多糖、总生物碱。

4 Disperse Sweling and Relieve Pain

Banxia is externally applied to disperse swelling and relieve pains. Its efficacy is closely related to pharmacological effects of anti-inflammatory, antibacterial and analgesic, etc. The main material bases are polysaccharides and total alkaloids.

【应用】
[Applications]

一、主治病证
I Indications

1. 咳嗽痰多　治疗湿痰壅滞，咳嗽声重，痰多质粘者，常配伍橘红、白茯苓、甘草以燥湿化痰，理气和中，如《太平惠民和剂局方》二陈汤和现代制剂二陈丸；治咳嗽气喘，咯痰黄稠，常与陈皮、苦杏仁、枳实等同用以清热化痰，理气止咳，如《医方考》清气化痰丸；治眩晕头痛，胸膈痞满，恶心呕吐等，常与天麻、茯苓、白术等同用以化痰息风，健脾祛湿，如《医学心语》半夏白术天麻汤。

1 Cough with Profuse Sputum

For dampness phlegm, stagnation, heavy cough, and sticky sputum, it is always compatible with Juhong (Citri Grandis Exocarpium), Baifuling (Poria) and Gancao to dry and resolve phlegm, regulate qi and harmonize middle energizer such as Erchen Tang (Decoction) in *Taiping Huimin Hejiji Ju Fang (The Prescriptions of the Bureau of Taiping People's Welfare Pharmacy)* and Modern preparation Erchen Wan For asthmatic cough with thick and yellowish sputum, it is always compatible with Chenpi, Kuxingren and Zhishi to clear heat and resolve phlegm as well as regulate qi and relieve cough such as Qingqi Huatan Wan in *Yifangkao*; for dizziness headache, chest fullness, nausea and vomiting, it is always compatible with Tianma, Fuling and Baizhu to relieve phlegm and recuperate wind, strengthen the spleen and dampness such as Banxia Baizhu Tianma Tang (Decoction) in *Yixue Xinyu (Experience on Medical practices)* .

现代临床，半夏配伍常用于治疗梅尼埃病、梅核气等，如二陈汤。

In modern clinical practice, Banxia compatibility is always used to treat Meniere's disease and globus hystericus as in Erchen Tang (Decoction).

2. 呕吐　治疗胸脘痞闷，烦热，气逆欲呕者，可配黄连、甘草、桂枝等以寒热并调，和胃降逆，如《伤寒杂病论》黄连汤；治痰饮及胃寒呕吐，常配生姜，以和胃止呕，散饮降逆，如《金匮要略》小半夏汤。

2 Vomiting

For the epigastric stuffiness and obstruction ,

irritability and vomiting , it can be combined with Huanglian, Gancao and Guizhi, etc., to regulate the balance of the cold and the hot ,harmonize stomach and descend the rising of qi, such as Huanglian Tang (Decoction) from *Shanghan Zabing Lun*; For treating phlegm and water retention, vomiting due to stomach cold , it is often combined with ginger to relieve vomiting by harmonizing the stomach, relieving water retention and descending adverse qi, such as Xiaobanxia Tang (Decoction) in *Jingui Yaolue*.

现代临床，半夏配伍常用于治疗呕吐、妊娠呕吐、消化道疾病等，如小半夏汤。

In modern clinical practice, Banxia compatibility is always used to treat vomiting, pregnant vomiting and digestive tract diseases, such as Xiao Banxia Tang (Decoction).

3. 心下痞证　治疗心下痞满而不痛，或呕吐，肠鸣下利，常与干姜、黄芩、黄连等配伍以平调寒热、辛开苦降，如《伤寒杂病论》半夏泻心汤；治心下痞硬，干噫食臭，干呕，心烦不得安，可与生姜、甘草等配伍以和胃消痞，宣散水气，如《伤寒论》生姜泻心汤。

3 Epigastric Stuffiness Syndromes

For epigastric stuffiness and fullness, or vomiting, or borbormus with diarrhea, it is always combined with Ganjiang, Huangqin and Huanglian to achieve the effect of neutral balancing the cold and hot, with the pungent for dispersing and the bitter for descending, such as Banxia Xiexin Tang (Decoction) in *Shanghan Zabing Lun*. For epigastric stuffiness and rigidity, dry belching with food malodor, retching and vexation, it is always combined with Ganjiang and Gancao to harmonize the stomach and dissipate abdominal mass, diffuse the edema. Shengjiang Xiexin Tang (Decoction) in *Shanghan Zabing Lun* is an example.

现代临床，半夏配伍常用于治疗冠心病、心律失常、病毒性心肌炎等，如半夏泻心汤。

In modern clinical practice, Banxia compatibility is always used to treat coronary heart disease, arrhythmia and viral myocarditis, such as Banxia

Xiexin Tang (Decoction).

4. **瘿瘤、痰核、痈疽肿毒** 治瘿瘤痰核，常配昆布、海藻、贝母等；治痈疽发背、无名肿毒初起或毒蛇咬伤，可生品研末调敷或鲜品捣敷。

4 Goiter, Subcutaneous Nobule and Large Carbuncle

For goiter and subcutaneous nobule, it is used together with *Kunbu, Haizao and Beimu*, for large carbuncle, unknown swelling toxin or poisonous snake bite, directly apply the raw powder or pounded fresh medicinal on the affected area .

现代临床，半夏配伍常用于治疗恶性肿瘤、乳腺增生症、淋巴结核等，如海藻玉壶汤。

In modern clinical practice, Banxia compatibility is always used to treat malignant tumor, hyperplasia of mammary glands and lymphoid tuberculosis3, such as Haizao Yuhu Tang (Decoction).

二、用法用量
II Administration and Dosage

3~9g，煎汤，内服一般炮制后使用；外用适量，磨汁涂或研末以酒调敷患处。

3~9g processed Banxia is decocted for oral administration, appropriate amount of the raw is used externally and ground into juice or powder to mix with liquor for external application.

三、注意事项
III Precautions

1. 不宜与川乌、制川乌、草乌、制草乌、附子同用。

1 It is incompatible with Chuanwu, Zhichuanwu (processed), Caowu, Zhicaowu (processed) and Fuzi.

2. 生半夏有引起"麻舌而刺喉"的毒副作用，生品内服宜慎。阴虚燥咳、血证及孕妇慎用。

2 Banxia (kaw) has toxicity and side effects causing "stinging tongue and throat", so the raw products should be taken with caution. Patients with dry cough due to yin deficiency, hemorrhagic diseases and pregnant women should use it with cautions.

【知识拓展】
[Knowledge Extension]

半夏具有刺激性、神经系统和生殖系统的毒性，可通过选用正品药材、规范炮制、合理配伍、对证用药等控毒方法控制毒性和保证疗效。

Banxia is toxic, which may stimulate the nervous system and reproductive system. Its toxicity can be restrained and its curative effect can be retained through the selection of authentic medicinal materials, standard processing, rational compatibility, and medication based on syndromes.

川 贝 母
Chuanbeimu
(Fritillariae Cirrhosae Bulbus)

川贝母是著名的川产道地药材。川贝母味苦、甘，性微寒，归肺、心经，具清热润肺，化痰止咳，散结消痈的功效，主治肺热燥咳，干咳少痰，阴虚劳嗽，痰中带血，瘰疬，乳痈，肺痈等热痰、燥痰等证。川贝母中主要含生物碱类成分，有镇咳、祛痰、平喘、降血压、增强心肌收缩力、抗血小板聚集、抗肿瘤、抗菌、抗炎等药理作用，可用于治疗慢性支气管炎、咳嗽、哮喘、呼吸道感染。根据"十八反"，川贝母不宜与川乌、制川乌、草乌、制草乌、附子同用。

Chuanbeimu is a noted genuine regional medicinal in Sichuan province. Chuanbeimu is bitter and sweet in flavor and slightly cold in nature and it enters the lung and heart meridians. The effects of Chuanbeimu are clearing heart and moistening lung, dissolving phlegm and arresting cough, removing stasis and eliminating carbuncle. It is mainly indicated for heat and dry phlegm syndromes including dry cough due to the heat in the lung, dry cough with less phlegm, long time cough caused by yin deficiency, bloody phlegm, scrofula, mastitis and lung abscess. Chuanbeimu can be used to treat chronic bronchitis, cough, asthma, respiratory tract infection, because it mainly contains alkaloids which has antitussive, expectorant, asthmatic, lowering blood pressure, enhancing myocardial contractility, antiplatelet aggregation, antitumor, antibacterial, anti-inflammatory and other pharmacological effects. According to the "eighteen antagonisms", Chuanbeimu should not be used with Chuanwu, Zhichuanwu (processed), Caowu, Zhicaowu (processed) and Fuzi together.

【品种品质】
[Variety and Quality]

一、基原品种与品质
I Origin Varieties and Quality

1. **品种概况** 来源于百合科植物川贝母 *Fritillaria cirrhosa* D. Don、暗紫贝母 *Fritillaria unibracteata* Hsiao et K. C. Hsia、甘肃贝母 *Fritillaria przewalskii* Maxim.、梭砂贝母 *Fritillaria delavayi* Franch.、太白贝母 *Fritillaria taipaiensis* P. Y. Li 或瓦布贝母 *Fritillaria unibracteata* Hsiao et K. C. Hsia var. *wabuensis*（S. Y. Tang et S. C. Yue）Z. D. Liu, S. Wang et S. C. Chen 的干燥鳞茎。按性状不同分别习称"松贝"、"青贝"、"炉贝"和"栽培品"。

1 Variety

It is originated from the dried bulbs of *Fritillaria cirrhosa* D. Don *of Liliaceae, Fritillaria unibracteata Hsiao* et K.C.Hsia, *Fritillaria przewalskii Maxim., Fritillaria delavayi Franch., Fritillaria taipaiensis* P.Y. Li, *or tile Fritillaria unibracteata Hsiao* et K.C. Hsia var. *Wabuensis* (SY Tang et SC Yue) ZD Liu, S. Wang et S.C. Chen. According to different characteristics, they are referred to as "Songbei", "Qingbei", "Lubei" and "cultivation products".

贝母之名始见于《神农本草经》，而川贝母最早记载于明代的本草著作，且提出川产为优，如《本草从新》言"川产最佳，圆正底平，开瓣味甘"。随后各代本草对药用川贝母的品种描述十分不详，既有资料也较混乱，大致涵盖了古代川蜀地域的川贝母、暗紫贝母、甘肃贝母、梭砂贝母和太白贝母物种，中国药典在此基础上又增加了瓦布贝母作为基原植物。

Beimu was first appeared in the book of *Shennong Bencao Jing* and Chuanbeimu was first recorded in the herbal works of Ming Dynasty and proposed that the medicinals produced in Sichuan province is superior. As described in *Bencao Congxin (New Revised Materia Medica)*, "Beimu produced in Sichuan province is superior with the round shape, flat bottom, cracked shell and sweet flavor." The description of medicinal Chuanbeimu of the following generations of Chinese materia medica is much unknown, and the available data is also confusing. It roughly covers the species of *Fritillaria cirrhosa* D. Don *of Liliaceae, Fritillaria unibracteata Hsiao* et KCHsia, *Fritillaria przewalskii Maxim., Fritillaria delavayi Franch., Fritillaria taipaiensis* P.Y. Li in the ancient Chuanshu area. On the basis, *tile Fritillaria unibracteata* Hsiao et K.C. Hsia var. *Wabuensis* (S.Y. Tang et S.C. Yue) Z.D. Liu, S. Wang et SC Chen's dried bulbs have been added as a primitive plant in the pharmacopoeia.

2. **种植采收** 川贝母药材一般以人工种植为主，在四川阿坝、理县、小金等县，甘肃漳县，云南丽江等地均有种植，一般可通过种子、鳞茎繁殖，也有采用人工育种、搭棚种植方式进行基地化栽培。古代既有少量的不成熟栽培，主要限于"大"贝母,与野生品一起多在夏、秋季或积雪融化后杂草未长时采挖。

2 Planting and Harvesting

Chuanbeimu is mainly produced through artificial cultivation. At present, it has been cultivated in some areas including Aba, Lixian, Xiaojin, and other counties in Sichuan province, Zhangxian in Gansu province, Lijiang in Yunnan province and other places, and it can generally be propagated by seeds and bulbs, but also by artificial breeding and greenhouse cultivation. In ancient times, there were a small amount of immature cultivation, which was mainly "big" Beimu, and together with wild products, they were mostly dug out in summer, autumn or during snow melting and weeds growing.

3. **道地性及品质评价** 自古以来,四川是川贝母的道地产区。古代对川贝母的质量评价包含了形、色、味等多个方面。形态上以"开瓣"、"圆正底平"者为佳,颜色上以"色白"、"皮细白"者为佳,质量上以"体轻"者尤良,气味上以"味淡"、"味甘"者为佳。现代已完善了包含颜色、形状、粉性、气味等指标的性状评价方法以及醇溶物、总生物碱含量测定的化学评价方法。

3 Genuineness and Quality Evaluation

Since ancient times, Sichuan is the genuine regional producing area of Chuanbeimu. In ancient times, the quality evaluation of Chuanbeimu included many aspects such as shape, color, and taste. The morphology of "open flap" and "round positive bottom flat" is the best. It is better with "color white" and "thin white skin" in color, especially "light" in quality, and "light" and "sweet" in odor. What's more, the characteristics evaluation method on color, shape, mealiness, odour and other indicators, as well as the chemical evaluation method on alchohol soluble and total alkaloid content has been greatly improved in modern times.

川贝母主要含有生物碱,其他非生物碱类成分包括萜类、甾体、脂肪酸、嘌呤、腺苷、多糖和多酚类等,其中,西贝母碱、贝母辛、贝母素甲等为其镇咳平喘的主要物质基础,皂苷类成分是其祛痰的主要物质基础。《中国药典》规定川贝母药材中含西贝母碱不得少于 0.050%。

Chuanbeimu mainly contains alkaloids, and other non-alkaloids including terpenoids, steroids, fatty acids, purines, adenosine, polysaccharides, and polyphenols. Sipeimine, peimisine, peimine and others are considered as the main material basis of antitussive and antiasthmatic effects, and the content of saponins as the basis of eliminating phlegm for this kind of medicinal. According to the *Pharmacopoeia of the People's Republic of China*, the content of sipeimine of Chuanbeimu should not be less than 0.050%.

二、炮制品种与品质
II Processed Varieties and Quality

川贝母的临床常用品种 1 个,为生川贝母。川贝母以色白、粉性足、质坚实为佳。

At present, one of the common species in clinical practice is Shengchuanbeimu (raw) and the white, powdery and solid ones are considered to be the superior one.

三、中成药品种与品质
III Varieties and Quality of Chinese Patent Medicines

含有川贝母的中成药有 200 余个,《中国药典》收载含有川贝母的中成药 40 余个。以川贝母为君药或主药的品种有二母宁嗽丸、川贝止咳露、川贝枇杷糖浆、川贝雪梨膏等。在中成药的品质控制中多采用显微鉴别、薄层鉴别确定川贝母的存在,通过显微鉴别"淀粉粒广卵形或贝壳形,脐点短缝状、人字状或马蹄状,层纹可察见"确定含有川贝母。蛇胆川贝软胶囊,薄层色谱法以川贝母为对照药材,对药中的川贝母进行检测。

At present, there are more than 200 Chinese patent medicines containing Chuanbeimu and the *Pharmacopoeia of the People's Republic of China* (Part I) contains 40 of them. Chuanbeimu is used as sovereign medicinal or main medicinal, including Ermu Ningke Wan, Chuanbei Zhike Lu (Syrup), Chuanbei Pipa Tangjiang, Chuanbei Xueli Gao (Syrup) etc. In the quality control of Chinese patent medicine, the presence of Chuanbeimu was determined by microscopic identification and TLC identification. The presence of Chuanbeimu was determined by microscopic identification of "starch granule broad oval or conchoid, umbilical point short slit, herringbone or horseshoes, lamellar visible". TLC was used to detect Chuanbeimu in the Shedan Chuanbei Ruanjiaonang (Soft capsule) by taking Chuanbeimu as a reference medicinal.

【制药】
[Pharmacy]

一、产地加工
I Processing in Production Area

川贝母一般于春夏茎叶枯萎前，选晴天采挖，清除泥土，注意避免损伤，不能淘洗，及时将采回的新鲜贝母摊放竹席上晾干。干燥时不能堆沤，否则发黄变质，可以烘烤干燥。

Chuanbeimu is generally dug in sunny days before the stems and leaves wither in spring and summer with the soil removed but not damaging and washing them. The freshly collected Beimu should be spread out on bamboo mat to dry in time instead of being stacked. Otherwise, it will turn yellow and deteriorate. Or you can dry them by baking.

二、饮片炮制
II Processing of Decoction Pieces

为缓和川贝母的药性，便于有效成分煎出，方便制剂和服用，形成了米炒制、炒制等十余种炮制方法。现川贝母临床多用生品，除去杂质后，碾成细粉冲服或制剂用。

In order to moderate the medicinal properties of Chuanbeimu and to acquire the active ingredients as well as for easily preparing and taking, more than ten kinds of processing methods including stir-frying with rice and stir-frying has been formed. At present, the Chuanbeimu (raw) is mostly applied in the clinical practice. After removing the impurities, grind into fine powder, then mix with water and take it directly, or ready for the applying of making preparations.

三、中成药制药
III Pharmacy of Chinese Patent Medicines

含川贝母的中成药，剂型非常丰富，涵盖固体、液体和半固体剂型，具体包括片剂、糖浆剂、膏剂、丸剂、口服液、颗粒剂、散剂、合剂、胶囊剂、冲剂等。

The Chinese patent medicines containing Chuanbeimu are rich in pharmaceutical forms, covering solid, liquid and semisolid pharmaceutical forms, including tablets, syrups, ointments, pills, mixtures, granules, powders, mixtures, capsules, granules, etc.

含川贝母的传统中成药制剂多制成糖浆剂、膏剂等。现今为满足现代制剂处方成形性及减少服用剂量，一般制剂如片剂、颗粒剂等多以川贝母粉末入制剂中。

Chinese pharmaceutical preparations containing Chuanbeimu are mostly made into syrups, ointments, etc. Nowadays, in order to meet the requirements of modern preparation and reduce the dosage, the powder of Chuanbeimu is usually used in the tablets and granules preparations.

如二母宁嗽丸，用蜜泛丸，缓和了组方中川贝母、石膏、黄芩的寒凉之性，且蜂蜜能辅助温中补益，增强了该药的润肺止咳之效。

Take Ermu Ningsou Wan as example, it is made into honey pills to relieve the the cold and cool nature of Chuanbeimu, Shigao (Gypsum Fibrosum), Huangqin (Astragali seu Hedysari

Radix) in the prescription, and the honey can help warm and nourish, enhance the effect of this medicine in moisturizing the lungs and relieving cough.

【性能功效】
[Property and Efficacy]

一、性能
I Property

川贝母苦、甘, 微寒; 归肺、心经。

Chuanbeimu is bitter and sweet in flavor, slightly cold in nature, and enters the lung and heart meridians.

二、功效
II Efficacy

1. **清热润肺, 化痰止咳**　川贝母性寒可清热化痰止咳, 味甘性润能润化燥痰。其功效的发挥与川贝母祛痰、镇咳、平喘、抗菌等药理作用密切相关。川贝母祛痰、镇咳、平喘、抗菌的有效物质基础主要是皂苷类、生物碱类成分, 通过增加呼吸道的分泌量, 扩张支气管作用以及作用于中枢神经系统, 达到化痰止咳平喘的作用。

1 Clearing Heat and Moistening the Lung, Relieve Phlegm and Relieve Cough

Chuanbeimu with cold nature, can clear heat, reduce phlegm, relieve cough, and the sweetness nature could moisturize the lung and dry phlegm. Its effectiveness is closely related to pharmacological effects such as the expectorating, relieving asthma and cough, and antibacteria, etc. The effective material base of the expectorant, the antitussive, relieving asthma and antibacteria of Chuanbeimu is mainly saponins and alkaloids. Those materials can help increasing the amount of respiratory secretions, dilating the bronchus and work on the nervous system so that Chuanbeimu can reduce phlegm and relieve cough as well as asthma.

2. **散结消痈**　川贝母清化郁热, 化痰散结, 消痈。其功效的发挥与抗炎、抗肿瘤等药理作用密切相关。川贝母抗炎与抗肿瘤的主要物质基础为生物碱类成分。

2 Dissipating Mass and Eliminate Carbuncle

Chuanbeimu clears stagnation and heat, dissolves phlegm, dissolves sputum, and eliminates carbuncle. Its effectiveness is closely related to anti-inflammatory and anti-tumor pharmacological effects. The effective material basis of anti-inflammatory and anti-tumor of Chuanbeimu is mainly alkaloids.

【应用】
[Applications]

一、主治病证
I Indications

1. **虚劳咳嗽, 肺热燥咳**　治疗肺阴虚劳嗽, 久咳有痰者, 常配沙参、麦冬等以养阴润肺, 化痰止咳; 治肺热、肺燥咳嗽, 常配知母以清肺润燥, 化痰止咳, 如二母散《急救仙方》; 治痰热咳嗽, 可配黄芩、枇杷叶清热化痰, 止咳。

1 Cough of Consumptive Disease, Cough of Lung Heat

For the deficiency of lung yin and long-term cough with phlegm, Chuanbeimu is often combined with Shashen (*Adenophorae Radix*), *Maidong*, etc. to tonify yin to moisten the lung and resolve phlegm to suppress cough, similarly, for lung heat and coughing of lung dryness. It is often combined with Zhimu to clear the lung and moisten dryness, resolve phlegm to suppress cough, such as Ermu San (Powder) recorded in *Jijiu Xianfang (Xianfang First Aid)*. For coughing of phlegm-heat, and it can be used with Huangqin and Pipaye to clear heat and resolve phlegm, and relieve cough.

现代临床, 川贝母配伍常用于治疗急慢性支气管炎及上呼吸道感染、百日咳等, 如百合固金汤。

In modern clinical practice, Chuanbeimu compatibility is often used to treat acute and chronic bronchitis, upper respiratory tract infection, and pertussis, etc., such as Baihe Gujin Tang (Decoction).

2. 瘰疬，乳痈，肺痈　治疗痰火郁结之瘰疬，常配玄参、牡蛎等药用，如消瘰丸《医学心悟》；治热毒壅结之乳痈、肺痈，常配蒲公英、鱼腥草等以清热解毒，消肿散结；治肺痈咳唾浓痰，多与鱼腥草、鲜芦根、薏苡仁配伍，以清热解毒、化痰排脓。

2 Scrofula, Mastitis and Lung Abscess

Chuanbeimu can be combined with Xuanshen, Muli (Ostreae Concha) for the treatment of scrofula due to phlegm-fire depression usually, such as Xiaolei Wan recorded in *Yixue Xinwu (Comprehension of Medicine)*; it can also be combined with Pugongying (Taraxaci Herba), Yuxingcao to treat mastitis and lung abscess due to excessive heat and toxicity through clearing heat toxin, detumescence and lump dissipation. In addition, for the treatment of lung abscess with coughing and sticky phlegm, it is often combined with Yuxingcao, Xianlugen *(Phragmitis Rhizoma)*, Yiyiren to clear heat toxin, resolving phlegm to

discharging pus.

现代临床，川贝母配伍常用于治疗恶性肿瘤、乳腺增生症、淋巴结核等，如海藻玉壶汤。

In modern clinical, Chuanbeimu compatibility is often used to treat malignant tumor, hyperplasia of mammary glands and lymphoid tuberculosis, such as Haizao Yuhu Tang (Decoction).

二、用法用量
II Administration and Dosage

3~10g，煎汤；一次 1~2g，研粉冲服。

3~10g, water decoction; 1~2g at a time, grind to powder and take it.

三、注意事项
III Precautions

1. 不宜与川乌、制川乌、草乌、制草乌、附子同用。

1 It should not be used with Chuanwu, Zhichuanwu, Caowu, Zhicaowu and Fuzi.

2. 脾胃虚寒及有湿痰者不宜用。

2 It should be avoided being used for patients who are characterized by spleen and stomach deficiency with dampness phlegm.

苦 杏 仁

Kuxingren
(Armeniacae Semen Amarum)

苦杏仁是著名的山东产道地药材。常用炮制品为燀苦杏仁、炒苦杏仁。苦杏仁味苦，性微温，有小毒，归肺、大肠经，具降气止咳平喘、润肠通便的功效，主治咳喘证、肠燥便秘等。苦杏仁中主要含苷类、脂肪酸、蛋白质、各种游离氨基酸等，具有镇咳、平喘、祛痰、抗炎、镇痛、抗肿瘤、降血糖、降血脂等药理作用，可用于治疗咳喘、便秘等。苦杏仁有小毒，可通过依

法炮制、对证用药、合理配伍、控制剂量等控毒增效。

Kuxingren is a genuine regional medicinal in Shandong province. Commonly used processed products are Dankuxingren (scalding) and Chaokuxingren (stir-frying). Kuxingren is bitter in taste, mild in nature, mild in toxicity, enters to the lungs and large intestine meridians.It has the effects of descending qi, relieving cough and dyspnea and moistening intestines to relieve constipation, with indications for the syndromes of cough and asthma, constipation due to intestinal dryness and so on. Kuxingren mainly contains glycosides, fatty acids, proteins, various free amino acids, etc, which have extensive pharmacological effects on stopping cough and relieving asthmatic symptoms, anti-inflammation, relieving pain, antitumor, eliminating phlegm, reducing blood glucose, and reducing blood lipid. Kuxingren is slightly poisonous. Its toxicity can be controlled by stipulated processing, medicating based on the correct syndrome differentiation, rational combination and managed dosage, so as to increase its efficacy.

【品种品质】
[Variety and Quality]

一、基原品种与品质
I Origin Varieties and Quality

1. **品种概况**　来源于蔷薇科植物山杏 *Prunus armeniaca* L.var. *ansu* Maxim.、西伯利亚杏 *Prunus sibirica* L.、东北杏 *Prunus mandshurica*（Maxim.）Koehne 或杏 *Prunus armeniaca* L. 的干燥成熟种子。

1 Variety

Kuxingren is the dry mature seeds of *Prunus armeniaca* L.var. *ansu* Maxim. (Shanxing), *Prunus sibirica* L. (Xiboliyaxing), *Prunus mandshuric* (Maxim) (Dongbeixing), or Koehne *Prunus armeniaca* L (Xing) from the plants of Rosaceae.

苦杏仁首载于《神农本草经》。《临证指南医案》卷四首次将"苦杏仁"作为本草正名,《本草图经》曰：正品杏"其木高丈余,二月敷青,叶如梅叶,园而尖,三月开红花,四月结实,五六月熟,大如黄梅。其实有数种,黄而园者为金杏,相传云出济南郡之分流山,彼人谓之汉帝杏,今近都多种之,熟最早；其扁而青黄者为木杏,其仁入药,今以东来者为胜"。古代药用杏

仁均来源于蔷薇科 Prunus 属多种植物的种仁,并以家种杏仁为主,与现今药用品种基本一致。

Kuxingren was first recorded in the book of *Shennong Bencao Jing (Shennong's Classic of Materia Medica)*. In Volume 4 of *Linzheng Zhinan Yian*, "Kuxingren" was employed as the name of the medicinal for the first time. According to the book of *Bencao Tujing* in terms of genuine apricot, "the height of its trunk is more than 1 zhang. It is green in February, its leaves are like plum leaves, which are round and sharp. It blooms red flowers in March, and bears fruit in April. It is ripe in May and June, the fruit is as big as Huangmei (yellw plum). There are several kinds of apricots. The yellow and round apricot is called as golden apricot. According to legend, this species of apricot come out of the Fenliu Mountain in Jinan County, which is called Han Emperor Apricot. Nowadays, it is planted in many places near the capital, and it matures earliest, the flat and green yellow apricots are called wooden apricots, whose kernels are used as medicines. Nowadays, apricots from the east are considered with good quality." Ancient medicinal almonds were derived from the kernels of various plants of the genus Prunus of the Rosaceae family, and the main species were most home grown apricots, which are basically consistent with the current medicinal varieties.

2. **种植采收**　苦杏仁药材一般以人工种植为主,在内蒙古、吉林、辽宁、河北、山西、陕西等地均有种植。一般采用大垅播种或者嫁接繁殖。大垅春播于 3 月下旬,秋播于 11 月下旬；嫁接繁殖枝接于 3 月下旬,芽接于 7 月上旬至 8 月下旬进行。夏季成熟后采收果实,但由于气候与品种不同也有迟到秋季采收者。

2 Planting and Harvesting

The medicinal of Kuxingren are mainly planted artificially in Inner Mongolia, Jilin, Liaoning, Hebei, Shanxi, and Shanxi Provinces. Commonly, the cultivation methods are sowing or grafting breeding. As for big ridge seeding, it is planted in big ridge seeding in spring in late March, autumn in late November, grafting breeding is in late March, and budding is from early July to late August. Fruits are to be harvested after maturity in summer, or later time due to different climates and varieties.

3. 道地性及品质评价　苦杏仁道地性不明显，自古以来，苦杏仁均以"东来着"为胜，如今，苦杏仁主产三北地区（华北、东北、西北），以内蒙古、吉林、辽宁、河北、山西、陕西为多。以山东产者为佳。

3 Genuineness and Quality Evaluation

It is not well know for the genuine production region of Kuxingren. From ancient times to the present, it has been widely accepted that the best Kuxingren are "from the east". Today, Kuxingren are mainly produced in the three northern regions (North China, Northeast China, and Northwest China). The majority are from Inner Mongolia, Jilin, Liaoning, Hebei, Shanxi, and Shaanxi provinces, those produced in Shandong are preferred.

苦杏仁主要含有苦杏仁苷，脂肪油，杏仁酶等化学成分。其中，苦杏仁苷是其止咳平喘的主要物质基础，苦杏仁油是润肠通便的主要物质基础。《中国药典》规定苦杏仁药材中苦杏仁苷含量不得少于 3.0%。

Kuxingren mainly contains chemical components including amygdalin, fatty oil and cellas, among which amygdalin is the material basis for the effects of relieving cough and asthma and laxative function is depended on bitter almond oil. The *Pharmacopoeia of the People's Republic of China* stipulates that the content of amygdalin in the medicinal materials of Kuxingren should not be less than 3.0%.

二、炮制品种与品质
II Processed Varieties and Quality

苦杏仁的炮制品有 4 个，临床常用品种有近 10 种，如苦杏仁、燀苦杏仁、炒苦杏仁等。燀苦

杏仁以表面乳白色，有特殊香气为佳。炒苦杏仁以表面微黄色，偶带有焦斑，具香气者为佳。炒苦杏仁以形如燀苦杏仁，表面黄色至棕黄色，微带焦斑。有香气，味苦为佳。《中国药典》规定燀苦杏仁中苦杏仁苷含量不得少于 2.4%，而炒苦杏仁中苦杏仁苷含量不得少于 2.1%。

There are 4 processed products of Kuxingren, among them, 10 varieties are available clinically, such as Kuxingren, Dankuxingren (scalding), Chaokuxingren (stir-frying) etc. Dankuxingren (scalding) with milky white color and unique fragrance are considered to have better quality. Chaokuxingren (stir-frying) with yellowish skin, burnt spot are considered to have better quality. Chaokuxingren (stir-frying) is like Dankuxingren (scalding) in shape, with brown and yellow color and burnt spot occasionally are considered to have better quality. In the *Pharmacopoeia of the People's Republic of China*, it is stipulated that the content of amygdalin in Dankuxingren (scalding) should not be less than 2.4%, while the content of amygdalin in Chaokuxingren (stir-frying) must not be less than 2.1%.

三、中成药品种与品质
III Varieties and Quality of Chinese Patent Medicines

含有苦杏仁或其炮制品的中成药有 200 余个，其中药典收载有 88 余个。以苦杏仁为君药或主药的品种有三拗片、三仁合剂、杏苏止咳颗粒等。在中成药的品质控制中多采用显微鉴别确定苦杏仁的存在，采用薄层鉴别和含量测定法进行指标成分限量。如三拗片中以苦杏仁为君药，含量测定法限定每个最小规格（片）中有效成分苦杏仁苷含量的下限以保证作用；非以苦杏仁为君药的制剂石斛夜光丸、四方胃片等通过显微鉴别"石细胞橙黄色、贝壳形，壁较厚，较宽一边纹孔明显"确定含有苦杏仁。咳喘顺丸制剂中薄层色谱法检测苦杏仁苷的含量。

There are two hundred kinds of Chinese patent medicines contain Kuxingren or their processed products, more than 88 of which are included in the pharmacopoeia. Prescriptions with Kuxingren as sovereign medicinal are as follows: San'ao Pian (Ttablets), Sanren Heji, Xingsuzhike Keli and so on. In the quality control of Chinese patent medicines, the existence of Kuxingren is mostly determined by microscopic identification, and the index composition was limited by TLC identification and content determination. For example, Kuxingren act as a sovereign medicinal in San'ao Pian (Tablets), the content determination method sets the lowest quantity of amygdalin, the active ingredient in each minimum specification (tablets), to ensure its effect. The preparations like Shihuyeguang Wan and and Sifangwei Pian (tablets) with Kuxingren as no-sovereign medicinal, were identified the containing of Kuxingren by microscopic identification on "the stone cells are orange yellow, shell-shaped, with thick wall and wide side striation". TLC was used to detect contents of amygdalin in Kechuanshun Wan.

【制药】
[Pharmacy]

一、产地加工
I Processing in Production Area

一般将杏采收后除去果肉，击破果核，取出种子经过晾晒至干或阴干即可。

Generally, after collecting apricots, remove the flesh, break the shell, and take out the seeds to dry in the air.

二、饮片炮制
II Processing of Decoction Pieces

为杀酶保苷，自唐代以来，逐渐形成了"净制→燀制→剥皮→切片→干燥"工艺，饮片以颗粒均匀、饱满、味苦者为佳。由此加工的燀苦杏仁、炒苦杏仁成为商品规格中的主流。

In order to destroy the enzymes and protect glycosides, complicated processing methods have been formed since ancient times. Since the Tang dynasty, the processing technology has been formed, which is of "cleansing →decoction →peeling →slicing → drying" and the decoction pieces are preferably those with uniform, full, and bitter taste. The Dankuxingren (scalding) and Chaokuxingren (stir-frying) have become the mainstream in product specifications.

苦杏仁炮制的原理是杀酶保苷。苦杏仁经蒸、煮、蝉、炒等加热处理，酶被破坏，使苦杏仁苷在体内胃酸的作用下，缓缓分解，产生适量的氢氰酸。苦杏仁苷溶于水，用冷水煎煮虽能将其提取出来，但因冷水可激发其酶的活性，使苦杏仁苷分解成氢氰酸和苯甲醛，挥发损失。

The principle of Kuxingren processing is to destroy the enzymes and protect the glycosides. After the bitter almond is heated by steaming, boiling, decoction, stir-frying, etc., the enzyme is destroyed, and the amygdalin is slowly decomposed under the action of gastric acid in the body to generate an appropriate amount of hydrocyanic acid. Amygdalin is soluble in water. Although it can be extracted by boiling in cold water, the amygdalin can be decomposed into hydrocyanic acid and benzaldehyde because of its enzymatic activity.

三、中成药制药
III Pharmacy of Chinese Patent Medicines

含苦杏仁的中成药，剂型十分丰富，涵盖了固体、液体剂型，具体包括丸剂、颗粒剂、胶囊剂、片剂、合剂（口服液）、冲剂、糖浆剂等剂型。成药制剂中，若饮片需煎煮提取入药，可选择生品；若入丸散剂，选择炮制品安全性更高。

There are various kinds of Chinese patent medicines containing Kuxingren, covering the solid and liquid pharmaceutical forms, including pills, granules, capsules, tablets, mixtures (oral liquids), granules, syrups and other pharmaceutical forms. In the pharmaceutical preparations, if the decoction pieces need to be boiled and extracted for use as medicines, raw products can be selected, if being used into pills or powders, processed products are safer.

例如三拗片，其制备过程采用苦杏仁入药，利用高温条件入煎，实现杀酶保苷，确保疗效。在杏苏止咳糖浆制剂工艺中，因苦杏仁中氢氰酸为有毒成分，且易溶于水，因此采用水蒸气蒸馏法对苦杏仁进行提取，并用90%乙醇进行稀释，限定氢氰酸的含量，保证制剂的安全性。

Take San'ao Pian (Tablets) as the example, the preparation process uses Kuxingren into the medicines, using high temperature to make the decoction, so to destroy the enzyme to protect glycosides and ensure the efficacy. In the preparation process of Xingsu Zhike Tangjiang, because hydrocyanic acid in Kuxingren is toxic and soluble in water, the bitter almond is extracted by steam distillation and diluted with 90% ethanol to limit the content of hydrocyanic acid and ensure the safety of the preparation.

【性能功效】
[Property and Efficacy]

一、性能
I Property

苦杏仁苦、微温，质润，有小毒，归肺、大肠经。

Kuxingren is slightly poisonous, bitter in flavor, warm and moist in nature, and enters the lung and large intestine meridians.

二、功效
II Efficacy

1. 降气止咳平喘　苦杏仁主入肺经，味苦

降泄，肃降兼宣发肺气而能止咳平喘，为治"咳喘之要药"。其功效的发挥与苦杏仁与镇咳、平喘等作用密切相关。苦杏仁的镇咳、平喘作用的有效物质基础主要是苦杏仁苷成分，通过抑制咳嗽中枢而起镇咳平喘作用。

1 Descending Qi, Relieving Cough and Asthma

Kuxingren mainly enters the lungs meridian, tastes bitter and descends qi so that it can relax the depressed lung qi to relieve cough and asthma, which is an important medicinal to treat for "cough and asthma". Its effectiveness is closely related to the effects of the antitussive and relieving asthma. The main effective material basis of antitussive and antiasthmatic effect is amygdalin, which plays an antitussive and antiasthmatic role by inhibiting cough nerve center.

2. 润肠通便　苦杏仁质润多脂、下气、润肠通便。其功效的发挥与通便等药理作用密切相关。主要物质基础是苦杏仁油成分。

2 Moistening Intestines to Relieve Constipation

Kuxingren are moist and fatty, with the functions of descending qi, moistening intestines to relieve constipation. The exertion of the effect is closely related to pharmacological effects of defecation, and its main material basis is bitter almond oil.

【应用】
[Applications]

一、主治病证
I Indications

1. 咳喘证　治疗咳喘证之风寒咳喘，胸闷气逆，苦杏仁常与麻黄、甘草配伍，以散风寒宣肺平喘，如《伤寒杂病论》三拗汤和现代中成药三拗片等；若治疗风热咳嗽，发热汗出，常配散风热宣肺的桑叶、菊花，如《温病条辨》桑菊饮和现代中成药桑菊感冒丸；若燥热咳嗽，配桑叶、贝母、沙参，以清肺润燥止咳，如《温病条辨》桑杏汤、《医门法律》清燥救肺汤；肺热咳喘，配石膏等以清肺泄热宣肺平喘，如《伤寒论》麻杏

石甘汤。

1　Cough and Asthma Syndrome

In the treatment of cough and asthma syndrome, for the wind cold cough, chest tightness and qi reversal, Kuxingren is often used combined with Mahuang and Gancao to dispel wind and cold, dispersing the lungs to relieve asthma, such as San'ao Tang (Decoction) in *Shanghan Zabing Lun* and modern Chinese medicines San'ao Pian (Tablets), etc. In the treatment of wind heat cough, fever sweat, Sangye (Mori Folium) and Juhua for dispelling the wind and diffusing the lung are often used together with Kuxingren, such as Sangju Yin (Decoction) in *Wenbing Tiaobian*, and modern Chinese patent medicines Sangju Ganmao Wan; if for hot dry cough , Kuxingren is often used combined with Sangye, Beimu, and Shashen to clear lung-heat and moisten dryness and relieve panting, such as Sang Xing Tang (Decoction) in *Wenbing Tiaobian*, Qingzao Jiufei Tang (Decoction) in *Yimen Falv*, As for cough and panting due to lung heat, Kuxingren is often combined with Shigao to clear lung-heat and diffuse the lung to calm panting, such as Ma Xing Shi Gan Tang (Decoction) in *Shanghan Zabing Lun*.

在现代临床苦杏仁配伍常用于治疗肺结核、支气管炎、肺脓肿等属于风寒犯肺或痰热阻肺者。如三拗汤、桔梗杏仁煎。

In modern clinical practice, Kuxingren compatibility such as in San'ao Tang (Decoction) and Jiegeng Xingren Tang (Decoction) is commonly applied to treat the syndromes of wind-cold invading the lungs or phlegm heat obstructing the lungs, such as tuberculosis, bronchitis, and pulmonary abscesses.

2.　**肠燥便秘**　治疗肠燥便秘，苦杏仁常与柏子仁、郁李仁配伍，如《世医得效方》五仁丸。用于老年人或产后大便秘结，常与火麻仁、当归、枳实等同用，如润肠丸。

2　Intestinal Dryness and Constipation

Kuxingren is often combined with Baiziren

and Yuliren such as Wuren Wan from *Shiyi Dexiao Fang*. For the elderly or postpartum constipation, it is often compatible with Huomaren, Danggui, and Zhishi, such as Runchang Wan.

在现代临床苦杏仁配伍常用于治疗急性胃肠炎、胃炎、消化不良、便秘和胆囊炎属于湿温初起及暑温夹湿之湿重于热者。如三仁汤。

In modern clinical practice, its compatibility is often used for the treatment of gastroenteritis, gastritis, poor digestion, constipation, and cholecystitis, whose patients are inflicted by the initial dampness warmth or summer warmth with dampness or dampness more than heat, such as Sanren Tang (Decoction).

二、用法用量
II　Administration and Dosage

5~10g，煎汤，生品入煎剂后下。

5~10g, decoction, the raw products should be added into decoction later.

三、注意事项
III　Precautions

1.　本品有小毒，用量不宜过大；婴儿慎用（儿童10~20粒，成人40~60粒可引起中毒反应）。

1　This product is slightly toxic, so the dosage should not be too large, use it with caution for infants (10 to 20 grains for children, 40 to 60 grains for adults can cause poisoning reactions).

2.　苦杏仁苷水解产物氢氰酸，具有较大的毒性，临床需炮制后应用。阴虚咳喘及大便溏泻者忌用。

2　A product of amygdalin hydrolysate named Hydrocyanic acid is highly toxic, for clinical application it needs to be processed first. Avoid use for those with yin deficiency, cough, asthma and loose stools.

第二十章 安 神 药
Chapter 20　Tranquilization Medicinals

凡以宁心安神为主要功效，常用以治疗心神不宁证的药物，称为安神药。此类药物多味甘、性偏寒凉，滋补清热，主归心、肝经而能宁心安神、养心益肝，某些药物还有镇心安神、平肝潜阳的功效，用于治疗心神不宁证和肝阳上亢证，体现了《素问·至真要大论》"惊者平之"的治疗法则。安神药多属对症治标之品，尤其矿石类安神药，只宜暂用，不可久服，且伤胃耗气，故脾胃虚弱者慎用。现代药理研究表明，安神药多具有镇静、催眠、抗惊厥、抗焦虑、改善学习记忆力、抗心律失常、改善心肌缺血、保护心肌细胞、提高耐缺氧能力、降血压、降血脂、抗衰老、抑制血小板聚集、增强免疫力等药理作用。常见的安神药有酸枣仁、柏子仁、远志、合欢皮等。

Tranquilization medicinals refer to medicinals that can nourish the heart to tranquilize and treat restless spirit syndrome. They have cold nature and sweet taste, which nourishing and clearing away heat, acting on the heart and liver meridians, so as to calm and soothe the mind, nourish the heart and the liver. Besides, some medicinals have the effect of setting heart and calming mind, pacifying liver and suppressing yang. And it also can be used for syndrome of restlessness and hyperactivity of liver yang, which reflect the Chinese medicine treatment principle of "treating fright by calming" in *Suwen · Zhizhenyao Dalun (Inner Canon of Huangdi · Plain Conversation)*. Tranquilization medicinals are mainly target at symptoms, among which especially mineral medicines can easily hurt the stomach and consumes qi, so it can't be taken for a long time, only for temporary use. Thus, patients with weak spleen and stomach should use them with cautions. Modern pharmacological studies have shown that tranquilization medicinals have pharmacological effects such as the sedative, hypnotic, anticonvulsant, anxiolytic, improving learning and memory, antiarrhythmia, improving myocardial ischemia, protecting myocardial cells, increasing hypoxia resistance, lowering blood pressure and blood lipids, anti-aging, inhibiting platelet aggregation, enhancing immunity and so on. Tranquilization medicinals including *Suanzaoren*, *Baiziren*, *Yuanzhi*, Hehuanpi (Albiziae Cortex), are commonly used.

酸 枣 仁

Suanzaoren
(Ziziphi Spinosae Semen)

酸枣仁为河北产道地药材。临床常用生酸枣仁、炒酸枣仁。酸枣仁味甘、酸，性平，归肝、胆、心经，具养心补肝、宁心安神、敛汗、生津功效，主治心神不宁证、体虚自汗、盗汗。酸枣仁中主要含皂苷类、黄酮类、生物碱类、三萜类、甾体类、脂肪酸和挥发油等成分，有镇静、催眠、改善心肌缺血、降血脂及提高免疫力等药理作用，临床用于治疗神经衰弱、老年轻度认知障碍及前列腺增生等属心神不宁证、心肾亏虚证及肾阳虚证者。

Suanzaoren is agenuine regional medicinal produced in Hebei. The raw and Chaosuanzaoren (stir-frying) is often used in clinical practice. Suanzaoren is sweet and sour in flavor, neutral in nature, and it enters the liver, gallbladder and heart meridian. It has the effects of nourishing the heart and replenishing the liver, calming the nerves, inhibiting sweating, engendering liquid. It can treat the symptoms of restlessness, weakness and spontaneous sweating, night sweats. Suanzaoren mainly contains saponin, flavonoids, alkaloids, triterpenes, steroids, fatty acids and volatile oils, which possess various pharmacological effects, such as calming spirit, hypnotizing, improving myocardial ischemia, decreasing blood lipids and improving immunity. It can be used for the treatment of neurasthenia, mild cognitive impairment in the elderly, prostatic hyperplasia which belongs to the syndrome of restless spirit, heart and kidney deficiency and kidney-yang deficiency.

【品种品质】
[Variety and Quality]

一、基原品种与品质
I Origin Varieties and Quality

1. **品种概况**　来源于鼠李科植物酸枣 *Ziziphus jujuba Mill. var. spinosa (Bunge) Hu ex H. F. Chou* 的干燥成熟种子。

1 Variety
Suanzaoren are the dry mature seeds of *Ziziphus jujuba MILL. var. spinosa (Bunge.) Hu ex H. F. Chou* from the family of Rhamnaceae.

酸枣仁首载于《神农本草经》，梁·陶弘景

《本草经集注》称其："子似武昌枣而味极酸，东人啖之以醒睡"，《本草图经》谓："似枣木而皮细，其木心赤色，茎叶俱青，花似枣花，八月结实，紫红色，似枣而圆小味酸"。上述本草所指"酸枣仁"基原植物与鼠李科植物酸枣一致，但其药用部位最初以果实入药，唐代以后逐渐演变为种子入药，沿用至今。

Suanzaoren was firstly recorded in *Shennong Bencao Jing. Bencaojing Jizhu* made by Tao Hongjing in Liang dynasty, called that "Suanzaoren" is similar to Wuchang zao. It is very sour, so that people eat it to wake up". *Bencao Tujing* recorded it as "the tree of Suanzaoren and Zao are similar. But the bark of Suanzaoren is fine, the centers of trees are crimson, its stems and leaves are green, the flowers of Suanzaoren is similiar to that of Zao, and its fruit is fuchsia and mature in August, looks like that of Zao, but more round and small ". Materia Medica has shown that the original plants of "Suanzaoren" are consistent with those of Rhamnaceae. However, its medicinal parts —— fruits, which were originally used as a medicine, and gradually evolved into a seed as a medicine from the Tang Dynasty to the present.

2. **种植采收**　酸枣仁以野生为主，主产于河北、山西、内蒙古、陕西、山东等地。主产地也有栽培，在栽培上有有性繁殖和无性繁殖两种方法，并建立了种子繁殖和分株繁殖等新技术。酸枣仁栽种后第二年开花结果，多于 9~10 月果熟后采收。

2 Planting and Harvesting
Suanzaoren are mainly wild, produced in Hebei, Shanxi, Inner Mongolia, Shaanxi, Shandong provinces and other places. In the main producing area, there are also cultivated Suanzaoren. There are two cultivation methods of sexual propagation and asexual propagation, and new technologies such as seed reproduction and branch propagation have been established. Suanzaoren blossoms and yields fruit in the second year after planting and is generally harvested from September to October after the fruit is ripe.

3. 道地性及品质评价 历代本草记载，河北邢台是酸枣仁的道地产区。酸枣仁形态上以"粒大""饱满"为佳，颜色上以"紫红"为佳，质感"光华油润""无杂质"为佳。

3 Genuineness and Quality Evaluation

According to historical records of Materia Medica, Xingtai of Hebei province is a genuine producing area of Suanzaoren. The good Suanzaoren should be "large" and "full seeds" in shape, "purplish red" in color, with "smooth and oily" texture and "no impurities".

酸枣仁主含皂苷类（如酸枣仁皂苷 A、酸枣仁皂苷 B）、黄酮类（如斯皮诺素）和生物碱类（如酸枣仁碱 A）。皂苷类、黄酮类及生物碱类是发挥镇静催眠作用的主要药效物质基础，皂苷类成分还对心血管有作用。此外酸枣仁中还含有三萜类、多糖等化合物。《中国药典》规定酸枣仁中酸枣仁皂苷 A 不得少于 0.030%，斯皮诺素不得少于 0.080%。

Suanzaoren mainly contains saponins (e.g. Jujuboside A, Jujuboside B), flavonoids (e.g. spinosin) and alkaloids (e.g. jujube saponine A). The saponins, flavonoids and alkaloids are the main medicinal material basis for sedative and hypnotic effects. And saponins also have the cardiovascular effects. In addition, Suanzaoren also contains compounds such as triterpenoids and polysaccharides. *The Pharmacopoeia of the People's Republic of China* stipulates that the Jujuboside A should not be less than 0.030% and the spinosin should not be less than 0.080%.

二、炮制品种与品质
II Processed Varieties and Quality

目前，酸枣仁的炮制品种有生酸枣仁、炒酸枣仁 2 种。酸枣仁以浅黄色，富油性为佳；炒酸枣仁以表面微鼓起，微具焦斑，略有焦香气为佳。酸枣仁及炒酸枣仁中酸枣仁皂苷 A 及斯皮诺素含量规定同药材。

At present, there are two types of processed-products of Suanzaoren, including Shengsuan

zaoren (raw) and Chaosuanzaoren (stir-frying). Suanzaoren is preferably of light yellow and rich oil. Chaosuanzaoren (stir-frying) with slightly bulging surface, slightly scorched spots, and a slightly burnt aroma is better. The content regulation of jujuboside A and spinosin in Suanzaoren and fried Suanzaoren is the same as that of medicinal materials.

三、中成药品种与品质
III Varieties and Quality of Chinese Patent Medicines

含酸枣仁或其炮制品的中成药有 140 余个，其中药典收载 35 个。以酸枣仁为君药或主药的品种有安神宝颗粒、安神胶囊、枣仁安神胶囊、枣仁安神颗粒等。在中成药的品质控制中多采用薄层色谱法、显微鉴别来确定酸枣仁的存在，采用含量测定法进行指标成分限量以保证药效。如安神宝颗粒采用薄层色谱法以酸枣仁皂苷 A、B 对照品为对照，确定酸枣仁的存在；天王补心丸、柏子养心丸等通过显微鉴别"内种皮细胞棕黄色，表面观长方形或类方形，垂周壁连珠状增厚"确定含有酸枣仁；枣仁安神颗粒（胶囊）采用高效液相色谱法测定其中斯皮诺素的含量来保证药效。

There are more than 140 Chinese patent medicines containing Suanzaoren or its processed products, of which 35 are contained in the *Pharmacopoeia of the People's Republic of China*. Among them, prescriptions with Suanzaoren as sovereign are as follows: Anshenbao Keli, Anshen Jiaonang, Zaoren Anshen Jiaonang, Zaoren Anshen Keli, etc. In terms of quality control, TLC and microscopic identification are often used to determine the existence of Suanzaoren, and the content determination method is used to limit the index components to ensure the efficacy. For example, In Anshenbao Keli uses the jujuboside A and B reference to determine the existence of Suanzaoren by TCL. The preparations like Tianwang Buxin Wan and Baizi Yangxin Wan, etc. have the characteristic of "inner seed coat cells are brownish-yellow, surface are oblong or rectangular-like, and peripheric walls pearls-like thickening" through microscopic identification to determine Suanzaoren. In Zaoren Anshen Jiaonang (Capsule), HPLC is used to determine the content of spinosin to ensure the efficacy.

【制药】
[Pharmacy]

一、产地加工
I Processing in Production Area

秋末冬初采收成熟果实，过早采收种仁偏瘦，质量差，出仁率低。趁鲜净皮肉，将枣核洗净晒干，用机械碾核壳，筛除核壳，收集枣仁，晒干。

The ripe fruits of Suanzaoren are harvested in late autumn and early winter. Pre-harvest fruits are thinner, poor quality, with low kernel yield. Then clear off the flesh, wash it clean and dry it, remove the shell mechanically, collect then and dry in Sunshine.

二、饮片炮制
II Processing of Decoction Pieces

在古代，酸枣仁的炮制方法就多达 10 余种。现代形成了净制、捣碎、炒制的工艺，由此加工成酸枣仁、炒酸枣仁。

In ancient times, there were more than 10 kinds of processing methods for Suanzaoren. In modern times, the process techniques of cleaning, mashing and stir-frying is formed, by which they are processed into Suanzaoren and fried Suanzaoren.

酸枣仁炒制可使种皮开裂，易于粉碎和有效成分溶出，同时能起到杀酶保苷的作用。

The process of Stir-frying makes the seeds Suanzaoren cracked and easy to be crushed, which facilitate dissolving the effective ingredients.

Meanwhile, it can play a role in killing enzymes and protecting glycosides.

三、中成药制药
III Pharmacy of Chinese Patent Medicines

含酸枣仁的中成药，剂型丰富，涵盖固体、液体制剂。具体包括片剂、丸剂、胶囊剂、颗粒剂、合剂。含酸枣仁的传统中成药制剂多制成蜜丸，以酸枣仁细粉入药。现代制剂除了多以酸枣仁细粉或水煎液入制剂外，还有部分以乙醇提取有效成分入制剂。

There are various kinds of Chinese patent medicines containing Suanzaoren, covering solid, liquid preparations, including tablets, pills, capsules, granules, and mixtures (oral liquid). Chinese patent medicine pills containing Suanzaoren are mostly made into honey pills, and the fine powder of Suanzaoren is used as medicine. Suanzaoren in form of water extracted or powder is made into preparations and in some preparations, the active ingredients extracted with ethanol are applied.

如以酸枣仁入药的天王补心丸，其制备过程采用炒酸枣仁入药，制成蜜丸在体内溶散缓慢，达到缓释目的。而在天王补心丸（浓缩丸）、女珍颗粒等制剂，多采用水煎煮法提取以保证皂苷类有效物质的充分提取；枣仁安神胶囊、参乌健脑降囊、参芪五味子片等制剂中则采用乙醇提取镇静有效物质。

Tianwang Buxin Wan, which uses Suanzaoren as medicine, use fried Suanzaoren in the preparation process, and the prepared honey pill dissolves slowly in the body to achieve the purpose of sustained release. And Suanzaoren are mostly extracted by water in Tianwang Buxin Nongsuowan and Nvzhen Keli to ensure the full extraction of saponins. In Zaoren Anshen Jiaonang (Capsules), Shenwu Jiannao Jiaonang (Capsule), Shenqi Wuweizi Pian (Pills), ethanol is used to extract sedative and effective substances of

Suanzaoren.

【性能功效】
[Property and Efficacy]

一、性能
I Property

酸枣仁甘、酸，平；归肝、胆、心经。

Suanzaoren is sweet and acid in flavor, neutral in nature, and enters the liver, gallbladder and heart meridians.

二、功效
II Efficacy

1. **养心补肝** 酸枣仁善滋养心、肝之阴血，而达养心补肝之效，因而具有抗心律失常、抗心肌缺血、保护心肌细胞等药理作用。酸枣仁的抗心律失常、抗心肌缺血、保护心肌细胞作用的有效物质基础主要是皂苷类成分，通过抑制心肌组织 Bcl-2 降低和 Bax 表达的升高、缩小心肌梗死面积、抑制线粒体信号通路中 caspase-3 及 caspase-9 的活性等发挥作用。

1 Nourishing Heart and Liver

Suanzaoren is good at nourishing the yin blood of the heart and liver, and has the effect of nourishing heart and liver, so it has the pharmacological effects such as anti-arrhythmia, anti-myocardial ischemia, and protecting myocardial cells. The effective substance basis for its pharmacological action is mainly saponins, and it inhibits the decrease of Bcl-2 and the increase of Bax expression, reduces myocardial infarction area, and inhibits the activity of caspase-3 and caspase-9 in the mitochondrial signaling pathway.

2. **宁心安神** 酸枣仁长于安神，达宁心安神之效，因而具有镇静、催眠、抗惊厥、抗抑郁等药理作用，主要的物质基础有皂苷类、黄酮类、生物碱类成分。

2 Relieving Mental Stress

Suanzaoren is good at tranquilizing and has the effects of calming the nerves, so it has sedative, hypnotic, anticonvulsant and antidepressant effects, the main material basis is saponin, flavonoid, and alkaloid.

3. **敛汗，生津** 酸枣仁味酸能敛，善敛汗生津，其功效的发挥可能与调节中枢神经系统等药理作用密切相关。

3 Gathering Sweat and Promoting Production of Body Fluid

Suanzaoren is acid and can collect sweat and promote fluid. Its effectiveness may be closely related to regulating the central nervous system and other pharmacological effects.

此外，现代研究显示其还有降血压、降血脂、抗衰老、抗肿瘤等作用。

In addition, modern research shows that it also has the effects of lowering blood pressure and blood lipid, anti-aging, and anti-tumor.

【应用】
[Applications]

一、主治病证
I Indications

1. **心神不宁证** 治疗心神不宁证，酸枣仁常与甘草配伍治疗肝虚有热之虚烦不眠，如《金匮要略》酸枣仁汤；若心肾不交，心悸失眠，健忘梦遗者，可配伍柏子仁补气养血，如《体仁汇编》柏子养心丸；若心脏亏虚，神志不守，恐怖惊惕，常多恍惚，易于健忘，睡卧不宁者，可与人参等配伍以补血安神，如《太平惠民和剂局方》宁志膏。

1 Restless Mind

For the treatment of restless syndrome, Suanzaoren is often combined with Gancao to treat liver deficiency and heat deficiency and insomnia, such as Suanzaoren Tang (Decoction) in *Jingui Yaolue*; For treating the non-interaction between heart and kidney, insomnia and palpitations, forgetfulness and dreaming with nocturnal emission, Suanzaoren is combined with

Boziren (Platycladi Semen) can tonify qi and nourish blood, such as Baizi Yangxin Wan in *Tiren Huibian (Body Kernel Compilation)*. Suanzaoren combined with Renshen have nourishing blood and tranquilization effects which can be used to treat that the heart deficiency, unconsciousness, horrified and alarmed, stunned, forgetful, sleepless syndrome, such as Ning Zhi Gao (Cream) in *Taiping Huimin Heji Ju Fang*.

现代临床，酸枣仁配伍常用于治疗神经衰弱失眠、神志恍惚、中枢神经系统兴奋所致的惊厥属于心神不宁证者，如酸枣仁汤、枣仁安神液、柏子养心丸、解郁安神颗粒；亦多用于治疗老年轻度认知障碍属于心肾亏虚的记忆减退、头昏目眩，如参乌健脑胶囊、健脑丸等；还常用于治疗心律失常、心肌缺血属于心阴血亏虚者，如枣仁安神液、安神宝颗粒、天王补心丸等。

In modern clinical practice, Suanzaoren compatibility is often used to treat neurasthenia insomnia, unconsciousness caused by mental depression, and convulsions caused by central nervous system excitement, which belongs to restlessness mind syndrome, such as in Suanzaoren Tang (Decotion), Zaoren Anshen Ye (Mixture), Baizi Yangxin Wan, and Jieyu Anshen Jiaonang (Granules). It is also used for the treatment of cognitive impairment in old and young people with memory loss caused by heart and kidney deficiency and dizziness, such as in Shenwu Jiannao Jiaonang (Capsules), Jiannao Wan, etc. It is also commonly used in the treatment of arrhythmias and myocardial ischemia that are deficient in heart *yin* blood, such as in Zaoren Anshen Ye (Mixture), Anshenbao Keli, Tianwang Buxin Wan, etc.

2. **体虚自汗，盗汗**　对体虚自汗、盗汗者，可与固表止汗药配伍；对津伤口渴，咽干口燥者，常与知母等配伍以清热生津，如《金贵要略》酸枣仁汤。

2 Spontaneous Sweating Due to Deficiency of Body, Night Sweat

Suanzaoren can be used with exterior-securing anhidrotic medicinal to treat someone who is spontaneous sweating due to deficiency of body, night sweats. The Suanzaoren Tang (Decotion) in *Jingui Yaolue*, Suanzaoren combined with Zhimu has the effects of clearing heart and promoting fluid production, which is commonly used to treat thirst due to fluid deficiency and dry throat.

现代临床，酸枣仁配伍常用于治疗月经失调、不孕症、遗精属于肾精亏虚者及前列腺增生等属于肾阳虚证者，前者如天紫红女金胶囊等，后者如补肾益脑丸等。

In addition, it is commonly used in the treatment of menstrual disorders, infertility, and nocturnal emission, which belong to kidney essence deficiency, and prostate hyperplasia of yang deficiency. The former one uses Tianzihong Nujin Jiaonang (Capsules), the latter one uses Bushen Yinao Wan.

二、用法用量
II Administration and Dosage

10~15g。
10~15g. water decoction.

三、注意事项
III Precautions

凡有实邪郁火及患有滑泄症者慎服。
Anyone who has excessive pathogen and suppressed fire and suffers from lingering diarrhea should use it with caution.

第二十一章　平肝息风药
Chapter 21　Liver-soothing and Wind-extinguishing Medicinals

凡以平肝息风、制止痉挛、治疗肝风内动，惊厥抽搐为主要作用的药物，称为平肝息风药，又叫息风止痉药。肝风内动证有寒热之不同，故此类药物药性亦有寒凉和温热区别。平肝息风药多药性寒凉，质重沉降，主入肝经，能平肝潜阳，息风止痉。某些药物还可入心经，善降上逆之气火，故能凉血止血。体现了《黄帝内经》之"热者寒之"和《神农本草经》之"疗热以寒药"的中医治则。平肝息风药多苦寒质重，如做丸散服用，易伤脾胃。药物药性有寒凉和温燥不同，证因不同应区别使用。某些药物还具有毒性，孕妇应慎用。现代研究表明，平肝息风药多具有镇静、抗惊厥、抗癫痫、降血压、抗炎、抗菌、抗氧化、增强免疫力等药理作用。部分药物还具有保肝、止血等药理作用。常见的平肝熄风药有牛黄、天麻、石决明、牡蛎等。

The medicinals which soothing the liver to stop wind, are also called extinguishing wind to arrest convulsions medicinals, refer to the medicinals that can extinguish wind to pacify liver and arrest convulsions for the treatment of liver wind and convulsions. Liver-wind internal movement syndrome is different from cold and heat, so the medicinal properties of this kind of medicines also differ in cold and warm. Generally, the medicinal properties of liver-pacifying and wind-extinguishing medicinals are cold, heavy and hard in texture, which enter into the liver meridian and can pacify the liver to subdue *yang* and extinguish wind to arrest convulsions. Some medicinals can enter into the heart meridian and descend *qi* and fire ascending counterflow, thereby cooling the blood to stop bleeding. This remedy reflects the Chinese medicine treatment principles of "treating heat with cold" in *Huangdi Neijing* and "healing heat with cold medicines" in *Shennong Bencao Jing*. Because of their bitter, cold nature and heavy texture, they are easy to impair the spleen and stomach if made into pill or powder. Medicinals should be used properly in line with the syndrome due to the differentiation of cold and warm medicinal properties. Pregnant women should use it with caution for some toxic medicinals. Modern research indicates that liver-pacifying and wind-extinguishing medicinals possess various pharmacological effects such as sedation, anti-convulsion, antiepileptic, lowering blood pressure, anti-inflammation, anti-bacteria, antioxidating and boosting the immune system. Some medicinals can also protect liver and stanch bleeding. The liver- soothing and wind-extinguishing medicinals such as Niuhuang, Tianma, Shijueming, and Muli, are commonly used.

牛　黄

Niuhuang

(Bovis Calculus)

牛黄主产于西北、华北、东北、西南等地。临床常用炮制品主要为牛黄粉末。牛黄味甘，性凉，归心、肝经，具有清心、豁痰、开窍、凉肝、息风、解毒的功效，主治肝风内动证、热闭神昏证、热毒疮疡、咽喉肿痛。牛黄主要含胆红素、胆汁酸、胆汁酸盐、胆甾醇类、麦角甾醇等成分，有解热、镇咳、祛痰、平喘、镇静、抗惊厥、抗脑缺血、保肝、利胆、抗炎、抗菌、抗病毒、增强免疫功能等药理作用，可用于治疗热病神昏、中风痰迷、惊痫抽搐、癫痫发狂、咽喉肿痛、口舌生疮、痈肿疔疮等。牛黄性凉，非实热证忌用，孕妇慎用。

Niuhuang is mainly produced in the regions of northwest, northeast, southwest and north of China. The powder of Niuhuang is the most commonly used processed product in clinic. The medicinal properties of Niuhuang are sweet, cold and enter heart and liver meridians. Niuhuang possesses various effects such as clearing away the heart-fire, eliminating phlegm, opening the orifices, cooling the liver, calming the endogenous wind and detoxifying. Niuhuang mainly contains bilirubin, bile acid, bile salts, cholesterols, ergosterol and other ingredients. It has antipyretic, antitussive, expectorant, antiasthmatic, sedation, anticonvulsant, anti-cerebral ischemia, liver protection, cholagogic, anti-inflammation, antibacterial, anti-virus, enhancing innmune function and beneficial effects. The compatibilities of Niuhuang are commonly used in clinics for the treatment of heat-induced loss of consciousness, wind stroke and phlegmatic coma, epilepsy and convulsions, delirium, sore throat, aphtha of the mouth and tongue, abscess and furuncle. Due to the cold medicinal property of Niuhuang, patients of non-excess heat syndrome should be contraindicated and pregnant women should use it with cautions.

【品种品质】
[Variety and Quality]

一、基原品种与品质
I Origin Varieties and Quality

1. 品种概况　来源于牛科动物牛 *Bos taurus domesticus* Gmelin 的干燥胆结石。

1 Variety

Niuhuang is the dried gallstones of *Bos taurus domesticus* Gmelin.

牛黄首载于《神农本草经》。《吴普本草》载："牛出入呻者有之。"后载于《重修政和经史证类备用本草》，列为兽部上品。除天然牛黄外，市场还流通着人工牛黄、体外培植牛黄等品种。

Niuhuang is firstly recorded in *Shennong Bencao Jing*. As recorded in *Wupu Bencao*, those cattle like moaning while walking and their horn lighting in the night, there are yolklike Niuhuang can be seen in gallbladder after they dying. In *Chongxiu Zhenghe Jingshi Zhenglei Beiyong Bencao (Revision of the Administrative System and Spare Materia Medica of Classics, History and Evidence)*, Niuhuang are classified as an superior medicine among the animal medicinal products. In addition to natural Niuhuang, the market also circulates artificial Niuhuang and in vitro cultivated Niuhuang.

2. 养殖采收　牛黄主产于我国西北、华北、东北、西南等地。产于北京、天津者称为"京牛黄"；产于西北地区者称为"西牛黄，西黄"；产于东北地区者称为"东牛黄"。宰牛时，如发现有牛黄，即滤去胆汁，将牛黄取出，除去外部薄膜，阴干。

2 Farming and Harvesting

Niuhuang is mainly produced in the regions of northwest, northeast, southwest and north of China. Those produced in Beijing and Tianjin are usually called "Jing Niuhuang". "Xi Niuhuang, Xihuang" and "Dongniuhuang" are produced in the regions of northwest and northeast, respectively. When slaughtering the cattle, once Niuhuang is found, filter the bile and take out Niuhuang immediately ,dry in shade after peeling the outer membrane.

3. 道地性及品质评价　历代本草记载，牛黄在全国各地均有分布。现主产于西北、华北、东北、西南等地区。

3 Genuineness and Quality Evaluation

According to historical records, Niuhuang is distributed all over the country. It is mainly produced in the north, northwest, northeast and southeast of China.

古人从颜色、质地等方面进行牛黄的品质评价。牛黄以呈卵形、类球形、三角形或四方形，大小不一，气清香，味苦而后甘，有清凉感，嚼之易碎，不粘牙为佳。与水调和，涂于指甲上，染面成黄色，俗称"挂甲"。以完整、色棕黄、质酥脆、断面层纹清晰而细腻者为佳。牛黄中主要含胆酸、脱氧胆酸、胆甾醇等；主要以胆酸、胆红素为化学评价指标。《中国药典》规定牛黄中含胆酸不得少于4.0 %，含胆红素不得少于25.0 %。

The ancients have proposed the quality evaluation indexes of Niuhuang from the aspects of color and texture. The superior Niuhuang is ovoid, spherical, triangular or quadrangular, which has different sizes, and has a pleasant smell and tastes bitter subsequently sweet. Moreover, it possesses a cool feeling and is easy to chew but not sticking. The modern evaluation method of Niuhuang is to mix it with water and apply the mixture on the nail, then the nail is dyed yellow, which is commonly known as "Guajia". The one complete, brown-yellow, crisp, with clear and delicate cross-section are better. Niuhuang mainly contains cholic acid, deoxycholic acid and cholesterols, etc. Cholic acid and bilirubin are the main chemical evaluation indexes of Niuhuang. The *Pharmacopoeia of the People's Republic of China* stipulates that Niuhuang should contain no less than 4.0% cholic acid and no less than 25.0% bilirubin.

二、炮制品种与品质
II Processed Varieties and Quality

牛黄多以生品入药，牛黄炮制品的含量测定要求同牛黄药材。

Niuhuang is usually used in the form of raw material. The content detemination requirment for the processed product is the same as required for the raw medicinal above.

三、中成药品种与品质
III Varieties and Quality of Chinese Patent Medicines

据统计，《中国药典》收载含有牛黄（人工牛黄）的中成药有90个。以牛黄为君药或主药的品种有安宫牛黄丸、牛黄解毒丸、牛黄上清丸等。为确保制剂的安全性、有效性，含有牛黄的中成药常采用薄层色谱法和含量测定法进行指标成分限量检查。如以牛黄为主药的安宫牛黄丸（散），用薄层色谱法限定胆酸的含量，含量测定法限定 一次口服剂量中胆红素不得少于限定量，以确保药效。

According to statistics, there are more than 90 Chinese patent medicines containing Niuhuang or artificial Niuhuang in *Pharmacopoeia of the People's Republic of China*, among which, prescriptions with Niuhuan as sovereign medicinal are as follows: Angong Niuhuang Wan, Niuhuag Jiedu Wan, Niuhuag Shangqing Wan. In order to ensure the safety and effectiveness of preparations, Chinese patent medicines containing Niuhuang often use TLC and content determination to check the limit of index components. Taking Angong Niuhuang Wan (Pills)/ San (Podwers) as an example, in which Niuhuang as the main medicinal, It uses TLC to limit the content of cholic acid, and the content determination method restricts the bilirubin in an oral dose to no less than stipulated limit to ensure the efficacy.

【制药】
[Pharmacy]

一、产地加工
I　Processing in Production Area

宰牛时注意检查胆囊、胆管及肝管，如有结石，立即取出，除尽附着的薄膜，用灯心草或棉花等包上，外用毛边纸或纱布包好，置阴凉处，至半干时用线扎好，以防裂开，阴干。

When slaughtering the cattle, the gall bladder, bile duct and hepatic duct should be seriously noticed. Once the gallstone is found, take it out immediately, remove the attached diaphragm and wrap it with rushes or cotton. Subsequently, wrap it with raw-edged paper or gauze and put it in a cool place until half-dried, then tie it with thread to avoid cracking and keep on drying it in the shade.

二、饮片炮制
II　Processing of Decoction Pieces

牛黄一般以生品研细呈粉末后入药。

Niuhuang is commonly used as a medicinal after being ground into a fine powder.

三、中成药制药
III　Pharmacy of Chinese Patent Medicines

含牛黄的中成药，剂型十分丰富，涵盖固体和液体剂型。传统中药制剂中，由于牛黄资源匮乏，价格昂贵且受热成分易受破坏，故牛黄多入丸、散剂。现代中药制剂中，为满足临床急症使用、药效迅速的需求，还开发成注射剂。如将安宫牛黄丸演化改进，制备成清开灵注射液，注射给药，发挥疗效更快。

There are various kinds of Chinese patent medicines containing Niuhuang, covering preparations of solid and oral liquid. Due to the shortage, high price and unstable components of Niuhuang, it is generally used in pills and powders in Chinese pharmaceutical preparations. In modern Chinese pharmaceutical preparations, in order to meet the needs of clinical emergency use and rapid medicinal effect, injections have also been developed. For instance, Angong Niuhuang Wan is improved and prepared into Qingkailing Zhusheye, which exhibits quick curative effects after administration.

如安宫牛黄丸，全方由牛黄、郁金、犀角、麝香、珍珠、栀子、黄连、黄芩、朱砂、雄黄、冰片 11 味药组成，是我国传统药物中最负盛名的急症用药。牛黄直接研细粉入药，避免药物提取受热破坏，降低治疗价值。

Angong Niuhuang Wan, the whole prescription is composed of 11 medicinals including Niuhuang, Yujin, Xijiao, Shexiang, Zhenzhu, Zhizi, Huanglian, Huangqin, Zhusha, Xionghuang, Bingpian. It is the most famous prescription for emergency treatment in Chinese medicine. Niuhuang is directly used in the form of superfine powder, which can be free from heat damage of extraction to reduce the therapeutic value.

【性能功效】
[Property and Efficacy]

一、性能
I　Property

牛黄苦、凉，归心、肝经。

Niuhuang is biter in flavor, cold in nature, and enters the heart and liver Meridians.

二、功效
II Efficacy

1. 息风止痉 牛黄苦、凉，气味芳香，长于清心凉肝，息风止痉。其功效的发挥与镇静、抗惊厥、保肝、利胆等作用密切相关。牛黄能增加中枢抑制药的镇静作用，也可拮抗中枢兴奋药的兴奋作用，同时可延长惊厥潜伏期，对戊四氮所致惊厥的治疗效果最强。牛磺酸可能是这些作用的物质基础。

1 Extinguishing Wind to Arrest Convulsion

The medicinal property of Niuhuang is bitter, cold and has a fragrant smell. It has fwnctions of clearing heart and liver hot, and extinguishing wind to arrest convalsions. The efficacy of Niuhuang is closely related to its sedation, anti-convulsion, liver protection, and cholagogic effects. Niuhuang can increase the sedative effects of central inhibitory medicinals, antagonize the excitatory effect of central stimulants, and prolong the incubation period of convulsions. It has the strongest therapeutic effect on convulsion caused by pentylenetetrazole. Taurine may be the material basis for these effects.

2. 化痰开窍 牛黄性凉气香入心，能清心而化痰开窍。其功效的发挥与镇咳、祛痰、平喘、抗脑缺血等作用有关。牛黄镇咳作用的物质基础可能是牛磺酸和去氧胆酸。牛黄中的胆酸钠能扩张支气管，对抗组织胺和毛果芸香碱所致支气管痉挛，胆酸有效抑制支气管痉挛。牛黄能显著改善缺血再灌注大鼠神经功能缺损症状。

2 Dissipating Phlegm for Resuscitation

The cool scent of Niuhuang enters the heart, can clear the heart and dispel phlegm and resuscitation. Its effect is related to antitussive, expectorant, antiasthmatic, anti-cerebral ischemia and other effects. The material basis of the antitussive effect of Niuhuang may be taurine and deoxycholic acid. The sodium cholate in Niuhuang can dilate the bronchi and resist bronchospasm caused by histamine and pilocarpine. Cholic acid can effectively inhibit bronchospasm.

Niuhuang can significantly improve the symptoms of neurological deficit in rats with ischemia-reperfusion.

3. 清热解毒 牛黄味苦性凉，为清热解毒要药，单用内服外用均可。其功效的发挥与解热、抗炎、抗菌、抗病毒、增强免疫功能等有关。牛黄对多种热证及炎症模型都有显著的抑制作用，对革兰氏阳性菌、乙型脑炎病毒有较强抑制作用。牛磺酸和去氧胆酸可能是其解热的有效成分。胆汁酸是抗菌的主要有效成分。

3 Clearing Heat and Detoxification

Niuhuang tastes bitter, cold and is a main medicine for heat clearing and detoxification relieving heat, administered alone in internal or externaluse. which is related to its relieving heat, anti-inflammatory, anti-bacterial, anti-virus and enhancing immune function effects. It has a significant inhibitory effect on a variety of heat syndromes and inflammation models. Taurine and deoxycholic acid may be the effective ingredients for antipyretic. Bile acid is the main effective component for the antibacterial effect of Niuhuang.

【应用】
[Applications]

一、主治病证
I Indications

1. 肝风内动证 治肝风内动证，牛黄常与其他清热解毒、息风开窍之品配伍以增效，如《痘疹世医心法》万氏牛黄清心丸和现代中成药万氏牛黄清心丸；若治小儿急惊风壮热神昏，痉挛抽搐，牛黄可与清热息风药同用，如《医学入门》牛黄抱龙丸和现代中成药小儿百寿丸。

1 Syndrome of Internal Stirring of Liver Wind

Niuhuang is often combined with heat-clearing and detoxicating medicines and wind-extinguishing and orifices-opening medicines to enhance its efficacy, such as Wanshi Niuhuang Qingxin Wan in *Douzhen Shiyi Xinfa (Psychological Method of Pox and Rash)* and modern Chinese patent medicine. It can also be used for the treatment of acute infantile convulsion, high fever and loss of consciousness, spasm and convulsions in children when combined with heat-clearing and wind-extinguishing medicinal, such as Niuhuang Baolong Wan in *Yixuerumen (Introduction to Medicine)* and Xiaoer Baishou Wan in modern Chinese patent medicine.

现代临床，牛黄配伍常用于治疗小儿高热惊厥、急性感染性疾病高热惊厥、乙型脑炎、肝性脑病及肺性脑病昏迷惊厥等属肝风内动证者，如安宫牛黄丸。

In modern clinical practice, Niuhuang compatibility is often used to treat children with high fever convulsions, acute infectious diseases, high fever convulsions, Japanese encephalitis, hepatic encephalopathy, and pulmonary encephalopathy, coma and convulsions belonging to internal stiring of liver wind, etc, such as Angong Niuhuang Wan (Pills).

2. **热闭神昏证**　治温热病热入心包，神昏谵语，或痰热闭阻心包所致神昏口噤、不省人事等症，牛黄常与麝香、冰片、朱砂配伍，以增强其清心开窍之力，如《温病条例》安宫牛黄丸。

2 Syndrome of Heat Block and Loss of Consciousness

Niuhuang is often used with Shexiang, Bingpian, Zhusha to enhance the efficacy of clearing the heart and opening the orifices, which can be used for the treatment of pericardial heat from febrile disease, delirium, or faintness and unconsciousness caused by phlegm-heat blocking closure, such as Angong Niuhuang Wan in *Wenbing Tiaobian.*

现代临床，牛黄配伍可治疗脑缺血、高血压、出血性脑卒中、脑损伤、流行性乙型脑炎等疾病，如牛黄降压丸。

In modern clinical applications, Niuhuang-based prescriptions can be used to treat cerebral ischemia, hypertension, hemorrhagic stroke, brain injury, Japanese encephalitis and other diseases, such as Niuhuang Jiangya Wan.

3. **热毒疮疡、咽喉肿痛**　治咽喉肿痛、溃烂，口舌生疮，牛黄可与他药配伍内服或外用，如《绛囊撮药》珍珠散，《咽喉脉证通论》牛黄解毒丸。治痈疽、乳岩、疔毒、瘰疬等，牛黄可与麝香、乳香、没药等合用，如《外科证治全生集》犀黄丸。

3 Heat Toxin and Sore and Ulcer, Swelling in the Throat

Niuhuang can be used in combination with other medicines for internal or external use to treat sore throat, ulceration and sore in mouth and tongue, such as Zhenzhu San (Powders) in *Jiangnang Cuoyao (Crimson Sac Pinch of Medicine)* and Niuhuang Jiedu Wan in *Yanhou Maizheng Tonglun (General Theory of Throat Pulse Syndrome)*. It can also be used with Shexiang, Ruxiang and Moyao for the treatment of carbuncle, breast cancer, furunculosis and scrofula, such as Xihuang Wan in *Waike Zhengzhi Quansheng Ji.*

现代临床，牛黄配伍常用于治疗上呼吸道感染、支气管炎、流行性感冒及肺炎等属于热证者，如小儿牛黄清心散。

In modern clinical practice, Niuhuang compatibility such as Xiaoer Niuhuang QingXin San is usually used to treat patients with heat syndromes, such as upper respiratory tract infection, bronchitis, influenza and pneumonia.

二、用法用量
II Administration and Dosage

0.15~0.35g，多入丸散用；外用适量，研末敷患处。

It is commonly used in pill and powder (0.15~0.35g). For external use, a proper amount of Niuhuang is ground into powder and applied to the wound.

三、注意事项
III Precautions

孕妇慎用，非实热证忌用。

Pregnant women should use it with caution and patients without excess heat syndrome should be contraindicated.

天　麻

Tianma
(Gastrodiae Rhizoma)

天麻是贵州、云南及四川的道地药材。云南昭通天麻，贵州大方天麻和四川金口河乌天麻获得国家地理标志保护产品。天麻味甘，性平，归肝经，具有息风止痉，平抑肝阳，祛风通络的功效，主治小儿惊风，癫痫抽搐，破伤风，头痛眩晕，手足不遂，肢体麻木，风湿痹痛等。天麻中主要含有天麻素、香荚兰醇、天麻苷元、对羟基苯甲醛、琥珀酸及多种微量元素等成分，有镇静、抗惊厥、抑制中枢神经系统、镇痛、保护神经元细胞、抗氧化、降血压、抗眩晕、抗心肌缺血、抗炎、调节免疫功能等药理作用。

Tianma is a genuine regional medicinal in Guizhou, Yunnan and Sichuan province. Tianma in Zhaotong, Yunnan Province, Tianma in Dafang, Guizhou Province, and Wu Tianma in Jinkouhe, Sichuan Province are awarded as the protective products of national geographical indication. The medicinal properties of Tianma are sweet and neutral, which enters into the liver meridian. Tianma (Gastrodiae Rhizoma) possesses various pharmacological effects such as extinguishing wind to arrest convulsions, suppressing liver yang and dispelling wind to free the collateral vessels. Tianma is used for the treatment of infantile convulsion, epilepsy and convulsions, tetanus, headache and dizziness, paralysis of the extremities, numbness of the limbs and rheumatic arthralgia etc. Tianma mainly contains gastrodin, vanilla alcohol, gastrodigenin, P-hydroxybenzaldehyde, succinic acid and various trace elements, which exhibit multi-pharmacological effects such as sedation, anti-convulsion, inhibition of central nervous system, analgesia, protection of neuron cells, antioxidation, antihypertension, anti-vertigo, anti-myocardial ischemia, anti-inflammatory and regulation of immune function etc.

【品种品质】
[Variety and Quality]

一、基原品种与品质
I Origin Varieties and Quality

1. 品种概况　来源于兰科植物天麻 *Gastrodia elata* Bl. 的干燥块茎。

1 Variety

Tianma is the dry stem tuber of *Gastrodia elata* Bl. of Orchidaceae.

天麻首载于《神农本草经》，记载为赤箭芝。宋代《开宝本草》始收载天麻之名。明代《本草纲目》中将二者合并称"天麻赤箭"。甄权《药性论》和沈括《梦溪笔谈》所描述的赤箭即为兰科天麻。

Tianma was firstly recorded as "Chijianzhi" in *Shennong Bencao Jing*. The name of Tianma was first recorded in *Kaibao Bencao* in Song Dynasty. The two together were then called "Tianmachijian" in *Bencao Gangmu* in Ming Dynasty. "Chijian" recorded in *Yaoxing Lun (Theory of Property)* written by Zhen Quan and *Mengxi Bitan (Dream Creek Essays)* written by Shen Kuo is exactly Tianma of Orchidaceae.

2. 种植采收　现今主产于贵州、云南及四川等地。天麻是和蜜环菌形成的共生植物。种植分有性繁殖和无性繁殖两种方法，均采用林下规范化种植，于每年冬至前后采收。栽培时，菌材选用壳斗科、桦木科、蔷薇科树木，营养菌种为优质蜜环菌。

2 Planting and Harvesting

Nowadays, Tianma is mainly produced in Guizhou, Yunnan and Sichuan provinces etc. Tianma is a symbiotic plant formed with armillaria. The cultivation of Tianma can be divided into 2 categories: sexual propagation and vegetative propagation, both of which are planted under the forest and collected around the winter solstice every year. During cultivation, fagaceae, betulaceae and rosaceae are selected and high-quality armillaria is used as the nutritious strain.

3. 道地性及品质评价 天麻的道地性与品质优势在东汉末年即有论述，并开始人工栽培。《药材出产辨》记载"四川、云南、陕西汉中产者均佳"。由此可见，四川、云南所产天麻品质较优。形态以"质坚""鹦哥嘴"者为佳，颜色以"断面明亮"为佳。除此之外，现代还认为，天麻以质地坚实沉重、无空心者（冬麻）质佳；质地轻泡、有残留茎基、断面色晦暗、空心者（春麻）质次。天麻素是天麻的主要成分，现在主要以天麻素和对羟基苯甲醇作为其化学评价指标。《中国药典》规定天麻药材中含天麻素和对羟基苯甲醇的总量不得少于0.25%。

3 Genuineness and Quality Evaluation

The genuineness and quality advantages have been discussed at the end of the Eastern Han Dynasty and artificial cultivation has been conducted. According to *Yaocai Chuchan Bian*, the quality of Tianma produced in Sichuan, Yunnan province is the best, which indicates the optimal quality of Tianma produced in these areas. Tianma with hard and "Parakeet's beak" in shape and bright color in section has the best quality. In addition, it is believed that the quality of Tianma is better if it is solid , heavy and no hollow (Dongtianma), while the light one with dark section , residual stem base cand being hollow

(Chuntianma) , is considered as inferior in quality. Gastrodin is the main component of Tianma. At present, gastrodin and p-hydroxybenzyl alcohol are the main chemical evaluation indexes of Tianma. The *Pharmacopoeia of the People's Republic of China* stipulates that the total amount of gastrodin and p-hydroxybenzyl alcohol in gastrodia elata should not be less than 0.25%.

二、炮制品种与品质
II Processed Varieties and Quality

《中国药典》收载的天麻的炮制方法为润制或蒸制后切片，市场还流通有酒炙天麻、煨天麻、麸炒天麻等炮制品种。天麻以呈不规则的薄片，角质样，半透明，有光泽，表面黄白色或淡棕色，无纤维点，质脆，气微，味淡，味甘为佳。《中国药典》规定天麻片的含量测定同药材。

The processing method of Tianma included in the *Pharmacopoeia of the People's Republic of China* is moistening or steaming and then slicing. The market also circulates processed Tianma which is stir-fried with liquor, roasted or stir-fried with bran. The optimal one of Tianma presents an irregular flake, keratinous, translucent, glossy, yellow-white or light brown on the surface, without fiber points, crisp in texture with tiny odor, and bland and sweet flavor. *Pharmacopoeia of the People's Republic of China* stipulates that the content determination of Tianma tablets is the same as that of medicinal materials.

三、中成药品种与品质
III Varieties and Quality of Chinese Patent Medicines

据统计，《中国药典》收载含有天麻的中成药共计54个，以天麻为君药或主药的品种有天麻丸、天麻钩藤颗粒、天麻头痛片、天麻丸、全天麻胶囊等。在中成药的品质控制中多采用显微鉴别确定天麻的存在，采用薄层色谱法和含量测定法进行指标成分限量。如天麻头痛片的显微鉴定中规定见"含糊化多糖类物薄壁细胞"代表含有天麻，另明确限定了每片中天麻素的含量。

A total of 54 Chinese patent medicines containing Tianma is recorded in *Pharmacopoeia of the People's Republic of China*, among which Chinese patent medicines with Tianma as main medicine are Tianma Wan, Tianma Gouteng Keli, Tianma Toutong Pian (Tablets) and Quantianma Jiaonang (Capsules) etc. In the quality control of Chinese patent medicines, the existence of Tianma is determined by microscopic identification, and the index components are determined by TLC and content determination. For example, in the microscopic identification of Tianma Toutong Pian, it is specified that "parenchyma cells containing gelatinized polysaccharides" represent the existence of Tianma, and the content of gastrodin in each tablet is clearly defined.

【制药】
[Pharmacy]

一、产地加工
I Processing in Production Area

天麻一般收获后要趁鲜分级洗净，蒸至透心，低温干燥，晾干水气，烘干。

After harvest, Tianma should be freshly graded and cleaned, steamed with circulating steam till fully ripe. Then it is dried at low temperature and baked after drying.

二、饮片炮制
II Processing of Decoction Pieces

现代天麻炮制逐渐形成了"润透-切片-蒸煮-酒炙"工艺，由此加工的天麻成为商品规格的主流。鲜天麻蒸制后干燥，天麻素含量较直接晒干或烘干明显增加，天麻苷含量减少。这是因为天麻中的天麻素在一定条件下会发生酶解，通过蒸制可灭活酶活性，使天麻素不被分解成容易氧化损失的天麻苷元。

In modern times, the technology of "moistening, slicing, steaming and stir-frying with liquor" has gradually been applied in the processing of Tianma and the processed Tianma has become the mainstream of commodity specifications. The content of gastrodigenin in the fresh Tianma processed by drying directly or baking is decreased but the content of gastrodin is increased. The reason is that gastrodin in Tianma can be enzymolysised under certain conditions. The enzyme that could decompose gastrodin can be inactivated by steaming, so as to protect gastrodin from decomposition.

三、中成药制药
III Pharmacy of Chinese Patent Medicines

在中成药中，天麻主要与其他药物以复方配伍形式应用，也有以天麻单味药物制成的制剂，如全天麻胶囊。含天麻的中成药，剂型十分丰富，涵盖了固体、液体与半固体剂型。天麻是名贵的药食同源药材之一，口服和外用都多用生品。现代中药制剂中，若用于平肝息风止痉，多选用天麻；若用于祛风通络止痛，多选用酒炙天麻。

The compatibilities of Tianma and other medicines are commonly applied in Chinese patent medicines. While there are also preparations made from the single medicinal of Tianma, such as Quantianma Jiaonang (Capsule). There are various Chinese patent medicines containing Tianma, covering solid, liquid and semi-solid pharmaceutical forms. Tianma is one of the precious medicinal materials with prominent safety and is usually used in raw material for oral and external applications. In modern Chinese pharmaceutical preparations, Tianma is often used for the treatment of pacifying liver and extinguishing wind to arrest convulsions, while JiuzhiTianma (stir-frying with liquor) is recommended to dispel wind to free the collateral and relieve pain.

天麻素及其苷元是天麻的主要药效物质。天麻素既溶于水，也溶于醇；而天麻苷元水溶性较差，醇溶性好。加之天麻系贵细药材，粉碎后粉性强，辅以淀粉等填充剂，全粉入药后能保证药材的综合利用。因此，中成药中天麻一般以粉碎、醇提或醇水双提入药。如全天麻胶囊和天麻钩藤颗粒中天麻均直接粉碎入药，以最大限度保留有效成分。在天舒片、天舒胶囊的现代制剂过程中，采用醇水双提的工艺路线，先用90%乙醇提取脂溶性成分和挥发油，再用水提取水溶性成分，实现对各类成分的综合提取，确保临床疗效。

Gastrodin and gastrodigenin are the main therapeutic medicinal materials of Tianma. Gastrodin is soluble both in water and alcohol, while gastrodigenin has poor water solubility and good alcohol solubility. In addition, Tianma is a precious medicinal and contains plenty of powder after being crushed, filling agents such as starch are often added to ensure the comprehensive utilization of medicinal materials of the whole powder. Therefore, in Chinese patent medicines, Tianma is generally used by grinding, alcohol extraction or alcohol and water extraction. For example, Quantianma Jiaonang and Tianma Gouteng Yin are both use Tianma by crushing it into powder. In the process of modern improvement of Tianshu Pian and Tianshu Jiaonang, the alcohol and water double extraction method is adopted. Firstly, 90% alcohol is used to extract liposoluble components and volatile oil, and then water-soluble components are extracted by water to realize the comprehensive extraction of various components and ensure the clinical efficacy.

【性能功效】
[Property and Efficacy]

一、性能
I Property

天麻甘，平；归肝经。

Tianma is sweet in flavor, neutral in nature, and enters the liver meridian.

二、功效
II Efficacy

1. 息风止痉　天麻性平缓，入肝经，息肝风，止痉挛。其功效的发挥，与镇静催眠、抗惊厥等药理作用密切相关。天麻素及其苷元、香草醇等是其镇静催眠和抗惊厥的有效成分。

1 Extinguishing Wind to Arrest Convulsion

Tianma is neutral and enters into the liver meridian, which can extinguish the wind of liver and arrest convulsions that is closely related to the pharmacological effects of sedation, hypnosis and anti-convulsion etc. Gastrodin, gastrodigenin, vanillyl alcohol, etc are the effective components for its sedative and hypnotic anti-convulsion activity.

2. 平抑肝阳　天麻质重沉降，入肝经，平肝潜阳。其功效的发挥与降血压、抗眩晕等药理作用密切相关。天麻素、天麻苷元等是其降血压的有效成分。天麻多糖、天麻苷元是其抗眩晕的有效成分。

2 Suppression of Liver Yang

Tianma is heavy in texture and enters into the liver meridian and can pacify the liver to subdue yang, which is closely related to its antihypertension and anti-vertigo effects. Gastrodiae polysaccharide, gastrodigenin, etc. are its effective ingredients for lowering blood pressure. Gastrodiae polysaccharide and gastrodigenin are the effective components for its anti-vertigo activity.

3. 祛风通络　天麻味甘，性平，祛外风，通经络。其功效的发挥与其抗炎、抗衰老、抗血小板聚集、抗血栓等药理作用密切相关。天麻苷元是其抗炎的有效成分。天麻多糖是其抗衰老的有效成分。天麻素是其镇痛的有效成分。天麻素、天麻苷元和天麻多糖是其血小板凝聚、抗血栓的有效成分。

3 Dispelling Wind to Free the Collateral Vessels

The medicinal properties of Tianma are

sweet, neutral and can dispel external wind to free the meridian and collateral, which is closely related to its pharmacological effects of anti-inflammation, anti-aging, anti-platelet aggregation and anti-thrombosis etc. Gastrodigenin is its anti-inflammatory active ingredient; gastrodiae polysaccharide is its anti-aging active ingredient; gastrodin is its analgesic active ingredient. gastrodin, gastrodigenin and gastrodiae polysaccharide are the effective components for its antiplatelet aggregation and antithrombosis effects.

【应用】
[Applications]

一、主治病证
I Indications

1. 肝风内动，惊痫抽搐　治疗小儿急惊风，天麻常与他药配伍以增效，如《医宗金鉴》钩藤饮；治疗小儿脾虚慢惊，与人参、白术、白僵蚕等药配伍，如《普济本事方》醒脾丸；治小儿诸惊，与全蝎、制天南星、制僵蚕配伍，如《魏氏家藏方》天麻丸；治破伤风痉挛抽搐、角弓反张，又与天南星、白附子、防风等药配伍，如《外科正宗》玉真散。

1 Internal Stirring of Liver Wind and Convulsions

Tianma is often used with other medicines to treat acute infantile convulsions, such as Gouteng Yin (Decoction) in *Yizong Jinjian*. It is combined with Renshen, Baizhu and Jiangcan (*Bombyx Batryticatus*) for the treatment of spleen deficiency of chronic infantile convulsion such as Xingpi Wan in *Puji Benshifang (Experiential Prescriptions for Universal Relief)*. In the combination with Quanxie, Zhitiannanxing (*Arisaematis Rhizoma Preparatum*) and Jiangcan, it is used to treat infantile panic, such as Tian Ma Wan in *Weishi Jiacang Fang (Treasure Prescription of Wei's Family)*. It is also compatible with Tiannanxing, Baifuzi and Fangfeng to treat tetanus, spasm,

convulsions and opisthotonos such as Yuzhen San (Powder) in *Waike Zhengzong*.

现代临床，天麻配伍常用于治疗癫痫、轻型破伤风、流脑、乙脑、小儿急惊风、小儿慢惊风等属于肝风内动或热极生风者，如小儿抗痫胶囊。

In modern clinical practice, Tianma based prescriptions are often used to treat epilepsy, mild tetanus, meningitis, encephalitis B, infantile acute convulsion and infantile chronic convulsion with liver and extreme heat engendering wind such as Xiaoer KangXian Jiaonang.

2. 眩晕，头痛　治疗多种原因导致的眩晕、头痛，天麻与它药配伍治疗，如《杂病证治新义》天麻钩藤饮、《医学心悟》半夏白术天麻汤。若头风攻注，偏正头痛，头晕欲倒者，可配等量川芎为丸，如《普济方》天麻丸。

2 Vertigo and Headache

The compatibilities of Tianma and other medicines can be used for the treatment of various factors induced vertigo and headache, such as TianmMa Gouteng Yin (Drink) in *Zabing Zhengzhi Xinyi* and Banxia Baizhu Tianma Tang (Decotion) in *Yixue Xinwu (medical Revelation)*. It can be made into pills with equivalent amount of Chuanxiong for the treatment of wind attack in head, headache and dizziness, such as Tian Ma Wan in *Puji Fang*.

现代临床，以天麻配伍常用于治疗高血压、神经官能症等属于肝阳上亢者，如天麻头痛片。

In modern clinical applications, Tianma based prescriptions such as Tianma Toutong Pian are often used to treat hypertension and neurosis with ascendant hyperactivity of liver yang.

3. 肢体麻木，手足不遂，风湿痹痛　治中风手足不遂，筋骨疼痛，风湿痹痛，关节屈伸不利等证，天麻与多药配伍使用，如《圣济总录》天麻丸、《十便良方》天麻酒、《医学心悟》秦艽天麻汤等。

3 Numbness of Limbs, Paralysis of the Limbs, Rheumatism and Arthralgia

The compatibilities of Tianma and other

medicines can be used to treat wind stroke induced paralysis of the limbs, arthralgia and myalgia, rheumatic arthralgia and flexor extensor adverse, such as Tianma Wan in *Sheng Ji Zonglu*, Tian Ma Jiu in *Shibian Liangfang* (*Ten Effective Prescription*) and Qinjiao Tianma Tang in *Yixue Xinwu* medical Revelations.

现代临床，天麻配伍常用于治疗脑血管意外及其后遗症、风湿性关节炎、类风湿性关节炎等，如天麻丸。

In modern clinical applications, Tianma based prescriptions such as Tian Ma Wan are often used to treat cerebrovascular accident and its sequelae, rheumarthritis and rheumatoid arthritis, etc.

二、用法用量
II Administration and Dosage

3~10g，煎汤。

3~10g, water decoction.

三、注意事项
III Precautions

对天麻过敏人群禁用。

It is forbidden for patients allergic to Tianma.

第二十二章 开 窍 药
Chapter 22　Resuscitation Medicinals

凡以开窍醒神、治疗闭证神昏为主要作用的药物，称为开窍药。此类药物多味辛性温，辛香行散，性善走窜，主入心经，故可治疗闭证神昏。开窍药辛香走窜，为治标之品，易耗伤正气，故应用不能过量，且只宜暂服，不可久用。药物芳香成分易挥发，故一般不入煎剂。现代研究表明，开窍药多具有调节中枢神经、促进胃肠运动、促消化、抗心律失常、抗肿瘤、抗心肌缺血、抗炎等药理作用。常见的开窍药有麝香、苏合香、冰片、蟾酥等。

Resuscitation medicinals refer to the medicinals that can open the orifices and awaken the spirit, and treat unconsciousness and block syndromes. The medicinal nature of resuscitation medicinals is pungent and warm. The pungent flavor has the characteristics of diffusion, so it is good at mobile and penetrating. The resuscitation medicinals mainly enter the heart meridian. Thus, this kind of medicinals can treat unconsciousness and block syndromes. The resuscitation medicinals are mainly used to treat incidental aspect. They can be just used to temporarily, and they have the tendency of hurting healthy qi, so they should not be used for a long time. Thus, patients are not allowed to take them overdose. There are many volatile chemical components in the resuscitation medicinals, so they are generally not used in decoctions. Modern researches showed that the resuscitation medicinals have many pharmacological effects, such as regulating central nervous system, promoting gastrointestinal movement, promoting digestion, anti-arrhythmia, anti-tumor, anti-myocardial ischemia, and anti-inflammation. Resuscitation medicinals including Shexiang (Moschus), Suhexiang (Styrax), Bingpian (Borneolum Syntheticum) and Chansu (Bufonis Venenum) are commonly used.

麝　香

Shexiang
(Moschus)

麝香是著名的川产道地药材。麝香味辛，性温，归心、脾经，有开窍醒神，活血通经，消肿止痛的功效，主治闭证神昏、瘀血诸证、疮痈、咽喉肿痛。麝香主要含大环酮类、甾体类、吡啶类、氨基酸等成分，有强心、耐缺氧、抗内毒素、保护脑缺血再灌注损伤、抗心肌缺血缺氧损伤、抗神经细胞缺血缺氧损伤、抗炎、镇痛等药理作用，可用于治疗冠心病心绞痛、老年糖尿病合并心绞痛、心力衰竭、心肌梗死等所属气滞血瘀所致的胸痹证。本品有兴奋子宫之效，孕妇禁用。

Shexiang is a noted genuine regional

medicinal in Sichuan. Shexiang is acid and warm in nature; it enters the heart and spleen meridians. It has the effects of opening the orifices to awaken the spirit, activating blood and pass through meridians, disperse swelling and relieve pain, and it can treat unconsiousenss and block syndrome, stagnant blood syndrome, sores and swelling and pain in throat. Shexiang mainly contains macrocyclic ketones, steroids, pyridine, amino acids and other components, which possess various pharmacological effects, such as strengthen the heart, hypoxic tolerance, anti-endotoxin, protection of cerebral ischemia reperfusion injury, anti-myocardial ischemia and hypoxic injury, anti-neuronal cell injury by ischemic hypoxia, anti-inflammatory and analgesic etc. Shexiang can be used for the treatment of coronary heart disease, angina pectoris, elderly diabetes combined with angina pectoris, heart failure, myocardial infarction, etc. These symptoms belong to chest discomfort caused by qi stagnation and blood stasis. This medicine has the effect of stimulating the uterus, so it is forbidden used for pregnant women.

【品种品质】
[Variety and Quality]

一、基原品种与品质
I Origin Varieties and Quality

1. **品种概况**　来源于鹿科动物林麝 *Moschus berezovskii* Flerov、马麝 *Moschus sifanicus* Przewalski 或原麝 *Moschus moschiferus* Linnaeus 成熟雄体香囊中的干燥分泌物。成熟雄麝在脐和阴茎之间的腹部有特殊的囊状麝香腺，囊内分泌麝香。

1 Variety

Shexiang is dry secretions from mature male sachets of *Moschus berezovskii* Flerov, *Moschus sifanicus* Przewalski, or *Moschus moschiferus* Linnaeus. The mature male musk deer has a special cystic musk gland in the abdomen between the umbilicus and the penis, which secretes Shexiang.

　　麝香始载于《神农本草经》,《本草经集注》云 "麝形似獐，常食柏叶，又啖蛇，五月得香……其香正在麝阴茎前皮内，别有膜裹之"。《本草纲目》言 "麝之香气远，故谓之麝香"。《本草崇原》又云 "麝形似獐而小，色黑，常食柏叶及蛇虫，其香在脐，故名麝脐香"。上述本草中记载 "麝香" 的基原动物应为鹿科动物林麝与马麝，而现今还包括了东北地区的原麝。

Shexiang was firstly recorded in *Shennong Bencao Jing*. *Bencaojingjizhu (Collective Commentaries on Classics of Materia Medica)* notes: Musk deer grow like roe deer; often eat cypress leaves and snakes. Musk deer began to produce Shexiang in May... There is a membrane inside the front skin of the musk penis... *Bencao Gangmu* noted: The fragance of musk is far, so it's called Shexiang. *Bencao Chongyuan (Materia Medica Believe in the Source)* notes: Musk deer is like roe deer. It is small and black in shape. Musk deer often eats cypress leaves, snakes and insects. Shexiang is located in navel, so Shexiang is also called Sheqixiang. According to these notes of the books, the source animals of "Shexiang" should be *Moschus berezovskii* Flerov and *Moschus sifanicus* Przewalski, which now also includes *Moschus moschiferus* Linnaeus from the northeast.

2. **养殖采收**　四川、陕西、甘肃、青海、云南、黑龙江、吉林等地有野生或饲养。现代林麝养殖技术已有突破，市场上天然麝香与人工麝香均在使用。林麝对养殖环境要求较高，以安静、清洁、高海拔地区为宜，一般活体取香，每年1次。

2 Farming and Harvesting

Musk is wild or breeding in Sichuan, Shanxi, Gansu, Qinghai, Yunnan, Heilongjiang, Jilin and other regions. There has been a breakthrough in modern *Moschus bere zovskii* Flerov breeding technology. Both natural Shexiang and artificial Shexiang are used in the market. *Moschus berezovskii* Flerov has a higher requirement on the breeding environment, which is suitable for quiet, clean and high-altitude areas. Generally, Shexiang is taken in vivo once a year.

3. 道地性及品质评价　历代本草记载，四川是麝香的道地产区之一，并延续至今。古代主要从质地对麝香进行品质评价，认为香结实者佳。现代麝香性状评价指标更为丰富，实际流通中主要以外形自然、富于弹性、手捏之微软，内香仁易聚易散，放手仍复原状，即属真品，且颗粒色紫黑、粉末色棕褐色、质柔、油润、香气浓烈者为佳。

3 Genuineness and Quality Evaluation

According to historical records, Sichuan is one of the genuine producing areas of Shexiang, and still in use. In ancient times, the quality of Shexiang was evaluated mainly from the aspect of texture. It was considered that those with strong fragrance are better. At present, Shexiang character evaluation indicators are more abundant. Shape of authentic Shexiang is natural and flexible. The fragrant kernel in the capsule is easy to gather and scattered, and it can be restored without hand. It is better to have purplish black particles, brown powder, soft and oily texture, and rich fragrance.

麝香主要含大环酮类（麝香酮、麝香醇、降麝香酮、麝香吡喃等）、甾体类（胆甾醇、胆甾-4烯-3-酮等）、吡啶类（麝香吡啶、羟基麝香吡啶A和B等）及氨基酸类等成分。其中麝香酮是其脑保护、双向调节中枢神经系统等多种药理作用的主要物质基础，此外，麝香还含有多肽、无机盐、微量元素等。《中国药典》规定麝香中麝香酮的含量不得少于2.0%。

Shexiang mainly contains macrocyclic ketones (Musk ketone, Musk alcohol, Normusketone, Muskpyran, etc.), steroids (Cholsesterel, Cholest-4-en-3-one, etc.), pyridine class (Muscopyridine, Hydroxymuscopyridine A and B, etc.) and amino acids. Among them, musk ketone is the main material basis of protecting brain, two-way regulation of central nervous system and other pharmacological actions. In addition, Shexiang also contains polypeptides, inorganic salts, trace elements, etc. The *Pharmacopoeia of the People's Republic of China* stipulates that the content of musk ketone in Shexiang should not be less than 2.0%.

二、炮制品种与品质
II Processed Varieties and Quality

麝香历来均应用生品。目前，麝香的炮制品种为生麝香。麝香以饱满、皮薄、仁多，捏之有弹性、香气浓烈者为佳。饮片的品质评价同药材。

From ancient times to now, Shexiang has been used in raw products. At present, the processed varieties of Shexiang are also raw. Shexiang in fullness, thin skin, many kernel, elasticity, strong aroma is better. The quality evaluation of its decoction pieces was the same as that of medicinals.

三、中成药品种与品质
III Varieties and Quality of Chinese Patent Medicines

含麝香的中成药有460余个，其中药典收载70余个。以麝香为君药或主药的品种有麝香保心丸、片仔癀（胶囊）、安宫牛黄丸等。在质量控制多采用气相色谱法确定麝香的存在，采用含量测定法进行有效成分限量以保证药效。如安宫牛黄丸、麝香保心丸、麝香通心滴丸、贝羚胶囊等制剂，均通过气相色谱法鉴别麝香酮来确定麝香的存在；麝香风湿胶囊、片仔癀（胶囊）以麝香酮含量的低限来保证其质量。

At present, there are more than 460 Chinese patent medicines containing Shexiang, of which more than 70 Chinese patent medicines are recorded in *Pharmacopoeia of the People's Republic of China*. Among which, prescriptions with Shexiang as sovereign are as follows: Shexiang Baoxin Wan, Pianzaihuang Jiaonang (Capsules), AngongNiuhuang Wan, etc. In the quality control, GC is often used to determine the presence of Shexiang, and the content determination method is used to limit the effective components to ensure the efficacy in the following prescriptions: Angong Niuhuang Wan, Shexiang Baoxin Wan, ShexiangTongxin Diwan, Beiling Jiaonang (Capsules), etc. The existence of Shexiang was determined by the identification of musk ketone by GC. The quality of Shexiang Fengshi Jiaonang (Capsules) and Pianzaihuang Jiaonang (Capsules) was guaranteed by the low content of musk ketone.

【制药】
[Pharmacy]

一、产地加工
I Processing in Production Area

野麝多在冬季至次春猎取，猎获后，割取香囊，阴干，习称"毛壳麝香"；剖开香囊，除去囊壳，习称"麝香仁"。

Wild musk deer is mostly hunted from winter to the next spring. Then the sachets are cut and dried in the shade. The dried sachet is called "Maoke Shexiang". When the sachets are opened and the shells are removed, it is commonly called "ShexiangRen".

家麝直接从其香囊中取出麝香仁，阴干或用干燥器密闭干燥。

In musk deer, musk kernels are taken directly from the sachet, and dried in the shade or in a tight-sealed desiccator.

二、饮片炮制
II Processing of Decoction Pieces

麝香多以净制、研碎为工艺，由此加工成生麝香。

Purifying and grinding are the mainly processing technologies of Shengshexiang (raw).

三、中成药制药
III Pharmacy of Chinese Patent Medicines

含麝香的中成药，剂型十分丰富。多选用生麝香，打粉入药。同时，因天然麝香资源匮乏，目前，也有以人工麝香替代麝香入药者，在一定程度上减少了对天然麝香的需求。

There are various kinds of Chinese patent medicines containing Shexiang. In the patent medicine preparation, raw Shexiang is directly powdered into medicine. At the same time, there is also use of artificial Shexiang instead of Shexiang in medicine, which reduces the demand on natural Shexiang to some extent.

如麝香保心丸，选用人工麝香代替麝香入药，与人参提取物等共研成细粉后，再与苏合香、适量白酒泛丸，可使麝香有效成分如麝香酮快速溶出，从而迅速发挥药效作用。而在麝香祛痛搽剂制剂工艺中，因麝香中的有效成分麝香酮可溶于乙醇，故采用 50% 的乙醇提取有效成分以达到搽剂的制备要求。

For example, Shexiang Baoxin Wan, using artificial Shexiang instead of Shexiang, grinding it into fine powder with Ginseng extract, and then it is prepared with Suhexiang (Styrax) and appropriate amount of liquor to make pills. In this way, the active components of Shexiang, such as musk ketone, can be rapidly dissolved out, so as to quickly play the role of pharmacodynamics. In the process of Shexiang Qutong Chaji (Liniment) preparation, since its effective ingredient musk ketone is soluble in ethanol, 50% ethanol is used to extract the effective ingredient to meet the preparation requirements of the liniment.

【性能功效】
[Property and Efficacy]

一、性能
I Property

麝香辛，温；归心、脾经。

Shexiang is pungent in flavor, warm in nature, and enters the heart and spleen meridians.

二、功效
II Efficacy

1. 开窍醒神 麝香芳香走窜，开窍通闭，开通心脉，为醒神回苏之要药。其功效的发挥与其脑保护、中枢双向调节、强心、耐缺氧等药理作用密切相关。麝香的脑保护、中枢双向调节、耐缺氧作用的有效物质基础主要是麝香酮成分，通过抗脑组织氧化损伤和调节 VEGF、MMP-9 等血管和细胞凋亡相关物质而保护神经组织。

1 Open the Orifices to Arouse the Spirit

Shexiang has the function of moving and penetrating for the aromatic nature, opening the orifices to free block, and opening the heart and vessels. It is the core medicine to revive the spirit-mind. The function of Shexiang is closely related to its pharmacological effects such as brain protection, central pivot two-way regulation, heart strengthening, and hypoxia tolerance. Musk ketone is the effective material basis of brain protection, two-way regulation of central pivot and hypoxia tolerance.It can protect nervous tissue by antioxidative damage and regulating VEGF, MMP-9 and other related substances of vascular and cell apoptosis.

2. 活血通经 麝香味辛能散，可行血之瘀滞，开经络之壅遏，具活血通经之功。其功效的发挥与其抗凝血、扩张血管、改善微循环、兴奋子宫平滑肌等作用密切相关。主要物质基础是麝香酮。

2 Promote Bloood Circulation and Dredge Channels

Shexiang is pungent in flavor, which can disperse the blood stasis, move the obstruction of meridians and collaterals, with the function of promoting the blood circulation and dredge the meridians and collateral. Its effect is closely related to anticoagulation, vasodilation, improvement of microcirculation and stimulation of uterine smooth muscle. Its main material basis is musk ketone.

3. 消肿止痛 麝香活血散结，破瘀消癥，具消肿止痛之功。其功效的发挥，与其抗炎、镇痛等作用密切相关。主要物质基础是多肽。

3 Relieve Swelling and Pain

Shexiang has blood-quickening and stasis-dissipating functions, it can break blood stasis and eliminate masses, as well as disperse swelling and relieve pain. Its efficacy is closely related to its anti-inflammatory and analgesic function. The main material basis is polypeptides.

此外，现代研究显示麝香具有抗肿瘤、升血压、增强呼吸功能、增加免疫功能等作用。

In addition, modern studies have shown that Shexiang has the effects of anti-tumor, raising blood pressure, enhancing respiration and increasing immune function.

【应用】
[Applications]

一、主治病证
I Indications

1. 闭证神昏 治疗热闭神昏者，常与牛黄、冰片、朱砂等配伍，清热开窍，如《温病条辨》安宫牛黄丸、《太平惠民和剂局方》至宝丹；若兼痉挛抽搐者，可配伍羚羊角、朱砂、磁石等以清热解毒、息风止痉，如《外台秘要》紫雪丹；若中风卒昏、阻闭清窍之寒闭神昏，面青、身凉、脉沉、四肢厥逆者，可与苏合香、檀香、安息香配伍以行气、芳香开窍，如《太平惠民和剂局方》苏合香丸。

1 Unconsciousness and Block Syndromes

Shexiang is often combined with Niuhuang, Bingpian and Zhusha to clear away heat and open the orifices to treat the patient of warm febrile diseases, such as Angong Niuhuang Wan in *Wenbing Tiaobian* and Zhibao Dan (Elixir) in *Taiping Huimin Heji Ju Fang*. In addition, for the accompanied spasm and convulsion, Shexiang can be combined with Lingyangjiao (Saigae Tataricae Cornu), Zhusha (Cinnabaris) and Cishi (Magnetitum) to clear heat and remove toxin, relieve spasm by calming endogenous wind, such as Zixue Dan (Elixir) in *Waitai Miyao*. For the treatment of wind stroke with coma , or dizziness and loss of conscious caused by cold closure characterized by bluish complexion, cool body, deep pulse, and extreme cold limbs, Shexiang is combined with Suhexiang (Styrax), Tanxiang and Anxixiang to promote the flow of qi and open the orifices with aroma, such as Suhexiang Wan in *Taiping Huimin Heji Ju Fang*.

现代临床，麝香配伍常用于治疗流行性脑脊髓膜炎、乙型脑炎、肝昏迷、脑出血、败血症等属于热闭神昏者，如安宫牛黄丸、至宝丹、紫雪丹；还可与他药配伍用于治疗急性脑血管疾病、癔症性昏厥、冠心病心绞痛、心肌梗死等属于寒闭与寒凝气滞者，如苏合香丸。

In modern clinical practice, Shexiang compatibility is often used to treat epidemic cerebrospinal meningitis, Japanese encephalitis, hepatic coma, hematencephalon, sepsis, etc, which belong to warm febrile diseases, such as Angong Niuhuang Wan, Zhibao Dan, Zixue Dan; Shexiang is also combined with other medicines for the treatment of acute cerebrovascular disease, hysteric syncope, angina pectoris of coronary heart disease, myocardial infarction, etc., which belong to cold closure and cold coagulation stagnation, such as Suhexiang Wan.

2. 瘀血诸证　对厥心痛者，常配伍桃仁、木香等，行气止痛，如《圣济总录》麝香汤；对经闭、痛经，常与桃仁、红花、川芎等配伍，如《医林改错》通窍活血汤；对瘀肿疼痛者，配伍乳香、没药、红花等，活血定痛，如《良方集腋》七厘散和现代中成药七厘散。

2 Stagnant Blood Syndromes

To treat the patients with heart pain caused by heart blood stasis and obstruction, Shexiang is often combined with Taoren and Muxiang for moving qi to relieve pain, such as Shexiang Tang (Decoction) in *Sheng Ji Zonglu*. To treat the women's disease of amenorrhea and dysmenorrheal, Shexiang can be combined with Taoren, Honghua and Chuanxiong for activating blood and resolving stasis, such as Tongqiaohuoxue Tang (Decoction) in *Yilin Gaicuo (Correction of the Errors of Medical Works)*. To treat the patients with stasis swelling of painful, Shexiang can be combined with Ruxiang, Moyao and Honghua for activating blood to relieve pain, such as Qili San (Powder) in *Liangfang Jiye (A good Combination of Armpit)* and the Chinese patent medicine Qili San.

现代临床，麝香配伍常用于治疗冠心病、心绞痛、老年糖尿病合并心绞痛、心力衰竭、心肌梗死等属于气滞血瘀所致的胸痹证，如麝香保心丸、麝香通心滴丸。

At present, Shexiang compatibility is often used in the treatment of coronary heart disease, angina pectoris, senile diabetes combined with angina pectoris, and heart failure and myocardial infarction which belong to chest impediment caused by qi stagnation and blood stasis, such as Shexiang Baoxin Wan and She XiangTongxin Diwan.

3. 疮痈，咽喉肿痛　对痈疽发背、恶疮者，配伍雄黄、矾石等，如《备急千金要方》麝香膏；对痰核、流注、瘰疬者，与乳香、没药等配伍以散结活血，如《外科证治全生集》小金丹；对热毒疮痈者，可配伍雄黄、乳香、没药等，如《外科证治全生集》醒消丸；对咽喉肿痛者，常配伍珍珠粉、牛黄、蟾酥等，如《雷公上诵芳堂方》六神丸。

3 Toxic Swellings, Painful and Swollen Throat

Shexiang can be combined with Xionghuang and Fanshi to treat the patients of toxic swellings inforearm and malign sore, such as She Xiang

Gao (Paste) in *Beiji Qianjin Yaofang (Essential Recipes for Emergent Use Worth A Thousand Gold)*. Shexiang is combined with Ruxiang, Moyao for treating deep multiple abscess and scrofula by invigorating the blood and dissipating nodule, such as Xiao Jin Dan from the *Waike Zhengzhi Quansheng Ji (Life-For-An Compendium of External Medicine Patterns and Treatment)*. To treat heat toxin and toxic swellings, Shexiang can be combined with Xionghuang, Ruxiang and Moyao, such as Xingxiao Wan in *Waike Zhengzhi Quansheng Ji*. To treat painful and swollen throat, Shexiang can be combined with Zhenzhufen (Margarita), Niuhuang, Chansu for clearing heat and removing toxin, such as Liushen Wan in *Leigong Shangsong Fangtang Fang (Lei Gong Recites Fang Tang Fang)*.

二、用法用量
II Administration and Dosage

0.03~0.1g，多入丸散。外用适量。

0.03~0.1g, and it is mostly prepared into pills and powder. For external use, proper dose should be applied.

三、注意事项
III Precautions

1. 孕妇禁用。

1 Pregnant women should not use it.

2. 本品辛香走窜开通，易于耗气伤阳，夺血伤阴，脱证忌用，虚证亦当慎用。

2 Shexiang is pungent and easy to open, which is easy to consume qi and yang, cause the loss of blood and yin. Therefore, it is forbidden to use for patients with collapse syndrome. For patients with deficiency syndrome should be used with cautions.

第二十三章 补 益 药
Chapter 23　Tonifying Medicinals

凡以补虚扶弱、纠正人体气血阴阳虚衰的病理偏向为主要功效，主治人体气血阴阳不足，脏腑功能衰退所致的虚证的药物，称为补虚药，因皆有补益作用，又叫补益药。因补虚功效有补气、补血、补阴、补阳之异，又可分为补气药、补血药、补阴药、补阳药。补气药与补阳药以补气与温阳为主，多具温热之性；补阴药多以滋养阴液为主、具清热之功，多有寒凉之性。根据"甘能补"的理论，补益药多味甘。因气血阴阳之间在生理上相互依存，在病理上相互影响，故补益药多配伍使用，如补气药与补阳药合用，补血药和补阴药合用等。不得盲目使用补益药，若邪实而正不虚者，误用补虚药有"闭门留寇"之弊。服用补益药需注意顾护脾胃，并正确处理祛邪与扶正的关系。现代研究表明，补益药多对非特异性及特异性免疫功能有增强作用，可增强机体对各种有害刺激的抵抗能力；某些对肾上腺皮质系统有兴奋作用；具有调节糖、脂肪代谢的作用、强心作用，能够提高机体工作能力、改善睡眠和食欲，并能降低疲劳、增加体重，有滋补强壮作用。常见的补益药有人参、麦冬、甘草、当归、黄芪、鹿茸等。

Medicinals, with the main effects of tonifying the deficiency, strengthening the weakness, and correcting the pathological trend in the qi-blood deficiency, and yin-yang deficiency, are called tonifying medicinals. They are usually used to treat the syndrome of weakness due to qi-blood deficiency, yin-yang deficiency, and the degeneration of viscera and bowels function, so they are called deficiency-tonifying medicinals. Due to the effect of tonifying, it is also called buyiyao in Chinese. Since the effects of tonifying deficiency are different in types of tonifying qi, blood, yin and yang, tonifying medicinals can be divided into qi-tonifying medicinals, blood-tonifying medicinals, yin-tonifying medicinals and yang-tonifying medicinals correspondingly. The functions of qi-tonifying medicinals and yang-tonifying medicinals mainly focus on tonifying qi and warming yang, so most of both kinds of medicinals have warm nature. Yin-tonifying medicinals mostly nourish yin fluid and have the function of clearing heat, so they mostly have cold nature. According to the theory of "Sweet medicinals are tonic", the flavor of most tonic medicinals is sweet. Since qi, blood, yin and yang are interdependent physiologically and interactive pathologically, tonic medicinals are often used in combination. For example, qi-tonifying medicinals are combined used with yang-tonifying medicinals, and blood-tonifying medicinals are used with yin-tonifying medicinals. Tonifying medicinals should not be used rashly. If the pathogen in the body is strong and vital qi is not weak, misuse of the tonifying medicinals have the disadvantages of "closing the door resulting in the bandit being stuck inside", which means keeping the pathogens inside the body. When taking the tonifying medicinals, patients should take care of the spleen and stomach, and correctly deal with the relationship between the eliminating pathogens and strenthing the vital qi. Modern researches show that tonic medicinals enhance the non-specific and specific immune functions, which can enhance the body's resistance to various harmful substances;

some have excitatory effects on the adrenal cortex system. It has regulatory effects on sugar and fat metabolism, and a cardio tonic function. It also has effects on improving the working ability of human body, improving sleep quality and appetite, and is able to reduce fatigue, increase weight, nourish and strengthen human body. Common tonifying medicinals include Renshen, Maidong, Gancao, Danggui, Huangqi and Lurong.

人　参

Renshen
(Ginseng Radix et Rhizoma)

人参为东北名贵道地药材。常用炮制品为生晒参、红参。人参味甘、微苦，性微温，归脾、肺、心、肾经，有大补元气，复脉固脱，补脾益肺，生津养血，安神益智的功效，治疗体虚欲脱、肢冷脉微，脾虚食少，肺虚喘咳，津伤口渴，内热消渴，气血亏虚，久病虚羸，惊悸失眠，阳痿宫冷等。人参主要含人参皂苷、多糖、挥发油等成分，有增强记忆力、提高免疫力、改善心血管、延缓衰老和抗肿瘤等药理作用，可治疗心脑血管疾病、心悸、失眠、健忘、阳痿、遗精等属气虚证者。人参不宜与藜芦、五灵脂、莱菔子同用。

Renshen is a valuable genuine regional medicinal in Northeast China. Commonly used processed products include Shengshaishen and Hongshen. Renshen is sweet and slightly bitter in flavor, slightly warm in nature, and the meridian entries are spleen, lung, heart and kidney. It has the effects of tonifying original qi, invigorating the veins, and stop collapse, tonifying the spleen and lungs, generating fluid and nourishing blood, tranquilizing the mind and improving mental health. It is often used to treat the syndromes of physical depletion, limb coldness, weak pulse, spleen deficiency and eating less, lung deficiency and cough, thirst due to insufficiency of body fluid, internal heat and diabetes, deficiency of qi and blood, weakness due to long-time illness, palpitation and insomnia, impotence and cold womb, etc. Renshen mainly contains ginsenosides, polysaccharides, volatile oil and other components, which has pharmacological effects such as memory enhancement, immunity improvement, cardiovascular improvement, anti-aging and anti-tumor effects. It can treat cardiovascular and cerebrovascular diseases, palpitations, insomnia, amnesia, impotence and nocturnal emission that belong to qi deficiency syndrome. Renshen should not be used together with Lilu, Wulingzhi and Laifuzi.

【品种品质】
[Variety and Quality]

一、基原品种与品质
I Origin Varieties and Quality

1. 品种概况　来源于五加科植物人参 *Pananx ginseng* C. A. Mey 的干燥根和根茎。栽培者称"园参"，野生者称"山参"；播种在山林野生状态下自然生长者称"林下山参"，习称"籽海"。

1 Variety
Renshen is the dried root and rhizome of *Pananx Renshen* C.A.Mey of Araliaceae. The artificially cultivated ones are called "Yuanshen", while the wild ones are called "Shanshen". Those growing naturally in wild forests are called

"Linxiashanshen", and they are generally called "Zihai".

人参首载于《神农本草经》。《本草图经》描述上党人参 "其根状如防风而润实，春生苗，多于深山中背阴近椴漆下湿润处，初生小者三四寸许，一桠五叶；四五年后生两桠五叶，未有花茎；至十年后生三桠；年深者生四桠，各五叶，中心生一茎，俗名百尺杆。三月、四月有花，细小如粟，蕊如丝，紫白色。秋后结子，或七八枚，如大豆，生青熟红，自落"，与今人参形态基本相符。

Renshen was firstly recorded in the book of *Shennong Bencao Jing*. According to *Bencao Tujing*, the root shape of Shangdang Renshen is like Fangfeng, and it is plump. It grows in spring and often grows in the dampness place under lindens in the shadow of the mountain. The newborn of Shangdang Renshen is three or four inches in size, with five leaves a fork. Four or five years later, there will be two forks and five leaves, but no flower stems. There will be three forks in ten years. The older trees grow four forks, each with five leaves and a stem in the center, commonly known as Baichigan (100 feet pole). Flowering in March and April, it is as small as millet, and its purple and white pistils are like filaments. When autumn falls, there will be about seven or eight seeds which are like soybeans. The color is green when they are raw, and become red when they are ripe. They fall down when growing ripe. They are basically consistent with the form of Renshen today.

2. 种植采收　人参主产于吉林、辽宁、黑龙江，以人工栽培为主，野生资源为辅。主要采用伐林栽参为主、非林地栽参和林下参并存的栽培方式。产区多数在六年生收获参根，一般于9~10月中旬挖取，以 "边起、边选、边加工" 为原则，应避免支根或须根受损伤。根据鲜参质量可加工成生晒参或红参。

2 Planting and Harvesting

Renshen is mainly produced in Jilin province, Liaoning province and Heilongjiang province. The majority of Renshen is artificially cultivitated, with wild Renshen as supplement. Renshen is cultivated mainly in the deforested land, co-existing with cultivated Renshen in non-forest land and Linxiashen. The harvest of Renshen in the producing area is mostly conducted after it is planted in six years, and generally it is dug out during September to mid-October. The work of digging goes under the principle of "digging and selecting go with processing" in order to avoid the injuries of branches or fibrous roots. The quality of fresh Renshen determines whether it is processed into Shengshaishen (raw and dried Renshen) or Hongshen (red Renshen).

3. 道地性及品质评价　据本草记载，野生人参产地最早源于山西上党潞州，今山西省东南部。灭绝后，产区逐渐向东向北转移。现以吉林抚松所产人参为道地药材，习称 "吉人参"。传统人参以 "条粗、质硬、完整者" 为佳，形态上以支大、芦长、体灵、皮细、色嫩黄、纹细密、饱满、浆水足、无破伤者为佳，实际流通中主要以 "重量、皂苷含量" 为评价指标。

3 Genuineness and Quality Evaluation

According to the records of Materia Medica, the earliest wild Renshen originated in Shangdang area of Luzhou which is in the southeast of Shanxi province nowadays. After the extinction of wild Renshen in the above place, the plant area gradually moved from east to north. These days, Renshen planted in Fusong, Jilin is used as genuine regional medicinals, which is commonly called "Jirenshen". It is believed that Renshen with thick body, hard texture and intact appearance is preferred. In terms of morphology, those with large branches, long reeds, graceful shape, tender skin, slight yellow color, fine lines, fullness and juicy figure without injuries are regarded as high-quality ones. The evaluation indexes "weight, the contents of saponins" is mainly used in actual circulations.

人参主要含有皂苷类成分，《中国药典》规定人参药材中含人参皂苷 Rg_1 和人参皂苷 Re 的总量不得少于 0.30%、人参皂苷 Rb_1 不得少于 0.20%。一般认为，人参皂苷类成分是人参的药效物质基础。此外，人参还含有有机酸、挥发油、多糖、黄酮、氨基酸等成分。

The main component of Renshen is saponin. According to the *Pharmacopoeia of the People's Republic of China*, the total amount of ginsenoside Rg_1 and ginsenoside Re in ginseng herbs should not be less than 0.30% and ginsenoside Rb_1 should not be less than 0.20%. It is generally believed that ginsenosides are the therapeutic material basis of Renshen. In addition, Renshen also contains the components of organic acids, volatile oils, polysaccharides, flavones, amino acids and so on.

二、炮制品种与品质
II Processed Varieties and Quality

人参的炮制品种有 10 余种，临床常用有人参片、红参片等。人参片以体轻，质脆，香气特异，味微苦、甘为佳。红参片以类圆形或椭圆形薄片，外表皮红棕色，半透明，切面平坦，角质样，质硬而脆，气微香而特异，味甘、微苦为佳。《中国药典》规定人参片中含人参皂苷 Rg_1 和人参皂苷 Re 的总量不得少于 0.27%、人参皂苷 Rb_1 不得少于 0.18%；红参片中含人参皂苷 Rg_1 和人参皂苷 Re 的总量不得少于 0.22%、人参皂苷 Rb_1 不得少于 0.18%。

There are more than 10 kinds of processed products of Renshen, among which the commonly used ones in clinic are Renshen slices, Hongshen slices, etc. Renshen slices with special aroma which are light, crisp, slightly bitter in taste and sweet in flavor are preferred. Hongshen slices are round or oval in shape, with a reddish-brown and translucent surface. The cut surface is flat, horny, hard and brittle. The slice which is slightly and specifically fragrant, sweet and bitter in flavor is preferred. The *Pharmacopoeia of the People's Republic of China* stipulates that the total contents of ginsenoside Rg_1 and ginsenoside Re in slices should not be less than 0.27%, and ginsenoside Rb_1 should not be less than 0.18%; the total content of ginsenoside Rg_1 and ginsenoside Re in Hongshen slices should not be less than 0.22%, and the ginsenoside Rb_1 should be not less than 0.18%; the total contents of ginsenoside Rg_1 and ginsenoside Re in slices should not be less than 0.22%, and ginsenoside Rb_1 should not be less than 0.18%.

三、中成药品种与品质
III Varieties and Quality of Chinese Patent Medicines

含有人参或其炮制品的中成药有 620 余个，其中《中国药典》收载 116 个。以人参为君药或主药的品种有人参归脾丸、十一味参芪片等。在中成药的品质控制中多采用显微鉴别及薄层色谱法确定人参的存在，采用含量测定法进行指标成分限量。如十一味参芪片以人参为君药，通过显微鉴别"草酸钙簇晶直径 20~68μm，棱角锐尖"确定含有人参，以薄层色谱法检测人参皂苷 Rg_1、Re 的存在，以 HPLC 法测定人参皂苷 Rg_1、人参皂苷 Re 的总量以限定每片含人参的量以保证作用。

There are more than 620 Chinese patent medicines containing Renshen or its processed products, among them there are 116 included in the *Pharmacopoeia of the People's Republic of China*. Prescriptions with Renshen as sovereign are Renshen Guipi Wan, Shiyiwei Shenqi Pian (Tablets) and so on. In the quality control of Chinese patent medicines, the existence of Renshen is mainly determined by microscopic identification and TLC, and the index composition is limited by content determination. For example, the existence of Renshen in Shiyiwei Shenqi Pian which uses Renshen as sovereign is determined by microscopic identification of "calcium oxalate clusters with a diameter of 20~68 μm and sharp edges". People use TLC to identify the existence of ginsenoside Rg_1 and Re, and use HPLC to measure the total amounts of ginsenoside Rg_1 and

Re to ensure the amount contained in each tablet, so that the efficacy can be ensured.

【制药】
[Pharmacy]

一、产地加工
I Processing in Production Area

鲜人参采收后，抖净泥土，水洗，下须（或不下须），于阳光下晾晒 1~2 天后，35~45℃ 烘干或水洗后蒸至深黄色稍显红，质地柔软时出锅，65~70℃ 烘干，至参根含水量 13% 以下时，取出回潮，整形固定，得生晒参或红参。

After harvested, fresh Renshen is shaken to get rid of the soil and then washed. If necessary, the whiskers are removed. Being aired under the sunlight for 1 to 2 days, it should be dried at 35 ~ 45℃ or steamed to deep yellowish red after being washed. It should be removed from the pot when its texture is soft, and dried at 65 ~ 70℃. When the water content of the Renshen root is below 13%, it should be taken out, gotten dampness, shaped and fixed in order to get the Shengshaishen or Hongshen.

二、饮片炮制
II Processing of Decoction Pieces

从古至今，人参以生用或蒸制后用为主，逐渐形成了"润透 - 蒸煮 - 切制"工艺，由此加工的人参片、红参片成为商品规格中的主流。

Since ancient times, Renshen has been mainly used raw or steamed. The processing technology of "moisturizing-cooking-cutting" has gradually formed. Renshen slices and Hongshen slices processed by this technology have become the mainstream in commodity specifications.

人参炮制的目的在于清洁药材，防止发霉变质和虫蛀，利于贮存和运输，抑制酶活性，减少在自然干燥过程中酶对有效成分的破坏，以保存药性，增强补益作用。人参不同炮制品在某些药理活性的性质及作用强度上存在一定差异。如人参蒸制成红参后生成的人参皂苷 Rh_2 和麦芽酚及其苷类等特有成分，在鲜人参及生晒参中没有，因此，红参较生晒参抗衰老作用强。

The purpose of Renshen processing is to clean the medicinal materials, prevent mildew and moth damage, facilitate storage and transportation, inhibit the enzyme activity, and reduce the damage of enzyme to effective ingredients during the process of natural drying, so as to preserve the medical efficacy and enhance the tonic effect. Some pharmacological activities of different processed products of Renshen have differences in properties and efficacy. For example, after Renshen is steamed into Hongshen, ginsenoside Rh_2, maltol and its glycosides of Hongshen are formed and these unique components which are not contained in fresh Renshen and fried fresh Renshen. Therefore, Hongshen has stronger anti-aging effect than that of fried fresh Renshen.

三、中成药制药
III Pharmacy of Chinese Patent Medicines

在中成药中，人参一般可单独入药，也与其他药物以复方配伍形式应用。含人参的中成药，剂型十分丰富，涵盖固体和液体剂型。人参为贵细药材，为提高药材的利用率，入成药一般打粉直接入药，如人参归脾丸是在归脾汤基础上进行剂型改良，将人参与其他药材共粉碎成细粉制成的大蜜丸。除直接打粉外，由于人参采用水煎煮法提取皂苷类成分如 Rg_1、Re 会发生降解，因此部分制剂可采用乙醇回流法、浸渍、渗漉等方法。

In Chinese patent medicines, Renshen can generally be used as medicine alone or as compound combined with other medicinals. Chinese patent medicines containing Renshen are very rich in pharmaceutical forms, covering solid and liquid pharmaceutical forms. Renshen is a precious medicinal material, in order to improve the utilization rate; it is usually ground into fine powder and used directly. For example, Renshen Guipi Wan is modified on the basis of the Guipi Tang (Decoction), and the method is to grind Renshen and other medicinal materials into fine powder to get Dami wan. In addition to direct powdering, ethanol refluxing, immersion and percolation are often used in some preparations due to the fact that saponin components such as Rg_1 and Re may degrade in the extraction process of the decoction.

【性能功效】
[Property and Efficacy]

一、性能
I Property

人参甘、微苦，微温。归脾、肺、心、肾经。

Renshen is sweet and slightly bitter in flavor, slightly warm in nature and enters the spleen, lung, heart and kidney meridians.

二、功效
II Efficacy

1. 大补元气、补脾益肺　人参大补元气，补五脏气，尤善补脾气，益肺气。其功效的发挥与人参抗疲劳、增强免疫功能、促进造血功能、保护急性肺损伤等药理作用密切相关。人参的抗疲劳、增强免疫功能作用的有效物质基础主要是人参皂苷、多糖类、蛋白类成分，通过调节中枢神经系统、抗自由基、调节糖代谢和减少乳酸堆积等发挥作用。

1 Tonifying Original Qi, Invigorating the Spleen and Benefiting the Lungs

Renshen is greatly capable of tonifying original qi and five zang qi, especially good at nourishing spleen qi and benefiting lung qi. The function of Renshen is closely related to its pharmacological effects such as anti-fatigue, enhancing immune function, promoting

hematopoiesis, protecting from acute lung injury etc. Ginsenosides, polysaccharides and proteins are the effective substances for anti-fatigue and immune function enhancement of Renshen, which play a role by regulating the central nervous system, fighting free radicals, regulating sugar metabolism and reducing lactic acid accumulation.

2. 复脉固脱　人参善大补元气，能复脉固脱。其功效的发挥与抗心肌缺血损伤、抗休克等药理作用密切相关。人参抗心肌损伤、抗休克作用的主要物质基础为人参皂苷类成分，通过保护心肌、抗氧化、增加造血功能、改善微循环等发挥作用。

2 Invigorating the Pulse and Relieving Desertion

Renshen is good for tonifying the original qi and invigorating the pulse and relieving desertion. The function of Renshen is closely related to its pharmacological effects such as anti-myocardial ischemic injury and anti-shock. The main material basis of the anti-myocardial injury and anti-shock effect of Renshen is ginsenoside, which plays a role in protecting myocardium, anti-oxidation, increasing hematopoietic function and improving microcirculation.

3. 生津止渴　人参甘温不燥，补益脾肺，助运化，输精微，布津液，使气旺津生，而达益气生津止渴之效。其功效的发挥与降血糖等作用密切相关。人参降血糖作用的主要物质基础是人参皂苷、多糖类成分，通过降低血糖水平、抑制α-淀粉酶活性、调节物质代谢中血糖与甘油三酯的相互转化等发挥作用。

3 Promoting Fluid Production and Quenching Thirst

Renshen, sweet in flavor and warm in nature, doesn't dryness. It can nourish and benefit the spleen and lung, boost transformation, deliver essence, and distribute body fluid, which acts for flourishing qi and generating fluid, obtaining the effect of invigorating qi, engendering body fluid and quenching thirst. The function of Renshen is closely related to its hypoglycemic effect. Since the ginsenosides and polysaccharides in Renshen are the main material basis of the hypoglycemic effect, they play a role by lowering blood glucose level, inhibiting and regulating α-amylase, and regulating the mutual transformation of blood glucose and serum triglycerides in metabolism.

4. **安神益智**　人参补益心气，安神益智。其功效的发挥与人参增强记忆、调节中枢神经系统、保护脑缺血再灌注损伤等药理作用密切相关。人参增强记忆、调节中枢神经系统作用的主要物质基础是人参皂苷、多糖类成分，通过调节淀粉样前体蛋白水解过程、降低海马氧化应激水平、保护神经细胞和细胞线粒体功能等发挥作用。

4 Tranquilizing the Mind and Promoting Intelligence

The functions of Renshen to benefit the heart and qi, tranquillize the mind and promote intelligence are closely related to its pharmacological effects of enhancing memory, regulating the central nervous system, and protecting against cerebral ischemia-reperfusion injury. The main material basis of Renshen to enhance memory and regulate the central nervous system is ginsenosides and polysaccharides, which play a role by regulating the process of amyloid precursor protein hydrolysis, reducing the level of hippocampal oxidative stress, protecting nerve cells and cellular mitochondrial function, etc.

此外，现代研究显示人参具有抗过敏、抗利尿、抗溃疡、抗肿瘤等作用。

In addition, modern research shows that Renshen has the functions of anti-allergy, anti-diuresis, anti-ulcer, anti-tumor, etc.

【应用】
[Applications]

一、主治病证
I Indications

1. **气虚欲脱证**　治疗元气虚极欲脱，脉微欲绝重症者，人参可单味重用，如《景岳全书》独参汤；对兼见亡阳征象者，可与附子等配伍以补气固脱、回阳救逆，如《正体类要》参附汤；若兼见亡阴征象者，可与麦冬、五味子等配伍以补气养阴、敛汗固脱，如《内外伤辨惑论》生脉散。

1 Qi Deficiency Syndrome

When Renshen being used to treat patients with extreme deficiency of original qi, and serious patients with minimal pulse, it can be used alone in large dosage, for example Dushen Tang recorded in *Jingyue Quanshu*. And for those who have the signs of yang depletion at the same time, it can be compatible with Fuzi to invigorate qi for relieving desertion, restore yang and rescue patients from collapse, such as Shenfu Tang (Decoction) recorded in *Zhengti Leiyao*. For patients who have signs of yin depletion, Renshen can be used with Maidong, Wuweizi to invigorate qi, nourish yin, reduce sweat and relieve desertion, such as Shengmai San (Powder) recorded in Neiwaishang Bianhuolun.

现代临床，人参配伍常用于休克、急性心力衰竭、急性哮喘等气虚欲脱等危急证候，如参附注射液。

In modern clinical practice, Renshen compatibility (eg. Shenfu Zhushe Injection) is often used to treat shock, acute heart failure, acute asthma and other critical symptoms due to qi deficiency.

2. **脾肺气虚证**　治疗脾气虚衰倦怠乏力，食少便溏者，可与白术、茯苓等配伍以健脾利湿，如《太平惠民和剂局方》四君子汤；对脾气亏虚，中气下陷者，可与黄芪、升麻等配伍以补气升阳，如《脾胃论》补中益气汤；对脾气虚弱，不能统血而致失血者，可与黄芪、白术等配伍以益气摄血，如《济生方》归脾汤；对脾气虚之短气喘促、懒言声微等症，可与五味子、苏子等配伍以补益肺气、止咳平喘，如《备急千金要方》补肺汤。

2 Spleen and Lung Qi Deficiency Syndrome

Renshen can be used in combination with

Baizhu, Fuling and other medicinals through invigorating spleen and dispelling dampness to treat patients with fatigue, lack of appetite and loose stools caused by spleen qi deficiency, such as Sijunzi Tang (Decoction) recorded in *Taiping Huimin Heji Jufang (The Prescriptions of the Bureau of Taiping People's Welfare Pharmacy)*. When Renshen being used together with Huangqi, Shengma and other medicinals to treat spleen qi deficiency and middle qi depression, it has the effects of yang qi supplement, such as Buzhong Yiqi Tang (Decoction) recorded in *Piwei Lun*; for those with the weak spleen and blood coagultion, and being liable to have haemorrhage, Renshen can be used in combination with Huangqi, Baizhu and other medicinals to benefit qi and control blood, such as Guipi Tang in *Jisheng Fang (Prescriptions for helping people)*. Renshen can be used together with Wuweizi, Suzi and other medicinals through tonifying and replenishing the lung qi, suppressing cough and calming panting to treat expiratory dyspnea and weakness in lung qi deficiency, etc, such as Bufei Tang (Decoction) recorded in *Beiji Qianjin Yaofang (Essential Recipes for Emergent Use Worth A Thousand Gold)*.

现代临床，人参配伍常用于治疗慢性胃炎、肠易激综合征、十二指肠球部溃疡等属于脾气虚、气阴两虚者，如四君子汤、人参健脾丸等。

In modern clinical practice, Renshen compatibility eg. Sijunzi Tang, Renshen Jianpi Wan is often used to treat chronic gastritis, irritable bowel syndrome, duodenal ulcer , and so on due to deficiency of spleen qi and qi-yin deficiency.

3. **气津两虚之口渴，消渴证** 对热病气津两伤之口渴、脉大无力者，可与知母、石膏等配伍以清热泻火，如《伤寒论》白虎加人参汤；对气阴两虚之消渴证，可与麦冬、五味子等配伍以养阴生津，如《内外伤辨惑论》生脉散。

3 Thirst Due to Qi and Fluid Deficiency, Consumptive Thirst Syndrome

Renshen can be used in combination with Zhimu, Shigao and other medicinals to treat thirst and pulse weakness due to qi-fluid deficiency, such as Baihu Renshen Tang recorded in *Shanghan Zabing Lun (Treatise on Cold Damage Diseases)*; for those with qi- yin deficiency, it can be combined with Maidong and Wuweizi to nourish yin and fluid, such as Shengmai San in *Neiwaishang Bianhuolun (Differentiation on Endogenous)*.

现代临床，人参配伍常用于治疗糖尿病属于气津两伤之消渴证者，如参芪消渴胶囊。

In modern clinical practice, Renshen compatibility such as Shenqi Xiaoke Jiaonang is often used to treat diabetes with consumptive thirst syndrome due to qi-yin deficiency.

4. **血虚证** 治疗气血两虚证，可与白术、当归等配伍以补益气血，如《景岳全书》参归汤、《正体类要》八珍汤。

4 Blood Deficiency Syndrome

In the treatment of qi-blood deficiency syndromes, Renshen can be combined with Baizhu, Danggui and other medicinals to enrich qi and blood, such as Shengui Tang (Decoction) recorded in *Jingyue Quanshu* and Bazhen Tang (Decoction) in *Zhengti Leiyao*.

现代临床，人参配伍常用于治疗贫血属于气血两虚证者，如八珍丸、人参养荣丸。

In modern clinical practice, Renshen compatibility (eg. Bazhen Wan and Renshen Yangrong Wan) is often used to treat anemia due to qi-blood deficiency.

5. **心悸、失眠、健忘** 治疗心气不足、血虚心失所养所致的心悸、失眠、健忘者，可与酸枣仁、柏子仁等配伍以养心安神，如《摄生秘剖》天王补心丹；对心气虚之心悸怔忡、脉结代者，可与炙甘草等配伍，如《伤寒论》炙甘草汤。

5 Palpitations, Insomnia and Forgetfulness Syndrome

For patients with palpitations, insomnia and forgetfulness caused by qi-blood deficiency, Renshen can be combined with Suanzaoren, Baiziren and other medicinals to nourish the heart and calm the mind, such as Tianwang Buxin Wan recorded in *Shesheng Mipou (Secret of Health-Preservation)*; Renshen together with Zhigancao be used for those with heart palpitations, and intermittent pulse duo to heart qi deficiency, such as Zhigancao Tang (Decoction) recorded in *Shanghan Zabing Lun (Treatise on Cold Damage Diseases)*.

现代临床，人参配伍常用于治疗心肌营养不良、慢性心力衰竭，心肌梗死等属于心气虚者，如天王补心丹。

In modern clinical practice, Renshen compatibility (eg. Tianwang Buxin Wan) is often used to treat the diseases such as myocardial dystrophy, chronic heart failure, myocardial infarction due to heart qi deficiency.

二、用法用量
II Administration and Dosage

3~9g，另煎兑服；也可研粉吞服，一次 2 g，一日 2 次。

3~9g decoction alone for blending; or swallow 2g powder after being grinded, twice a day.

三、注意事项
III Precautions

1. 人参不宜与藜芦、五灵脂、莱菔子同用，不宜同时吃萝卜或喝茶，以免影响补益作用。

1. Renshen should not be used with Lilu, Wulingzhi, Laifuzi, and it should not be taken with radish or tea at the same time which may weaken the nourishing effects.

2. 实证、热证而正气不虚者忌服。

2. It is forbidden for patients without vital qi deficiency and those suffering from excess syndrome and heat syndrome.

【知识拓展】
[Knowledge Extension]

人参被誉为"百草之王"，人参茎叶、花、果、芦、皮等部位也被证实可进一步被综合利用与开发。人参目前已作为新资源食品、保健食品被广泛应用，由于人参具有显著抗衰老作用，对皮肤病及老化、损伤具有一定治疗和修复作用，为化妆品的开发提供有力条件。

Renshen is known as the "King of Herbs", thus the stems, leaves, flowers, fruits, head and peel of Renshen have been confirmed to be further comprehensively utilized and developed. Renshen has been widely used as a new resource of food and healthy food. Because of the significant anti-aging effect, it has certain therapeutic and repairing function for skin diseases, aging skin and skin injuries, which provides advantages for the development of cosmetics.

麦 冬
Maidong
(Ophiopogonis Radix)

麦冬为浙江道地药材，习称为"杭麦冬"；另有四川产者习称为"川麦冬"，主产于四川绵阳、三台等地。麦冬味甘、微苦，性微寒，归心、肺、胃经，有养阴生津、润肺清心的功效，主治肺燥干咳、阴虚痨嗽、喉痹咽痛、津伤口渴、内热消渴、心烦失眠、肠燥便秘。麦冬中主要含甾体皂苷、高异黄酮类、各种类型的多聚糖，以及单萜糖苷、色原酮等，有抗疲劳、清除自由基、提高细胞免疫功能、降血糖等药理作用，临床上用于治疗心律失常、心绞痛、糖尿病、萎缩性胃炎等属阴虚证者。

Known as "Hangmaidong" produced in Zhejiang province, Maidong is a traditionally recognized genuine regional medicinal. Besides, "Chuanmaidong" produced in Sichuan is mainly produced in Mianyang, Santai and other places. The medicinal properties of Maidong are sweet, slightly bitter, and slightly cold. The meridian entries of Maidong are the stomach, lung and heart. It has the effects of tonifying yin to engender fluid, moistening the lung and clearing the heart. Maidong is often used to treat dry cough due to lung deficiency, overstrain cough due to yin deficiency, pharyngalgia due to throat impediment, thirsty due to fluid depletion, wasting-thirst due to internal heat, insomnia due to vexation, astriction due to intestinal dryness. Maidong contains steroidal saponins, high isoflavones, various types of polysaccharides, monoterpene glycosides and chromogens, and has pharmacological effects such as anti-fatigue, scavenging free radicals, improving cellular immune function, and lowering blood glucose. Clinically, Maidong is often used to treat arrhythmia, angina, diabetes and atrophic gastritis, which belong to yin deficiency syndrome.

【品种品质】
[Variety and Quality]

一、基原品种与品质
I Origin Varieties and Quality

1. 品种概况　来源于百合科多年生草本植物麦冬 Ophiopogon ja ponicus (L. f.) Ker-Gawl. 的干燥块根。

1 Variety

Maidong is derived from the dried roots of *Ophiopogon ja ponicus* (L.f.) Ker-Gawl.

麦冬始载于《神农本草经》，原名麦门冬。《本草拾遗》曰："出江宁小润，出新安大白。其大者苗如鹿葱，小者如韭叶，大小有三四种，功

用相似，其子圆碧"。可见，古代药用麦冬不止一种，今只留一种。

Maidong was first listed in *Shennong Bencao Jing*, formerly known as Maimendong. *Bencao Shiyi* recorded that is small and moistening from Jiangning, big and white from Xinan. The large seedlings of Maidong were like Lycoris squamigera, while the small ones were like leek leaves. There were three or four sizes, but their efficacy and usage were similar. Maidong had an oval shape and a shiny surface. It can be inferred that there was more than one type of Maidong in ancient times. Only one breed is retained today.

2. 种植采收　当前麦冬主产于浙江、四川。在栽培上麦冬采用分株繁殖进行栽种，浙江于立夏至芒种，于栽培后第3年立夏时采挖，称"杭麦冬"；四川于清明前后栽种，栽培第2年清明后采挖，称"川麦冬"。野麦冬多在清明后挖取，习称"土麦冬"。

2 Planting and Harvesting

Today, Maidong is mainly produced in Zhejiang and Sichuan. Maidong is planted by branch propagation during the period from Beginning of summer to Grain in Ear (Zhejiang) or around Qingming (Sichuan). In terms of cultivation, Maidong is cultivated by means of division propagation. In Zhejiang, Maidong is carried out during the third years at the Beginning of summer, which is called "Hangmaidong". In Sichuan, the second year of cultivated Maidong is excavated after Qingming, and it is called "Chuanmaidong". Wild Maidong is excavated after Qingming, which is customarily called "Tumaidong".

3. 道地性及品质评价　产自浙江的麦冬称"杭麦冬"，栽培于杭州慈溪、余姚、萧山等市，为传统公认的道地药材；产自四川麦冬称"川麦冬"，主产于涪江流域的绵阳、三台等县市，亦为道地药材。形态上以"纺锤形"者为佳，颜色上以"黄白""淡黄"为佳，质地上认为"质柔软、半透明"为佳。现代对于麦冬性状评价指标均以表面淡黄白色、身干、个肥大、质软、半透

明、有香气、嚼之发黏者为佳；瘦子、色棕黄、嚼之黏性小者为次。麦冬中含多种甾体皂苷、高异黄酮、多糖、氨基酸等成分，主要有效成分是麦冬皂苷、麦冬多糖。

3 Genuineness and Quality Evaluation

Maidong from Zhejiang is called "Hangmaidong" and it is cultivated in Cixi, Yuyao, Xiaoshan and other cities in Hangzhou. It is a traditionally recognized genuine regional medicinal. "Chuanmaidong" is mainly produced in Mianyang, Santai, etc. of the Fujiang River Basin in Sichuan, and it is also a genuine regional medicinal.It is better to be "spindle" in shape, "yellow and white" and "light yellow" in color, and "soft and translucent" in texture. Modern evaluation indicators for Maidong traits are pale yellowish white, dry, bulky, soft, translucent, fragrant and chewy, while the skinny, brownish-yellow, and chewy stickiness ones are secondary. Maidong contains a variety of steroidal saponins, high isoflavones, polysaccharides, amino acids and other components. The main active ingredients are Maidong saponins and Maidong polysaccharides.

二、炮制品种与品质
II Processed Varieties and Quality

目前麦冬的炮制品种有 1 个，即生麦冬，在中医临床上麦冬多使用生品。《中国药典》规定，按干燥品计算，含麦冬总皂苷以鲁斯可皂苷元（$C_{27}H_{42}O_4$）计，不得少于 0.12%。

At present, there is only one type of processed Maidong, namely Shengmaidong (raw). In clinical practice of Chinese medicine, Maidong mostly uses raw products. According to the *Pharmacopoeia of the people's Republic of China*, calculated on the basis of dry products, the total saponin content of Ophiopogon cannot be less than 0.12% in terms of ruscogenin ($C_{27}H_{42}O_4$).

三、中成药品种与品质
III Varieties and Quality of Chinese Patent Medicines

据统计，《中国药典》收载含麦冬的中成药共计 120 余个。以麦冬为君药或主药的中成药有生脉饮、二冬膏等。质量控制多采用薄层色谱法确定麦冬的存在，如生脉饮，以麦冬为臣药，取麦冬对照药材用薄层色谱法鉴定麦冬的存在。

According to statistics, the *Pharmacopoeia of the people's Republic of China* contains more than 120 Chinese patent medicines containing Maidong. The Chinese patent medicines that use Maidong as the sovereign medicinal include Shengmai Yin (Drink), Erdong Gao (Cream) and so on. In terms of quality control, TLC is often used to determine the presence of Maidong. For example, Shengmai Yin takes Maidong as sovereign medicinal. Taking Maidong as reference raw medicinal, TLC is performed to detect whether Shengmai Yin contained Maidong.

【制药】
[Pharmacy]

一、产地加工
I Processing in Production Area

夏季采挖，洗净，反复暴晒、堆置，至七八成干，除去须根，干燥。

Maidong is harvested in summer. Maidong is washed, repeatedly exposed to sunlight and piled up. When it is 70%~80% dry, the fibrous roots are removed and dried.

二、饮片炮制
II Processing of Decoction Pieces

仅在古代，麦冬炮制方法就多达 10 余种。现多采用净制、润制，由此加工的生麦冬也成为商品规格中的主流。

In ancient times, there were more than 10 methods for processing Maidong. Nowadays, the main processing steps of raw Maidong are cleansing and moistening, which are the mainstream commercial specifications.

三、中成药制药
III Pharmacy of Chinese Patent Medicines

含有麦冬的中成药制剂种类较多，主要包括口服液体、固体、半固体制剂。在现代制剂中，麦冬多经过提取后以提取物形式加适当辅料制备中成药制剂。

Maidong is involved in many kinds of Chinese patent medicines and preparation forms, which mainly include kinds of oral liquid preparations, oral solid and semisolid preparations. In most modern preparations, Maidong is often extracted and added with the appropriate pharmaceutical excipients to prepare Chinese patent medicines.

如二冬膏，其制备过程采用多次加水煎煮麦冬以提取其中的皂苷和多糖类成分。如十味消渴胶囊，其制备过程采用加水煎煮后，加入 60% 乙醇溶液沉淀提取物中的淀粉，蛋白质和糖类成分，从而富集皂苷和水溶解性多糖类成分，然后入制剂中。

Erdong Gao, for example, the raw herbal material is often extracted by boiling water for extraction of saponins and polysaccharides. For example, Shiwei Xiaoke Jiaonang (Capsules) is prepared by boiling with water, adding 60% ethanol solution to the precipitation of starch, proteins and parts of polysaccharides in Maidong extract. Through this process, the saponins and parts of water-soluble polysaccharides are enriched in the preparations.

【性能功效】
[Property and Efficacy]

一、性能
I Property

麦冬甘、微苦，微寒；归心、肺、胃经。有养阴生津，润肺清心之功。

Maidong is sweet, slightly bitter in flavor, slightly cold in nature, and enters the stomach, lung and heart meridians. It has the effects of nourishing yin, engendering fluid, moistening lung, and relieving vexation.

二、功效
II Efficacy

1. **养阴生津** 麦冬益胃养阴，清热生津。其功效的发挥与降血糖、增强免疫功能等药理作用密切相关，主要物质基础为麦冬多糖，通过保护胰岛细胞、抑制糖原分解、抑制碳水化合物转化、提高免疫功能等发挥作用。

1 Nourishing Yin and Engendering Fluid

Maidong is good for benefiting stomach and nourishing yin, clearing heat and engendering fluid, which is closely related to pharmacological effects such as lowering blood sugar and enhancing immune function. The main material basis is Maidong polysaccharide, which plays a role in protecting islet cells, inhibiting glycogen decomposition, inhibiting carbohydrates translation, and improving immune function.

2. **润肺清心** 麦冬养阴润肺，滋阴养心，清心除烦。其功效的发挥与抗心律失常、抗心肌缺血、抗炎、镇咳、抗肺损伤等药理作用密切相关。主要物质基础为麦冬皂苷、多糖（MDG-1），通过激活 S1P/Akt/ERK 信号通路、抑制 NF-κBp65/TNF-α/ NO/ 组织因子分泌、激活钾离子通路、减弱气管副交感神经节神经元的兴奋性等发挥作用。

2 Moistening Lung and Relieving Vexation

Maidong can moisten lung and nourish yin, enrich yin and nourish the heart, clear the heart and relieve restlessness, which is closely related to pharmacological effects such as anti-arrhythmia, anti-myocardial ischemia, anti-inflammatory, antitussive and anti-lung injury. The main material bases are ophiopogonin and ophiopogon polysaccharide (MDG-1), which can activate the S1P/Akt/ERK signaling pathway, inhibit NF-κBp65/TNF-α/NO tissue factor secretion, activate potassium ion transmission, and attenuate the excitability of tracheal parasympathetic ganglion neurons and soon.

【应用】
[Applications]

一、主治病证
I Indications

1. **胃阴虚证**　治热伤胃阴，口干舌燥及胃阴虚有热之胃脘隐痛，饥不欲食，本品与生地黄、玉竹、沙参等品同用，如《温病条辨》益胃汤；治消渴，可与乌梅等生津止渴之品同用。治胃阴不足之气逆呕吐，可与半夏等配伍，如《金匮要略》麦门冬汤。治热邪伤津之肠燥便秘，可与生地黄、玄参等配伍，如《温病条辨》增液汤。

1 Syndrome of Deficiency of Stomach Yin

When treating patients with hot tongue dry thirst, stomach pain, hunger without appetite, induced by stomach yin deficiency, Maidong is often compatible with Shengdihuang (Rehmanniae Recens Radix), Yuzhu (Polygonati Odorati Rhizoma), and Shashen, such as Yiwei Tang (Decoction) in *Wenbing Tiaobian*. When treating patients with wasting-thirst, Maidong can be used with Wumei and other medicinals with effects of fluid engendering and thirst quenching. For the treatment of patients with qi counterflow and vomit caused by stomach yin deficiency, Maidong can

be compatible with Banxia, such as Maimendong Tang (Decoction) in *Jingui Yaolue*. For patients with intestinal dryness and constipation due to exuberant heat damaging fluid, Maidong can be compatible with Shengdihuang, Xuanshen, etc, such as Zengye Tang (Decoction) in *Wenbing Tiaobian*.

现代临床，麦冬为主的复方常用于治疗慢性胃炎、急性胃炎、非溃疡性消化不良等属于阴虚胃热者，如麦门冬汤。

In modern clinical practice, Maidong compatibility such as Maimendong Tang can be often used to treat chronic gastritis, acute gastritis, non-ulcerative dyspepsia and so on which belong to yin deficiency and stomach heat.

2. **肺阴虚证**　治阴虚肺燥有热的鼻燥咽干、干咳痰少、咳血、咽痛音哑等症，宜与阿胶、石膏、桑叶、枇杷叶等配伍，如《医门法律》清燥救肺汤；治阴虚火旺，咽喉肿痛，宜与玄参、桔梗、甘草等滋阴降火、利咽止痛药配伍，如经验方玄麦甘桔汤。

2 Syndrome of Deficiency of Lung Yin

When treating patients with nasal dryness, dry throat, dry phlegm, coughing blood, and dull sore throat caused by yin deficiency, lung dryness and heat, Maidong can be compatible with Ejiao, Shigao, Sangye, Pipaye, and so on, such as Qingzao Jiufei Tang in *Yimen Falv*. For patients with sore throat due to yin deficiency with effulgent fire, Maidong can be compatible with nourishing yin to reduce pathogenic fire, soothing the throat to relieve pain such as Xuanshen, Jiegeng, and Gancao, such as the classical formula Xuanmai Ganjie Tang.

现代临床，麦冬配伍常用于治疗放射性肺炎、慢性咽喉炎等属于阴虚肺热者，如玄麦甘桔汤。

In modern clinical practice, Maidong compatibility such as Xuanmai Ganju Tang, etc. is often used to treat radiation pneumonia and chronic pharyngitis, which are yin deficiency with lung heat.

3. 心阴虚证 治心阴虚有热之心烦、失眠多梦、健忘、心悸怔忡，宜与生地黄、酸枣仁、柏子仁等合用以养阴、安神，如《摄生秘剖》天王补心丹。治热伤心营，神烦少寐者，宜与黄连、生地黄、玄参等清心凉血、养阴之品配伍，如《温病条辨》清营汤。

3 Syndrome of Deficiency of Heart Yin

Treatment of patients with heart yin deficiency with fever causing upset, insomnia, dreaminess, forgetfulness, palpitations, Maidong can be compatible with the products of nourishing yin and soothing nerves such as Shengdihuang, Suanzaoren, and Baiziren, such as Tianwang Buxin Wan in *Shesheng Mipou*. For patients suffering from annoyance and sleeplessness due to heat damaging heart nutrient, Maidong can be compatible with Huanglian, Shengdihuang, Xuanshen and other medicines for relieving vexation, cooling blood, and nourishing yin, such as Qingying Tang in *Wenbing Tiaobian*.

现代临床，麦冬配伍常用于可用于治疗冠心病、充血性心力衰竭属于气阴两虚者，如参麦注射液。

In modern clinical practice, Maidong compatibility (such as Shenmai Injections) is often used to treat coronary heart disease and congestive heart failure, which belong to syndrome of dual deficiency of qi and yin.

【用法用量】
II Administration and Dosage

6~12g。

6~12g decoction.

【注意事项】
III Precautions

凡脾胃虚寒泄泻，胃有痰饮湿浊及暴感风寒咳嗽者忌服。

Patients with diarrhea due to spleen-stomach deficiency cold, phlegm-dampness syndrome, and cough induced by wind-cold are avoided taking.

甘 草

Gancao
(Glycyrrhizae Radix et Rhizoma)

甘草以内蒙古伊盟的杭锦旗及甘肃、宁夏的阿拉善旗一带为其道地产区。临床常用炮制品主要为生甘草、炙甘草。甘草甘平，归心、肺、脾、胃经，具有补脾益气，清热解毒，祛痰止咳，缓急止痛，调和诸药的功效，主治心气不足、脾气虚证、咳喘证等。甘草主要含三萜类、黄酮类、挥发油等成分，有抗菌，抗病毒，抗炎，解毒，抗氧化，延缓衰老，抗肿瘤，抗突变等药理作用，可用于治疗慢性胃肠炎、消化性溃疡、慢性肝炎等属脾胃气虚证者。甘草有盐皮质类固醇样作用，不宜长期或短期大量服用。

Gancao is a noted genuine regional medicinal produced in Hang Jin Qi in Inner Mongolia province, A La Shan Qi in Ningxia province and Gansu province. The clinical processed products are Shenggancao (raw) and Zhigancao (processed). Gancao is sweet in flavor and neutral in nature, and enters the heart, lung, spleen and stomach meridians. It has the effect of invigorating spleen and replenishing qi, heat-clearing and detoxifying, dispelling phlegm to stop coughing, relieving spasm and pain, and harmonizing the properties of the medicine. That can treat the symptoms of heart qi deficiency, spleen qi deficiency, cough syndrome, etc. Gancao mainly contains triterpenoids, flavonoids, volatile oil, etc, which possesses various pharmacological effects, such as antibacterial, antiviral, anti-inflammatory, detoxifying, anti-oxidant, anti-aging, anti-tumor, anti-mutation, etc. It can be used for the treatment of chronic gastroenteritis, peptic ulcer, chronic hepatitis and other syndromes which belong to the syndrome of deficiency of spleen qi and stomach qi. Gancao has a corticosteroid effect, so it should not be used for a long time or in large doses.

【品种与品质】
[Variety and Quality]

一、基原品种与品质
I Origin Varieties and Quality

1. **品种概况**　来源于豆科植物甘草 *Glycyrrhiza uralensis* Fisch.、胀果甘草 *Glycyrrhiza inflata* Bat. 或光果甘草 *Glycyrrhiza glabra* L. 的干燥根及根茎。

1 Variety

Gancao is the dry roots and rhizomes of *Glycyrrhiza uralensis* Fisch., *Glycyrrhiza inflata* Bat. or *Glycyrrhiza glabra* L. of leguminous.

甘草始载于《神农本草经》。宋代苏颂《本草图经》云："春生青苗，高一二尺，叶如槐叶，七月开紫花似奈，冬结实作角子如毕豆。根长者三四尺，粗细不定，皮赤，上有横梁，梁下皆细根也"，文献中描述的"甘草"原植物与现代所用豆科甘草属植物无异。

Gancao was first recorded in the book of *Shennong Bencao Jing*. In the Book of *Bencao Tujing (Illustration of Meteria Medica)* by Su Song in the Song Dynasty, it reads: Seedlings grow in spring and are 30 to 60 centimeters in height. The leaves are like locust leaves. The purple flowers bloom in July, the fruit that bears in winter is like pea. The roots are 90 to 120 centimeters in length, some are thick and thin, the skin is red. There are beams on the top and thin roots under the beam. The original plant of "Gancao" is consistent with all modern leguminous plants.

2. **种植采收**　以野生为主，但新疆、内蒙古、甘肃、及宁夏部分地区也有种植。主要采用种子繁殖、根茎繁殖和分株繁殖三种方式于春季或秋季栽培。春、秋二季皆可采挖，春季由清明至夏至采收；秋季由白露至地冻采收；采收期因各地气候、土壤条件存在很大差异而不尽相同。刚采挖的甘草将外表栓皮削去，习称"粉草"。

2 Planting and Harvesting

Gancao is mainly wild, but it is also cultivated in Xinjiang, Inner Mongolia, Hexi corridor in Gansu province, Longxi and some areas of Ningxia province. It is mainly cultivated in spring or autumn by seed propagation, rhizome propagation and individual plant propagation. Gancao can be harvested in both spring and autumn; Spring from Qingming to the Summer Solstice harvest; Harvest from White Dew to the Frozen Ground, and the harvest period varies with the change of climate and soil condition. The surface of Gancao is cut off by emboli, commonly known as "Fen Cao".

3. **道地性及品质评价**　自古以来内蒙古伊盟的杭锦旗及甘肃、宁夏是甘草的道地产区。现代甘草性状评价标准是以外皮细紧、色红棕、质坚实、体重、断面黄白色、粉性足、味甜者为佳。

3 Genuineness and Quality Evaluation

According to historical records, Hangjinqi in Inner Mongolia, and A La Shan Qi in Gansu province and Ningxia are genuine production areas of Gancao. The morden evaluation criteria traits of superior Gancao characters are thin and tight outer skin, red-brown color, solid quality, weight, yellow-white cross section, abundant starch, and sweet taste.

甘草主要含有三萜类（甘草甜素、甘草次酸、甘草苷等）、黄酮类（异甘草苷、甘草利酮等）和多糖。一般认为，甘草甜素为其主要甜味物质，也是其多种药理作用的主要物质基础，甘草苷是其调节消化系统功能的主要物质基础，甘草多糖是其调节免疫功能的主要物质基础，甘草黄酮是其抗炎、抗病毒、保护肺组织的主要物质基础。此外，甘草还含有甾醇、微量元素等。《中国药典》规定甘草中甘草苷不得少于 0.50%、甘草酸不得少于 2.0%。

Gancao mainly contains triterpenes (glycyrrhizin, glycyrrhizic acid, liquiritin, etc.), flavonoids (isoliquiritin, licoricone) and polysaccharides. It is generally believed that glycyrrhizin as its main sweet substance, as well as the main material basis for its various pharmacological effects. Liquiritin is the major material basis of regulating the function of the digestive system. Glycyrrhizae polysaccharide is the major material basis of regulating immune function. Glycyrrhizae flavone is the main material basis of its anti-inflammatory, antiviral and lung tissue protection. In addition, Gancao also contains sterol, trace elements, etc. The *Pharmacopoeia of the people's Republic of China* stipulates that liquiritin in Gancao shall not be less than 0.50% and glycyrrhizin not less than 2.0%.

二、炮制品种与品质
II Processed Varieties and Quality

甘草的炮制品种有甘草片、炙甘草 2 种。甘草片长于清热解毒、化痰止咳；蜜炙后，长于补脾和胃、益气复脉。

At present, there are two processed products of Gancao, including Gancao slice and Zhigancao (processed). Gancao slice is good at heat-clearing and detoxicating, dispelling phlegm and relieving cough. After roasted with honey, it can tonify the spleen and stomach, replenishing qi and complex pulse.

甘草片以外表皮红棕色或灰棕色、切面中心黄白色、质坚实、具粉性、味甜而特殊者为佳；炙甘草以切面黄色至深黄色，略有黏性，具焦香气，味甜者为佳。《中国药典》规定甘草片中甘草苷不得少于 0.45%、甘草酸不得少于 1.8%；炙甘草中甘草苷不得少于 0.50%、甘草酸不得少于 1.0%。

Gancao slice with some characteristics such as the skin reddish-brown or grey-brown solid, weight, yellow-white cut center, abundant starch and sweet taste is considered for the superior product. Zhigancao (processed) has yellow to deep yellow cut surface, slightly viscous, with burnt fragrance, sweet taste for the characteristics of the best products. The *Pharmacopoeia of the people's Republic of China* stipulates that liquiritin in Gancao slice should not be less than 0.45% and glycyrhizin not less than 1.8%. The liquiritin in Zhigancao (processed) should not be less than 0.5% and glycyrhizin should not be less than 1.0%.

三、中成药品种与品质
III Varieties and Quality of Chinese Patent Medicines

含甘草或其炮制品的中成药有 2300 余个，其中药典收载 400 余个。以甘草为君药或主药的品种有炙甘草合剂（颗粒）、甘草附子丸等。在中成药的品质控制中一般采用显微鉴别、薄层色谱法确定其存在，采用含量测定法进行有效成分的限定。如银翘散采用显微鉴别法观察晶纤维来确定甘草的存在；三拗片、小建中片采用薄层色谱鉴别法，与对照药材在色谱中相应的位置上显相同颜色的荧光斑点以确定甘草的存在；四君子丸、理中丸除了采用薄层色谱鉴别法与对照药材对照来确定甘草的存在外，同时还采用高效液相色谱法测定甘草酸的含量以保证药效。

There are more than 2300 Chinese patent medicines containing Gancao or its processed products and more than 400 Chinese patent medicines are contained in the Chinese Pharmacopoeia. Gancao as sovereign or the main medicinal varieties are Zhigancao Heji (Mixture). Keli, Gancaofuzi Wan, etc. In the quality control of Chinese patent medicine is generally determined by microscopic identification and TLC to determine the existence of Gancao, and content determination is used to limit the effective ingredients. For example, Yinqiao San (Powder) uses microscopic identification method to observe the crystal fiber determine the existence of Gancao; Sanjiao Pian (Tablets) and Xiaojianzhong Pian (Tablets) control medicine of Gancao have shown the same color fluorescent spots at corresponding positions in the chromatography to determine the existence of Gancao by TLC. Sijunzi Wan and lizhong Wan not only used TLC to identify the presence of Gancao, but also used HPLC to determine the content of glycyrrhizic acid to ensure the efficacy.

【制药】
[Pharmacy]

一、产地加工
I Processing in Production Area

甘草采收后需除去残茎、须根，按规格要求切成段，晾至半干，然后按根的粗细、大小分等级，捆成小捆，继续晒至全干。

For removing impurities and non-medicinal parts, drying of medicinal materials and according to the quality of the price, after harvesting, the residual stems and fibrous roots should be removed, cut into sections according to the specifications, and then hang to semi-dry, and then according to the size and length of the root classification, bundled into small bundles, continue to dry.

二、饮片炮制
II Processing of Decoction Pieces

甘草的炮制方法在古代多达16种，而现代以净制、切制、蜜制为主要加工工序，由此加工的甘草片、炙甘草成为商品规格中的主流。

There are more than 16 processed methods of Gancao in ancient times, while the main processed process in modern time is cleaning, cutting and honey-processed. Gancao slice and Zhigancao (processed) in this way have become the mainstream in commercial specifications.

甘草蜜制后其补益作用增强，与蜂蜜本身具有补益作用可起协同效应有关。

Gancao roasted by honey can enhance the tonic effect; honey has the tonic effect which has a synergistic effect with Gancao.

三、中成药制药
III Pharmacy of Chinese Patent Medicines

含甘草的中成药，剂型十分丰富。各制剂入药方式主要为粉末和水煎液。

The pharmaceutical form of Chinese patent medicines of Gancao; is very rich. And the powder and decoction of Gancao is mainly used to make preparations.

如以炙甘草入药的补中益气丸，将其与他药粉碎制成蜜丸，除了较完全保留炙甘草的药效成分、满足蜜丸成形所需之外，还能起到缓释的作用。又如止咳喘颗粒，制备过程中将炙甘草水煎煮提取，既使炙甘草中亲水性有效成分如甘草酸最大限度被提取出，又能使其迅速发挥药效作用。多种合剂如杏仁止咳合剂，制备过程中多使用到采用水提醇沉制得的甘草流浸膏进行配制，除去部分醇不溶性成分及杂质，同时保留水溶性有效成分，达到合剂制剂要求。

For example, Buzhong Yiqi Wan contains Zhigancao (processed), crushing it with other medicines to make honey pills, in addition to retaining the effective ingredients of Zhigancao (processed) and completely to meet the needs of honey pills formation; it also has a slow-release effect. During the preparation of Zhikechuan Keli, Zhigancao (processed) is extracted by water, so that the hydrophilic effective components such as glycyrrhizicacid are extracted to the maximum, and also make it quickly play a medicinal effect. There are many mixtures of Gancao, such as Xingrenzhike Heji, Gancao stream extract prepared by water extraction and alcohol precipitation in the preparation process; it removes some alcohol-insoluble ingredients and impurities, while retaining water-soluble active ingredients to meet the requirements of the mixture preparation.

【性能功效】
[Property and Efficacy]

一、性能
I Property

甘草性甘，平；归心、肺、脾、胃经。

Gancao is sweet in flavor, neutral in nature, and it enters heart, lung, spleen and stomach meridians.

二、功效
II Efficacy

1. **补脾益气** 甘草温中益气，补益脾气，调和脾胃。其功效的发挥与其调节消化系统功能、调节机体免疫功能等药理作用密切相关。甘草调节消化系统和免疫功能的有效物质基础主要是甘草甜素、甘草次酸等成分，通过缩短胃排空时间、促进胰液分泌、增加白细胞和骨髓有核细胞数量等发挥作用。

1 Invigorating the Spleen and Replenishing Qi

Gancao has the functions of warming middle and replenishing qi, benefiting spleen qi and harmonizing the spleen and stomach. Its efficacy is closely related to its pharmacological effects such as regulating the function of the digestive system and regulating the immune function of the body. The effective material basis of Gancao for regulating the digestive system and regulating the body's immune function is mainly glycyrrhizic acid, glycyrrhetic acid, etc. It works by shortening gastric emptying time, promoting pancreatic juice secretion, and increasing the number of leukocytes and bone marrow nucleated cells.

2. **清热解毒** 甘草通经脉，利血气，清热邪，解热毒。其功效的发挥与抗菌、抗病毒、抗炎、抗应激等药理作用密切相关。甘草的抗菌、抗病毒、抗炎、抗应激等药理作用，主要的有效物质基础是甘草甜素、甘草次酸、总黄酮，通过

抑制大肠杆菌和金黄色葡萄球菌、抑制呼吸道合胞病毒（RSV）复制、抑制二甲苯致小鼠耳廓肿胀等发挥作用。

2 Clearing Heat and Removing Toxincity

Gancao can dredge the meridians, benefiting qi and blood, clearing the heat evil, and detoxifying heat poison. Its efficacy is closely related to pharmacological effects such as antibacterial, antiviral, anti-inflammatory and anti-stress, and the main effective material basis is glycyrrhizic acid, glycyrrhetic acid and flavones. It works by inhibiting E. coli, staphylococcus aureus, inhibiting respiratory syncytial virus (RSV) replication, and suppressing swelling caused by xylene.

3. **祛痰止咳** 甘草补益肺气，润肺止咳，祛痰平喘。其功效的发挥与镇咳、祛痰、保护肺组织等药理作用密切相关。主要物质基础是甘草次酸、甘草黄酮等，主要通过提高咳嗽的吸气时间、减轻长期被动吸烟小鼠肺部损伤，减轻博莱霉素肺纤维化大鼠肺泡炎症和纤维化的病变程度等发挥治疗作用。

3 Dispelling Phlegm to Stop Cough

Gancao has the function of replenishing and restoring lung qi, moistening lung to suppress cough, dispelling phlegm and calms wheezing. The function of Gancao is closely related to its pharmacological effects such as settling cough, dispelling phlegm, lung tissue protection and others. The main effective material basis is glycyrrhizic acid and flavones, and it mainly plays a therapeutic role by increasing the inhalation time of cough, reducing the lung injury in long-term passive smoking mice, and reducing the degree of alveolar inflammation and fibrosis in bleomycin-induced pulmonary fibrosis rats.

4. **缓急止痛** 甘草味甘，能益气，善走诸经，无处不到，能润燥养筋，缓急止痛。该功效的发挥与镇痛等药理作用密切相关，主要的物质基础是黄酮类成分。

4 Relieving Spasm and Pain

Gancao is sweet in flavor, so it can nourish qi and good at dredge the meridians, and also has the effect of moisturizing dryness and nourishing muscle, relieving spasm and pain. The effect is closely related to pharmacological effects such as analgesia. The main material basis is flavonoids.

5. 调和诸药　甘草有中和之性，缓和药物之峻烈，解百药之毒。其功效的发挥与其吸附毒物、沉淀毒物及延缓有毒成分的吸收、拮抗或减轻有毒成分的毒性、肾上腺皮质激素样作用、提高小鼠肝细胞色素 P_{450} 的含量等药理作用密切有关，有效物质基础是甘草甜素。

5 Harmonizing the Properties of Medicinals

Gancao has the properties of neutralizing and the stimulation of relief medicinals, and it can remove the toxicity of hundreds of medicinals. This effect is closely related to the pharmacological effects of absorption of toxic substances, precipitation of toxic substances, delaying the absorption of toxic substances, antagonizing or reducing the toxicity of toxic substances, adrenal corticosteroid-like effects, and increasing the content of cytochrome P_{450} in the liver of mice. The main material basis is glycyrrhizic acid.

【应用】
[Applications]

一、主治病证
I Indications

1. 脾气虚证　治疗脾气虚证，常配伍人参、白术等以补气、益气健脾，如《太平惠民和剂局方》四君子汤；若脾虚日久，中气下陷，内脏下垂者，配伍升麻、柴胡以补脾益气，如《脾胃论》补中益气汤。

1 Spleen Qi Deficiency Syndrome

Gancao can be combined with Renshen, Baizhu, etc, which has the effect of nourishing qi, replenishing qi to invigorate the spleen and treat deficiency of spleen qi, such as Sijunzi Tang in *Taiping Huimin Heji Ju Fang*. And combined with Shengma, Chaihu has invigorate spleen and replenish qi effect to treat someone is deficiency of

spleen a long time, sinking of middle energizer, visceral droop such as Buzhong Yiqi Tang in *Piwei Lun*.

现代临床，甘草配伍常用于治疗慢性胃肠炎、消化性溃疡、慢性肝炎等属于脾胃气虚证者，如四君子汤、小建中汤、甘草泻心汤等。

In modern clinicial practice, Gancao compatibility is often used in the treatment of chronic gastroenteritis, peptic ulcer and chronic hepatitis and other deficiency of spleen qi syndrome, such as Sijunzi Tang, Xiaojianzhong Tang, Gancao Xiexin Tang and so on.

2. 心气不足证　对气血两虚，可与阿胶、人参等配伍以气血双补，如《伤寒论》炙甘草汤；对心气不足之失眠、多梦等，选用《备急千金要方》甘草丸。

2 Heart Qi Deficiency Syndrome

Gancao can be used with Ejiao and Renshen to tonify qi and blood to treat qi and blood deficiency, such as Zhigancao Tang in *Shanghan Lun (Treatise on Cold Damage Diseases)*. Someone has insomnia and dreaminess caused by heart qi deficiency, which can be treated with the Gancao Wan in *Beiji Qianjin Yao Fang (Essential Recipes for Emergent Use Worth a Thousand Gold)*.

现代临床，甘草配伍常用于多种心律失常属于心气不足、心动悸，脉结代等证者，如炙甘草汤、桂枝甘草汤等。

In modern clinicial practice, Gancao compatibility is often applied to a variety of arrhythmias like heart qi deficiency, heart palpitations and pulse generation, such as Zhigancao Tang (Decoction), Guizhiganca Tang (Decoction), etc.

3. 咳喘证　对外感风寒之咳喘，可与麻黄等配伍，如《太平惠民和剂局方》三拗汤；对风热袭肺之咳喘者，与桑叶等配伍，如《温病条辨》桑菊饮；对寒痰咳喘者，常与干姜、五味子等配伍，如《伤寒论》小青龙汤；对肺燥干咳者，与麦冬、桑叶等配伍，如《医门法律》清燥救肺汤；对热毒而致肺痈咳唾腥臭脓痰及湿痰咳嗽者，还可配伍桔梗。

3 Cough and Asthma Syndrome

Gancao combined with Mahuang can be

used to treat cough and pant caused by exogenous wind-cold syndrome, such as San'ao Tang in *Taiping Huimin Heji Ju Fang*. When the cough and asthma are caused by wind-heat assailing the lung, Gancao is commonly used with Sangye, such as Sangju Yin in *Wenbing Tiaobian*. Cold-phlegm to cough and asthma can be used with Ganjiang, Wuweizi, such as Xiaoqinglong Tang in *Shanghan Lun (Treatise on Cold Damage Diseases)*. For lung dryness dry cough commonly used with Maidong, Sangye, such as Qingzhao Jiufei Tang in *Yimen Falv,* and can also be used with Jiegeng for the treatment of heat toxin caused by lung carbuncle cough smelly pus sputum and wet sputum cough.

现代临床，甘草配伍常用于治疗上呼吸道感染、急性扁桃体炎、急性支气管炎、肺炎、慢性肺部疾病等属于外感邪气犯肺或肺气不利等所致咳嗽痰多证者，如三拗汤、麻黄汤、麻黄杏仁甘草石膏汤、桔梗汤、玄麦甘桔汤等。

In modern clinical practice, Gancao compatibility is often applied to treat upper respiratory tract infection, acute tonsillitis, acute bronchitis, pneumonitis, chronic pulmonary diseases, which belong to cough and phlegm syndrome caused by exogenous evil invade lung or lung qi stoppage, such as San'ao Tang, Mahuang Tang, Mahuang Xingren Gancao Shigao Tang, Jiegen Tang and Xuanmai Ganjie Tang, etc.

4. 挛急痛证　对各种原因所致的脘腹、四肢拘挛疼痛，如中焦虚寒者，可配伍桂枝、饴糖等，如《金匮要略》小建中汤；对湿热痢疾腹痛，多配伍黄连、黄芩等，如《伤寒论》葛根芩连汤。

4 Hypertonicity to Pain Syndrome

For pain in the abdomens and limbs caused by various reasons, such as deficiency and cold of middle energizer, Gancao can treat it combined with Guizhi, Yitang, for example, Xiaojianzhong Tang in *Jingui Yaolue*. For stomachache caused by dysentery with dampness-heat, Gancao is used with Huanglian, Huangqin, etc. such as Gegen Qinlian Tang in *Shanghan Lun (Treatise on Cold Damage Diseases)*.

现代临床，甘草配伍常用于治疗胃痛、腹痛及腓肠肌挛急疼痛等属于肝郁筋急者，如芍药甘草汤。

In modern clinical practice, Gancao compatibility is used to treat stomachache, abdominal pain and gastrocnemius acute pain caused by the liver depression and sinew hypertonicity, such as Shaoyao Gancao Tang (Decoction).

5. 热毒疮疡，咽喉肿痛　对痈疽疮疡，常与金银花、连翘等配伍，如《校注妇人良方》仙方活命饮；对咽喉红肿疼痛不甚者，可单用本品，如《伤寒论》桔梗汤。

5 Toxic Heat Ulcer and Swollen Sore Throat

Gancao can be compatible with Jinyin hua, Lianqiao for treatment of toxic swellings and sores, such as Xianfang Huomin Yin in *Jiaozhu Furen Lian Fang (Revised Good Remedies for Women)*. It is also used in throat redness pain, such as Jiegen Tang in *Shanghan Lun (Treatise on Cold Damage Diseases)*.

现代临床甘草配伍常用于治疗用于多种热毒证、咽喉肿痛，如《伤寒论》甘桔汤。

In modern clinical practice, Gancao compatibility is used to treat various heat toxin syndromes, swollen sore throat, such as Ganjie Tang in *Shanghan Lun (Treatise on Cold Damage Diseases)*.

6. 调和药性、药味　对药物或食物中毒，可重用本品浓煎，亦可与绿豆同煎。甘草具有缓和药性，调和百药的作用。

6 Harmonizing the Medicine Property and Flavor

For poisoning by medicinal or food, Gancao can be used for thick decocting or decocted with Lvdou (Vigna Radiata). Gancao has an effect of alleviating the medicinal property, harmonizing hundreds of medicines.

现代临床，甘草重用本品浓煎或与绿豆同煎可防治药物、食物及重金属等中毒。

In modern clinical practice, the concentrated solution by decocting Gancao and decocting it with Lvdou can be used to treat poison by medicinal, food or heavy metal.

二、用法用量
II Administration and Dosage

2~10g。

2~10g, for decoction.

三、注意事项
III Precautions

1. 不宜与海藻、京大戟、红大戟、芫花、甘遂同用。

1 Gancao should not be used with Haizao, Jingdaji, Hongdaji (Knoxiae Radix), Yuanhua, Gansui.

2. 湿盛胀满、浮肿者不宜用。

2 Patients with excessive humidity and puffy swelling should not use Gancao.

3. 单味甘草或甘草的复方制剂，不宜长期或短期大量服用。

3 Gancao or Gancao's compound preparations are not suitable for long-term or short-term heavy use.

当 归

Danggui
(Angelicae Sinensis Radix)

甘肃岷县为当归道地产区。因入药部分不同，当归分为全当归、当归头、当归身、当归尾、当归须等，功用亦各有特点。当归味甘、辛，性温，归肝、心、脾经，有补血活血，调经止痛，润肠通便的功效，主治血虚萎黄，眩晕心悸，月经不调，经闭痛经，虚寒腹痛，风湿痹痛，跌打损伤，痈疽疮疡，肠燥便秘等。当归中主要含挥发油、有机酸、糖类、鞣质及微量元素等，有抗血小板聚集、抗血栓、抗心肌缺血、扩张血管、调节子宫平滑肌、调节免疫、抗炎、镇痛、保肝、抗氧化、抗辐射、延缓衰老等药理作用，可用于治疗慢性盆腔炎、月经不调、肌肉和关节疼痛及神经痛等属血虚气弱证和疼痛诸证者。

The genuine production area of Danggui is Minxian County of Gansu Province. It is divided into different parts to be used as medicine, functions of the Danggui head, body, tail and root of Danggui also play different roles. Danggui is sweet, pungent, warm in nature, and enters the liver, heart, and spleen medicines. It has the effects of tonifying and activating blood, regulating menstruation and relieving pain, moistening the intestines to relax the bowels. In Chinese medicine clinical practice, Danggui is often used to treat sallow complexion due to blood deficiency, dizziness and palpitations, menstrual irregularities, amenorrhea and dysmenorrhea, abdominal pain due to deficiency cold, numbing pain due to wind-dampness, injury such as contusion, sprain or fracture from falling and blow, carbuncle, gangrene, sore and ulcers, astriction due to intestinal dryness, and so on. Danggui mainly contains volatile oil, organic acids, sugars, tannins and trace elements. Danggui has pharmacological effects such as anti-platelet aggregation, anti-thrombosis, anti-myocardial ischemia, dilation of blood vessels, regulation of uterine smooth muscle, regulation of immunity, anti-inflammatory, analgesia, liver protection, antioxidant, anti-radiation and delaying aging, etc. Clinically, Danggui is used to treat chronic pelvic inflammatory disease, irregular menstruation, muscle, joint pain and neuralgia, which belong to blood and qi deficiency syndromes, pain and so on.

【品种品质】
[Variety and Quality]

一、基原品种与品质
I Origin Varieties and Quality

1. **品种概况**　来源于伞形科植物当归 *Angelica sinensis* (Oliv.) Diels 的干燥根。

1 Variety

Danggui is derived from the dried roots of *Angelica sinensis* (Oliv.) Diels of Umbelliferous plants.

当归始载于《神农本草经》。《本草图经》记载道："春生苗，绿叶有三瓣，七八月开花似时罗，浅紫色。根黑黄色。二月、八月采根阴干。然苗有二种，都类芎藭，而叶有大小为异，茎梗比芎藭甚卑下。根亦二种，大叶名马尾当归，细叶名蚕头当归"。所附文州（今甘肃文县）当归药图，与今用之植物当归 *Angelica sinensis* (Oliv.) Diels 一致。

Danggui was first published in *Shennong Bencao Jing*. *Bencao Tujing* recorded that Danggui grows in spring with three leaves, and blooms in July and August like light purple dill. The roots are dark yellow, harvested in February and August and placed in the shade to dry. There are two kinds of seedlings, both of which are similar to those of Chuanxiong, but the size of the leaves and roots are inconsistent, the stem is shorter than that of Chuanxiong. The kind with large leaves is called Mawei Danggui, and the kind with thin leaves is called Cantou Danggui (silkworm head Danggui). The attached map of Danggui in Wenzhou (Wenxian County, Gansu) in the book is consistent with *Angelica sinensis* (Oliv.) Diels.

2. **种植采收**　当归以人工种植为主，主产于甘肃，湖北、云南、四川等地亦产。采用种子育苗移栽繁殖，通常栽培至第二年秋末果实成熟，种子呈粉白色时即可采收。

2 Planting and Harvesting

Danggui is mainly planted artificially, mainly produced in Gansu. In addition, it is also produced in Hubei, Yunnan, Sichuan and other places. Danggui seeds were used for seedling, transplanting and propagation. Danggui can be harvested when the fruits are mature and the seeds are pink-white at the end of the second year of cultivation.

3. **道地性评价及品质评价**　据《本草经集注》记载魏晋时期便确立了陇西（今甘肃临洮）当归道地产区的地位。《新修本草》强调了甘肃马尾当归之质优；《本草纲目》评价："今陕、蜀、秦州（今甘肃）、汶州诸州人多栽莳为货，以秦归头圆，尾多色紫，气香肥润者名马尾归，最胜他处。"至此，甘肃产当归品质最优，后世公认。

3 Genuineness and Quality Evaluation

According to *Bencaojing Jizhu*, Longxi (now Lintong, Gansu) was identified as the genuine production area of Danggui. *Xinxiu Bencao* emphasized the superior quality of horsetail Danggui produced in Gansu. According to *Bencao Gangmu*, in Shaanxi, Sichuan, Gansu and other places, most of them use cultivated Danggui as their goods. Among them, the Danggui from Gansu has a round head, a light purple tail, a fragrant smell, and a plump body, which is called Mawei Danggui, and its quality is better than others. Since then, the quality of Danggui produced in Gansu is the best, later recognized.

当归形态上以主根肥大、身长、支根少、油润者为佳，颜色上以外皮色黄棕、断面色黄白为佳，气味上以香气浓厚为佳。当归主要含有挥发油、有机酸、多糖、黄酮、鞣质及微量元素等化学成分。《中国药典》规定，本品按干燥品计算，挥发油不得少于 0.4%（mg/g），阿魏酸（$C_{10}H_{10}O_4$）不得少于 0.05%。

It is better to have "large root", "long body", "few branch roots", and "oily" in shape, and "yellow-brown skin" and "yellow-white section" in color, and "strong aroma" in smell. Danggui mainly contains chemical components such as volatile oil, organic acids, polysaccharides, flavones, tannins and trace element, etc. The

Pharmacopoeia of the people's Republic of China stipulates in the evaluation of chemical indicators that the volatile oil in Danggui should not be less than 0.4% (mg/g), and the ferulic acid ($C_{10}H_{10}O_4$) should not be less than 0.05% by dry product.

二、炮制品种与品质
II Processed Varieties and Quality

《中国药典》收录的当归炮制品种有 2 个，包括生当归、酒当归。生当归长于补血调经，润肠通便，活血解毒；酒当归长于活血散瘀，补血调经。生当归饮片外表皮浅棕色至棕褐色，切面黄白色或淡棕黄色，平坦有裂隙，中间有浅棕色的形成环，并有多数棕色的油点，香气浓郁，味甘、辛、微苦者为佳；酒当归以表面深黄色或浅棕黄色，有部分焦斑，味甘、微苦，香气浓厚，有酒香气者为佳。

At present, there are 2 kinds of processed products in the *Pharmacopoeia of the people's Republic of China*, including Shengdanggui (raw product), Jiudanggui (liquor-processed product). Shengdanggui is good at nourishing blood and regulating menstruation, relaxing bowels, promoting the blood circulation and detoxifying, while Jiudanggui has a faculty of activating the blood to dissipate stasis, tonifying blood to regulate menstruation. Shengdanggui has a light brown to tan outer skin, a yellow-white or pale brown-yellow cut surface, flat and cracked, a light brown ring in the middle, and some brown oil spots. It is better to have a strong aroma, sweet, pungent, and slightly bitter taste. Jiudanggui with dark yellow or light brown surface, some focal spots, sweet and slightly bitter taste, and strong liquor aroma has a good quality.

三、中成药品种与品质
III Varieties and Quality of Chinese Patent Medicines

《中国药典》收载含当归的中成药共计 290 余个。以当归为君药或主药的品种有养血当归精（糖浆、颗粒、胶囊、软胶囊）、调经止痛片等。在质量控制多采用显微鉴别和薄层色谱法确定当归的存在，以高效液相色谱法进行指标成分限量。

The current edition of the *Pharmacopoeia of the People's Republic of China* contains more than 290 Chinese patent medicines containing Danggui. The varieties taking Danggui as a sovereign medicinal include Yangxue Danggui Jing (Tangjiang, keli, jiaonang, ruanjiaonang), Tiaojing Zhitong Pian and so on. In the quality control, micro-identification and TLC are used to determine the presence of Danggui, and HPLC is used to limit the index components.

如十一味参芪片，通过显微鉴别"薄壁细胞纺锤形，表面有极细微的斜向交错纹理"确定含有当归，同时采用薄层色谱法参照当归对照药材确定当归的存在。如调经止痛片，以薄层色谱法确定当归的存在，通过高效液相色谱法测定每片含当归、川芎总量以阿魏酸（$C_{10}H_{10}O_4$）计，不得少于 50 μg。

For example, Shiyiwei Shenqi Pian, microscopy was used to identify "Thin-walled cells are spindle-shaped and have a very fine diagonally staggered surface" to determine the presence of Danggui, and TLC was also used to determine the presence of Danggui with reference to Danggui controls. Another example is Tiaojing Zhitong Pian. The existence of Danggui was determined by TLC. The total amount of Danggui and Chuanxiong in each tablet was determined by HPLC, and it should not be less than 50μg calculated with ferulic acid ($C_{10}H_{10}O_4$).

【制药】
[Pharmacy]

一、产地加工
I Processing in Production Area

秋末采挖，需及时除去茎叶、须根及泥土，待水分稍蒸发后根变软时，捆成小把烘干或熏干。

Danggui is harvested at the end of autumn. The stems, leaves, fibrous roots, and soil need to be removed in time and placed until the water is slightly evaporated and the roots are softened. And then, they are bundled into small bales to dry or smoke.

二、饮片炮制
II Processing of Decoction Pieces

仅在古代，当归的炮制方法就多达25种。宋代以来，形成了润、切、酒浸、炒的炮制工艺，至此加工的当归、酒当归成为商品规格中的主流。

In ancient times, there were as many as 25 ways to prepare Danggui. Since the Song Dynasty, the processing technology of moistening, cutting, liquor dipping, and stir-frying has formed. So far, processed Danggui and Jiudanggui (liquor-processed) have become the mainstream in product specifications.

当归酒制后水溶物增加，阿魏酸几乎无降低，收敛成分鞣质最少，还原糖和水溶性糖的含量增加，其中多糖类成分具有增强免疫的作用，实现酒制后增强活血、补血、调经的作用。

After Danggui is processed by liquor, the water soluble is increased, ferulic acid is hardly decreased, tannins is reduced. The amount of reducing sugar and water-soluble sugar is increased, among which the polysaccharide component has the function of enhancing immunity, and realizes the functions of promoting the blood circulation, nourishing blood and regulating menstruation after liquor roasting.

三、中成药制药
III Pharmacy of Chinese Patent Medicines

由当归组成的中成药制剂种类和剂型较多，主要包括口服液体、固体制剂。除此以外，还包括一部分外用制剂，如膏剂，搽剂和酊剂等。在多数现代制剂中，当归多经过提取后以提取物形式加适当辅料制备中成药制剂。在部分丸剂的制备中，当归经过粉碎成细粉后制备成丸。

Danggui is involved in many kinds of Chinese patent medicines and pharmaceutical forms, which mainly include kinds of oral liquid preparations and solid preparations. Additionally, Danggui is also involved in some external preparations, such as paste preparation, liniments, and tinctures and so on. Danggui is often used through combination with other medicinals to form a compound formula into the preparation. Among many modern preparations, the extract of Danggui is often used with the appropriate pharmaceutical excipients to prepare Chinese patent medicines. In preparation of some pills containing Danggui, the raw herbal material can also be crushed into fine powder and then appropriate pharmaceutical excipients are added to complete the preparation.

如在含有当归的乌鸡白凤颗粒的制备过程中，当归通常先采用水蒸气蒸馏的方法以提取其挥发油类成分，然后再加水煎煮提取有机酸和多糖类成分。在当归注射液的制备过程中，通过加水煎煮提取有机酸和多糖类成分，然后加入70%和80%乙醇溶液两次沉淀杂质后制备得到。

For example, during the preparation process of Wuji Baifeng Wan, the volatile oil is extracted through steam distillation, which is followed by extraction of organic acids and polysaccharides in boiling water. In preparation of Danggui injection, the raw herbal material is boiled by water to extract the organic acids and polysaccharides, and subsequently precipitated by 70% and 80% ethanol solutions for two times, to sediment and clean up impurities.

【性能功效】
[Property and Efficacy]

一、性能
I Property

当归甘、辛，温；归肝、心、脾经。

Danggui is sweet and pungent in flavor, warm in nature, and enters the liver, heart, and spleen meridians.

二、功效
II Efficacy

1. 补血活血　当归补中有动，行中有补，是补血活血之要药。其功效的发挥与当归促进机体造血功能、抗血小板聚集和抗血栓、改善血液流变性、降血脂和抗动脉粥样硬化等作用密切相关，主要的物质基础有阿魏酸、当归多糖。另外，当归的补血作用也可能与其含有维生素B_2、烟酸、叶酸等有关。

1 Tonifying and Activating Blood

Danggui can promote circulation of blood while replenishing blood; it can also replenish blood while promoting circulation of blood. Danggui is an important medicinal for tonifying and activating blood. This is closely related to the role of Danggui in promoting hematopoietic function, anti-platelet focusing and anti-thrombosis, improving blood rheology, lowering blood lipids and anti-atherosclerosis. The main material bases are ferulic acid and angelica polysaccharide. In addition, Danggui's blood-enriching effect may also be related to its content of vitamin B_2, niacin, and folic acid.

2. 调经止痛　当归辛散温补，可活血调经，散寒止痛。其功效的发挥与当归调节子宫平滑肌收缩、抗炎、镇痛等作用密切相关。当归多糖、当归挥发油是当归抗炎镇痛的有效物质。

2 Regulating Menstruation and Relieving Pain

Danggui has a pungent medicinal property, is good at dissipating cold and warm tonigication,

so it can be used to promote blood circulation, regulate menstruation, dissipate cold and relieving pain. It is closely related to the effects of Danggui on regulating uterine smooth muscle contraction, anti-inflammatory and analgesia. Angelica sinensis polysaccharide and angelica volatile oil are effective substances of Danggui for its anti-inflammatory and analgesic effects.

3. 润肠通便　当归养血润燥以通便。其功效的发挥与当归舒张胃肠平滑肌等作用密切相关，通过升高小肠推进率，调节体内胆囊收缩素（CCK-8）、胃动素（MOT）的含量发挥作用，主要物质基础是当归多糖、阿魏酸、挥发油。

3 Moistening the Intestines to Relax the Bowels

Danggui has the effect of nourishing blood and moisturizing dryness, so it can be used for relaxing the bowels. Its effects are closely related to the effect of Danggui on relaxing gastrointestinal smooth muscle and other effects, increasing the rate of small intestine advancing, regulating the content of cholecystokinin (CCK-8) and motilin (MOT) in the body. Angelica polysaccharide, ferulic acid, and volatile oil are effective substances for relaxing gastrointestinal smooth muscle.

【应用】
[Applications]

一、主治病证
I Indications

1. 血虚证　治疗心血亏虚，常配伍酸枣仁、柏子仁、白芍等；治疗心气血虚，常配伍黄芪等补气之品；治肝血亏虚，当归常配熟地、白芍等，如《医宗金鉴》补肝汤，《杂病源流犀烛》补血养肝明目汤；治心脾两虚，当归常与人参、黄芪、白术、炙草等同用，如《严氏济生方》归脾汤。

1 Blood Deficiency Syndrome

When treating patients with heart-blood

depletion, Danggui is often compatible with Suanzaoren, Baiziren, Baishao and so on. For treating patients with fearful throbbing due to heart qi blood deficiency, Danggui is often used in combination with Huangqi and other qi-enhancing medicinals. When treating patients with liver-blood depletion, Danggui is often compatible with Shudihuang, Baishao and so on, such as Bugan Tang in *Yizong Jinjian*, Buxue Yanggan Mingmu Tang in *Zabing Yuanliu Xizhu (The Origin and Developmenr of Miscellaneous Diseases)*. When treating syndrome of dual deficiency of the heart and spleen, Danggui is often compatible with Renshen, Huangqi, Baizhu, Zhigancao (processed) and so on, such as Guipi Tang in *Yanshi Jisheng Fang*.

现代临床，以当归为主的复方（如四物汤、温经汤、当归芍药散等），常用于治疗原发性痛经、子宫内膜异位症、习惯性流产、人工流产、不孕症等属于血虚兼有瘀滞病证者。以当归为主的复方（如当归补血汤、当归饮子、八珍汤等），常用于治疗贫血、慢性发热、过敏性紫癜、荨麻疹、再生障碍性贫血、白血病等属血虚气弱者。

In modern clinical practice, Danggui compatibility (such as Siwu Tang, Wenjing Tang, Danggui Shaoyao San, etc.) is often used to treat primary dysmenorrhea, endometriosis, habitual abortion, abortion analgesia, infertility, etc. which belong to blood deficiency and stasis stagnation. Besides, Danggui-based compounds (such as Danggui Buxue Tang, Danggui Yinzi, Bazhen Tang, etc.) are used to treat anemia, chronic fever, allergic purpura, urticaria, aplastic anemia, leukemia and so on, which belong to blood deficiency and qi weakness.

2. 闭经，经行腹痛　治血虚月经后期，当归常配伍熟地黄、白芍、川芎等；治血崩偏于虚寒者，常配伍阿胶、艾叶等，如《金匮要略》胶艾汤；治气血两虚之崩漏，多配伍熟地、人参、黄芩、白术等，如《傅青主女科》固本止崩汤；治血滞经闭，可与延胡索等配伍使用；治气血虚弱之经行腹痛，可配以人参、地黄、黄芪、

赤芍等。

2 Amenorrhea and Dysmenorrhea

When treating patients with low blood volume in the late menstrual period caused by blood deficiency, Danggui is often compatible with Shudihuang, Baishao, Chuanxiong and so on. When treating patients with flooding and deficiency cold, Danggui is often compatible with Ejiao, Aiye (Artemisiae Argyi Folium) and so on, such as Jiaoai Tang in *Jingui Yaolue (Synopsis of the Golden Chamber)*. For patients with flooding caused by qi and blood deficiency, Danggui is often compatible with Shudihuang, Renshen, Huangqin, Baizhu, and so on, such as Guben Zhibeng Tang in *Fuqingzhu Nvke (Fuqing Lord Gymecology Department)*. Danggui is often compatible with Yanhusuo to treat blood stagnation and amenorrhea. For treating dysmenorrhea caused by qi and blood deficiency, Danggui can be used with Renshen, Dihuang, Huangqin and Chishao.

3. 疼痛诸证　治心痛，血虚者，可与芍药、橘皮、人参、桃仁等同用，如《外台秘要》引《广济方》当归汤。治血虚有寒之腹痛，本品与生姜、羊肉同用，如《金匮要略》当归生姜羊肉汤。治疗久寒宿疾，胸腹中痛，以本品与橘皮、附子、大黄、干姜等同用，如《备急千金要方》当归汤。治疗跌打损伤瘀血作痛，如《医学发明》复元活血汤。治风湿痹痛，本品可配伍桂枝、独活、川芎等。

3 Pain

For the treatment of heartache induced by blood deficiency, Danggui is often compatible with Baishao, Jupi, Renshen, Taoren, and so on, such as Danggui Tang in Waitai Miyao (Arcame Essentials from the Imperial library) quoted from *Guangji Fang (Guangji Prescription)*. For the treatment of abdominal pain induced by blood deficiency, Danggui is often compatible with Shengjiang, mutton, such as Danggui Shengjiang Yangrou Tang in *Jingui Yaolue*. To treat chest and abdominal pain, Danggui can be used with Jupi, Fuzi, Dahuang, Ganjiang and so on, such as Danggui Tang in *Beiji Qianjin Yaofang*. To treat the pain caused by injuries from falls, such as Fuyuan Huoxue Tang (Decoction) in *Yixue Faming*. For treating rheumatism and pain, Danggui is compatible with Guizhi, Duhuo and Chuanxiong.

现代临床，以当归为主的复方常用于治疗冠状动脉硬化性心脏病、心绞痛、心律失常、高血压、肋软骨炎、坐骨神经痛、血管炎、雷诺氏病、脉管炎等属于气血瘀滞证，如桃红四物汤、当归四逆汤、血府逐瘀汤等。

Clinically, Danggui-based compounds are often used to treat coronary heart disease, angina pectoris, arrhythmia, hypertension, rib chondritis, sciatica, vasculitis, Raynaud's disease, vasculitis, etc. that belong to qi-blood stagnation syndrome such as Taohong Siwu Tang, Danggui Sini Tang, Xuefu Zhuyu Tang, etc.

4. **痈疽疮疡**　治疗疮疡初起肿胀疼痛，可与金银花、赤芍、天花粉等解毒消痈药同用，如《妇人良方》仙方活命饮；治疗痈疮成脓不溃或溃后不敛，可与黄芪、人参等同用，如《太平惠民和剂局方》十全大补汤；治疗脱疽溃烂，亦可与金银花、玄参、甘草同用，如《验方新编》四妙勇安汤。

4 Sore and Ulcer

When treating swelling and pain at the beginning of sore, Danggui can be used together with Jinyinhua, Chishao, Tianhuafen and so on, such as Xianfang Huoming Yin (Drink) in *Furen Liangfang*. For treating sore and ulcer which are difficult to rupture and not converge for a long time after rupture, Danggui can be used with Huangqi, Renshen and so on, such as Shiquan Dabu Tang (Decoction) in *Taiping Huimin Heji Ju Fang*. When treating sore ulcerated, Danggui can be used with Jinyinhua, Xuanshen, Gancao and so on, such as Simiao Yong'an Tang (Decoction) in *Yanfang Xinbian (New Compilation of Proved Recipes)*.

5. **血虚肠燥便秘**　治老年血虚肾亏之肠燥便秘，常与肉苁蓉、牛膝、升麻等同用，如《景岳全书》济川煎；治痔漏便秘，脱肛疼痛出血，常与郁李仁、枳实等配伍以润下通便止血，如《兰室秘藏》当归郁李仁汤；治消渴津亏，大便燥结，常配伍熟地、知母等以清热生津，润肠通便，如《兰室秘藏》当归润燥汤。

5 Constipation Caused by Blood Deficiency and Intestinal Dryness

When treating dry intestine-induced constipation due to blood and kidney deficiency of elderly, Danggui is compatible with Roucongrong, Niuxi, Shengma, and so on, such as Jichuan Decoction in *Jingyue Quanshu (Jingyue's Complete Works)*. For treating patients with prolapsed anal bleeding, Danggui is compatible with Yuliren, Zhishi, such as Danggui Yuliren Tang in *Lanshi Micang (OrchidHouse Secret Collection)*. For treating stool defecation, Danggui is often compatible with Shudihuang, Zhimu, such as Danggui Runzao Tang in *Lanshi MiCang*.

6. **咳喘短气**　治咳嗽气短、痰涎壅盛，常与苏子、半夏等祛痰止咳平喘药同用，如《太平惠民和剂局方》苏子降气汤。治肺肾阴亏，水泛为痰所致咳嗽痰多，呕恶喘逆等，常与熟地、半夏等配伍奏补肺益肾，止咳化痰之功，如《景岳全书》金水六君煎。

6 Cough and Breath Shortness

For cough, breath shortness, phlegm and sputum salivation, Danggui is often compatible with Suzi, Banxia, such as Suzi Jiangqi Tang in *Taiping Huimin Heji Jufang*. For cough caused by lung yin deficiency, Danggui is often compatible with Shudi, Banxia and so on, such as Jinshui Liujun Tang in *Jingyue Quanshu (Jingyue's Complete Works)*.

二、用法用量
II Administration and Dosage

6~12g。

6~12g for decoction.

三、注意事项
III Precautions

湿盛中满、大便溏泻者忌服。

People who are exuberant dampness with fullness in the middle or sloppy diarrhea should be avoided taking.

黄　芪
Huangqi
(Astragali Radix)

山西浑源、应县所产的膜荚黄芪及内蒙古产的蒙古黄芪为道地药材。临床常用炮制品主要为生黄芪、蜜黄芪等。黄芪味甘，性微温，归肺、脾经，有补气升阳，固表止汗，利水消肿，生津养血，行滞通痹，托毒排脓，敛疮生肌的功效，治疗脾肺气虚、气虚自汗、气虚水肿、气血亏虚、痈疽难溃或久溃不敛等。黄芪中主要含皂苷类、黄酮类、多糖类、氨基酸、微量元素等，有增强免疫、保肝、抗疲劳、调血压等药理作用，可用于治疗心脑血管疾病、急性肾小球肾炎、糖尿病、重症肌无力等属脾虚气陷证、气虚自汗、内热消渴及气血亏虚者。

Huangqi produced in Hunyuan and Yingxian of Shanxi and Mongolian Huangqi from Inner Mongolia are genuine medicinal materials. In clinical practice, Shenghuangqi (raw) and Mihuangqi (honey-processed) are mainly used. The nature of Huangqi is sweet and slightly warm. The meridians it entered are lung and spleen. Its key characteristics are tonifying qi and invigorating yang, securing the exterior to check sweating, inducing diuresis to alleviate edema, engendering fluid to tonify blood, relieving stagnation to dredge impediment, expelling toxin to evacuate pus, promoting tissue re-generation and wound healing. In traditional Chinese medicine clinical practice, Huangqi is often used to treat spleen and lung qi deficiency, spontaneous sweating, edema, depletion of qi and blood, and ulcer. Huangqi mainly contains saponins, flavones, polysaccharides, amino acids, trace elements, etc. Huangqi has pharmacological effects such as enhancing immunity, protecting liver, anti-fatigue, and regulating blood pressure, can be used to treat cardiovascular and cerebrovascular diseases, acute glomerulonephritis, diabetes, and myasthenia gravis, which belong to the spleen deficiency and qi sinking syndrome, exterior deficiency and spontaneous sweating, internal heat and wasting-thirst, qi and blood deficiency and so on.

【品种品质】
[Variety and Quality]

一、基原品种与品质
I Origin Varieties and Quality

1. **品种概况**　来源于豆科植物蒙古黄芪 *Astragalus membranaceus* (Fisch.) Bge. var. *mongholicus* (Bge.) Hsiao 或膜荚黄芪 *Astragalus membranaceus* (Fisch.) Bge. 的干燥根。

1 Variety

Huangqi is derived from the dried roots of the legume plant *Astragalus membranaceus* (Fisch.) Bge. var. *mongholicus* (Bge.) Hsiao or *Astragalus membranaceus* (Fisch.) Bge.

黄芪原名"老者"，首载于《神农本草经》。唐代《新修本草》开始有了黄芪原植物的最早描述："此物叶似羊齿，或如蒺藜，独茎，或作丛生"。《本草纲目》所载黄芪品种与现今药用的黄芪相符，所云栽培方法现今多用。

Huangqi was originally named "Laoqi", which was first listed in *Shennong Bencao Jing (Shennong's Classic of Materia Medica)*. According to *Xinxiu Bencao Newly Revised Materia Medica* of the Tang Dynasty, the original plants of Huangqi have leaves like goat teeth or the puncture vine, growing on single stems or in clusters. The varieties and cultivation methods of Huangqi in *Bencao Gangmu (Compendium of Materia Medica)* are consistent with the medicinal Huangqi.

2. 种植采收　黄芪以人工种植为主，以蒙古黄芪质量为佳。栽培多采用直接播种的方式，栽培品要求至少生长3~4年，以生长6~7年者质量最佳。采收时，将黄芪挖出后除净泥土、须根，切去根头，晒干。

2　Planting and Harvesting

Huangqi is mainly cultivated artificially. The quality of cultivated Mongolica Huangqi is best among them. Huangqi is cultivated mostly by sowing. The cultivated products are required to grow for at least 3 to 4 years, and the best quality is 6 to 7 years. When harvesting, Huangqi is excavated and fibrous roots and roots are removed and dried.

3. 道地性及品质评价　历代记载，唐代以甘肃为黄芪道地产区，宋代以后以山西产者为良，至清代又加内蒙古黄芪为道地药材。形态上以"身干，根条粗长，皱纹少"为佳、颜色上以"皮黄白色"为佳，味道上以"味微甜，嚼之微有豆腥味"为佳。现代黄芪除上述评价指标外认为粉性足，质硬而绵，不易折断，味甘，无黑心及空心者为佳。

3　Genuineness and Quality Evaluation

In the Tang Dynasty, Gansu is the genuine producing area of Huangqi. After the Song Dynasty, Shanxi producers were regarded as excellent varieties. To the Qing Dynasty, Huangqi in Inner Mongolia was also a genuine medicinal material. With dry body, thick and long roots, less wrinkles, yellow-white skin, slightly sweet taste, and slightly bean-flavored taste, Huangqi has a better quality. In addition to the above evaluation indicators, it is better to be powdery, hard and soft, not easy to break, sweet, and no black and hollow core.

黄芪主要含有多糖、黄酮及皂苷类成分，也是主要的药效物质基础。黄芪多糖主要有葡聚糖和杂多糖（如鼠李糖、阿拉伯糖、葡萄糖），黄酮类物质约30多种，包括槲皮素、山奈黄素、芦丁、毛蕊异黄酮等，皂苷有黄芪皂苷、异黄芪皂苷、乙酰基黄芪皂苷、大豆皂苷等四大类。不同地区的黄芪活性成分含量差异较大，黄芪主要以黄芪甲苷、毛蕊异黄酮葡萄糖苷为化学评价指标。

Huangqi mainly contains polysaccharides, flavonoids and saponins, which are the main medicinal substance basis. Astragalus polysaccharides are mainly dextran and heteropolysaccharides (such as rhamnose, arabinose, and glucose). There are more than 30 kinds of astragalus flavonoids, including quercetin, kaempferol, rutin, and isoflavones. There are four major types of saponins: astragalus saponin, isoflavone saponin, acetyl astragalus saponin and soybean saponin. The contents of active ingredients of Huangqi in different regions are quite different. Astragaloside IV and verbasil isoflavone glucoside are mainly used as the chemical evaluation indicators of Huangqi.

二、炮制品种与品质
II Processed Varieties and Quality

《中国药典》收录两种黄芪炮制品，包括生黄芪与蜜黄芪。生黄芪饮片以类圆形或椭圆形厚片为主，也有斜片、压制大片、马蹄片等规格。厚片以表面黄白色、中心深黄色，内层有棕色环纹及放射状纹理，外层有曲折裂隙，味甜，有粉性者为佳，含黄芪甲苷（$C_{41}H_{68}O_{14}$）不得少于0.040%，毛蕊异黄酮葡萄糖苷（$C_{22}H_{22}O_{10}$）不得少于0.020%。蜜黄芪形如黄芪片，以表面深黄色、滋润有光泽，味甜，有蜜糖香气，不粘手为佳，含黄芪甲苷不得少于0.030%，毛蕊异黄酮葡萄糖苷不得少于 0.020%。

In the *Pharmacopoeia of the People's Republic of China*, there are 2 types of processed products of Huangqi, including Shenghuangqi (raw) and Mihuangqi (honey-processed). Shenghuangqi slices are mainly round or oval thick tablets, and there are also oblique tablets, pressed large tablets, horseshoe tablets and other specifications. Thick tablets are yellow-white on the surface, browning and radial grains in the inner layer and circuitous crack in the outer layer, dark yellow in the core, sweet and powdery. Astragaloside IV ($C_{41}H_{68}O_{14}$) in raw Huangqi must be higher than 0.040%, and calycosin-7-glucoside ($C_{22}H_{22}O_{10}$) must be higher than 0.020%. As for Mihuangqi (honey-processed), it is better to have a dark yellow and shiny surface, taste sweet, honey aroma, and be not sticky. Astragaloside IV ($C_{41}H_{68}O_{14}$) in honey Huangqi must be higher than 0.030%, and calycosin-7-glucoside ($C_{22}H_{22}O_{10}$) must be higher than 0.020%.

三、中成药品种与品质
III Varieties and Quality of Chinese Patent Medicines

据统计,《中国药典》收载含有黄芪的中成药共计 166 个。以黄芪为君药或主药的品种有补中益气丸、归脾丸、玉屏风口服液等。以显微鉴别确定黄芪的存在,采用高效液相色谱法进行指标成分限量。如补中益气丸中以炙黄芪为君药,含量测定法限定以黄芪甲苷计。

At present, there are more than 166 Chinese patent medicines of Huangqi in the *Pharmacopoeia of the People's Republic of China*. The varieties taking Huangqi as a sovereign medicine include Buzhong Yiqi Wan, Guipi Wan, Yupingfeng Koufuye and so on. The existence of Huangqi is confirmed by microscopic identification, and the limit of index components is determined by HPLC. For example, Buzhong Yiqi Pills take Huangqi

as sovereign medicine, and their content is determined by astragaloside IV.

【制药】
[Pharmacy]

一、产地加工
I Processing in Production Area

春、秋二季采挖,除去须根和根头,晒干。

Huangqi was excavated in spring and autumn. The fibrous roots and root tip of Huangqi are removed. The roots of Huangqi were dried completely.

二、饮片炮制
II Processing of Decoction Pieces

从古至今,黄芪形成了多种炮制方法,逐渐形成了"润透-切片-蜜炙"工艺,由此加工的黄芪、蜜炙黄芪成为商品规格中的主流。

Since ancient times, there have been various methods for processing Huangqi, and gradually formed the "soaking-slicing-honey-roasted" process, Huangqi (raw product) and Mizhihuangqi (honey-processed product) have become the mainstream in product specifications.

蜜炙是使黄芪"增效"的重要手段,蜜炙后的黄芪,其黄芪多糖、黄芪皂苷含量增加,可能是因为蜜炙使皂苷成分的溶解性增加。

Honey roasted is an important means to "synergize" Huangqi. Astragalus polysaccharide and astragalus saponin contents increased in Huangqi processed by honey may be due to the increase of solubility of saponin components by honey.

三、中成药制药
III Pharmacy of Chinese Patent Medicines

含有黄芪的中成药制剂剂型丰富,包括液

体、固体制剂等。黄芪可以单独组方入制剂中，如黄芪颗粒；但是多和其他药物配伍入制剂中。在多数现代制剂中，黄芪多经过提取后以提取物形式加适当辅料制备中成药制剂。在部分丸剂的制备中，黄芪也可以粉碎成细粉后加辅料制备成丸。

Huangqi is involved in many kinds of Chinese patent medicines in various pharmaceutical forms, which mainly include kinds of oral liquid preparations and oral solid preparations. Huangqi can be formulated separately into the preparation, such preparation named as Huangqi Granules. This herbal medicine often used through combination with other herbal medicines to form a compound formula into preparation. Among many modern preparations, the extract of Huangqi is often used with the appropriate pharmaceutical excipients to prepare Chinese patent medicines. In preparation of some pills containing Huangqi, the raw herbal material can also be crushed into fine powder and then appropriate pharmaceutical excipients are added to complete the preparation.

如黄芪注射液制剂中，采用加水煎煮的方法提取三萜皂苷和多糖，为尽可能除去淀粉、蛋白质和糖类成分，采用 75% 和 85% 的乙醇溶液两次沉淀方法，从而主要得到三萜皂苷类成分。由于三萜皂苷类组分具有一定的酸性，为保证黄芪注射液的稳定性及提高皂苷类成分的溶解性等，加 20% 氢氧化钠溶液调节 pH 7.5。

For example, in the preparation of Huangqi injection, Huangqi is boiled with water to extract triterpenoid saponins and polysaccharide, and subsequently precipitated by 75% and 85% ethanol solutions respectively to remove starch, proteins and sugars as much as possible, and the triterpenoid saponins are mostly preserved. The triterpenoids possess a certain acidity, so to ensure the stability of astragalus injection and improve the solubility of saponins, the pH value of the solution is adjusted to 7.5 by adding 20% sodium hydroxide solution.

【性能功效】
[Property and Efficacy]

一、性能
I Property

黄芪甘、微温，归肺、脾经。

Huangqi is sweet in flavor, lukewarm in nature, and enters the lung and spleen meridians.

二、功效
II Efficacy

1. 补气升阳　黄芪善补肺脾之气，为补中益气要药。其功效的发挥与抗氧化、抗疲劳、抗寒冷、抗缺氧、改善胃肠道运动、保护中枢神经系统等药理作用有着密切的关系。有效物质基础主要是黄芪多糖、黄芪总黄酮、黄芪皂苷，通过作用于肾上腺轴、提高胃肠道兴奋性激素水平、改善心室收缩功能、降低海马神经元胞内钙离子水平等发挥作用。

1 Tonifying Qi and Elevating Yang

Huangqi is good for invigorating the lung and spleen, tonifying and strengthening qi and is called key drug for middle jiao. It is closely related to pharmacological effects such as anti-oxidation, anti-fatigue, anti-cold, anti-hypoxia, improving gastrointestinal movement and protecting the central nervous system. The main effective material bases are astragalus polysaccharide, astragalus total flavonoids, astragalus saponin. They work by acting on the adrenal axis, increasing gastrointestinal excitatory hormone levels, improving ventricular systolic and diastolic function, and reducing hippocampal neuron cytosolic calcium.

2. 固表止汗　黄芪能补脾肺之气，益卫固表止汗。此功效的发挥与增强免疫功能密切相关。有效物质基础主要是黄芪多糖和黄芪皂苷，通过增加脾脏、胸腺重量，增加免疫细胞（巨噬细胞、中性粒细胞、淋巴细胞）数量与活力而发挥作用。

2 Securing the Exterior to Check Sweating

Huangqi can nourish the spleen and lung qi, and can solidify antiperspirant, which is closely related to the effects on enhancing immune function. The main effective material bases are astragalus polysaccharide and astragalus saponin, which play a role by increasing the weight of the spleen and thymus and increasing the number and vitality of immune cells (macrophages, neutrophils, lymphocytes).

3. 利水消肿　黄芪善补气利水消肿。其功效的发挥与利尿等药理作用密切相关，主要的物质基础有黄芪乙酸乙酯组分和正丁醇组分，通过提高 Na^+、Cl^- 排出量，减少血清中醛固酮含量以及增加心房钠尿肽含量等发挥作用。

3 Inducing Diuresis to Alleviate Edema

Huangqi is good at nourishing qi and diuretic swelling. Its effect is closely related to pharmacological effects of diuresis. The main effective material bases are ethyl acetate component and n-butanol component, which can significantly increase Na^+、Cl^- excretion, reduce serum aldosterone (ALD), and increase atrial natriuretic peptide (ANP) content.

4. 生津养血　黄芪能补脾肺之气以养血，统行血脉。其功效的发挥与促进造血功能和血管生成、防治糖尿病等药理作用密切相关，主要物质基础为黄芪多糖，通过促进造血干细胞的分化增殖、降低内质网损伤、促进胰岛素信号蛋白的合成、升高糖原合成酶活性等发挥作用。

4 Engendering Fluid and Nourishing Blood

Huangqi can be used to promote hematopoietic function and angiogenesis, and prevent diabetes. The main material basis is astragalus polysaccharide, which plays a role by promoting the differentiation and proliferation of hematopoietic stem cells, reducing endoplasmic reticulum damage, promoting the synthesis of insulin signaling proteins, and increasing the enzyme activity of glycogen synthesis.

5. 行滞通痹　黄芪补气，气生则血行，能行滞通痹。其功效的发挥与改善血液流变学、缓解动脉粥样硬化、抗血栓、调节血压、降脂保肝等作用密切相关。主要物质基础有黄芪皂苷、黄芪多糖，通过降低血液黏稠度、降低炎症因子水平、抑制血小板聚集、调节心血管、降低肝脏的脂质沉积并提高其抗氧化能力等发挥作用。

5 Moving Stagnation

Huangqi can dredge retardant by enriching qi, which correlates with the effects of improving blood rheology, alleviating atherosclerosis, antithrombotic, regulating blood pressure, and lowering lipid and protecting liver. The main material bases are astragalus saponin and astragalus polysaccharide, which play a role by reducing blood viscosity, reducing inflammatory transmitter levels, inhibiting platelet aggregation, regulating cardiovascular, reducing liver lipid deposition and improving its antioxidant capacity.

此外，黄芪中含有微量元素硒，能提高谷胱甘肽过氧化物酶活性，激活解毒酶系，从而对肝细胞起到保护作用。

In addition, Huangqi contains trace element selenium, which can increase the activity of glutathione peroxidase and activate the detoxifying enzyme system, thereby protecting liver cells.

6. 托疮排脓，敛疮生肌　黄芪能补气托毒，温养脾胃而敛疮生肌。其功效的发挥与黄芪抗菌、抗病毒、增强免疫功能等作用密切相关，通过抑制感染病毒后的细胞病变，诱生干扰素，提高 NK 细胞的活性，减少心肌 Ca^{2+} 内流，抑制感染细胞中病毒核酸复制发挥作用。

6 Expelling Pus of Sores, Healing up Sore and Promoting Granulation

The effect of Huangqi on discharging pus, converging wounds, and promoting granulation is related to antibacterial, antiviral, and immune function enhancement. Huangqi plays a role by inhibiting the cytopathy after infection with virus, inducing interferon, increasing the activity of NK cells, reducing myocardial Ca^{2+} influx, and inhibiting viral nucleic acid replication in infected cells.

【应用】
[Applications]

一、主治病证
I Indications

1. **脾虚气陷证** 治脾气虚弱，黄芪常与人参等补气健脾药相须为用，如现代中成药参芪口服液、参芪十一味颗粒等。治脾虚中气下陷，当与人参、升麻、柴胡配伍以补中益气、升阳举陷，如《脾胃论》补中益气汤；治脾虚水湿失运，可配伍白术、茯苓等健脾利水药；治脾虚不能统血所致失血证，常与人参、白术等补气摄血药同用，如《济生方》归脾汤。

1 Syndrome of Sinking of Qi Due to Spleen Deficiency

For patients with weak spleen qi, fatigue, and loose stools, they could compare with qi-tonifying and spleen-strengthening medicinals such as Renshen. For example, modern Chinese patent medicines include Shenqi Koufuye, Shenqi Eleven Keli, and so on. For the treatment of qi depression caused by spleen deficiency, it can be used in combination with Renshen, Shengma, Chaihu and other medicinals to supplement qi and promote yang depression, such as Buzhong Yiqi Tang in *Piwei Lun*. When treating patients with water transport disorder, edema and oliguria due to spleen deficiency, Huangqi can be compatible with spleen invigorating and diuresis medicinals such as Baizhu and Fuling. For the treatment of blood loss caused by the inability of the spleen to govern the blood, Huangqi is often used with tonifying qi and controlling bleeding medicinals (Renshen and Baizhu), such as Guipi Tang in *Jisheng Fang (Prescriptions to Aid the Living)*.

2. **脾气虚证，表虚自汗** 治肺气虚弱，黄芪常配伍人参、紫菀、五味子等，如《备急千金要方》补肺汤；治疗卫虚不顾，表虚自汗，易感风邪者，常配伍白术、防风等益气固表、祛风散邪药，如《丹溪心法》玉屏风散；治脾肺气虚所致卫气不固，常配伍牡蛎、麻黄根，如《太平惠民和剂局方》牡蛎散；治阴虚盗汗，须与生地黄、黄柏等同用以滋阴降火，如"治盗汗之圣药"《兰室秘藏》当归六黄汤。

2 Spleen Qi Deficiency Syndrome, Exterior Deficiency and Spontaneous Sweating

For patients with lung qi deficiency, Huangqi is often used with Renshen, Ziwan, Wuweizi, etc., such as Bufei Tang (Decoction) in *Beiji Qianjin Yaofang (Essential Recipes for Emergent Use Worth A Thousand Gold)*. When treating patients with spontaneous sweating and susceptibility to the wind pathogen, Huangqi is often used in combination with Baizhu and Fangfeng to invigorate qi for consolidating exterior, and eliminate the wind pathogen, such as Yupingfeng San (Powder) from *Danxi Xinfa (Danxi Mental Method)*. For patients with spontaneous sweating caused by deficiency of spleen and lung qi, Huangqi is used together with Muli and Mahuanggen, such as Muli San in *Taiping Huimin Heji Jufang (The Prescriptions of the Bureau of Taiping People's Welfare Pharmacy)*. When treating patients with night sweating caused by yin deficiency, Huangqi should be used with nourishing yin and lowering fire medicinals such as Shengdihuang and Huangbo including the "Holy medicine for night sweats"—Danggui Liuhuang Tang from *Lanshi Micang (Orchid House Secret Collection)*.

现代临床，黄芪配伍常用于治疗胃溃疡等属脾肺气虚者，如参芪膏。

In modern clinical practice, Huangqi compatibility [such as Shenqi Gao, etc.] is often used to treat gastric ulcers and other diseases with spleen and lung deficiency.

3. **气虚水肿** 治气虚不运，水湿停聚之浮肿尿少，常与防己、白术、茯苓等同用，如《金匮要略》防己黄芪汤。

3 Edema Caused by Qi Deficiency

For patients with water retention and edema due to qi deficiency, Huangqi is often used with Fangji, Baizhu, Fuling, etc, such as Fangji

Huangqi Tang from *Jingui Yaolue (Synopsis of Prescriptions of The Golden Chamber)*.

现代临床，黄芪配伍常用于治疗慢性肾炎属于脾肾阳虚、血瘀湿阻者，如肾康宁胶囊、防己黄芪汤等。

In modern clinical practice, Huangqi compatibility (such as Shenkangning Jiaonang, Fangji Huangqi Tang, etc.) is often used to treat chronic nephritis caused by spleen and kidney yang deficiency and the blood stasis and dampness.

4. **血虚萎黄** 治血虚及气血两虚所致面色萎黄、神倦脉虚，常与当归配伍，如《兰室秘藏》当归补血汤和现代中成药当归补血口服液。

4 Sallow Complexions Caused by Blood Deficiency

When treating patients with withered-yellowish face, listlessness, feeble and weak pulse result from asthenia of qi and blood, Huangqi can be compatible with Danggui, such as Danggui Buxue Tang from *Lanshi Micang (Orchid House Secret Collection)* and Chinese patent medicine Danggui Buxue Koufuye.

现代临床，黄芪配伍常用于治疗各种贫血症、过敏性紫癜等属于血虚发热证者，如黄芪桂枝五物。

In modern clinical practice, Huangqi compatibility (such as Huangqi Guizhi Wuwu Tang) is often used to treat all kinds of anemia, allergic purpura, etc. for those with blood deficiency fever symptom.

5. **内热消渴** 治气津不足，内热消渴，常配伍天花粉、葛根等生津止咳药，如《医学衷中参西录》玉液汤。

5 Internal Heat and Wasting-thirst

In treating this condition, Huangqi is often combined with Tianhuafen, Gegeng, such as Yuye Tang from *Yixue Zhongzhong Canxi Lu*.

现代临床，黄芪配伍常用于治疗糖尿病，如玉液汤、七味消渴胶囊、七味糖脉舒胶囊等。

In modern clinical practice, Huangqi compatibility (such as Yuye Tang, Qiwei Xiaoke Jiaonang, Qiwei Tangmaishu Jiaonang, etc.) is often used to treat diabetes.

6. **气血亏虚证，半身不遂，痹痛麻木** 治气虚血滞不行的痹痛、肌肤麻木者，常配伍桂枝、芍药等，如《金匮要略》黄芪桂枝四物汤。治中风后遗症，常配伍当归、川芎、地龙等活血通络药，如《医林改错》补阳还五汤；治风寒湿痹、气虚血滞之肢体麻木、疼痛，常与人参、当归、肉桂等配伍，如《太平惠民和剂局方》十全大补汤。

6 Deficiency of Qi and Blood, Causing Hemiplegia Numbness, Painful Impediment and Numbness

For those who suffer from pain and numbness due to qi deficiency and blood stagnation, Huangqi is often combined with Guizhi and Shaoyao, such as Huangqi Guizhi Siwu Tang from *Jingui Yaolue (Synopsis of Prescriptions of The Golden Chamber)*. For the treatment of the sequelae of stroke, Huangqi is often used in combination with Danggui, Chuanxiong, Dilong and other promoting the blood circulation and removing obstruction in channel medicinals, such as Buyang Huanwu Tang from *Yilin Gaicuo (Correction on of the Errors of Medical Works)*. For treating numbness and pain in the limbs caused by wind cold and dampness, qi deficiency and blood stagnation, Huangqi is usually compatible with Renshen, Danggui, Rougui, such as Shiquan Dabu Tang from *Taiping Huimin Heji Jufang*.

现代临床，黄芪配伍常用于体虚及肿瘤患者的免疫调节剂，以改善放疗时白细胞下降，亦可用于治疗神经末梢炎、中风后遗症等属气血虚滞者，前者如固元片、养阴生血合剂，后者如黄芪桂枝五物。

In modern clinical practice, Huangqi compatibility is often used as immune modulators for patients with physical deficiencies and tumors to improve white blood cells decline during radiotherapy (such as Guyuan Pian, Yangyin Shengxue Ji, etc.). Besides, the compounds such as Huangqi Guizhi Wuwu Tang can also be used to treat patients with nerve stagnation and stagnation of qi and blood due to nerve ending inflammation and stroke sequelae.

7. 疮疡难溃，溃久不敛 治痈疽气血亏损，正虚毒盛不能托毒外达，脓成难溃者，常与人参、白术、穿山甲、白芷等补益气血、解毒排脓药配伍，如《医宗金鉴》托里透脓散。治疮疡后期，气血亏虚，疮口难敛者，常配伍人参、当归、肉桂等药，如《太平惠民和剂局方》十全大补汤。

7 Sore and Ulcer Difficult to Rupture and not Astringing for a Long Time

For patients with this condition, it is often compatible with Renshen, Baizhu, Chuanshanjia, Baizhi and other nourishing qi and blood, such as Tuoli Tounong San from *Yizong Jinjian*. In the late stage of skin and external diseases, Huangqi is often compatible with Renshen, Danggui, Rougui

for those who are difficult to converge, such as Shiquan Dabu Tang.

二、用法用量
II Administration and Dosage

9~30g。
9~30g for decoction.

三、注意事项
III Precautions

疮疡初起，表实邪盛及阴虚阳亢等证忌用。
From the beginning of the sore, symptoms such as excess of exterior and pathogenic, and yang hyperactivity due to yin deficiency are contraindicated.

鹿 茸
Lurong
(Cervi Cornu Pantotrichum)

鹿茸是"血精"，为补阳药之首，分为"花鹿茸"（黄毛茸）和"马鹿茸"（青毛茸）。花鹿茸以东北吉林双阳、辽宁西丰为道地产区；马鹿茸以新疆、内蒙古等为道地产区。花鹿茸品质优于马鹿茸。鹿茸临床常用炮制品主要为鹿茸片与鹿茸粉等。鹿茸味甘、咸，温，入肾、肝经，有壮肾阳、益精血、强筋骨、调冲任、托疮毒的功效，主治肾阳虚证、精血亏虚证、筋骨不健证、崩漏带下证、疮疡塌陷不起或溃久不敛证。鹿茸主要含氨基酸类、蛋白质、脂类等成分，有增强免疫功能、促进性功能、抗衰老、抗疲劳、改善睡眠等药理作用，可用于再生障碍性贫血、放疗后白细胞减少属于肾阳虚者及房室传导阻滞属于精血俱虚证者。鹿茸宜从小量开始，缓缓增加剂量，不可骤用大量；凡阴虚有热、实热证、外感热证均禁用。

Lurong is regarded as "blood essence", the best medicinal for tonifying yang. It can be divided into "Hualurong" (yellow velvet) and "Malurong" (green velvet). The genuine Hualurong is produced in Shuangyang of Jilin and Xifeng of Liaoning in northeast China; and so are the Malurong in Xinjiang and Inner Mongolia. The quality of Hualurong is better than Malurong. Lurong slices and Lurong powder are the main processed products of Lurong in clinical. Lurong is sweet and salty in flavor, and warm in nature. The meridian entries are kidney and liver. It has the effects of strengthening kidney yang, benefiting blood and essence, strengthening bones and muscles, regulating Chong and Ren meridians, and decreasing toxicity. It can be used to treat kidney yang deficiency, blood-essence deficiency, muscle and bone weakness, syndrome of metrorrhagia, disunion and slow recovery of sore and ulcer. Lurong is rich in amino acids, proteins, lipids and other components which can pharmacologically enhance immunity function, promote sexual function, improve anti-aging, reduce the fatigue, improve sleeping quality and so on. It can be used to treat kidney yang deficiency patients with aplastic anemia, or the leukopenia after radiotherapy. And it can also be used to treat blood-essence deficiency patients with the atrioventricular block. It is better for Lurong to be taken with small doses at the beginning, and it should be increased little by little. It is dangerous to take a large amount once or increase the dose all of sudden. It is forbidden to use Lurong to treat syndromes of yin deficiency with heat, syndromes of excess heat, and syndromes of exogenous heat.

【品种品质】
[Variety and Quality]

一、基原品种与品质
I Origin Varieties and Quality

1. 品种概况　来源于鹿科动物梅花鹿 *Cervus nippon* Temminck 或 马鹿 *Cervus elaphus* Linnaeus. 的雄鹿未骨化的幼角。

1 Variety

Lurong is the young antler from the male *Cervus nippon* Temminck or *Cervus elaphus* Linnaeus before it is ossified.

鹿茸首载于《神农本草经》,《图经本草》云:"以形如小紫茄子者为上,或云茄子茸,太嫩血气犹未具,不若分歧如马鞍形者有力。茸不可嗅,其气能伤人鼻",所附郓州鹿与今用梅花鹿 *Cervus nippon* Temminck 无异。

Lurong was first recorded in *Shennong Bencaojing*. According to *Tujing Bencao (Identification of Drug Production)*, Lurong, with the similar shape of a small purple eggplant, is regarded as a good one, so it is also called Qiezirong (eggplant antler). If the antler is too tender, the blood is not yet available, and it is not as strong as the one with saddle shaped antlers. Don't smell antlers, because it hurts people's noses. There is no difference between Yingzhou deer recorded in *Tujing Bencao (Identification of Drug Production)* and sika deer (*Cervus Nippon* Temminck) today.

2. 养殖采收　梅花鹿主要分布在吉林、辽宁、黑龙江;马鹿主要分布在新疆、内蒙古等地。现今鹿茸多采自于人工养殖之鹿,根据收茸规格要求不同,夏、秋二季锯取梅花鹿的二杠茸、三岔茸,马鹿的三岔茸、四岔茸。

2 Raising and Harvesting

Sika deer can be seen in Jilin, Liaoning and Heilongjiang. Red deer is mainly in the Xinjiang, Inner Mongolia and so on. Nowadays, Lurong are mostly collected from deer in artificial breeding. According to the different requirements of specifications, Ergangrong (Lurong with one lateral branch) and Sancharong (Lurong with two lateral branches) of sika deer Sancharong (Lurong with three lateral branches) and Sicharong (Lurong with four lateral branches) of red deer are harvested by saw in summer and autumn.

3. 道地性及品质评价　花鹿茸以吉林双阳、辽宁西丰为道地产区,品质优。马鹿茸以黑龙江林口、辽宁抚顺、内蒙古赤峰、新疆伊犁为道地产区,品质较优。现今,品质评价均以茸形粗壮、饱满、皮毛完整、质嫩、油滑、无骨棱、无钉者为佳。

3 Genuineness and Quality Evaluation

Shuangyang of Jilin, and Xifeng of Liaoning are the genuine producing areas of Hualurong, which has excellent quality. Malurong with superior quality is usually produced in Linkou of Heilongjiang, Fushun of Liaoning, Chifeng of Inner Mongolia, and Yili of Xinjiang. Nowadays, quality evaluation is based on the characteristics of Lurong, the one with thick and plump shape, intact fur, tender texture, and smooth surface without arris or nail is preferred.

鹿茸主要含有氨基酸、蛋白质、多肽、胆固醇等,一般认为,溶血磷脂酰胆碱是其降压的主要物质基础，次黄嘌呤、鸟嘌呤、磷脂类物质是其抑制单胺氧化酶的主要物质基础，多肽类化合物是促进核酸和蛋白质合成的主要物质基础。此外，鹿茸还含有甾体类、多胺类、糖类、微量元素等成分。《中国药典》采用性状、理化鉴别和薄层色谱方法对鹿茸进行鉴别，并未有指标成分限定量及等级质量划分标准。等级评定一般多通过观察鹿茸的形状、外观是否饱满、分枝情况、质量、皮毛颜色、茸毛触感及气味等来进行划分。

Lurong is rich in amino acids, proteins, peptides, cholesterol and so on. It is generally believed that lysophosphatidylcholine is the main material basis for the medicine of blood pressure reduction; hypoxanthine, guanine and phospholipids are the main material basis for its inhibition of monoamine oxidase; and polypeptide compounds are the main material basis for the promotion of nucleic acid and protein synthesis. In addition, Lurong also contains steroids, polyamines, sugars, trace elements, etc. According to the *Pharmacopoeia of the People's Republic of China*, the identification of Lurong can be carried out by methods of morphological identification, physical and chemical identification and TLC. There is no content limitation of indicator components and classfication standard for grade quality. Grading is generally based on the shape, appearance, branching, quality, the fur color, fuzz, and odor of the antler.

二、炮制品种与品质
II Processed Varieties and Quality

目前鹿茸的炮制品有鹿茸片与鹿茸粉。临床常用的鹿茸片常以蜡片、粉片、纱片、骨片形式进行商品流通，品质参差不齐。

At present, the processed products of Lurong include Lurong slices and Lurong powder. The commonly used Lurong slices in the clinic are usually circulated in the forms of wax, powder, yarn and bone, with uneven quality.

三、中成药品种与品质
III Varieties and Quality of Chinese Patent Medicines

含有鹿茸或其炮制品的中成药有 220 余个，其中《中国药典》收载 19 个。以鹿茸为君药或主药的品种有强肾片、鹿茸精注射液等。在中成药的品质控制中多采用显微、理化鉴别及薄层色谱法确定鹿茸的存在，以分光光度法测定样品吸收光谱特征。如在强肾片中通过显微鉴别"未骨化的骨组织淡灰色或近无色"确定鹿茸的存在；鹿茸精注射液中用理化鉴别和薄层色谱法鉴别鹿茸，以分光光度法测定样品最大吸收与最小吸收以判断鹿茸的真伪优劣。

At present, there are more than 220 kinds of Chinese patent medicines containing Lurong or its processed products, and 19 of them are recorded in the *Pharmacopoeia of the People's Republic of China*, among which, prescriptions with Lurong as sovereign include Qiangshen Tablets, Lurongjing Injection and so on. In terms of quality control, microscopic identification, physical and chemical identification, and TLC are adopted to identify the existence of pilose antler, and the absorption spectral characteristics of samples are determined by spectrophotometry. For example, the existence of pilose antler in Qiangshen Tablets is determined by microscopic identification of "light gray or nearly colorless bone tissue without ossification". The composition of pilose antler in Lurongjing Injection is identified by the method of physical-chemical identification and the method of TLC. Measurement of the maximum and minimum absorption of pilose antler by means of spectrophotometry is used to judge the quality of Lurong.

【制药】
[Pharmacy]

一、产地加工
I Processing in Production Area

鹿茸产地加工以锯茸（砍茸）、排血、洗茸、煮烫、干燥为主要工序。马鹿茸加工方法不同之处是煮烫时不要求排血，煮烫和干燥时间比花鹿茸长。

The main processing procedures of Lurong production are sawing Lurong (chopping Lurong), blood discharging, washing, boiling and drying. But it is different to process Malurong since it does not require blood discharging during boiling, and the time spent in cooking and drying is longer than Hualurong.

二、饮片炮制
II Processing of Decoction Pieces

传统鹿茸的炮制方法较多，包括羊脂制、黄精汁制、酒制、酥制、蜜制、熬膏等多种方法。目前，逐渐形成了"锯茸 - 排血 - 干燥"工艺，由此加工的鹿茸片、鹿茸粉成为商品规格中的主流。

There are many traditional Lurong processing methods, including processing with suet, Huangjing (*Polygonati Rhizoma*) juice, liquor, butter, honey, ointment and so on. At present, the process of "sawing-discharging-drying" has gradually been formed, and the processed tablets and powder have become major products in Lurong medicine market.

鹿茸炮制的目的是脱水干燥，防腐消毒，便于保存。然而，鹿茸作为动物药，多肽、氨基酸、脂质类、甾体类、核酸等主要活性成分经过长时间加热不利于药效的保留。鹿茸直接"劈成碎块，研成细粉"制成的鹿茸粉质量较优。

The purpose of processing Lurong is dehydration, antiseptic and disinfection in order to make it easy for preservation. However, as the medicine made from animals, the main active ingredients of Lurong such as peptides, amino acids, lipids, steroids, and nucleic acids are not conducive to the preservation of efficacy after long-term heating. The quality of Lurong powder directly made by "cuting into pieces and grinding into fine powder" is of better quality.

三、中成药制药
III Pharmacy of Chinese Patent Medicines

含鹿茸的中成药，剂型十分丰富，涵盖了固体、液体与半固体剂型。鹿茸有效成分受热易损失，在中成药中，多以全粉或酒提方式入药。如参茸多鞭酒制备过程中以 60° 以上高粱酒回流制备；人参鹿茸丸中的药材粉碎成细粉，制成的蜜丸在体内缓慢溶散使方中的有效成分发挥缓慢而持久的滋肾生津，益气、补血作用。

Chinese patent medicines containing Lurong are very rich in pharmaceutical forms, including the forms of solid, liquid and semi-solid. The effective components of Lurong tend to lose when heated, so in the preparation of Chinese patent medicine, Lurong is mostly used in the way of powdering or liquor extraction. For example, Lurong Duobian Jiu (Wine) is prepared by refluxing sorghum liquor over 60 ℃. In the production of, the medicinal mate- rials in Renshen Lurong Wan are crushed into fine powder, and the honey pills are slowly disolved and dispersed in the body, so that the effective components in the prescription play a slow and lasting role in nourishing the kidney, promoting fluid production, benefiting qi and enriching blood.

【性能功效】
[Property and Efficacy]

一、性能
I Property

鹿茸甘、咸，温；归肾、肝经。

Lurong is sweet and salty in flavor, warm in nature, and enters the kidney and liver meridians.

二、功效
II Efficacy

1. 壮肾阳，益精血　鹿茸有较强的补肾阳、益精血功效，为峻补元阳之品。其功效的发挥与增强免疫功能、抗氧化、抗衰老、抗疲劳等药理作用密切相关。鹿茸增强免疫功能、抗氧化、抗衰老、抗疲劳的有效物质基础主要是多肽及水提物，通过提高巨噬细胞吞噬能力，增加红细胞和白细胞数量，调控单胺氧化酶与过氧化物歧化酶的活性等发挥作用。

1 Strengthening the Kidney Yang and Benefiting Essence and Blood

Lurong has strong effects of invigorating kidney yang and replenishing blood and essence, and thus it is a product for tonifying kidney yang. The exertion of its efficacy is closely related to the pharmacological effects of enhancing immune function, anti-oxidation, anti-aging and anti-fatigue. The effective substance basis of the above effects is mainly polypeptide and water extract, which plays a role by improving phagocytic capacity of macrophages, increasing the number of red blood cells and white blood cells, regulating the activities of monoamine oxidase and peroxidase dismutase.

2. 强筋骨　鹿茸补肾阳以强筋骨。其功效的发挥与鹿茸促进骨折愈合、抗骨质疏松等作用密切相关。鹿茸促进骨折愈合、抗骨质疏松的主要物质基础为多肽类成分，通过促进成骨细胞增殖、抑制破骨细胞的活性等发挥作用。

2 Strengthening Bones and Muscles

Lurong tonifies kidney yang to strengthen bones and muscles. Its effectiveness is closely related to the role of Lurong in promoting fracture healing and anti-osteoporosis. The main substance of Lurong, which promotes fracture healing and anti-osteoporosis, is the polypeptide, which plays an important role in promoting the proliferation of osteoblasts and inhibiting the activity of osteoclasts.

3. 调冲任　鹿茸甘温，可固冲任、调带脉。其功效的发挥与增强性功能等药理作用密切相关。鹿茸增强性功能与其含有多种激素，具有性激素样作用有关，其物质基础主要是水提物，可通过调节下丘脑 - 垂体 - 性腺轴影响性器官，进而改善生殖机能。

3 Regulating Chong and Ren Meridians

The warm nature of Lurong has functions of strengthening and regulating the Chong and Ren meridians. Its efficacy is closely related to the pharmacological action of enhancing sexual function. The enhancement of sexual function of Lurong is related to the presence of a variety of hormones which have sex hormone like effects. The material basis is mainly water extract, which can affect the sexual organs by regulating the hypothalamus-pituitary-gonadal axis, thus improving the reproductive function.

4. 托疮毒　鹿茸补阳气、益精血以扶助正气而托疮毒。其功效的发挥与促进伤口愈合等药理作用密切相关。鹿茸促进伤口愈合的主要物质基础是多肽类物质，可通过促进表皮细胞和成纤维细胞增殖，加速皮肤创伤的修复。

4 Promoting the Recovery of Sores

Lurong tonifies yang qi and replenishes blood and essence to support vital qi and quicken the recovery of sore. Its efficacy is closely related to its pharmacological action of promoting wound healing function. The main material basis of Lurong to promote wound healing is the polypeptide, which can accelerate the repair of skin wounds by promoting the proliferation of epidermal cells and fibroblasts.

此外，现代研究显示鹿茸具有神经保护、抗肿瘤等作用。

Additionally, modern research shows that Lurong has neuroprotective and antitumor effects.

【应用】
[Applications]

一、主治病证
I Indications

1. **肾阳不足，精血亏虚证** 治疗肾脏虚弱，足膝软弱，小便不利，腰脊疼痛证，鹿茸常与熟地黄、山药等配伍以补肾益精，如《普济方》鹿茸酒。

1 Deficiency of the Kidney Yang and Deficiency of Blood and Essence

For the treatment of the kidney deficiency, weakness of feet and knees, inhibited urination, and lumbar pain, Lurong combined with other medicinalss like Shudihuang and Shanyao is often used to tonify the kidney and essence, such as Lurong Jiu (Wine) recorded in *Puji Fang*.

现代临床，鹿茸配伍常用于治疗房室传导阻滞属于精血俱虚者及再生障碍性贫血、放化疗后白细胞减少属于肾阳虚者，如鹿茸精注射液和如鹿茸血酒。

In modern clinical practice, Lurong compatibility is often used to treat atrioventricular block due to blood-essence deficiency. It is also used to treat patients with aplastic anemia and leukopenia after radiotherapy due to kidney yang deficiency, such as Lurongjing injection and Lurong blood liquor.

2. **肾虚筋骨痿软，小儿五迟** 对肾阳虚，筋骨不健之腰膝酸软或小儿发育不良，五迟五软者，单用或与其他补肾阳、强筋骨药同用；治骨折后期，久不愈合者，常与续断、骨碎补等配伍以强筋骨，如《医宗金鉴》补肾地黄丸。

2 Kidney Deficiency, Weakness in Bones and Muscles, and Five Delays of Children

Lurong can be used for those with soreness of the waist and knees or infantile dysplasia due to kidney yang deficiency and weak bones and muscles. It can be used alone or in combination with other medicinals for tonifying kidney yang and strengthening bones and muscles. Lurong

combined with Xuduan (*Dipsaci* Radix) and Gusuibu (*Drynariae* Rhizoma) can be used to strengthen muscles and bones for patients who do not heal after a long time in the late stage of fracture treatment, such as Bushendihuang Wan in *Yizong Jinjian (Golden Mirror of Medicine)*.

现代临床，鹿茸配伍常用于治疗骨质疏松属于肝肾虚损者，如鹿茸壮骨胶囊。

In modern clinical practice, Lurong compatibility (eg. Lurong Zhuanggu Jiaonang) is often used to treat patients who suffer from osteoporosis with liver-kidney deficiency.

3. **冲任虚寒，崩漏带下** 对肝肾亏虚的崩漏不止，白带量多清稀者，常与川断、乌贼骨、盐菟丝子、盐沙苑子、桑螵蛸配伍以补肾固精止带，如《女科切要》内补丸。

3 Deficiency and Cold in Chong and Ren Meridians, Uterine Bleeding

Lurong can be used in combination with Chuanduan, Wuzeigu (*Cleistocactus* sepium), Tusizi (Cuscutae Semen) by salting, Shayuanzi (*Astragali Complanati* Semen) by salting, *Sangpiaoshao* to treat patients with metrorrhagia and excessive leucorrhea by tonifying the kidney, strengthening essence and eliminating leucorrhea, such as Neibu Wan in *Nvke Qieyao (Critical Tips for Women Diseases)*.

现代临床，鹿茸配伍常用于治疗妇科疾病属于肾虚不固之崩漏、带下属虚寒者，如定坤丹。

In modern clinical practice, Lurong compatibility (eg. Dingkun Wan) can be used to treat gynecological diseases such as metrorrhagia due to kidney deficiency and leukorrheal diseases due to deficient cold of kidney.

4. **疮疡难腐难溃，久溃不敛** 对气血不足，疮疡难腐难溃，或溃久不敛、脓水清稀者，常与黄芪、当归等配伍以增内补托毒之效。

4 Slow Recovery of Sore and Ulcerate

Lurong combined with other medicinals, such as Huangqi, Danggui, can be used to treat sores and ulcers that do not decay, or festering for a long time without healing and with clear and thin purulence. In this way, the effect of promoting pus discharge can be increased.

现代临床，鹿茸配伍常用于恶疮和乳腺炎、脓性疾患治愈迟缓等属于阴疽内陷者。

In modern clinical practice, Lurong compatibility is often used in the treatment of obstinate sore, mastitis, and slow recovery of purulent diseases caused by inward collapse of carbuncle toxin.

二、用法用量
II Administration and Dosage

1~2g，研末冲服。

1~2g, administered after being grinded into powder and dissolving.

三、注意事项
III Precautions

1. 鹿茸宜从小剂量开始，缓缓加量，不可骤用大量，以免阳升风动致头晕、目赤、昏厥，或助火动血而致衄血。

1 It's better to take Lurong from a small dose and add the amount gradually. It is dangerous to take a large amount once or increase the dose all of sudden, or it will cause the rise of yang and wind that may cause diseases such as dizziness, conjunctival congestion, fainting, and bleeding caused by fire accumulation.

2. 凡阴虚有热、实热证、外感热证均禁用鹿茸。

2 Patients with yin deficiency with heat, syndrome of excessive heat, and syndrome of external contraction of wind-heat should be not allowed to use Lurong.

【知识拓展】
[Knowledge Extension]

鹿全身都是宝，不仅鹿茸入药用，鹿角、鹿心、鹿血、鹿尾、鹿肾、鹿胎、鹿胆、鹿鞭、鹿筋、鹿肉、鹿骨、鹿皮等均可入药，具有很高的养生保健功能及药用价值。

The whole body of deer is full of treasures. Not only is Lurong used for medicine, but the horn, heart, blood, tail, kidney, fetus, gall, genitals, tendon, venison, bone skin and so on can be used as medicines. They have great medical value and function of health care.

附录一　中　药　名　称

序号	药名	拼音	拉丁名
1	艾叶	Aiye	Artemisiae Argyi Folium
2	安息香	Anxixiang	Benzoinum
3	巴豆	Badou	Crotonis Fructus
4	巴戟天	Bajitian	Morindae Officinalis Radix
5	白豆蔻	Baidoukou	Amomi Kravanh Fructus
6	白茯苓	Baifuling	Poria
7	白附子	Baifuzi	Typhonii Rhizoma
8	白花蛇	Baihuashe	Bungarus Parvus
9	白芨	Baiji	Bletlilae Rhizoma
10	白及	Baiji	Bletillae Rhizoma
11	白僵蚕	Baijiangcan	Bombyx Batryticatus
12	白蔹	Bailian	Ampelopsis Radix
13	白茅根	Baimaogen	Imperatae Rhizoma
14	白芍	Baishao	Paeoniae Radix Alba
15	白术	Baizhu	Atractylodis Macrocephalae Rhizoma
16	白菀	Baiwan	Aster ericoides
17	白薇	Baiwei	Cynanchi Atrati Radix Et Rhizoma
18	白芷	Baizhi	Angelicae Dahuricae Radix
19	百部	Baibu	Stemonae Radix
20	柏子仁	Baiziren	Platycladi Semen
21	斑蝥	Banmao	Mylabris
22	板蓝根	Banlangen	Isatidis Radix
23	半夏	Banxia	Pinelliae Rhizoma
24	薄荷	Bohe	Menthae Haplocalycis Herba
25	薄荷脑	Bohenao	l-menthol
26	北沙参	Beishashen	Glehniae Radix
27	鳖甲	Biejia	Trionycis Carapax
28	槟榔	Binglang	Arecae Semen

续表

序号	药名	拼音	拉丁名
29	冰片	Bingpian	Borneolum Syntheticum
30	补骨脂	Buguzhi	Psoraleae Fructus
31	苍耳子	Cangerzi	Xanthii Fructus
32	苍术	Cangzhu	Atractylodis Rhizoma
33	草乌	Caowu	Aconiti Kusnezoffii Radix
34	柴胡	Chaihu	Bupleuri Radix
35	蝉蜕	Chantui	Cicadae Periostacum
36	蟾蜍	Chanchu	Bufo bufo gargarizans Cantor
37	蟾酥	Chansu	Bufonis Venenum
38	蟾衣	Chanyi	Bufonis Periostracum
39	菖蒲	Changpu	Acori Tatarinowii Rhizoma
40	常山	Changshan	Dichroae Radix
41	车前子	Cheqianzi	Plantaginis Semen
42	沉香	Chenxiang	Aquilariae Lignum Resinatum
43	陈皮	Chenpi	Citri Reticulatae Pericarpium
44	赤芍	Chishao	Paeoniae Radix Rubra
45	川贝母	Chuanbeimu	Fritillariae Cirrhosae Bulbus
46	川楝子	Chuanlianzi	Toosendan Fructus
47	川木香	Chuanmuxiang	Vladimiriae Radix
48	川乌	Chuanwu	Aconiti Radix
49	川芎	Chuanxiong	Chuanxiong Rhizoma
50	川续断	Chuanxuduan	Dipsaci Radix
51	穿山甲	Chuanshanjia	Squama Manitis
52	磁石	Cishi	Magnetitum
53	刺五加	Ciwujia	Acanthopanacis Senticosi Radix et Rhizoma Seu Caulis
54	葱白	Congbai	Allii Fistulosi Bulbus
55	大豆黄卷	Dadouhuangjuan	Sojae Semen Germinatum
56	大黄	Dahuang	Rhei Radix et Rhizoma
57	大蓟	Daji	Cirsii Japonici Herba
58	大蒜	Dasuan	Allii Sativi Bulbus
59	大枣	Dazao	Jujubae Fructus
60	丹参	Danshen	Salviae Miltiorrhizae Radix et Rhizoma
61	丹皮	Danpi	Moutan Cortex
62	胆矾	Danfan	Blue Vitriol
63	淡竹叶	Danzhuye	Lophatheri Herba

续表

序号	药名	拼音	拉丁名
64	当归	Danggui	Angelicae Sinensis Radix
65	党参	Dangshen	Codonopsis Radix
66	地肤子	Difuzi	Kochiae Fructus
67	地骨皮	Digupi	Lycii Cortex
68	地黄	Dihuang	Rehmanniae Radix
69	地龙	Dilong	Pheretima
70	地榆	Diyu	Sanguisorbae Radix
71	丁香	Dingxiang	Caryophylli Flos
72	冬虫夏草	Dongchongxiacao	Cordyceps
73	独活	Duhuo	Angelicae Pubescentis Radix
74	杜仲	Duzhong	Eucommiae Cortex
75	阿胶	Ejiao	Asini Corii Colla
76	莪术	Ezhu	Curcumae Rhizoma
77	儿茶	Ercha	Catechu
78	番泻叶	Fanxieye	Sennae Folium
79	防风	Fangfeng	Saposhnikoviae Radix
80	防己	Fangji	Stephaniae Tetrandrae Radix
81	粉葛	Fenge	Puerariae Thomsonii Radix
82	蜂蜜	Fengmi	Mel
83	茯苓	Fuling	Poria
84	浮小麦	Fuxiaomai	Tritici aestivi Semen
85	附子	Fuzi	Aconiti Lateralis Radix Praeparata
86	覆盆子	Fupenzi	Rubi Fructus
87	甘草	Gancao	Glycyrrhizae Radix et Rhizoma
88	甘遂	Gansui	Kansui Radix
89	干姜	Ganjiang	Zingiberis Rhizoma
90	干漆	Ganqi	Toxicodendri Resina
91	藁本	Gaoben	Ligustici Rhizoma
92	葛根	Gegen	Puerariae Lobatae Radix
93	钩藤	Gouteng	Uncariae Ramulus Cum Uncis
94	狗脊	Gouji	Cibotii Rhizoma
95	枸杞	Gouqi	Lycium barbarum L.
96	骨碎补	Gusuibu	Drynariae Rhizoma
97	瓜蒂	Guadi	Melo Pedicellus
98	瓜蒌	Gualou	Trichosanthis Fructus

续表

序号	药名	拼音	拉丁名
99	瓜蒌皮	Gualoupi	Trichosanthis Pericarpium
100	瓜蒌子	Gualouzi	Trichosanthis Semen
101	关白附	Guanfuzi	Aconiti Radix
102	关黄柏	Guanhuangbo	Phellodendri Amurensis Cortex
103	关木通	Guanmutong	Aristolochiae Manshuriensis Caulis
104	广防己	Guangfangji	Aristolochiae Fangchi Radix
105	广藿香	Guanghuoxiang	Pogostemonis Herba
106	龟甲	Guijia	Testudinis Carapax Plastrum
107	桂枝	Guizhi	Cinnamomi Ramulus
108	蛤蚧	Gejie	Gecko
109	海金沙	Haijinsha	Lygodii Spora
110	海藻	Haizao	Sargassum
111	诃子	Hezi	Chebulae Fructus
112	合欢皮	Hehuanpi	Albiziae Cortex
113	何首乌	Heshouwu	Polygoni Multiflori Radix
114	红参	Hongshen	Ginseng Radix et Rhizoma Rubra
115	红花	Honghua	Carthami Flos
116	厚朴	Houpo	Magnoliae Officinalis Cortex
117	湖北贝母	Hubeibeimu	Fritillariae Hupehensis bulbus
118	虎杖	Huzhang	Polygoni Cuspidati Rhizoma Et Radix
119	花蕊石	Huaruishi	Ophicalcitum
120	滑石	Huashi	Talcum
121	槐花	Huaihua	Sophorae Flos
122	黄柏	Huangbo	Phellodendri Chinensis Cortex
123	黄花蒿	Huanghuahao	Artemisia annua L.
124	黄精	Huangjing	Polygonati Rhizoma
125	黄连	Huanglian	Coptidis Rhizoma
126	黄芪	Huangqi	Astragali Radix
127	黄芩	Huangqin	Scutellariae Radix
128	火麻仁	Huomaren	Cannabis Fructus
129	鸡内金	Jineijin	Galli Gigerii Endothelium Corneum
130	姜黄	Jianghuang	Curcumae Longae Rhizoma
131	降香	Jiangxiang	Dalbergiae Odoriferae Lignum
132	金钱草	Jinqiancao	Lysimachiae Herba
133	金银花	Jinyinhua	Lonicerae Japonicae Flos

续表

序号	药名	拼音	拉丁名
134	京大戟	Jingdaji	Euphorbiae Pekinensis Radix
135	荆芥	Jingjie	Schizonepetae Herba
136	桔梗	Jiegeng	Platycodonis Radix
137	菊花	Juhua	Chrysanthemi Flos
138	橘红	Juhong	Citri Grandis Exocarpium
139	橘皮	Jupi	Citri Reticulatae Pericarpium
140	枯矾	Kufan	Alumen
141	苦参	Kushen	Sophorae Flavescentis Radix
142	苦杏仁	Kuxingren	Armeniacae Semen Amarum
143	款冬花	Kuandonghua	Farfarae Flos
144	昆布	Kunbu	Laminariae Thallus Eckloniae Thallus
145	莱菔子	Laifuzi	Raphani Semen
146	兰草	Lancao	Orchida Herba
147	雷公藤	Leigongteng	Tripterygium wilfordii
148	雷丸	Leiwan	Omphalia
149	藜芦	Lilu	veratrum Nigrum
150	荔枝核	Llizhihe	Litchi Semen
151	连翘	Lianqiao	Forsythiae Fructus
152	羚羊角	Lingyangjiao	Saigae Tataricae Cornu
153	硫黄	Liuhuang	Sulfur
154	龙胆	Longdan	Gentianae Radix et Rhizoma
155	龙胆	Longdan	Gentianae Radix et Rhizoma
156	龙骨	Longgu	Draconis Os
157	漏芦	Loulu	Rhapontici Radix
158	芦根	Lugen	Phragmitis Rhizoma
159	芦荟	Luhui	Aloe
160	鹿角	Lujiao	Cervi Cornu
161	鹿角胶	Lujiaojiao	Cervi Cornus Colla
162	鹿茸	Lurong	Cervi Cornu Pantotrichum
163	罗布麻叶	Luobumaye	Apocyni Veneti Folium
164	绿豆	Lüdou	Vigna Radiata
165	葎草	Lücao	Humulus scandens
166	麻黄	Mahuang	Ephedrae Herba
167	麻仁	Maren	Cannabis Fructus
168	马兜铃	Madouling	Aristolochiae Fructus

续表

序号	药名	拼音	拉丁名
169	马钱子	Maqianzi	Strychni Semen
170	麦冬	Maidong	Ophiopogonis Radix
171	麦门冬	Maimendong	Ophiopogonis Radix
172	麦芽	Maiya	Hordei Fructus Germinatus
173	曼陀罗	Mantuoluo	Datura stramonium Linn.
174	芒硝	Mangxiao	Natrii Sulfas
175	茅香	Maoxiang	Cymbopogon citratus (DC.) Stapf.
176	没药	Moyao	Myrrha
177	虻虫	Mengchong	Tabanus
178	牡丹皮	Mudanpi	Moutan Cortex
179	牡蛎	Muli	Concha Ostreae
180	木瓜	Mugua	Chaenomelis Fructus
181	木通	Mutong	Akebiae Caulis
182	木香	Muxiang	Aucklandiae Radix
183	南五味子	Nanwuweizi	Schisandrae Sphenantherae Fructus
184	牛蒡子	Niubangzi	Arctii Fructus
185	牛黄	Niuhuang	Bovis Calculus
186	牛膝	Niuxi	Achyranthis Bidentatae Radix
187	炮姜	Paojiang	Zingiberis Rhizoma Praeparatum
188	佩兰	Peilan	Eupatorii Herba
189	砒霜	Pishuang	Arsenicum Sablimatum
190	枇杷叶	Pipaye	Eriobotryae Folium
191	平贝母	Pingbeimu	Fritillariae Ussuriensis Bulbus
192	蒲公英	Pugongying	Taraxaci Herba
193	蒲黄	Puhuang	Typhae Pollen
194	千里光	Qianliguang	Senecionis Scandentis Hebra
195	牵牛子	Qianniuzi	Pharbitidis Semen
196	前胡	Qianhu	Peucedani Radix
197	茜草	Qiancao	Rubiae Radix Et Rhizoma
198	羌活	Qianghuo	Notopterygii Rhizoma Et Radix
199	秦艽	Qinjiao	Gentianae Macrophyllae Radix
200	青黛	Qingdai	Indigo Naturalis
201	青蒿	Qinghao	Artemisiae Annuae Herba
202	青礞石	Qingmengshi	Chloriti Lapis
203	青木香	Qingmuxiang	Aristolochiae Radix

续表

序号	药名	拼音	拉丁名
204	青皮	Qingpi	Citri Reticulatae Pericarpium Viride
205	轻粉	Qingfen	Calomelas
206	全蝎	Quanxie	Scorpio
207	人参	Renshen	Ginseng Radix et Rhizoma
208	人参叶	Renshenye	Ginseng Polium
209	肉苁蓉	Roucongrong	Cistanches Herba
210	肉桂	Rougui	Cinnamomi Cortex
211	乳香	Ruxiang	Olibanum
212	三棱	Sanleng	Sparganii Rhizoma
213	三七	Sanqi	Notoginseng Radix et Rhizoma
214	桑寄生	Sangjisheng	Taxilli Herba
215	桑螵蛸	Sangpiaoxiao	Mantidis OÖtheca
216	桑叶	Sangye	Mori Folium
217	沙参	Shashen	Adenophora Radix
218	沙苑子	Shayuanzi	Astragali Complanati Semen
219	砂仁	Sharen	Amomi Fructus
220	山药	Shanyao	Dioscoreae Rhizoma
221	山楂	Shanzha	Crataegi Fructus
222	山茱萸	Shanzhuyu	Corni Fructus
223	商陆	Shanglu	Phytolaccae Radix
224	芍药	Shaoyao	Paeonia lactiflora Pall.
225	蛇床子	Shechuangzi	Cnidii Fructus
226	麝香	Shexiang	Moschus
227	神曲	Shenqu	Massa Medicata Fermentata
228	升麻	Shengma	Cimicifugae Rhizoma
229	生姜	Shengjiang	Zingiberis Rhizoma recens
230	生山药	Shengshanyao	Dioscoreae Rhizoma
231	石膏	Shigao	Gypsum Fibrosum
232	石斛	Shihu	Dendrobii Caulis
233	石决明	Shijueming	Haliotidis Concha
234	柿蒂	Shidi	Kaki Calyx
235	熟地黄	Shudihuang	Rehmanniae Radix Praeparata
236	水蓼	Shuiliao	Polygonum hydropiper L.
237	水牛角	Shuiniujiao	Bubali Cornu
238	水银	Shuiyin	Hydrargyrum

续表

序号	药名	拼音	拉丁名
239	水蛭	Shuihzi	Hirudo
240	苏合香	Suhexiang	Styrax
241	苏木	Sumu	Sappan Lignum
242	酸枣仁	Suanzaoren	Ziziphi Spinosae Semen
243	太子参	Taizishen	Pseudostellariae Radix
244	檀香	Tanxiang	Santali Albi Lignum
245	桃仁	Taoren	Persicae Semen
246	天冬	Tiandong	Asparagi Radix
247	天花粉	Tianhuafen	Trichosanthis Radix
248	天麻	Tianma	Gastrodiae Rhizoma
249	天南星	Tiannanxing	Arisaematis Rhizoma
250	甜杏仁	Tianxingren	Sweet almond
251	铁皮石斛	Tiepishihu	Dendrobii officinalis Caulis
252	土鳖虫	Tubiechong	Eupolyphaga Steleophaga
253	土茯苓	Tufuling	Smilacis glabrae Rhizoma
254	土瓜根	Tuguagen	Trichosanthes Radix
255	土木香	Tumuxiang	Inulae Radix
256	菟丝子	Tusizi	Cuscutae Semen
257	威灵仙	Weilingxian	Clematidis Radix Et Rhizoma
258	乌梅	Wumei	Mume Fructus
259	乌头	Wutou	Aconite Main Root
260	乌药	Wuyao	Linderae Radix
261	乌贼骨	wuzeigu	Cleistocactus Sepium
262	巫山淫羊藿	Wushan Yinyanghuo	Epimedii wushanense T.S.Ying
263	吴茱萸	Wuzhuyu	Euodiae Fructus
264	蜈蚣	Wugong	Scolopendra
265	五倍子	Wubeizi	Galla Chinensis
266	五加皮	Wujiapi	Acanthopanacis Cortex
267	五灵脂	Wulingzhi	Trogopterori Faeces
268	五味子	Wuweizi	Schisandrae Chinensis Fructus
269	西瓜	Xigua	Aconitum carmichaelii Debx.
270	西红花	Xihonghua	Croci Stigma
271	西洋参	Xiyangshen	Panacis Quinquefolii Radix
272	犀角	Xijiao	Rhinoceros Unicornis
273	细辛	Xixin	Asari Radix Et Rhizoma

续表

序号	药名	拼音	拉丁名
274	夏枯草	Xiakucao	Prunellae Spica
275	仙鹤草	Xianhecao	Agrimoniae Herba
276	仙茅	Xianmao	Curculiginis Rhizoma
277	鲜芦根	Xianlugen	Phragmitis Rhizoma
278	香附	Xiangfu	Cyperi Rhizoma
279	香加皮	Xiangjiapi	Periplocae Cortex
280	小茴香	Xiaohuixiang	Foeniculi Fructus
281	辛夷	Xinyi	Magnoliae Flos
282	雄黄	Xionghuang	Bealgar
283	徐长卿	Xuchangqing	Cynanchi Paniculati Radix Et Rhizoma
284	续断	Xuduan	Dipsaci Radix
285	玄参	Xuanshen	Scrophulariae Radix
286	旋覆花	Xuanfuhua	Inulae Flos
287	血竭	Xuejie	Draconis Sanguis
288	血余炭	Xueyutan	Crinis Carbonisatus
289	鸦胆子	Yadanzi	Bruceae Fructus
290	鸭蛋子	Yadanzi	Bruceae Fructus
291	延胡索	Yanhusuo	Corydalis Rhizoma
292	羊胆	Yangdan	Sheep gallbladder
293	羊踯躅花	Yangzhizhuhua	Rhododendri Flos
294	洋金花	Yangjinhua	Daturae Flos
295	伊贝母	Yibeimu	Fritillariae Pallidiflorae Bulbus
296	饴糖	Yitang	Saccharum Granorum
297	益母草	Yimucao	Leonuri Herba
298	薏苡仁	Yiyiren	Coicis Semen
299	茵陈	Yinchen	Artemisiae Scopariae Herba
300	淫羊藿	Yinyanghuo	Epimedii Folium
301	鱼腥草	Yuxingcao	Houttuyniae Herba
302	禹白附	Yubaifu	Typhonii Rhizoma
303	禹州漏芦	Yuzhouloulu	Echinopsis Radix
304	玉竹	Yuzhu	Polygonati Odorati Rhizoma
305	郁金	Yujin	Curcumae Radix
306	郁李仁	Yuliren	Pruni Semen
307	芫花	Yuanhua	Genkwa Flos
308	远志	Yuanzhi	Polygalae Radix

续表

序号	药名	拼音	拉丁名
309	月季花	Yuejihua	Rosae Chinensis Flos
310	皂矾	Zaofan	alum soap
311	皂荚	Zaojia	Gleditsiae Fructus
312	皂角刺	Zaojiaoci	Gleditsiae Spina
313	泽泻	Zexie	Alismatis Rhizoma
314	浙贝母	Zhebeimu	Fritillariae Thunbergii Bulbus
315	珍珠	Zhenzhu	Margarita
316	珍珠粉	Zhenzhufen	Margarita
317	珍珠母	Zhenzhumu	MArgaritifera Concha
318	知母	Zhimu	Anemarrhe Naerhizoma
319	栀子	Zhizi	Gardeniae Fructus
320	枳椇子	Zhijuzi	Hoveniae Semen
321	枳壳	Zhiqiao	Aurantii Fructus
322	枳实	Zhishi	Aurantii Fructus Immaturus
323	朱砂	Zhusha	Cinnabaris
324	猪胆	Zhudan	Pig gallbladder
325	猪胆汁	Zhudanzhi	Sus scrofa domestica Brisson
326	猪苓	Zhuling	Polyporus
327	竹沥	Zhuli	Bamboo Leaches
328	竹茹	Zhuru	Bambusae Caulis In Taenias
329	竹叶	Zhuye	Lophatheri Herba
330	紫河车	Ziheche	Placenta Hominis
331	紫花地丁	Zihuadiding	Violae Herba
332	紫石英	Zishiying	Fluoritum
333	紫苏	Zisu	Perillae Folium
334	紫苏梗	Zisugeng	Perillae Caulis
335	紫苏叶	Zisuye	Perillae Folium
336	紫苏子	Zisuzi	Perillae Fructus
337	紫菀	Ziwan	Asteris Radix et Rhizoma

附录二 方 剂 名 称

序号	方剂名称	拼音	英文名称
1	安宫牛黄丸	Angong Niuhuang Wan	Angong Niuhuang Pill
2	安神定志丸	Anshen Dingzhi Wan	Anshen Dingzhi Pill
3	安胎丸	Antai Wan	Antai Pill
4	安血饮	Anxue Yin	Anxue Decoction
5	安中散	Anzhong San	Anzhong Powder
6	八珍汤	Bazhen Tang	Bazhen Decoction
7	八正散	Bazheng San	Bazheng Powder
8	白虎加苍术汤	Baihu Jia Cangzhu Tang	Baihu plus Cangzhu Decoction
9	白虎加人参汤	Baihu Jia Renshen Tang	Baihu Plus Renshen Decoction
10	白虎汤	Baihu Tang	Baihu Decoction
11	白通汤	Baitong Tang	Baitong Decoction
12	百合地黄汤	Baihe Dihuang Tang	Baihe Dihuang Decoction
13	百合固金汤	Baihe Gujin Tang	Baihe Gujin Decoction
14	百合知母汤	Baihe Zhimu Tang	Baihe Zhimu Decoction
15	半夏白术天麻汤	Banxia Baizhu Tianma Tang	Banxiao Baizhu Tianma Decoction
16	半夏泻心汤	Banxia Xiexin Tang	Banxia Xiexin Decoction
17	补肺汤	Bufei Tang	Bufei Decoction
18	补肝汤	Bugan Tang	Bugan Decoction
19	补肾地黄丸	Bushen Dihuang Wan	Bushendihuang Pills
20	补阳还五汤	Buyang Huanwu Tang	Buyang Huanwu Decoction
21	补中益气汤	Buzhong Yiqi Tang	Buzhong Yiqi Decoction
22	补中益气丸	Buzhong Yiqi Wan	Buzhong Yiqi Dripping Pills
23	参贝陈皮丸	Shen Bei Chenpi Wan	Shen Bei Chenpi Pill
24	参附汤	Shenfu Tang	Shenfu Decoction
25	参归汤	Shengui Tang	Shengui Decoction
26	参苓白术散	Shenling Baizhu San	Shenling Baizhu Powder
27	苍术汤	Cangzhu Tang	Cangzhu Decoction
28	苍术丸	Cangzhu Wan	Cangzhu Pill
29	柴葛解肌汤	Chaige Jieji Tang	Chaige Jieji Decoction

续表

序号	方剂名称	拼音	英文名称
30	柴葛青蒿汤	Chaige Qinghao Tang	Chaige Qinghao Decoction
31	柴胡疏肝散	Chaihu Shugan San	Chaihu Shugan Powder
32	川升麻散	Chuanshengma San	Chuanshengma Powder
33	川芎茶调丸	Chuanxiong Chatiao Wan	Chuanxiong Chatiao Pill
34	川芎调茶散	Chuanxiong Chatiao San	Chuanxiong Chatiao Powder
35	磁朱丸	Cizhu Wan	Cizhu pill
36	大补阴丸	Dabuyin Wan	Dabuyin Pill
37	大承气汤	Da chengqi Tang	Da chengqi Decoction
38	大黄附子汤	Dahuang Fuzi Tang	Dahuang Fuzi Decoction
39	大黄牡丹汤	Dahuang Mudan Tang	Dahuang Mudan Decoction
40	大黄汤	Dahuang Tang	Dahuang Decoction
41	大建中汤	Dajianzhong Tang	Dajianzhong Decoction
42	大香连丸	Da Xianglian Wan	Da Xianglian Pill
43	丹参散	Danshen San	Danshen Powder
44	丹参饮	Danshen Yin	Danshen Decoction
45	当归补血汤	Danggui Buxue Tang	Danggui Buxue Decoction
46	当归六黄汤	Danggui Liuhuang Tang	Danggui Liuhuang Dection
47	当归龙荟丸	Danggui Longhui Wan	Danggui Longhui Pill
48	当归润燥汤	Danggui Runchang Tang	Danggui Runchang Decoction
49	当归散	Danggui San	Danggui Powder
50	当归芍药散	Danggui Shaoyao San	Danggui Shaoyao Powder
51	当归生姜羊肉汤	Danggui Shengjiang Yangrou Tang	Danggui Shengjiang Mutton Decoction
52	当归四逆汤	Danggui Sini Tang	Danggui Sini Decoction
53	当归汤	Danggui Tang	Danggui Decoction
54	当归饮子	Danggui Yinzi	Danggui Yinzi
55	当归郁李仁汤	Danggui Yuliren Tang	Danggui Yuliren Decoction
56	导气汤	Daoqi Tang	Daoqi Powder
57	抵圣散	Disheng San	Disheng Powder
58	颠倒木金散	Diandiao Mujin San	Diandiao Mujin Powder
59	定坤丹	Dingkun Dan	Dingkun Pellet
60	独参汤	Dushen Tang	Dushen Decoction
61	独活寄生汤	Duhuo Jisheng Tang	Duhuo Jisheng Decoction
62	独活细辛汤	Duhuo Xixin Tang	Duhuo Xixin Decoction
63	莪术散	Ezhu San	Ezhu Powder
64	莪术丸	Ezhu Wan	Ezhu Pill

续表

序号	方剂名称	拼音	英文名称
65	二陈汤	Erchen Tang	Erchen Decoction
66	二姜丸	Erjiang Wan	Erjiang Pill
67	二妙散	Ermiao San	Ermiao Powder
68	二妙丸	Ermiao Wan	Ermiao Pill
69	二母散	Ermu San	Ermu Powder
70	二香散	Erxiang San	Erxiang Powder
71	防风通圣散	Fangfeng Tongsheng San	Fangfeng Tongsheng Powder
72	防己黄芪汤	Fangji Huangqin Tang	Fangji Huangqi Decotion
73	肺肾两益汤	Feishen Liangyi Tang	Feishen Liangyi Decoction
74	茯苓升麻汤	Fuling Shengma Tang	Fuling Shengma Decoction
75	腐尽生肌散	Fujin Shengji San	Fujin Shengji Powder
76	附子理中丸	Fuzi Lizhong Wan	Fuzi Lizhong Pill
77	附子丸	Fuzi Wan	Fuzi Pill
78	复方丹参丸	Fufang Danshen Wan	Fufang Danshen Pill
79	复元活血汤	Fuyuan Huoxue Tang	Fuyuan Huoxue Decoction
80	甘草附子汤	Gancao Fuzi Tang	Gancao Fuzi Decoction
81	甘草麻黄汤	Gancao Mahuang Tang	Gancao Mahuang Decoction
82	甘草丸	Gancao Wan	Gancao Pill
83	甘桔汤	Ganjie Tang	Ganjie Decoction.
84	甘露消毒丹	Ganlu Xiaodu Dan	Ganlu Xiaodu Pill
85	干姜附子汤	Ganjiang Fuzi Tang	Ganjiang Fuzi Decoction
86	膈下逐瘀汤	Gexia Zhuyu Tang	Gexia Zhuyu Decoction
87	葛根芩连汤	Gegen Qinlian Tang	Gegen Qinlian Decoction
88	葛根汤	Gegen Tang	Gegen Decoction
89	钩藤饮	Gouteng Yin	Gouteng Decoction
90	固本止崩汤	Guben Zhibeng Tang	Guben Zhibeng Decoction
91	归脾汤	Guipi Tang	Guipi Decoction
92	桂枝茯苓丸	Guizhi Fuling Wan	Guizhi Fuling Pill
93	桂枝附子汤	Guizhi Fuzi Tang	Guizhi Fuzi Decoction
94	桂枝甘草汤	Guizhi Gancao Tang	Guizhi Gancao Decoction
95	桂枝加桂汤	Guizhi Jiagui Tang	Guizhi Jiagui Decoction
96	桂枝加厚朴杏子汤	Guizhi jiahoupo Xingzi Tang	Guizhi jiahoupo Xingzi Decoction
97	桂枝芍药知母汤	Guizhi Shaoyao Zhimu Tang	Guizhi Shaoyao Zhimu Decoction
98	桂枝汤	Guizhi Tang	Guizhi Decoction
99	海藻玉壶汤	Haizao Yuhu Tang	Haizao Yuhu Decoction
100	蒿豉丹	Haochi Dan	Haochi Pill

续表

序号	方剂名称	拼音	英文名称
101	荷叶丸	Heye Dan	Heye Pill
102	厚朴温中汤	Houpo Wenzhong Tang	Houpo Wenzhong Decoction
103	化血丹	Huaxue Dan	Huaxue Pellet
104	黄柏丸	Huangbai Wan	Huangbai Pill
105	黄连解毒汤	Huanglian Jiedu Tang	Huanglian Jiedu Decoction
106	黄连汤	Huanglian Tang	Huanglian Decoction
107	黄连丸	Huanglian Wan	Huanglian Pill
108	黄龙汤	Huanglong Tang	Huanglong Decoction
109	黄芪桂枝五物汤	Huangqi Guizhi Wuwu Tang	Huangqi Guizhi Wuwu Decoction
110	黄芩滑石汤	Huangqin Huashi Tang	Huangqin Huashi Decoction
111	黄芩散	Huangqin San	Huangqin Powder
112	黄芩汤	Huangqin Tang	Huangqin Decoction
113	回生散	Huisheng San	Huisheng Powder
114	回阳三建汤	Huiyang Sanjian Tang	Huiyang Sanjian Decoction
115	活血祛瘀汤	Huoxue Quyu Tang	Huoxue Quyu Decoction
116	活血止痛汤	Huoxue Zhitong Tang	Huoxue Zhitong Decoction
117	藿朴苓夏汤	Huopo Lingxia Tang	Huopo Lingxia Decoction
118	藿香安胃散	Huoxiang Anwei San	Huoxiang Anwei Powder
119	藿香和中汤	Huoxiang Hezhong Tang	Huoxiang Hezhong Decoction
120	藿香散	Huoxiang San	Huoxiang Powder
121	藿香正气散	Huoxiang Zhengqi San	Huoxiang Zhengqi Powder
122	济川煎	Jichuan Jian	Jichuan Decoction
123	加味葛根芩连汤	Jiawei Gegen Qinlian Tang	Jiawei Gegen Qinlian Decoction
124	胶艾汤	Jiaoai Tang	Jiaoai Decoction
125	金不换正气散	Jinbuhuan Zhengqi San	Jinbuhuan Zhengqi Powder
126	金铃子散	Jinlingzi San	Jinlingzi Powder
127	金水六君子煎	Jinshui Liujunzi Jian	Jinshui Liujun Decoction
128	九味羌活汤	Jiuwei Qianghuo Tang	Jiuwei Qianghuo Decoction
129	桔梗汤	Jiegeng Tang	Jiegeng Decoction
130	桔梗杏仁煎	Jiegeng Xingren Jian	Jiegeng Xingren Decoction
131	橘皮汤	Jupi Tang	Jvpi Decoction
132	橘皮竹茹汤	Jupi Zhuru Tang	Jvpi Zhuru Decoction
133	宽中丸	Kuanzhong Wan	Kuanzhong Pill
134	理苓汤	Liqing Tang	Liqing Decoction
135	理中散	Lizhong San	Lizhong Powder
136	理中汤	Lizhong Tang	Lizhong Decoction

续表

序号	方剂名称	拼音	英文名称
137	理中丸	Lizhong Wan	Lizhong Pill
138	利胆丸	Lidan Wan	Lidan Pill
139	连理汤	Lianli Tang	Lianli Decoction
140	连梅汤	Lianmei Tang	Lianmei Decoction
141	凉膈散	Liangge San	Liangge Powder
142	苓甘五味姜辛汤	Ling Gan Wuwei Jiang Xin Tang	Ling Gan Wuwei Jiang Xin Decoction
143	苓桂阿胶汤	Linggui Ejiao Tang	Linggui Ejiao Decoction
144	苓桂术甘汤	Linggui Zhugan Tang	Linggui Zhugan Decoction
145	六神丸	Liushen Wan	Liushen Pill
146	麻黄连翘赤小豆汤	Mahuang Lianqiao Chixiaodou Tang	MahuangLianqiao Chixiaodou Decoction
147	麻黄汤	Mahuang Tang	Mahuang Decoction
148	麻杏石甘汤	Maxing Shigan Tang	Maxing Ganshi Decoction
149	麻子仁丸	Maziren Wan	Maziren Pill
150	麦门冬汤	Maimendong Tang	Maimendong Decoction
151	牡蛎散	Muli San	Muli Powder
152	木香槟榔丸	Muxiang Binglang Wan	Muxiang Binglang Pill
153	木香顺气汤	Muxiang Shunqi Tang	Muxiang Shunqi Decoction
154	宁坤至宝丹	Ningkun Zhibao Dan	Ningkun Zhibao Pellet
155	宁志膏	Ningzhi Gao	Ningzhi Emplastrum
156	牛黄抱龙丸	Niuhuang Baolong Wan	Niuhuang Baolong Pill
157	平肝开郁止血汤	Pinggan Kaiyu Zhixue Tang	Pinggan Kaiyu Zhixue Decoction
158	平胃散	Pingwei San	Pingwei Powder
159	七味白术散	Qiwei Baizhu San	Qiwei Baizhu Powder
160	羌活胜湿汤	Qianghuo Shengshi Tang	Qianghuo Shengshi Decoction
161	秦艽天麻汤	Qinjiao Tianma Tang	Qinjiao Tianma Decoction
162	青蒿鳖甲汤	Qinghao Biejia Tang	Qinghao Biejia Decoction
163	青蒿丸	Qinghao Wan	Qinghao Pill
164	清胆汤	Qingdan Tang	Qingdan Decoction
165	清肝活瘀汤	Qinggan Huoyu Tang	Qinggan Huoyu Decoction
166	清骨散	Qinggu San	Qinggu Powder
167	清金散	Qingjin San	Qingjin Powder
168	清金丸	Qingjin Wan	Qingjin Pill
169	清凉涤暑汤	Qingliang Dishu Tang	Qingliang Dishu Decoction
170	清气化痰丸	Qingqi Huatan Wan	Qingqi Huatan Pill
171	清胃散	Qingwei San	Qingwei Powder

续表

序号	方剂名称	拼音	英文名称
172	清瘟败毒饮	Qingwen Baidu Yin	Qingwen Baidu Decoction
173	清营汤	Qingying Tang	Qingying Decoction
174	清燥救肺汤	Qingzao Jiufei Tang	Qingzao Jiufei Decoction
175	琼玉膏	Qiongyu Gao	Qiongyu Paste
176	润肠丸	Runchang Wan	Runchang Pill
177	三拗汤	Sanao Tang	Sanao Decoction
178	三仁汤	Sanren Tang	Sanren Decoction
179	桑菊饮	Sangju Yin	Sangju Decoction
180	桑杏汤	Sangxing Tang	Sangxin Decoction
181	芍药甘草汤	Shaoyao Gancao Tang	Shaoyao Gancao Decoction
182	芍药汤	Shaoyao Tang	Shaoyao Decoction
183	少腹逐瘀汤	Shaofu Zhuyu Tang	Shaofu Zhuyu Decoction
184	麝香汤	Shexiang Tang	Shexiang Decoction
185	身痛逐瘀汤	Shentong Zhuyu Tang	Shentong Zhuyu Decoction
186	神术散	Shenzhu San	Shenzhu Powder
187	升麻葛根汤	Shengma Gegen Tang	Shengma Gegen Decoction
188	升麻芷葛汤	Shengma Zhige Tang	Shengma Zhige Decoction
189	生地黄煎	Shengdihuang Jian	Shengdihuang Decoction
190	生地黄汤	Shengdihuang Tang	Shengdihuang Decoction
191	生化汤	Shenghua Tang	Shenghua Decoction
192	生姜泻心汤	Shengjiang Xiexin Tang	Shengjiang Xiexin Decoction
193	生脉散	Shengmai San	Shengmai Powder
194	十全大补汤	Shiquan Dabu Tang	Shiquan Dabu Decoction
195	石膏知母汤	Shigao Zhimu Tang	Shigao Zhimu Decoction
196	顺气活血汤	Shunqi Huoxue Tang	Shunqi Huoxue Decoction
197	四君子汤	Sijunzi Tang	Sijunzi Decoction
198	四妙散	Simiao San	Simiao Powder
199	四妙勇安汤	Simiao yong'an Tang	Simiao Yong'an Decoction
200	四逆加人参汤	Sini Jia Renshen Tang	Sini Jia Renshen Decoction
201	四逆散	Sini San	Sini Powder
202	四逆汤	Sini Tang	Sini Decoction
203	四生丸	Sisheng Wan	Sisheng Pill
204	四顺散	Sishun San	Sishun Powder
205	四物汤	Siwu Tang	Siwu Decoction
206	苏合香丸	Suhexiang Wan	Suhexiang Pill
207	苏叶黄连汤	Suye Huanglian Tang	Suye Huanglian Decoction

续表

序号	方剂名称	拼音	英文名称
208	苏子降气汤	Suzi Jiangqi Tang	Suzi Jiangqi Decoction
209	酸枣仁汤	Suanzaoren Tang	Suanzaoren Decoction
210	桃核承气汤	Taohe Chengqi Tang	Taohe Chengqi Decoction
211	桃红四物汤	Taohong Siwu Tang	Taohong Siwu Decoction
212	桃仁红花煎	Taoren Honghua Jian	Taoren Honghua Decoction
213	天台乌药散	Tiantai Wuyao San	Tiantai Wuyao Powder
214	天王补心丹	Tianwang Buxin Dan	Tianwang Buxin Pill
215	调营散	Tiaoying San	Tiaoying Powder
216	通窍活血汤	Tongqiao Huoxue Tang	Tongqiao Huoxue Decoction
217	通瘀煎	Tongyu Jian	Tongyu Decoction
218	托里透脓散	Tuoli Tounong San	Tuoli Tounong Powder
219	托里消毒散	Tuoli Xiaodu San	Tuoli Xiaodu Powder
220	完肤续命汤	Wanfu Xuming Tang	Wanfu Xuming Decoction
221	胃苓汤	Weiling Tang	Weiling Decoction
222	温经汤	Wenjing Tang	Wenjing Decoction
223	温脾汤	Wenpi Tang	Wenpi Decoction
224	乌梅丸	Wumei Wan	Wumei Pill
225	五苓散	Wuling San	Wuling Powder
226	五仁丸	Wuren Wan	Wuren Pill
227	五味消毒饮	Wuwei Xiaodu Yin	Wuwei Xiaodu Decoction
228	犀黄丸	Xihuang Wan	Xihuang Pill
229	犀角地黄汤	Xijiao Dihuang Tang	Xijiao Dihuang Decoction
230	下瘀血汤	Xiayuxue Tang	Xiaxueyu Decoction
231	仙方活命饮	Xianfang Huoming Yin	Xianfang Huoming Decoction
232	香砂六君子汤	Xiangsha Liujunzi Tang	Xiangsha Liujunzi Decoction
233	香砂平胃丸	Xiangsha Pingwei Wan	Xiangsha Pingwei Powder
234	逍遥散	Xiaoyao San	Xiaoyao Powder
235	消瘰丸	Xiaoluo Wan	Xiaoluo Pill
236	消乳汤	Xiaoru Tang	Xiaoru Decoction
237	小半夏汤	Xiao banxia Tang	Xiao banxia Decoction
238	小柴胡汤	Xiaochaihu Tang	Xiaochaihu Decoction
239	小建中汤	Xiaojianzhong Tang	Xiaojianzhong Decoction
240	小金丹	Xiaojin Dan	Xiaojin Pellet
241	小青龙汤	Xiaoqinglong Tang	Xiaoqinglong Decoction
242	小温经汤	Xiaowenjing Tang	Xiaowenjing Decoction
243	泻心汤	Xiexin Tang	Xiexin Decoction

续表

序号	方剂名称	拼音	英文名称
244	新伤续断汤	Xinshang Xuduan Tang	Xinshang Xuduan Decoction
245	醒脾丸	Xingpi Wan	Xingpi Pill
246	醒消丸	Xingxiao Wan	Liushen Pill
247	玄麦甘桔汤	Xuanmai Ganjie Tang	Xuanmai Ganjie Decoction
248	血府逐瘀汤	Xuefu Zhuyu Tang	Xuefu Zhuyu Decoction
249	异功散	Yigong San	Yigong Powder
250	益胃汤	Yiwei Tang	Yiwei Decoction
251	益元散	Yiyuan San	Yiyuan Powder
252	薏苡仁汤	Yiyiren Tang	Yiyiren Decoction
253	茵陈白芷汤	Yinchen Baizhi Tang	Yinchen Baizhi Decoction
254	茵陈蒿散	Yinchen Hao San	Yinchen Hao Powder
255	茵陈蒿汤	Yinchenhao Tang	Yinchenhao Decoction
256	银翘散	Yinqiao San	Yinqiao Powder
257	引杨石林方	Yin Yangshilin Fang	Yin Yangshilin Fang
258	玉屏风散	Yupingfeng San	Yupingfeng Powder
259	玉液汤	Yuye Tang	Yuye Decoction
260	玉真散	Yuzhen San	Yuzhen Decoction
261	元胡止痛方	Yuanhu Zhitong Fang	Yuanhu Zhitong Powder
262	越婢加术汤	Yuebijiazhu Tang	Yuebijiazhu Decoction
263	越鞠丸	Yueju Wan	Yueju Pill
264	匀气散	Yunqi San	Yunqi Powder
265	增液承气汤	Zengye Chengqi Tang	Zengye Chengqi Decoction
266	增液汤	Zengye Tang	Zengye Decoction
267	珍珠散	Zhenzhu San	Zhenzhu Powder
268	真武汤	Zhenwu Tang	Zhenwu Decoction
269	正柴胡饮	Zhengchaihu Yin	Zhengchaihu Decoction
270	知母鳖甲汤	Zhimu Biejia Tang	Zhimu Biejia Decoction
271	止红肠澼丸	Zhihong Changpi Wan	Zhihong Changpi Pill
272	止痛接骨散	Zhitong Jiegu San	Zhitong Jiegu Powder
273	枳实薤白桂枝汤	Zhishi Xiebai Guizhi Tang	Zhishi Xiebai Guizhi Decoction
274	至宝丹	Zhibao Dan	Zhibao Pellet
275	炙甘草汤	Zhigancao Tang	Zhigancao Decoction
276	紫雪丹	Zixue Dan	Zixue Pellet

附录三 古籍名称

序号	古籍名称	拼音	英文名
1	《百一选方》	Baiyi Xuanfang	One Hundred and Qne Choice
2	《备急千金要方》	Beiji Qianjin Yaofang	Essential Recipes for Emergent Use Worth A Thousand Gold
3	《本草备要》	Bencao Beiyao	Compendium of Materia Medica
4	《本草崇原》	Bencao Chongyuan	Materia Medica Believe in the Source
5	《本草从新》	Bencao Congxin	New Revised Materia Medica
6	《本草发挥》	Bencao Fahui	Elaboration of Materia Medica
7	《本草纲目》	Bencao Gangmu	Compendium of Materia Medica
8	《本草纲目拾遗》	Bencaogangmushiyi	Supplement to the Compendium of Materia Medica
9	《本草汇》	Bencao Hui	Treasury of Words on Materia Medica
10	《本草汇言》	Bencao Huiyan	Materia Medica Huiyan
11	《本草经集注》	Bencaojing Jizhu	Collective Commentaries on Classics of Materia Medica
12	《本草蒙荃》	Bencao Mengquan	Enlightening Primer of Materia Medica
13	《本草品汇精要》	Bencaopinhuijingyao	Compendium of Materia Medica
14	《本草求真》	Bencao Qiuzhen	Seeking Truth from the Grass
15	《本草拾遗》	Bencaoshiyi	Supplement to Materia Medica
16	《本草述》	Bencao Shu	Description of Materia Medica
17	《本草述钩元》	Bencao Shu Gouyuan	Delving into the Description of Materia Medica
18	《本草图经》	Bencaotujing	Illustration of Meteria Medica
19	《本草新编》	Bencao Xinbian	Renew Materia Medica
20	《本草衍义》	Bencao Yanyi	The Meaning of Materia Medica
21	《本草衍义补遗》	Bencaoyanyibuyi	Addendum of Materia Medica
22	《本草易读》	Bencao Yidu	Easy Read Materia Medica
23	《辨证录》	Bianzhenglu	Syndrome Differentiation to Record
24	《兵部手集方》	Bingbushoujifang	Hand Set Square of the Ministry of War
25	《产孕集》	Chanyun Ji	Maternity and Pregnancy Collection
26	《成方便读》	Chengfang Biandu	Easy to Read

续表

序号	古籍名称	拼音	英文名
27	《此事难知》	Cishi Nanzhi	This Matter is Difficult to Know
28	《丹溪心法》	Danxi Xinfa	Danxi Mental Method
29	《滇南本草》	Dian Nan Ben Cao	Materia Medica of South Yunnan
30	《痘疹世医心法》	Douzhen Shiyi Xinfa	Psychological Method of Pox and Rash
31	《妇人良方大全》	Furen Liangfang Daquan	Women's Recipe
32	《傅青主女科》	Fuqingzhunvke	Fuqing Lord Gynecology Department
33	《古今医统》	Gujinyitong	Ancient and Modern Medical System
34	《广济方》	Guangjifang	Guangji Prescription
35	《国语》	Guoyu	Discourses of the States
36	《海药本草》	Haiyao Bencao	Oversea Materia Medica
37	《汉书》	Hanshu	History of the Han Dynasty
38	《洪氏集验方》	Hongshijiyanfang	Hong's Prescription
39	《黄帝内经》	Huang Di Nei Jing	Huangdi's Internal Classic
40	《鸡峰普济方》	Jifeng Pujifang	Jifeng Prescription for Universal Relief
41	《急救仙方》	Jijiu Xianfang	Xianfang First Aid
42	《济生方》	Jisheng Fang	Prescriptions for Helping People
43	《嘉佑补注本草》	Jiayou Buzhu Bencao	Remarks on Shennong's Classic of Materia Medica in Jiayou Year
44	《简易方议》	Jianyifangyi	A Brief Prescription of Discussion
45	《绛囊撮药》	Jiangnangcuoyao	Crimson Sac Pinch of Medicine
46	《金境内台方义》	Jinjing Neitai Fangyi	Taiwan Justice in the Teritory of Jin
47	《金匮要略》	Jingui Yaolue	Synopsis of the Golden Chamber
48	《金匮要略方论衍义》	Jingui Yaolue Fanglun Yanyi	Synopsis of Prescriptions of the Golden Chamber
49	《金匮玉函经》	Jingui Yuhan Jing	Golden Chamber Yuhan Classic
50	《经史证类备急本草》	Jingshi Zhenglei Beiji Bencao	Classified Materia Medica from Historical Classics for Emergency
51	《经验良方》	Jingyanliangfang	Good Experience
52	《景岳全书》	Jingyue Quanshu	Jingyue's Complete Works
53	《救荒本草》	Jiuhuang Bencao	Herbal Medicine for Famine Relief
54	《救伤秘旨》	Jiushangmizhi	Secret Purpose of Rescuing Injuries
55	《开宝重定本草》	Kaibao Chongding Bencao	Revised Materia Medica by Song Kaibao
56	《兰室秘藏》	Lanshi Micang	Orchid House Secret Collection
57	《雷公炮炙论》	Leigong Paozhi Lun	Leigong Treatise on the Preparation
58	《雷公上诵芳堂方》	Leigong Shansong Fangtang Fang	Lei Gong Recites Fang Tang Fang
59	《类证活人书》	Leizheng Huorenshu	Class of the Living Book

续表

序号	古籍名称	拼音	英文名
60	《类证治裁》	Leizheng Zhicai	Syndrome Differentiation and Treatment
61	《礼记》	Liji	Book of Rites
62	《良方集腋》	Liangfang Jiye	A Good Combination of Armpit
63	《临证指南医案》	Linzhengzhinanyian	Lin Zheng's Guide Medical Cases
64	《刘涓子鬼遗方》	Liu Juanzi Guiyi Fang	Liu Juanzi's Ghost Prescription
65	《六科准绳》	Liuke Zhunsheng	Six Principles
66	《马培之医案》	Mapeizhiyian	Ma Peizhi Medical Case
67	《梦溪笔谈》	Mengxi Bitan	Mengxi Essays
68	《名医别录》	Mingyi Bielu	Miscellaneous Records of Famous Physicians
69	《难经》	Nanjing	Classic of Questioning
70	《内外伤辨惑论》	Neiwaishang Bianhuolun	Differentiation on Endogenous
71	《女科切要》	Nüke Qieyao	Critical Tips for Women Diseases
72	《炮炙大法》	Paozhidafa	Main Solution of Processing
73	《脾胃论》	Piwei Lun	Treatise on Spleen and Stomach
74	《普济本事方》	Puji Benshi Fang	Effective Prescriptions for Universal Relief
75	《普济方》	Puji Fang	Preions for Universal Relief
76	《千金翼方》	Qianjin Yifang	Supplement to Prescriptions Worth a Thousand Gold Pieces
77	《儒门事亲》	Rumen Shiqin	Confucian Family Affairs
78	《山海经》	Shanhai Jing	The Book of Mountains and Seas
79	《伤寒六书》	Shanghan Liushu	Six books on Febrile Diseases
80	《伤寒论》	Shanghanlun	Treatise on Cold Damage Diseases
81	《伤寒杂病论》	Shanghan Zabing Lun	Treatise on Cold Damage and Miscellaneous Diseases
82	《伤科大成》	Shangkedacheng	Traumatology Department Recording
83	《摄生秘剖》	Sheshengmipou	Secret of Health-Preservation
84	《神农本草经》	Shennong Bencao Jing	Shennong's Classic of Materia Medica
85	《神农本草经百种录》	Shennong Bencaojing Baizhonglu	Shennong Herbal Classic 100 Kinds of Records
86	《沈氏尊生书》	Shenshi Zunsheng Shu	Shen's Book that Honors Life
87	《沈尧封女科辑要》	Shen Yaofeng Nüke Jiyao	Shen Yaofeng's Collection of Women's Studies
88	《审视瑶涵》	Shenshi Yaohan	Look at Yaohan
89	《圣济总录》	Sheng Ji Zonglu	General Records of Holy Universal Relief
90	《诗经》	Shi Jing	The Book of Songs
91	《十便良方》	Shibianliangfang	Ten Effective Prescription
92	《十药神书》	Shiyao Shenegshu	Miraculous Book of Ten Recipes

序号	古籍名称	拼音	英文名
93	《食疗本草》	Shiliao Bencao	Materia Medica for Dietotherapy
94	《世医得效方》	Shiyi Dexiaofang	World Medicine Effective Recipe
95	《寿世保元》	Shoushi Baoyuan	Longevity and Life Preservation
96	《蜀本草》	Shubencao	Shu Materia Medica
97	《素庵医案》	Su'an Yian	Su'an Medical Records
98	《素问病机气宜保命集》	Suwen Bingji Qiyi Baomingji	Simple Questions about Pathogenesis, Qi Should Protect Life
99	《太平惠民和剂局方》	Taiping Huimin Heji Ju Fang	The Prescriptions of the Bureau of Taiping People's Welfare Pharmacy
100	《太平圣惠方》	Taiping Shenghui Fang	Taiping Holy Prescriptions for Universal Relief
101	《汤液本草》	Tangye Bencao	Materia Medica for Decoctions
102	《汤液经》	Tangye Jing	The Classicals on Decoction
103	《体仁汇编》	Tiren Huibian	Body Kernel Compilation
104	《外科全生集》	Waike Quansheng Ji	Surgical whole life collection
105	《外科十三方考》	Waike Shisan Kao	Thirteen Prescriptions of Surgery
106	《外科正宗》	Waike Zhengzong	Orthodox Manual of External Medicine
107	《外科证治全生集》	Waike Zhengzhi Quansheng Ji	The Whole Life Collection of Surgical Treatment
108	《外台秘要》	Waitai Miyao	Arcane Essentials from the Imperial Library
109	《卫生鸿宝》	Weisheng Hongbao	Health Hongbao
110	《卫生家宝产科备要》	Weisheng Jiabao Chanke Beiyao	Treasured Household Prescriptions for Health
111	《卫生家宝方》	Weisheng Jiabao Fang	Treasured Household Prescriptions for Health
112	《魏氏家藏方》	Weishi Jiacang Fang	Treasure Prescription of Wei's Family
113	《温病条辨》	Wenbing Tiaobian	Detailed Analysis of Warm Diseases
114	《温热经纬》	Wenre Jingwei	Compendium on Epidemic Febrile Disease
115	《温热论》	Wenre Lun	Treatise on Warm-Heat Diseases
116	《吴普本草》	Wupu Bencao	Wu Pu's Materia Medica
117	《五十二病方》	Wushier Bingfang	Prescriptions for Fifty-two Diseases
118	《仙授理伤续断秘方》	Xianshou Lishang Xuduan Mifang	Monograph on Orthopedics and Traumatology of Traditional Chinese Medicine
119	《小儿药证直诀》	Xiao Er Yao Zheng Zhi Jue	Key to Diagnosis and Treatment of Children's Diseases
120	《校注妇人良方》	Jiaozhu Furen Liang Fang	Revised Good Remedies for Women
121	《新修本草》	Xinxiu Bencao	Newly Revised Materia Medica
122	《修事指南》	Xiushi Zhinan	Bibliography on Medicinal Processing

续表

序号	古籍名称	拼音	英文名
123	《咽喉脉证通论》	Yanhou Maizheng Tonglun	General Theory of Throat Pulse Syndrome
124	《延年方》	Yannian Fang	Macrobiotic Prescription
125	《严氏济生方》	Yanshi Jisheng Fang	Yan's Saving Prescription
126	《阎氏小儿方论》	Yanshi Xiaoer Fanglun	Yanshi Children's Prescription
127	《验方新编》	Yanfang Xinbian	New Compilation of Proved Recipes
128	《药品化义》	Yaopinhuayi	Meaning of Medicine
129	《药物出产辨》	Yaowu Chuchan Bian	Differentiation on Materia Medica and Their Producing Areas
130	《药性歌》	Yaoxingge	Verse of Medicinal Properties
131	《药性论》	Yaoxinglun	Theory of Property
132	《医方集解》	Yifang jijie	Collection of Medical Prescriptions
133	《医方考》	Yifangkao	Textual Research of Medical Prescriptions
134	《医经小学》	Yijing Xiaoxue	Medical Classics Primary School
135	《医林改错》	Yilin Gaicuo	Correction of the Errors of Medical Works
136	《医门法律》	Yimen Falü	Principles for Medical Profession
137	《医学发明》	Yixue Faming	Medical Invention
138	《医学金针》	Yixuejinzhen	Medical Golden Needle
139	《医学六书》	Yixue liushu	Six Books of Medicine
140	《医学入门》	Yixuerumen	Introduction to Medicine
141	《医学心悟》	Yixue Xinwu	Medical Revelations
142	《医学心语》	Yixuexinyu	Experience on Medical Practices
143	《医学源流论》	Yixue Yuanliulun	On the Origin and Development of Medicine
144	《医学衷中参西录》	Yixue Zhongzhong Canxi Lu	Records of traditional Chinese and western medicine in combination
145	《医原》	Yiyuan	Medicine Source
146	《医宗金鉴》	Yizong Jinjian	Golden Mirror of Medicine
147	《异物志》	Yiwu Zhi	Foreign Body Records
148	《疫疹一得》	Yizhenyide	A Case of Epidemic Rash
149	《酉阳杂俎》	Youyangzazu	YawYang Essays
150	《幼幼新书》	Youyou Xinshu	Young and Young New Book
151	《杂病源流犀烛》	Zabingyuanliuxizhu	The Origin and Development of Miscellaneous Diseases
152	《彰明附子记》	Zhangming Fuzi Ji	Zhangming's Aconite Biography
153	《珍珠囊》	Zhenzhunang	Pouch of Pearls
154	《珍珠囊补遗药性赋》	Zhenzhunang Buyi Yaoxingfu	The Supplement of the Pearl Capsule and the Fu of Medicine

续表

序号	古籍名称	拼音	英文名
155	《正体类要》	Zhengti Leiyao	Orthopedics and Traumatology
156	《症因脉治》	Zhengyin Maizhi	Syndrome Identification, Pathogeny, Pulse Diagnosis and Treatment
157	《直指方》	Zhizhi Fang	Zhizhi Prescription
158	《植物名实图考》	Zhiwu Mingshi Tukao	Illustrated Reference of Botanical Nomenclature
159	《重广补注神农本草并图经》	Zhongguang Buzhu Shennong Bencao bing Tujing	Heavy and Extensive Supplementary Note of Shennong Herbal and Map Classics
160	《重修政和经史证类备用本草》	Chongxiu Zhenghe Jing Shi-zhenglei Beiyong Bencao	Revision of the Administrative System and Spare Materia Medica of Classics, History and Evidence
161	《杂病证治新义》	Zabing Zhengzhi Xinyi	New Meanings of Diagnosis and Treatment of Miscellaneous Diseases
162	《肘后备急方》	Zhouhou Beiji Fang	Handbook of Prescriptions for Emergency

附录四　炮制方法

序号	炮制方法	拼音	英文
1	熬膏法	Aogaofa	ointment boiling
2	鳖血制	Biexuezhi	processing with soft-shelled turtle blood
3	燀制	Danzhi	blanching
4	炒焦	Chaojiao	stir-frying to brown
5	炒炭	Chaotan	stir-frying to scorch
6	炒制	chaozhi	stir frying
7	醋炒	Cuchao	stir-frying with vinegar
8	醋炙	Cuzhi	vinegar broiling
9	煅制	Duanzhi	calcining
10	发酵法	Fajiaofa	fermentation
11	发芽法	Fayafa	sprouting
12	麸炒	Fuchao	stir-frying with bran
13	复制	Fuzhi	complex producing
14	甘草汁制	Gancaozhizhi	processing with Gancao juice
15	蛤粉炒	Gefenchao	stir-frying with clam meal powder
16	烘焙	Hongbei	baking
17	黄精汁制	Huangjingzhizhi	processing with Huangjing juice
18	姜制	Jiangzhi	stir-frying with ginger
19	浸渍	Jinzi	soaking
20	酒拌蒸	Jiubanzheng	steaming with liquor mixture
21	酒炒	jiuchao	stir-frying with liquor
22	米炒制	Michaozhi	stir-frying with rice
23	米泔水制	Miganshuizhi	processing with rice swill
24	蜜炙	Mizhi	roasting with honey
25	漂洗	Piaoxi	rinsing
26	润制	Runzhi	moistening
27	砂烫	Shatang	scalding with sand

序号	炮制方法	拼音	英文
28	水飞法	Shuifeifa	grinding with water
29	水制	Shuizhi	processing with saline
30	酥制	Suzhi	processing with butter
31	土炒	Tuchao	stir-frying with earth
32	煨制	Weizhi	roasting
33	吴茱萸制	Wuzhuyuzhi	processing with Wuzhuyu
34	羊脂制	Yangzhizhi	processing with suet
35	淫羊藿制	Yinyanghuozhi	processing by Yinyanghuo
36	油制	Youzhi	processing with oil
37	蒸法	Zhengfa	steaming
38	蒸制	Zhengzhi	steaming
39	制露法	Zhilufa	dew making
40	制霜法	Zhishuangfa	crystallizing
41	猪血炒	Zhuxuechao	stir-frying with pig's blood
42	煮法	Zhufa	cooking
43	煮制	zhuzhi	decocting

附录五 制剂类型

序号	制剂类型	拼音	英文
1	巴布膏剂	Babugaoji	cataplasm
2	饼剂	Bingji	medicinal cake
3	茶剂	Chaji	medicated tea
4	搽剂	Chaji	liniment
5	冲剂	Chongji	granule
6	丹剂	Danji	pellet
7	滴鼻剂	Dibiji	nasal drop
8	滴丸	Diwan	dropping pill
9	滴眼剂	Diyanji	eye drop
10	酊剂	Dingji	tincture
11	钉剂	Dingji	nail preparation
12	锭剂	Dingji	pastille
14	膏药	Gaoyao	plaster
15	糕剂	Gaoji	medicinal cake
16	灌肠剂	Guanchangji	enema
17	海绵剂	Haimianji	sponge
18	含漱剂	Hanshuji	gargle
19	合剂	Heji	mixture
20	糊丸	Huwan	paste pill
21	煎膏剂	Jiangaoji	soft extract
22	胶囊剂	Jiaonangji	capsule
23	浸膏剂	Jingaoji	extract
24	灸剂	Jiuji	moxa-preparation
25	酒剂	Jiuji	vinum
26	颗粒剂	Keliji	granule
27	口服液	Koufuye	mixture
28	蜡丸	Lawan	wax pill
29	流浸膏剂	Liujingaoji	fluid extract

续表

序号	制剂类型	拼音	英文
30	露剂	Luji	distillate medicinal water
31	蜜丸	Miwan	honey pill
32	膜剂	Moji	film agent
33	凝胶剂	Ningjiaoji	gel-forming agent
34	浓缩丸	Nongsuowan	concentrated pill
35	喷雾剂	Penwuji	spray
36	片剂	Pianji	tablet
37	气雾剂	Qiwuji	aerosol
38	曲剂	Quji	fermented medicine
39	乳剂	Ruji	emulsion
40	软膏剂	Ruangaoji	ointment
41	散剂	Sanji	powder
42	栓剂	Shuanji	suppository
43	水蜜丸	Shuimiwan	water-honeyed pill
44	水丸	Shuiwan	water pill
45	汤剂	Tangji	decoction
46	糖浆剂	Tangjiangji	syrup
47	条剂	Tiaoji	medicinal roll
48	贴膏剂	Tiegaoji	emplastrum
49	涂膜剂	Tumoji	coating agent
50	丸剂	Wanji	pill
51	洗剂	Xiji	lotion
52	线剂	Xianji	medicated thread
53	橡胶膏剂	Xiangjiaogaoji	rubber patche
54	烟剂	Yanji	fumicant
55	药熏剂	Yaoxunji	Chinese herb fumigation
56	药浴剂	Yaoyuji	medicinal bath
57	药熨剂	Yaoyunji	traditional Chinese medicine ironing
58	油剂	Youji	oiling agent
59	熨剂	Yunji	medicated ironing
60	注射液	Zhusheye	injection